W9-AGB-914

O

Mammary Tumor Cell Cycle, Differentiation, and Metastasis

Cancer Treatment and Research

Emil J Freireich, M.D., D.Sc.(Hon.), *Series Editor*

Lippman ME, Dickson R (eds): Breast Cancer: Cellular and Molecular Biology. 1988. ISBN 0-89838-368-4
Kamps WA, Humphrey GB, Poppema S (eds): Hodgkin's Disease in Children: Controversies and Current Practice. 1988. ISBN 0-89838-372-2
Muggia FM (ed): Cancer Chemotherapy: Concepts, Clinical Investigations and Therapeutic Advances. 1988. ISBN 0-89838-381-1
Nathanson L (ed): Malignant Melanoma: Biology, Diagnosis, and Therapy. 1988. ISBN 0-89838-384-6
Pinedo HM, Verweij J (eds): Treatment of Soft Tissue Sarcomas. 1989. ISBN 0-89838-391-9
Hansen HH (ed): Basic and Clinical Concepts of Lung Cancer. 1989. ISBN 0-7923-0153-6
Lepor H, Ratliff TL (eds): Urologic Oncology. 1989. ISBN 0-7923-0161-7
Benz C, Liu E (eds): Oncogenes. 1989. ISBN 0-7923-0237-0
Ozols RF (ed): Drug Resistance in Cancer Therapy. 1989. ISBN 0-7923-0244-3
Surwit EA, Alberts DS (eds): Endometrial Cancer. 1989. ISBN 0-7923-0286-9
Champlin R (ed): Bone Marrow Transplantation. 1990. ISBN 0-7923-0612-0
Goldenberg D (ed): Cancer Imaging with Radiolabeled Antibodies. 1990. ISBN 0-7923-0631-7
Jacobs C (ed): Carcinomas of the Head and Neck. 1990. ISBN 0-7923-0668-6
Lippman ME, Dickson R (eds): Regulatory Mechanisms in Breast Cancer: Advances in Cellular and Molecular Biology of Breast Cancer. 1990. ISBN 0-7923-0868-9
Nathanson L (ed): Malignant Melanoma: Genetics, Growth Factors, Metastases, and Antigens. 1991. ISBN 0-7923-0895-6
Sugarbaker PH (ed): Management of Gastric Cancer. 1991. ISBN 0-7923-1102-7
Pinedo HM, Verweij J, Suit HD (eds): Soft Tissue Sarcomas: New Developments in the Multidisciplinary Approach to Treatment. 1991. ISBN 0-7923-1139-6
Ozols RF (ed): Molecular and Clinical Advances in Anticancer Drug Resistance. 1991. ISBN 0-7923-1212-0
Muggia FM (ed): New Drugs, Concepts and Results in Cancer Chemotherapy 1991. ISBN 0-7923-1253-8
Dickson RB, Lippman ME (eds): Genes, Oncogenes and Hormones: Advances in Cellular and Molecular Biology of Breast Cancer. 1992. ISBN 0-7923-1748-3
Humphrey G, Bennett, Schraffordt Koops H, Molenaar WM, Postma A (eds): Osteosarcoma in Adolescents and Young Adults: New Developments and Controversies. 1993. ISBN 0-7923-1905-2
Benz CC, Liu ET (eds): Oncogenes and Tumor Suppressor Genes in Human Malignancies. 1993. ISBN 0-7923-1960-5
Freireich EJ, Kantarjian H (eds): Leukemia: Advances in Research and Treatment. 1993. ISBN 0-7923-1967-2
Dana BW (ed): Malignant Lymphomas, Including Hodgkin's Disease: Diagnosis, Management, and Special Problems. 1993. ISBN 0-7923-2171-5
Nathanson L (ed): Current Research and Clinical Management of Melanoma. 1993. ISBN 0-7923-2152-9
Verweij J, Pinedo HM, Suit HD (eds): Multidisciplinary Treatment of Soft Tissue Sarcomas. 1993. ISBN 0-7923-2183-9
Rosen ST, Kuzel TM (eds): Immunoconjugate Therapy of Hematologic Malignancies. 1993. ISBN 0-7923-2270-3
Sugarbaker PH (ed): Hepatobiliary Cancer. 1994. ISBN 0-7923-2501-X
Rothenberg ML (ed): Gynecologic Oncology: Controversies and New Developments. 1994. ISBN 0-7923-2634-2
Dickson RB, Lippman ME (eds): Mammary Tumorigenesis and Malignant Progression. 1994. ISBN 0-7923-2647-4
Hansen HH (ed): Lung Cancer. Advances in Basic and Clinical Research. 1994. ISBN 0-7923-2835-3
Goldstein LJ, Ozols RF (eds): Anticancer Drug Resistance. Advances in Molecular and Clinical Research. 1994. ISBN 0-7923-2836-1
Hong WK, Weber RS (eds): Head and Neck Cancer. Basic and Clinical Aspects. 1994. ISBN 0-7923-3015-3
Thall PF (ed): Recent Advances in Clinical Trial Design and Analysis. 1995. ISBN 0-7923-3235-0
Buckner CD (ed): Technical and Biological Components of Marrow Transplantation. 1995. ISBN 0-7923-3394-2
Muggia FM (ed): Concepts, Mechanisms, and New Targets for Chemotherapy. 1995. ISBN 0-7923-3525-2
Klastersky J (ed): Infectious Complications of Cancer. 1995. ISBN 0-7923-3598-8
Kurzrock R, Talpaz M (eds): Cytokines: Interleukins and Their Receptors. 1995. ISBN 0-7923-3636-4
Sugarbaker P (ed): Peritoneal Carcinomatosis: Drugs and Diseases. 1995. ISBN 0-7923-3726-3
Sugarbaker P (ed): Peritoneal Carcinomatosis: Principles of Management. 1995. ISBN 0-7923-3727-1

Mammary Tumor Cell Cycle, Differentiation, and Metastasis

Advances in Cellular and Molecular Biology of Breast Cancer

edited by

Robert B. Dickson
Marc E. Lippman
Lombardi Cancer Research Center
Washington, D.C.

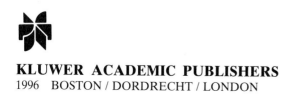

KLUWER ACADEMIC PUBLISHERS
1996   BOSTON / DORDRECHT / LONDON

Distributors for North America:
Kluwer Academic Publishers
101 Philip Drive
Assinippi Park
Norwell, Massachusetts 02061 USA

Distributors for all other countries:
Kluwer Academic Publishers Group
Distribution Centre
Post Office Box 322
3300 AH Dordrecht, THE NETHERLANDS

Library of Congress Cataloging-in-Publication Data

Mammary tumor cell cycle, differentiation, and metastasis : advances
   in cellular and molecular biology of breast cancer / edited by
   Robert B. Dickson, Marc E. Lippman.
      p. cm. -- (Cancer treatment and research ; v. 83)
   Includes bibliographical references and index.
   ISBN 0–7923–3905–3 (alk. paper)
     1. Breast--Cancer--Molecular aspects. 2. Cancer cells. 3. Cell
differentiation. 4. Metastasis. 5. Cell transformation.
I. Dickson, Robert B. (Robert Brent), 1952-   . II. Lippman, Marc
E., 1945-   . III. Series.
   [DNLM: 1. Breast Neoplasms. 2. Cell Differentiation. 3. Neoplasm
Metastasis. W1 CA693 v.83 1995 / WP 870 M262 1995]
   RC280.B8M265 1995
   616.99′449071--dc20
   DNLM/DLC
for Library of Congress   96-4654
                                       CIP

Copyright © 1996 by Kluwer Academic Publishers

All rights reserved. No part of this publication may be reproduced, stored in a retrieval system or transmitted in any form or by any means, mechanical, photo-copying, recording, or otherwise, without the prior written permission of the publisher, Kluwer Academic Publishers, 101 Philip Drive, Assinippi Park, Norwell, Massachusetts 02061

Printed on acid-free paper.

PRINTED IN THE UNITED STATES OF AMERICA

Contents

ROUYER, MARIA SANTAVICCA, ISABELLE STOLL,
CATHERINE WOLF, and MARIE-CHRISTINE RIO

Contributing Authors

RAMASAWAN ANBAZHAGA, Section of Cell Biology and Experimental Pathology, Institute of Cancer Research, London, SMZ 5 NG, UK

PATRICK ANGLARD, PHD, Institut de Genetigue et de Biologie Moleculaire at Cellulaire (IGBMC), CNRS/INSERM/ULP, P.P. 163, 67404 Illkirch Cedex, C.N. de Strasbourg, France

AMANDA ATHERTON, PHD, Johns Hopkins University, Baltimore, MD 21205, USA

PAUL BASSETT, PHD, Institut de Genetique et de Biologie Moleculaire et Cellulaire (IGBMC), CNRS/INSERM/ULP, P.P. 163, 67404 Ilkirch Cedex, C.N. de Strasbourg, Cedex, France

JEAN PIERRE BELLOCQ, MD, Service d'Anatomic Pathologique Generale, Centre Hospitalier Universitaire, Hopital de Hautepierre, 1 Avenue Moliere, 67098 Strasbourg, Cedex, France

MARIE-PIERRE CHENARD, MD, Service d'Anatomic Pathologique Generale, Centre Hospitalier Universitaire, Hopital de Hautepierre, 1 Avenue Molier, 67098 Strasbourg, Cedex, France

DAVID L. DANKORT, PHD, Institute for Molecular Biology and Biotechnology, Department of Biology, McMaster University, 1280 Main Street W., Hamilton, Ontario, L85 4K1 Canada

NANCY E. DAVIDSON, MD, The Johns Hopkins Oncology Center, 422 North Bond St., Baltimore, MD 21231-1001, USA

ROBERT B. DICKSON, PHD, Departments of Cell Biology and Pharmacology, Lombardi Cancer Center, The Research Building, 3970 Reservoir Road, Washington, DC 20007, USA

DON DUBIK, PHD, Department of Physiology, University of Manitoba, Winnipeg, MB, R3E OW3, Canada

PAUL A. EDWARDS, PHD, Division of Cellular Pathology, Department of Pathology, University of Cambridge, Tennis Court Road, Cambridge CB2 1QP, UK

WALTER J. ESSELMAN, PHD, Department of Microbiology, Michigan State University, East Lansing, MI 48824, USA

S.C. FONTAINE, PHD, AMC Cancer Research Center, Lakewood, CO 80214, USA

R.R. FRIIS, PHD, Laboratory of Clinical and Experimental Research, University of Berne, Berne, Switzerland CH-3004

K.H. FRITZEMEIER, PHD, Experimental Oncology, Research Laboratories of Schering AG, Berlin, FRG

BARRY GUSTERSON, PHD, MRCPATH, Section of Cell Biology and Experimental Pathology, Institute of Cancer Research, London, SMZ 5NG, UK

GLORIA H. HEPPNER, PHD, Breast Cancer Program, Karmanos Cancer Institute, 110 East Warren, Detroit, MI 48201, USA

TAHEREH KAMALATI, PHD, Section of Cell Biology and Experimental Pathology, Institute of Cancer Research, London, SMZ 5NG, UK

JASON D. KANTOR, PHD, Department of Surgery, Children's Hospital, and Program in Biological and Biomedical Sciences, Harvard Medical School, Boston, MA 02115, USA

M. JOHN KENNEDY, MB, FRCPI, The Johns Hopkins Oncology Center, 422 North Bond St., Baltimore, MD 21231-1001, USA

OLIVIER LEFEBVRE, PHD, Institut de Genetique et de Biologie Moleculaire et Cellulaire (IGBMC), CNRS/INSERM/ULP, p.p. 163, 67404 Illkirch Cedex, C.N. de Strasbourg, France

MARC E. LIPPMAN, MD, Departments of Medicine and Pharmacology, Lombardi Cancer Center, The Research Building, 3970 Reservoir Road, Washington, CD 20007, USA

P. MALONE, PHD, AMC Cancer Research Center, Lakewood, CO 80214, USA

DANIEL MEDINA, PHD, Department of Cell Biology, Baylor College of Medicine, One Baylor Plaza, Houston, TX 77030, USA

HORST MICHNA, PHD, Experimental Oncology, Research Laboratories of Schering AG, Berlin, FRG

FRED R. MILLER, PHD, Breast Cancer Program, Michigan Cancer Foundation, 110E. Warren Ave., Detroit, MI 48201, USA

WILLIAM J. MULLER, PHD, Institute for Molecular Biology and Biotechnology, Departments of Biology and Pathology, McMaster University, 1280 Main St. W., Hamilton, Ontario, L85 4K1, Canada

ELIZABETH A. MUSGROVE, PHD, Cancer Biology Division, Garvin Institute of Medical Research, St. Vincents Hospital, Sydney, N.S.W. 2010 Australia

BIRUNTHI NIRANJAN, PHD, Section of Cell Biology and Experimental Pathology, Institute of Cancer Research, London, SM2 5NG, UK

Y. NISHINO, PHD, Experimental Oncology, Research Laboratories of Schering AG, Berlin, FRG

AGNES NOEL, PHD, Institut de Genetique et de Biologie Moleculaire et Cellulaire (IGBMC), CNRS/INSERM/ULP, p.p. 163, 67404 Illkirch Cedex, C.N. de Strasbourg, France

AKIKO OKADA, PHD, Institut de Genetique et de Biologie Moleculaire et Cellulaire (IBBMC), CNRS/INSERM/ULP, p.p. 163, 67404 Illkirch Cedex, C.N. de Strasbourg, France

MALCOLM G. PARKER, PHD, Laboratory of Molecular Endocrinology, Imperial Cancer Research Fund, Lincoln's Inn Fields, London WC2A 3PX, UK

KIRTI V. PATEL, PHD, Institute of Cancer Research, The Haddow Laboratories, Cell Biology and Experimental Pathology, Belmont, Sutton, UK

KENNETH J. PIENTA, PHD, The University of Michigan Comprehensive Cancer Center and Division of Hematology/Oncology, Department of Internal Medicine, 5510 MS RB I, 1150 W. Medical Center Drive, Ann Arbor, MI 48109-0680, USA

K. PARCZYZK, PHD, Experimental Oncology, Research Laboratories of Schering AG, Berlin, FRG

WEI-PING REN, PHD, Department of Pharmacology, Wayne State University, 540 E. Canfield, Detroit, MI 48201, USA

TRACY S. REPLOGLE, PHD, The University of Michigan Comprehensive Cancer Center and Division of Hematology/Oncology, Department of Internal Medicine, 5510 MS RB I, 1150 W. Medical Center Drive, Ann Arbor, MI 48109-0680, USA

MARIE-CHRISTINE RIO, Institut de Genetique et de Biologie Moleculaire et Cellulaire (IGBMC), CNRS/INSERM/ULP, p.p. 163, 67404 Illkirch Cedex, C.N. de Strasbourg, France

NICOLAS ROUYER, MD, Institut de Genetique et de Biologie Moleculaire et Cellulaire (IGBMC), CNRS/INSERM/ULP, p.p. 163, 67404 Illkirch Cedex, C.N. de Strasbourg, France

MARIA SANTAVICC, PHD, Institut de Genetique et de Biologie Moleculaire et Cellulaire (IGBMC), CNRS/INSERM/ULP, p.p. 163, 67404 Illkirch Cedex, C.N. de Strasbourg, France

P.J. SCHEDIN, PHD, AMC Cancer Research Center, Lakewood, CO 80214, USA

MARTIN R. SCHNEIDER, PHD, Experimental Oncology, Research Laboratories of Schering AG, Berlin, FRG

ROBERT P.C. SHIU, PHD, Department of Physiology, University of Manitoba, Winnipeg, MB, R3E OW3, Canada

MICHAEL P. SCHREY, PHD, Unit of Metabolic Medicine, St. Mary's Hospital Medical School, Praed St., Paddington, London W2 1PG, UK

BONNIE F. SLOANE, PHD, Department of Pharmacology, Wayne State University, 540 E. Canfield, Detroit, MI 48201, USA

ROBERT STRANGE, PHD, AMC Cancer Research Center, Lakewood, CO 80214, USA

ISABELLE STOLL, PHD, Institut de Genetique et de Biologie Moleculaire et Cellulaire (IGBMC), CNRS/INERM/ULP, p.p. 163, 67404 Illkirch Cedex, C.N. de Strasbourg, France

ROBERT L. SUTHERLAND, PHD, Cancer Biology Division, Garvin Institute of Medical Research, St. Vincent's Hospital, Sydney, N.S.W. 2010 Australia

KIMBERLY J.E. SWEENEY, PHD, Cancer Biology Division, Garvin Institute of Medical Research, St. Vincent's Hospital, Sydney, N.S.W. 2010 Australia

L.B. THACKERY, PHD, AMC Cancer Research Center, Lakewood, CO 80214, USA

MARCELLA VENDITTI, PHD, Department of Physiology, Univeristy of Manitoba, Winnipeg, MB, R3E OW3, Canada

PETER H. WATSON, PHD, Department of Physiology, University of Manitoba, Winnipeg, MB, R3E OW3, Canada

COLIN K.W. WATTS, PHD, Cancer Biology Division, Garvin Institute of Medical Research, St. Vincent's Hospital, Sydney, N.S.W. 2010 Australia

WEI-ZEN WEI, PHD, Breast Cancer Program, Karmanos Cancer Institute, 110 East Warren, Detroit, MI 48201, USA

NOEL WEIDNER, MD, Department of Pathology, Box 0102, University of California, San Francisco, San Francisco, CA 94143-0102, USA

CLIFFORD W. WELSCH, PHD, Department of Pharmacolocy/Toxicology, Michigan State Univeristy, East Lansing, MI 48824, USA

JULIE J. WIRTH, PHD, Department of Microbiology, Michigan State University, East Lansing, MI 48824, USA

CATHERINE WOLF, PHD, Institut de Genetique et de Biologie Moleculaire et Cellulaire (IGBMC), CNRS/INSERM/ULP, p.p. 163, 67404 Illkirch Cedex, C.N. de Strasbourg, France

BRUCE R. ZETTER, PHD, Department of Surgery, Children's Hospital, and Program in Biological and Biomedical Sciences, Harvard Medical School, Boston, MA 02115, USA

YI-FAN ZHAI, PHD, Department of Pharmacology/Toxicology, Michigan State University, East Lansing, MI 48824, USA

Preface

This volume is the fifth since 1988 in a series designed to broadly examine current 'Advances in the Cellular and Molecular Biology of Breast Cancer.' As in previous volumes, we have asked recognized experts in cutting-edge topics to each provide a monograph focused on their areas of research. Again, we have turned to researchers to study rodent models of the disease and to those who study the cellular and molecular basis of human breast cancer. This is a time of unprecedented research advances in breast cancer, particularly in understanding the roles of receptors, signal transduction, the cell cycle, aberrant tumor host interactions in metastasis, and the development of more representative rodent models of the disease.

The first section of the book is devoted to new mouse models of mammary development and tumorigenesis. For breast cancer research to move forward, it is essential to use the mouse for better understanding of the roles of individual genes in development and neoplasia, and to establish better model systems for in vivo testing of new therapies for the disease. The first chapter, by R. Strange and his co-workers, introduces the fascinating topic of the regulation of cell death. This is an area of significant current progress that holds much promise for the development of new therapeutic approaches. In Chapter 2, by P.A.W. Edwards, a very promising technique is described for the rapid creation of a transgenic mammary gland. This technique is rapidly gaining utility for testing individual genes for their effects on mammary development and tumorigenesis. In Chapter 3, by D. Medina, a comprehensive view of preneoplastic changes in the mammary glands is presented. The ability to better understand early lesions leading to the disease is essential in our efforts to more accurately detect and prevent breast cancer. In Chapter 4, the final chapter of the section, D.L. Dankart and W.J. Muller describe their recent progress in establishing new transgenic mouse models of metastatic breast cancer. These studies are important both to better understand the metastic process and to provide the framework for testing new therapies with antimetastatic sites of action.

The second section of the book focuses on studies of human breast cancer and receptors, signaling, and the cell cycle. The first chapter of the section, by N.E. Davidson and M.J. Kennedy, discusses the signal transduction enzyme protein kinase C. Defective expression of this enzyme family occurs in breast cancer and provides a target for a new class of therapeutic agents directed against the disease. The second chapter, by C.W. Welsch and colleagues, deals with protein tyrosine phosphatases. These enzymes serve compensatory functions to attenuate the action of tryosine kinase–activating receptors. These enzymes potentially serve tumor suppressive roles in breast cancer. In the third chapter, T.S. Replogle and K.J. Pienta discuss the role of the nuclear matrix in organizing gene expression in the normal and malignant mammary epithelial cell. The fourth chapter, by R.L. Sutherland and his colleagues, describes regulation of the mammary epithelial cell cycle. Steroid and growth factor pathways converge to regulate positive and negative subunits of the cyclin-dependent protein kinases in the cell cycle. Mutations in the genes encoding these proteins are now understood to contribute to breast cancer progression. The fifth chapter, by R.P.C. Shiu and his colleagues, discusses nuclear oncogenes. Both steroid and growth factor pathways of cellular regulation regulate these genes; in addition, certain of these genes are commonly amplified or mutated in breast cancer. The sixth chapter, by H. Michna and colleagues, describes the role of progestins and antiprogestins in breast cancer. Antiprogestins appear to function by triggering cell death. The final chapter of the section, by M.G. Parker, discusses antiestrogen–estrogen receptor interactions. This is a very important topic for understanding the mechanisms whereby the disease becomes refractory to treatment with tamoxifen.

The final section of the book deals with defective tissue interactions in human breast cancer. Understanding this topic is essential in attacking or preventing metastasis of the disease. The first chapter of the section, by B. Gusterson and coworkers, provides a framework for understanding normal tissue architecture and the organization of diverse cell types. New data on differentiation antigens of the stromal and epithelial cells of normal and malignant gland are presented. The second chapter, by F.R. Miller, describes a new human model of preneoplasia. In addition, other mouse models of metastatic progression are presented. The third chapter, by N. Weidner, describes the process of tumor angiogenesis. Angiogenesis is a critical process in tumor growth and metastatic dissemination. The fourth chapter, by J.D. Kantor and B.R. Zetter, focuses on tumor cell mobility, another process critical to tumor metastasis. The fifth chapter, by W.P. Ren and B.F. Sloane, discusses the roles of cathepsins D and B in breast cancer. These enzymes, of the aspartyl and cysteine protease classes, respectively, have also been proposed to participate in metastasis. The sixth chapter, by P. Basset and coworkers, describes the metalloprotease subfamily of stromelysins. These enzymes may play roles both in stromal–epithelial interactions and tumor invasion. The seventh chapter, by K.V. Patel and M.P. Schrey, discusses the vasoactive peptide endothelin, a newly described growth factor in breast cancer. The final chapter of the section, by W.Z. Wei and G.H. Heppner, presents an introduction to breast cancer immunology. Perhaps this area, more than any other, holds significant promise for understanding the onset and suggesting modes for the prevention of the disease.

We are now in an extremely rapid period of acccumulating data on the molecular and cellular biology of breast cancer. These findings are highlighted by the chapters in this book. However, the real challenge is to translate these findings to new strategies of cancer prevention, control, and treatment. The readers of this volume share this responsibility with the authors and editors.

Mammary Tumor Cell Cycle,
Differentiation, and Metastasis

A

Mouse models of mammary development and tumorigenesis

1. Programmed cell death and mammary neoplasia

Pepper J. Schedin, Larissa B. Thackray, Patricia Malone, Susan C. Fontaine, Robert R. Friis, and Robert Strange

Introduction

Normal development and maintenance of tissue size is dependent on a balance between cell proliferation and cell death. Apoptosis, or programmed cell death, plays important roles in mammary gland development, from the embryonic development of sexual dimorphism to senescent involution of the mammary gland. The involution of secretory epithelium following pregnancy and lactation is the most dramatic example of the role of apoptosis in mammary gland development. This phase of mammary gland development provides an important physiological and pathological context in which to study the programmed death of epithelium, because a failure in cell death appears to contribute to neoplastic development [1–3]. Although considerable effort has been directed toward understanding the role of cell proliferation in neoplastic development, much less is known about the process of apoptotic cell death in either the control of normal tissue homeostasis or its potential influence on neoplastic development.

A perturbation in the balance between mitosis and apoptosis can contribute to the development of neoplasia [1–5]. For example, in rodent models of mammary tumorigenesis, conditions that permit or promote excessive cell proliferation permit the accumulation of mutations that contribute to subsequent development of mammary tumors [6–8]. In agreement with these experimental results, proliferative breast disease is also a significant risk factor for the development of breast cancer in humans [9–12]. However, prolonged cell survival can also permit the accumulation of mutations necessary for neoplastic transformation. It has been demonstrated that inhibition of apoptosis, which prolongs the cell life span, can contribute to neoplastic development [14–16]. In contrast, conditions that induce apoptosis, such as the involution of mammary epithelium following full-term pregnancy and lactation, are correlated with a reduced risk for developing breast cancer [17–23]. This suggests that apoptotic cell death of mammary epithelium during mammary gland involution may help explain the reduced risk for the development of breast cancer associated with pregnancy and lactation. In this chapter, we review some of the specific changes that occur during mammary gland involu-

R. Dickson and M. Lippman (eds.) MAMMARY TUMOR CELL CYCLE, DIFFERENTIATION AND METASTASIS. 1996. Kluwer Academic Publishers. ISBN 0-7923-3905-3. All rights reserved.

tion that identify the process of secretory epithelial cell deletion as a programmed cell death or apoptosis, examine some of the changes in gene expression that occur during the period of apoptosis, and present data from a chemoprevention study that suggest induction of apoptosis can inhibit mammary carcinogenesis.

Mammary gland involution

Following pregnancy and lactation, the mammary gland undergoes involution, a process involving dramatic tissue remodeling and massive epithelial cell death. The lactating breast, composed largely of epithelium committed to the secretion of milk proteins, regresses to a quiescent organ composed predominantly of fat cells surrounding a denuded mammary epithelial tree. In contrast to the inflammation and tissue disorder found in necrosis, mammary gland involution is an orderly, gene-mediated, physiological cell death process. The result is elimination of unwanted or potentially deleterious cells while maintaining overall tissue structure in the absence of an inflammatory response [24,25]. As reviewed later, morphological changes (including cytoplasmic and nuclear condensation and the appearance of apoptotic bodies), molecular changes (the nonrandom degradation of DNA into oligonucleosomal-length fragments), and gene expression seen during apoptosis in other developmental contexts provide evidence that secretory mammary epithelium undergoes apoptotic cell death during postlactational mammary gland involution. These changes are closely associated with a dramatic tissue remodeling that culminates in a reorganized mammary gland, ready for a new cycle of lactation.

Morphological changes observed during mammary gland involution

The virgin mouse mammary gland is a mostly ductal structure formed of one to two layers of epithelial cells (Figures 1 and 2A). At age 4–5 weeks, under the influence of ovarian hormones, the immature ducts branch and form lobular structures (Figure 1). During pregnancy (Figures 1 and 2B), these lobular units proliferate and differentiate into lobuloalveolar units composed of milk synthesizing cells. The lactating mammary gland (Figures 1 and 2C) has well-defined lobuloalveolar structures containing secretory material. The alveolar structures consist of a single layer of secretory epithelium with underlying myoepithelial cells and a well-defined basement membrane (Figure 2C). Very few adipocytes are detected in the lactating mammary gland. By 1 day after weaning, apoptotic cells can be found in the milk-filled lumen. Two days postweaning (Figure 2E), increased numbers of apoptotic cells are present in alveolar structures. Foci of collapsed alveoli are found interspersed among adipocytes. At 4 days after weaning (Figure 2F), lobuloalveolar structures are collapsed and cells showing the nuclear changes characteristic of apoptosis and

4

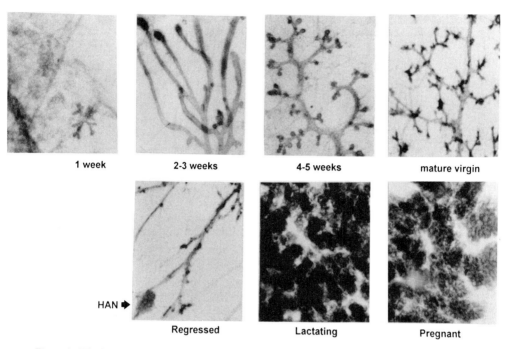

1 week   2-3 weeks   4-5 weeks   mature virgin

HAN ➡

Regressed   Lactating   Pregnant

Figure 1. Whole mount preparations of mouse mammary glands illustrate mammary gland development from early development through pregnancy, lactation, and regression. Mammary glands on glass slides were fixed in 10% buffered formaldehyde, defatted in acetone, stained with iron hematoxylin, cleared in methyl salicylate, mounted, and photographed.

apoptotic bodies are seen throughout sections of mammary glands. Six days after weaning (Figure 2G), the process of involution is well advanced, with little remaining evidence of apoptotic cells. Instead, a significant incursion of cellular stromal elements is seen surrounding areas of densely packed epithelial cells. The fully involuted and remodeled mammary gland (Figures 1 and 2H) consists mostly of adipocytes surrounding well-defined, but dramatically reduced, lobular structures reorganized for another cycle of lactation. As shown in Figures 1 and 2, most of the secretory mammary epithelium undergoes cell death. Although increased numbers of phagocytic cells are observed during involution, there is no massive infiltration of macrophages or granulocytes, as seen in inflammatory or necrotic processes [26–29,31–34]. Also shown in Figure 1 is a premalignant mammary lesion, or hyperplastic alveolar nodule (HAN), which, as will be discussed later, does not respond to signals for apoptosis during mammary gland involution.

Ultrastructural changes associated with mammary gland involution

Ultrastructural studies suggest that the process of involution begins shortly after weaning. The initial changes described include: incursion of the apical

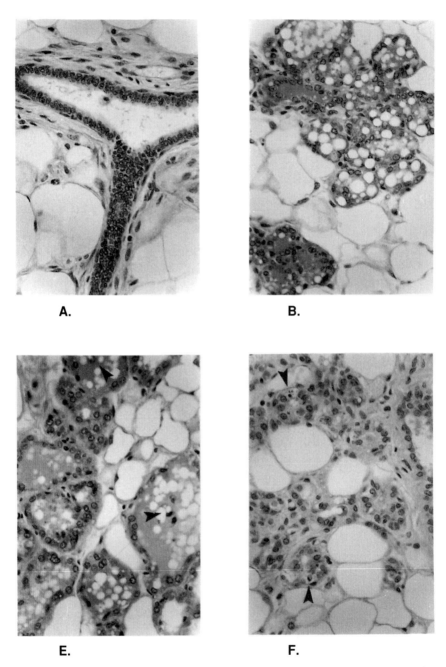

A.   B.

E.   F.

Figure 2. H&E stained sections of mouse mammary glands show changes at the cellular level from virgin through lactation and regression, including apoptotic cell death.

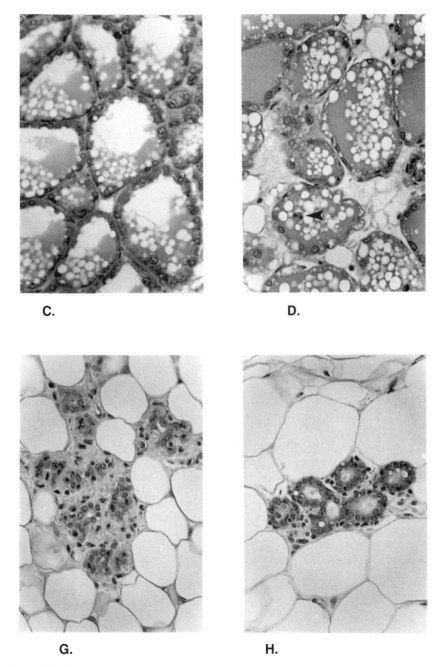

C.

D.

G.

H.

Figure 2 (continued)

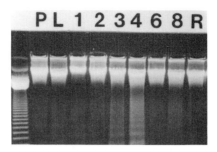

Figure 3. Electrophoretic analysis of nucleic acid integrity in DNA extracted from mouse mammary glands during pregnancy (P), lactation (L), 1, 2, 3, 4, 6 and 8 days after weaning and completion of repression (R). Oligonucleosomal fragments are detected faintly as early as 1 day after weaning of young. Ten microgram samples of DNA extracted from involuting mouse mammary glands were electrophoresed in 1% agarose gels containing 0.25 µg/ml ethidium bromide.

plasma membrane at various points along the cell surface of epithelial cells, depletion of organelles from this apical region, and the presence of numerous single membrane-bounded vacuoles that do not appear associated with secretory activity [26,28,31,32]. These effects are thought to be due to the increased intramammary pressure that occurs after weaning. Changes associated with induction of cell death are detectable by electron microscopy as early as 12 hours postweaning [26,28,31,32]. These changes include irregular branching and focal dilation of the endoplasmic reticulum and, within a few hours to 1 day after weaning, an increase in autophagic vacuoles [26,28,31,32] containing recognizable cellular organelles (mitochondria, endoplasmic reticulum, and cytoplasmic ground substance with free ribosomes). The number and size of these autophagic vacuoles increase by 2–3 days after weaning. Thereafter, the number decreases, but there is an increase in the number of membrane-bound cytoplasmic structures containing dense, irregular membrane-bounded bodies. These would appear to be the source of apoptotic bodies seen later in the process of apoptosis [24,26,28,29,31,32]. Consistent with the evidence of cellular changes observed as early as 12 hours after weaning by electron microscopy, we have detected molecular evidence of apoptosis. Fragmentation of DNA into oligonucleosomal-length fragments is detected within 24 hours after weaning is initiated (Figure 3). In addition, as discussed later, there are significant changes in gene expression within 24 hours after weaning [29,35,36].

Evidence of altered secretory epithelial cell–stromal interactions

Utilizing immunofluorescence analysis, we detected changes in basement membrane protein distribution between days 3–4 after weaning. There is marked thickening of the region in which basement membrane proteins are detected, suggesting that remodeling of the basement membrane occurs at this time. In Figure 4, immunofluorescence analysis of laminin expression during

8

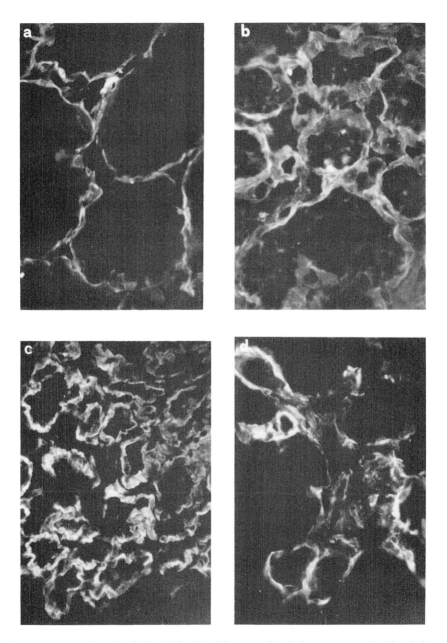

Figure 4. Immunohistochemical analysis of laminin expression during mammary gland involution. Tissue sections are from mouse mammary glands during lactation (a) and 2 (b), 6 (c) and 12 (d) days after weaning. Laminin was detected with a rabbit anti-laminin peptide sera. The secondary is FITC conjugated goat anti-rabbit IgG.

9

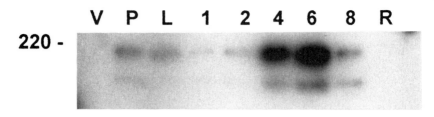

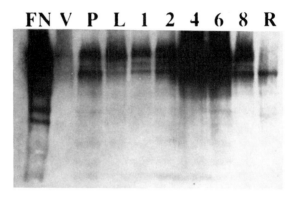

Figure 5. Immunoblot showing expression of laminin in protein samples from involuting mouse mammary glands with increased expression of laminin at days 4–6 after weaning. Protein samples are from virgin (V), pregnant (P), lactating (L), 1, 2, 4, 6 and 8 days after weaning and regressed (R). Rabbit antilaminin peptide is detected with ^{125}I-protein A.

Figure 6. Western analysis of fibronectin expression and integrity during mammary involution. Protein was extracted from mouse mammary glands. Virgin (V), pregnant (P), lactating (L), and 1, 2, 4, 6, and 8 days after weaning and regressed (R). FN is purified fibronectin.

mammary gland involution shows that laminin is detected as a very defined band in the lactating mammary gland. Two days after initiation of weaning, this band remains limited to a narrow band of basement membrane. At 6 days, however, the thickness of laminin is much increased. It also appears that laminin is present in increased amounts.

The role of this increased laminin expression is not clear. Immunoblot analysis also shows this increased expression of laminin (Figure 5). As involution proceeds, there is an increase in the deposition of connective tissue throughout collapsing lobuloalveolar units, and adipose cells reappear in interlobular areas [28,29,32,33,36]. Five to 6 days after weaning, alveolar structures have collapsed into knots of cells with little recognizable order. Immunofluorescence analysis of laminin expression shows a redundant and convoluted basement membrane surrounding collapsed remnants of alveolar epithelium at 6 days after weaning [33] (Figure 4). Although laminin appears to undergo modulation during remodeling of the mammary gland, it does not appear to be degraded. In contrast, between days 4 and 6 days after weaning, fibronectin appears to be induced and is partly degraded into smaller fragments (Figure 6). Of potential significance is the observation that fibronectin fragments, but not intact fibronectin, can induce the expression of metalloproteinases [39,40]. The expression of metalloproteinases is integral to remodeling during mammary involution and is perhaps important for the concomitant apoptotic cell death of mammary epithelium [30,41,42]. Involution in the mouse mammary gland is complete by about 14 days after weaning, at which time laminin and collagen IV expression is confined to tight bands surrounding the mammary epithelium (Figure 4) [26,31,33,35]. The fully involuted mammary gland resembles the mature virgin mammary gland. It is well organized with some lobular structure. In contrast to the mammary gland of a mature virgin, it also contains numerous riboncleoprotein particles. Thus, the bulk of tissue remodeling appears to accompany the peak of epithelial cell death, but apoptosis begins prior to detectable changes in stromal components.

Gene expression during mammary gland involution

Specific regulated changes in gene expression, reflecting the apoptotic cell death and tissue remodeling observed, are detected by Northern analysis of RNA extracted from involuting mammary glands [29,30,35,36]. In order to isolate and identify genes involved in mammary gland involution (particularly those involved in the apoptotic cell death, which plays an integral role in this process), we prepared cDNA libraries from lactating and involuting mouse mammary glands and employed them in a differential screening protocol. This screening and characterization was designed to detect genes that are strongly expressed at 1–2 days involution relative to lactation. Thus far, a large group of genes has been isolated or identified [36]. A number of these genes are associated specifically with (1) *apoptosis*: sulfated glycoprotein-2 (SGP-2) [43], tissue transglutaminase (tTG) [44], p53, c-*myc*, and TGFβ-1 [45–47], and (2) *tissue remodeling*: stromelysin 1 [48] and tissue inhibitor of metalloproteinase (TIMP) [49]. In addition, a number of *death-related cDNAs* were isolated [36]. Figure 7 shows the expression of some of these genes compared with the expression of whey acidic protein (WAP): *WDNM1*, a putative proteinase inhibitor associated with inhibition of mammary tumor metastasis [50]; *24p3/ NGAL*, a potential regulator of metalloproteinase activity [51,52]; *clone 4*, a cDNA related to *γ-fibrinogen* and *scabrous* [53,54], a *Drosophila* gene implicated in growth inhibition; *GlyCAM-1*, the ligand for L-selectin that is expressed in mouse and human milk [55]; *clone 121*, a cDNA related to osteopontin [56]; and *adipocyte differentiation related protein (ADRP)*, a gene cloned from cells induced to undergo adipocyte differentiation [57]. Northern blot analysis confirms specific regulation of expression of these genes during mammary gland involution (Figure 7). These patterns of expression, which have been confirmed in both the rat and mouse, give an indication of both the tight regulation and the complexity of gene expression associated with mammary gland involution. Thus, the execution and control of apoptotic cell death

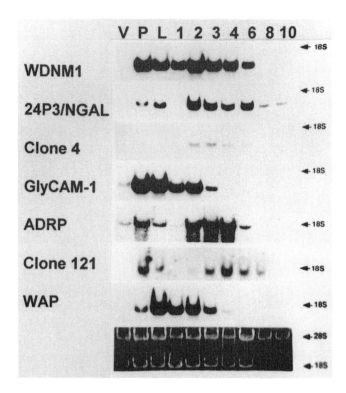

Figure 7. Northern analysis of expression of genes corresponding to cDNAs isolated from involuting mammary epithelium. RNA samples are from virgin (V), pregnant (P), lactating (L), 1, 2, 3, 4, 6, 8 and 10 days after weaning. Ten microgram samples of total RNA were used.

in involuting mammary epithelium appears to be linked to de novo gene expression. The number of genes associated with both apoptosis and tissue remodeling also suggests a close link between these processes.

Initiation and control of apoptosis during mammary gland involution

A number of studies have shown that the hormonal status of an animal has significant outcomes on the initiation and progression of mammary gland involution. Oxytocin, hydrocortisone, and prolactin have been found to inhibit the onset or to delay the progression of involution [27,32,58; Strange and Friis, unpublished observations]. These various studies suggest that the initiating event for involution is a cessation or decline of the hormonal stimulus necessary to maintain lactation. As previously discussed, both histological and ultrastructural indications of apoptotic cell death of mammary epithelium are detected as early as day 1 of mammary gland involution. This can be seen in Figure 2D and 2E showing apoptotic epithelial cells 1 and 2 days after the weaning of young is initiated. Electrophoretic analysis of nucleic acid integrity also reveals oligonucleosomal length fragments of DNA by 24 hours after weaning (Figure 3). Thus, some of the secretory epithelium responds rapidly to cessation of weaning. One interpretation of these observations is that these cells have undergone terminal differentiation, after which their survival is dependent upon lactogenic hormone stimulation.

After initiation of mammary gland involution, it becomes difficult to distinguish between the two major processes that occur during involution: epithelial cell death and tissue remodeling. These processes are so well coordinated during mammary gland involution that either process might induce or regulate the other. Immunohistochemical evidence of tissue remodeling is observed 2–3 days after initiation of weaning, as evidenced by changes in the expression and distribution of basement membrane proteins, as illustrated in Figures 4 and 5 [33–35,37,38]. Consistent with our studies, others have found that the basement membrane is significantly remodelled but that it remains within a defined region, suggesting some maintenance of order. In contrast to the disorder seen in secretory epithelium, immunohistochemical analysis reveals that the myoepithelium remains well organized and much less susceptible to apoptosis [28,29,34,37,38]. Perhaps the overall organization of the mammary gland is orchestrated by myoepithelial cells that are a major source of the proteolytic enzymes responsible for alteration of the basement membrane [29,33,38]. Other studies have suggested that the basement membrane becomes degraded and perhaps discontinuous [33,37]. Still others have found myoepithelial cells and basement membrane proteins exposed to luminal contents and have postulated that this results as dying epithelial cells are released into the lumen [26,31–33]. These observations are consistent with complementary roles for epithelial cell death and remodeling of the extracellular matrix (ECM) encompassing the mammary epithelium in the process of mammary gland involution.

Alterations of the expression and activity of proteinases

Evidence for the role of ECM in regulation of mammary epithelial cell function in vivo comes from studies that alter the balance between ECM degrading enzymes and their inhibitors [30,41,42]. Tissue remodeling during mammary involution has been transiently inhibited by implantation of pellets that release the matrix metalloproteinase inhibitor tissue inhibitor of metalloproteinases (TIMP) [30]. Premature involution in the mouse mammary gland has been induced by expression of an activated matrix degrading proteinase, stromelysin I [41]. During pregnancy, induction of a WAP-stromelysin I transgene in mouse mammary epithelium resulted in loss of basement membrane and a reduction both in gland complexity and biochemical differentiation of mammary glands in the mice bearing this transgene [41]. These data are consistent with the hypotheses that epithelial cell–matrix interactions are im-

13

portant for stabilizing the functional status of the mammary gland and that disruption of this interaction is an important component of the program that regulates apoptosis of epithelial cells during involution of the mammary gland.

The role of protease-mediated tissue remodeling is particularly interesting in the context of recent research focused on anoikis, apoptosis that is induced by the disruption of cell–matrix interactions. Results from in vitro studies of epithelial cells indicate that disruption of interactions between epithelial cells and extracellular matrix can induce apoptotic cell death of the epithelial cells [42,59–63]. These results present an interesting problem for determining the role of tissue remodeling during mammary gland involution. Modulation of cell–matrix interactions certainly has an important role in mammary gland development [64–66]. Mammary gland involution would not be completed without tissue remodeling. In addition, a failure in remodeling may contribute to initiation of neoplasia. The uncoupling of cell death from tissue remodeling could provide an environment that permits neoplastic development [35,41].

The exact role of tissue remodeling remains unclear. Does tissue remodeling induce apoptosis or is it a result of apoptosis? An increase in apoptotic cell death is seen early in involution when it is still reversible. At this point, there are no reported changes of basement membrane or cell–matrix interactions [26,28–34,37]. There is also little alteration in expression of genes that modulate or control tissue remodeling [29,30,35]. Thus, initial epithelial cell death following weaning appears to be a function of hormone ablation and the differentiated state of the cells [27]. However, in our studies of normal mammary gland involution in the mouse, the peak of apoptotic epithelial cell death comes 4 days after weaning, when alteration of the basement membrane appears greatest (Figures 4–6) [29]. This is consistent with in vitro studies suggesting that disruption of cell–matrix interactions induces apoptosis. The connection between these different forms of cell death will be important to define more clearly, particularly as they may be utilized to inhibit mammary tumorigenesis.

Model for complementary and interdependent roles for epithelial cell death and tissue remodeling during involution

Studies of mammary involution in vivo suggest that the apoptotic cell death of mammary epithelium initiated by weaning precedes and may generate the signals for initiation of tissue remodeling [26–29,31–32]. Epithelial cells undergoing apoptotic cell death and oligonucleosomal fragmentation of DNA are detected within 24 hours after weaning, but no changes in basement membrane integrity are seen until about 2 days postweaning [29,31–34]. Up to this time, mammary involution is also reversible. In addition, inhibition of proteinase activity involved in tissue remodeling is able to delay involution [30]. These

14

observations and experiments are consistent with the model that mammary involution and epithelial cell death are initiated by lactogenic hormone ablation due to weaning. This physiological hormone ablation directly causes apoptotic cell death of secretory epithelial cells. As these cells die, they retract from the surrounding matrix and are phagocytized. As long as this death remains at a low level, there is little induction of tissue remodeling enzymes. However, at some threshold level of cell death, sufficient fragmentation of basement membrane is caused to initiate a positive feedback loop, after which commitment to involution is irreversible. This could be caused by either the death and retraction of enough epithelial cells to release matrix fragments, or the local release of proteolytic enzymes by epithelial cells undergoing apoptosis to generate matrix fragments that would induce further proteinase expression [39,40]. Disruption of cell–matrix interactions accelerates the death process as secretory cells susceptible to cell death are released from their normal stromal and intercellular interactions. Some subset of cells, presumably those that have not undergone hormone-induced terminal differentiation, are not responsive to the cell death signals and remain protected from the remodeling process. These cells are the source of the mammary epithelium, in the regressed and reorganized mammary gland, that are ready for another cycle of lactation.

Why is pregnancy protective against breast cancer?

Mammary tumorigenesis is influenced by the developmental history of the mammary gland. In humans, pregnancy and lactation have been associated with protection against developing breast cancer, but the mechanism of this protection is not well understood [17–23]. This protection appears due, in part, to terminal differentiation and apoptotic cell death of secretory mammary epithelium [5,16,22,27,29]. Under the hormonal influence of pregnancy, resting mammary epithelium proliferates and differentiates into secretory epithelium committed to the synthesis of milk proteins. Weaning of young causes a physiological ablation of the lactogenic hormone stimulus, and secretory mammary epithelium undergoes apoptosis. This suggests that the apoptotic cell death that follows pregnancy and lactation is protective, in part, by removing a portion of the mammary epithelial cell that are at risk for neoplastic development. The secretory epithelium that is re-established during the next cycle of pregnancy and lactation is effectively depleted of cells carrying or susceptible to the accumulation of tumorigenic mutations. Consistent with this hypothesis, mammary epithelium that does not undergo involution, such as found in the breasts of nulliparous women, has a greater risk for developing breast cancer [17–23]. Induction of the normal program for cell death in premalignant or malignant mammary tissue presents a powerful potential means for prevention of the progression of mammary carcinogenesis.

Inhibition of apoptosis can contribute to mammary tumorigenesis

An important question to be answered is the contribution of a defect in or failure of apoptosis to initiation of mammary neoplasia. Prolonged cell survival is a characteristic of cells that fail to undergo apoptosis and of cells that comprise a premalignant mouse mammary lesion associated with increased tumor risk, the hyperplastic alveolar nodule (HAN) [7,8,67,68]. The HAN provides an experimental model for human breast hyperplasia. Hyperplastic alveolar nodules resemble mid-pregnant mammary epithelium but fail to fully regress following pregnancy and lactation. Figure 1 shows sections of normal mammary gland and a premalignant mammary hyperplasia from the same mouse 3 days after weaning. The failure of high risk mammary hyperplasias to regress suggests that a failure in the normal program for apoptosis contributes to initiation of neoplasia [7,8,16,22,29]. Support for this hypothesis is found in transgenic mouse studies of factors contributing to mammary tumorigenesis [16]. A transgenic mouse line, which constitutively expressed a growth hormone transgene in its mammary epithelium but did not develop mammary tumors, was crossed with a WAP-*Ha-ras* transgenic line that had a low mammary tumor incidence (2%) and normal postlactational involution. Expression of growth hormone in the mammary gland effectively blocked postlactational involution and, presumably, apoptotic cell death of mammary epithelium (this was not examined directly). The double transgenic mice had a dramatically increased incidence of mammary tumors, presumably due to the accumulation of mutations necessary to complement the weakly transforming oncogene [16]. Thus, mutation of a gene instrumental in the apoptotic death of mammary epithelium would be a likely contributor to mammary tumorigenesis.

Focal epithelial hyperplasias, morphologically similar to hormonally stimulated mammary epithelium that fail to regress fully during involution, are also observed in the human mammary gland and are recognized as significant risk factors for the development of breast cancer [4,9–13]. The persistence of differentiated epithelial hyperplasias in a hormonal environment that does not normally support such differentiation suggests that the epithelial cells fail to respond to normal signals to undergo apoptotic cell death or have a defect in the cascade of gene expression required for execution of apoptotic cell death. In a recent study of mammary hyperplasias in premenopausal women, a decrease in apoptosis relative to mitosis was found to accompany fibrocystic changes (including atypical ductal and lobular hyperplasia, lesions with increased risk for tumorigenesis) and carcinoma of the breast [4]. Similar observations have been made in studies of the factors contributing to B-cell and liver neoplasias [1–3,13–15]. The increased occurrence of neoplasia in breast epithelium of nulliparous women that does not undergo postlactational regression is also consistent with the hypothesis that a defect in apoptosis contributes to breast cancer in humans.

Can induction of apoptosis by altering cell–matrix interactions be utilized as a means of chemoprevention?

Treatment of rates and mice with difluoromethylornithine (DFMO) and retinyl acetate (RA), two important chemopreventive agents, is able to inhibit

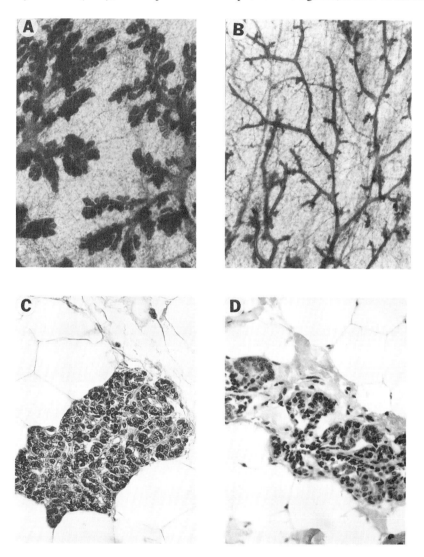

Figure 8. H&E stain of tissue sections from mammary glands of untreated (**A,C**) and treated (**B,D**) animals showing an increased presence of extracellular matrix and decreased complexity (a reduced epithelial cell compartment/component) in the mammary glands of animals treated with DFMO and RA (B,D). These animals were also protected from chemically induced mammary carcinogenesis.

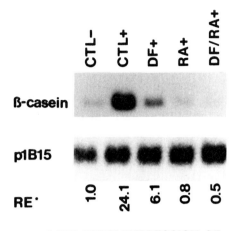

	CTL–	CTL+	DF+	RA+	DF/RA+
ß-casein					
p1B15					
RE*	1.0	24.1	6.1	0.8	0.5

*** RELATIVE EXPRESSION OF
STEADY STATE LEVELS**

Figure 9. Northern analysis of β-casein expression in mammary glands of treated versus control animals. Ten microgram samples of polyA⁺ RNA were used from untreated control (CTL–), hormone stimulated (E&P) control (CTL+), hormone stimulated with DFMO (DF+), hormone stimulated with RA (RA+), and hormone stimulated DFMO plus RA (DF/RA+).

the progression of mammary tumors [69–71]. Morphological studies of mammary glands of treated rats reveal pyknotic nuclei and a reduced epithelial cell compartment, a thickened ECM (Figure 8), and loss of functional differentiation (Figure 9). These features are consistent with apoptosis of mammary epithelium in the treated animals. Expression of genes associated with apoptosis of mammary epithelium is also detected. Northern blot analysis shows that tissue transglutaminase is increased to a level of induction comparable to that observed in involuting mouse and rat mammary glands (Figure 10) [29,72]. Northern analysis shows that tenascin expression is also increased. The decrease in gland complexity and induction of tenascin by DFMO and RA is consistent with published data that demonstrated tenascin can specifically inhibit functional differentiation of mammary epithelial cells in vitro [72].

Substrate gel analysis shows that various proteinases have increased expression in treated mammary glands [69]. In addition, we detected fragmentation of ECM proteins, including collagen IV and fibronectin. This provides an interesting possibility for induction of apoptosis by inhibiting epithelial cell attachment to factors or receptors in the basement membrane that are necessary for their continued survival. The observed increase in fibronectin fragments is consistent with this hypothesis because in other systems, fibronectin fragments have been shown to induce the expression of the matrix degrading proteinases collagenase, stromelysin I and matrilysin [39,40]. Induction of matrix metalloproteinases (MPPs) could generate a positive feedback loop in which fragmentation of ECM and basement proteins induces proteolytic activ-

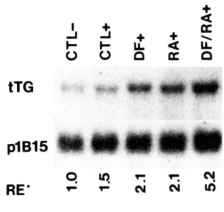

CTL– CTL+ DF+ RA+ DF/RA+

tTG

p1B15

RE*   1.0   1.5   2.1   2.1   5.2

* RELATIVE EXPRESSION OF
STEADY STATE LEVELS

Figure 10. Northern analysis of tissue transglutaminase (TGase) expression in mammary glands of treated versus control animals, as indiated in Figure 9. See Figure 9 for abbreviations.

ity that creates more fragmentation. The elevated levels of fibronectin fragments may provide a mechanistic link to the observed reduction in gland morphology in DFMO plus RA treated glands by inducing proteinases, which in turn degrade the basement membrane. While a cause-and-effect relationship between changes in ECM components and epithelial cell loss has not been established, the data are consistent with chemopreventive agent–related changes in ECM proteins and matrix degrading proteinases that result in degradation of ECM. The destruction of ECM could initiate epithelial cell loss by apoptosis (anoikis) by disrupting epithelial cell–basement membrane interactions [59–63].

References

1. Williams GT (1991) Programmed cell death: Apoptosis and oncogenesis. *Cell* 65:1097–1098.
2. Bursch W, Oberhammer F, Schulte-Hermann R (1992) Cell death by apoptosis and its protective role against disease. *Topics Pharm Sci* 13:245–251.
3. Raff MC (1992) Social controls, cell survival and cell death. *Nature* 356:397–399.
4. Allan DJ, Howell A, Poberts SA, Williams GT, Watson RJ, Coyne JD, Clarke RB, Laidlaw IJ, Potten CS (1992) Reduction in apoptosis relative to mitosis in histologically normal epithelium accompanies fibrocystic change and carcinoma of the premenopausal human breast. *J Pathol* 67:25–32.
5. Thompson HJ, Strange R, Schedin PJ (1992) Apoptosis in the genesis and prevention of cancer. *Cancer Epidemiol Biomarkers Prev* 1:597–602.
6. Barbacid M (1986) Oncogenes and human cancer: Cause or consequence? *Carcinogenesis* 7:1037–1042.
7. Medina D (1988) The preneoplastic state in mouse mammary tumorigenesis. *Carcinogenesis* 8:1113–1119.

19

8. Morris DW, Cardiff RD (1987) Multistep model of mouse mammary tumor development. *Adv Viral Oncol* 7:123–140.
9. Dupont WD, Page DL (1985) Risk factors for breast cancer in women with proliferative breast disease. *N Engl J Med* 312:146–151.
10. Wellings SR, Jensen HM, Marcum RG (1975) An atlas of subgross pathology of the human breast with special reference to precancerous lesions. *J Natl Cancer Inst* 30:231–273.
11. Dupont WD, Parl FF, Hartmann WH, Brinton LA, Winfield AC, Worrell JA, Schuyler PA, Plummer WD (1993) Breast cancer risk associated with proliferative breast disease and atypical hyperplasia. *Caner* 71:1258–1265.
12. London SJ, Connolly JL, Schnitt SJ, Colditz GA (1992) A prospective study of benign breast disease and the risk of breast cancer. *JAMA* 267:941–944.
13. Hockenberry D, Nuñez G, Milliman C, Schreiber RD, Korsmeyer SJ (1990) Bcl-2 is an inner mitochondrial membrane protein that blocks programmed cell death. *Nature* 348:334–336.
14. Willliams GT, Smith CA, Spooncer E, Dexter TM, Taylor DR (1990) Haemopoietic colony stimulating factors promote cell survival by suppressing apoptosis. *Nature* 343:76–79.
15. Schulte-Hermann R, Timmermann-Trosiener I, Barthel G, Bursch W (1990) DNA synthesis, apoptosis and phenotypic expression as determinants of growth altered foci in rat liver during phenobarbital promotion. *Cancer Res* 50:5127–5135.
16. Andres A-C, Bchini O, Schubar B, Dolder B, LeMeur M, Gerlinger P (1991) H-ras induced transformation of mammary epithelium is favored by increased oncogene expression or by inhibition of mammary regression. *Oncogene* 6:771–779.
17. Harris JR, Lippman ME, Veronesi U, Willett W (1992) Breast cancer. *N Engl J Med* 327:319–328.
18. Ewertz M, Duffy SW, Adami H-O, Kvale G, Loaned E, Meirik O, Mellengaard A, Soini I, Tulinius H (1990) Age at first birth, parity and risk of breast cancer: A meta-analysis of 8 studies from the Nordic countries. *Int J Cancer* 46:597–603.
19. Trichopoulos D, Hsieh CC, MacMahon B, Lin T-M, Lowe CR, Mirra AP, Ravnihar B, Salber EJ, Valaoras VG, Yuasa S (1983) Age at any birth and breast cancer risk. *Int J Cancer* 31:701–704.
20. Byers T, Graham S, Rzepka T, Marshall J (1985) Lactation and breast cancer: Evidence for a negative association in premenopausal women. *Am J Epidemiol* 121:664–674.
21. McTiernan A, Thomas DB (1986) Evidence for a protective effect of lactation on risk of breast cancer in young women. *Am J Epidemiol* 124:353–358.
22. Russo J, Rivera R, Russo IH (1992) Influence of age and parity on the development of the human breast. *Breast Cancer Res Treat* 23:211–218.
23. Yoo K-Y, Tajima K, Kurioshi T, Hirose K, Yoshida M, Miura S, Murai H (1992) Independent protective effect of lactation against breast cancer: A case-control study in Japan. *Am J Epidemiol* 135:726–733.
24. Wyllie AH, Kerr JFR, Currie AR (1980) Cell death: The significance of apoptosis. *Int Rev Cyt* 68:251–306.
25. Ucker DS (1991) Death by suicide: One way to go in mammalian cellular development? *N Biol* 3:103–109.
26. Helminen HJ, Ericsson JLE (1968) Studies on mammary gland involution II. Ultrastructural evidence for auto- and heterophagocytic pathways for cytoplasmic degradation. *J Ultrastruct Res* 25:214–227.
27. Ossowski L, Biegel D, Reich E (1979) Mammary plasminogen activator: Correlation with involution, hormonal modulation and comparsion between normal and neoplastic tissue. *Cell* 16:929–940.
28. Walker NI, Bennett RE, Kerr JFR (1989) Cell death by apoptosis during involution of the lactating breast in mice and rats. *Am Anat* 185:19–32.
29. Strange R, Li F, Saurer S, Burkhardt A, Friis RR (1992) Apoptotic cell death and tissue remodeling during mouse mammary gland involution. *Development* 115:49–58.
30. Talhouk RS, Bissell MJ, Werb Z (1992) Coordinated expression of extracellular matrix-

degrading proteinases and their inhibitors regulates mammary epithelial function during involution. *J Cell Biol* 118:1271–1282.

31. Wellings SR, DeOme KB (1963) Electron microscopy of milk secretion in the mammary gland in C3H/Crgl mouse. III. Cytomorphology of the involuting gland. *J Natl Cancer Inst* 30:241–248.

32. Lascelles AK, Lee CS (1978) Involution of the mammary gland. In *Lactation*, Vol IV. BL Larson (ed). New York: Academic Press, pp 115–177.

33. Warburton MJ, Mitchell S, Ormerod EJ, Rudland P (1982) Distribution of myoepithelial cells and basement membrane proteins in the resting, pregnant, lactating and involuting rat mammary gland. *J Histochem Cytochem* 30:667–676.

34. Dickson SR, Warburton MJ (1992) Enhanced synthesis of gelatinase and Stromelysin by myoepithelial cells during involution of the rat mammary gland. *J Histochem Cytochem* 40:697–703.

35. Li F, Strange R, Friis RR, Djonov V, Altermatt H-J, Saurer S, Niemann H, Andres A-C (1994) Expression of Stromelysin-1 and TIMP-1 in the involuting mammary gland and in early invasive tumors of the mouse. *Int J Cancer* 59:560–568.

36. Li F, Bielke W, Andres A-C, Friis RR, Bemis LT, Geske FJ, Strange R (1995) Isolation of cDNAs from mammary epithelium undergoing post-lactational apoptotic cell death. *Cell Death Differ* 2:108–117.

37. Martinez-Hernandez A, Fink LM, Pierce GB (1976) Removal of basement membrane in the involuting breast. *Lab Invest* 34:455–462.

38. Radnor CJP (1972) Myoepithelium in involuting mammary glands of the rat. *J Anat* 112:355–365.

39. Werb Z, Tremble PM, Behrendtsen O, Crowley E, Damsky CH (1989) Signal transduction through the fibronectin receptor induces collagenase and stromelysin gene expression. *J Cell Biol* 109:877–889.

40. Yamamoto H, Itoh F, Hinoda Y, Senota A, Yoshimoto M, Nakamura H, Imai K, Yachi A (1994) Expression of matrilysin mRNA in colorectal adenomas and its induction by truncated fibronectin. *Biochem Biophys Res Commun* 201:657–664.

41. Sympson C, Talhouk RS, Alexander CM, Chin JR, Clift SM, Bissell MJ, Werb Z (1994) Targeted expression of Stromelysin-1 in mammary gland provides evidence for a role of proteinases in branching morphogenesis and the requirement for intact basement membrane for tissue-specirfic gene expression. *J Biol Chem* 125:681–693.

42. Boudreau N, Sympson CJ, Werb Z, Bissell MJ (1995) Suppression of ICE and apoptosis in mammary epithelial cells by extracellular matrix. *Science* 267:891–893.

43. Buttyan R, Olsson CA, Pintar J, Chang C, Bandyk M, Ng P-Y, Sawczuk IS (1989) Induction of the TRPM-2 gene in cells undergoing programmed death. *Mol Cell Biol* 9:3473–3481.

44. Fesus L, Thomazy V, Falus A (1987) Induction and activation of tissue transglutaminase during programmed cell death. *FEBS Lett* 224:104–108.

45. Yonish-Rouach E, Renitzky D, Lotem J, Sachs L, Kimichi A, Oren M (1991) Wild-type p53 induces apoptosis of myeloid leukaemic cells that is inhibited by interleukin-6. *Nature* 352:345–347.

46. Evan GI, Wyllie AH, Gilbert CS, Littlewood TD, Land H, Brooks M, Waters CM, Penn LZ, Hancock DC (1992) Induction of apoptosis in fibroblasts by c-myc protein. *Cell* 69:119–128.

47. Martikianen P, Kyprianou N, Issacs JT (1990) Effect of transforming growth factor-β_1 on proliferation and death of rat prostatic cells. *Endocrinology* 127:2963–2968.

48. Matrisian LM, Glaichenhaus N, Gesnel M-C, Breathnach R (1985) Epidermal growth factor and oncogenes induce transcription of the same cellular mRNA in rat fibroblasts. *EMBO J* 4:1435–1440.

49. Gewert DR, Coulombe B, Castellino M, Skup D, Williams BRG (1987) Characterization and expression of a murine gene homologous to human EPA/TIMP: A virus-induced gene in the mouse. *EMBO J* 6:651–657.

50. Dear TN, Ramshaw IA, Kefford RF (1988) Differential expression of a novel gene, WDNM1, in nonmetastatic rat mammary adenocarcinoma cells. *Cancer Res* 48:5203–5209.

51. Triebel S, Bläser J, Reinke H, Tschesche H (1992) A 25 kDa α_2-microglobulin-related protein is a component of the 125 kDa form of human gelatinase. *FEBS Lett* 314:386–388.
52. Kjeldsen L, Johnsen AH, Sengeløv H, Borregaard N (1993) Isolation and primary structure of NGAL, a novel protein associated with human neutrophil gelatinase. *J Biol Chem* 268:10425–10432.
53. Baker NE, Mlodzik M, Rubin GM (1990) Spacing differentiation in the developing Drosophila eye: A fibrinogen-related lateral inhibitor encoded by scabrous. *Science* 250:1370–1377.
54. Rüegg C, Pytela R (1995) Sequence of a human transcript expressed in T-lymphocytes encoding a fibrinogen-like protein. *Gene* 160:257–262.
55. Dowbenko D, Kikuta A, Gillett N, Lasky L (1993) Glycosylation-dependent cell adhesion molecule 1 (GlyCAM-1) mucin is expressed by lactating mammary gland epithelial cells and is present in milk. *J Clin Invest* 92:952–960.
56. Senger DR, Perruzzi CA, Papadopoulos-Sergiou A, Van De Water L (1994) Adhesive properties of Osteopontin: Regulation by a naturally occurring thrombin-cleavage in close proximity to the GRGDS cell-binding domain. *Mol Biol Cell* 5:565–574.
57. Jiang H-P, Serrero G (1992) Isolation and characterization of a full-length cDNA coding for an adipose differentiaton-related protein. *Proc Natl Acad Sci USA* 89:7859–7860.
58. Schmidt GH (1971) *Biology of Lactation*. San Francisco: W.H. Freeman.
59. Meredith JE Jr, Fazeli B, Schwartz MA (1993) The extraellular matrix as a cell survival factor. *Mol Biol Cell* 9:953–961.
60. Frisch SM, Francis H (1994) Disruption of epithelial cell-matrix interactions induces apoptosis. *J Cell Biol* 124:619–624.
61. Bates RC, Buret A, van Helden DF, Horton MA, Burns GF (1994) Apoptosis induced by inhibition of intercellular contact. *J Cell Biol* 125:403–415.
62. Ruoslahti E, Reed JC (1994) Anchorage dependence, integrins and apoptosis. *Cell* 77:477–478.
63. Re F, Zanetti A, Sironi M, Polentarutti N, Lanfrancone L, Dejana E, Colotta F (1994) Inhibiton of anchorage-dependent cell spreading triggers apoptosis in cultures human endothelial cells. *J Cell Biol* 127:537–546.
64. Dürnberger H, Kratochwil K (1980) Specificity of tissue interaction and origin of mesenchymal cells in the androgen response to the embryonic mammary gland. *Cell* 19:465–471.
65. Haslam SZ (1991) Stromal-epithelial interactions in normal and neoplastic mammary gland. In *Regulatory Mechanisms in Breast Cancer*. M Lippman, R Dickson (eds). Boston: Kluwer Academic, pp 401–420.
66. Howlett AR, Bissell MJ (1993) The influence of tissue microenvironment (stroma and extracellular matrix) on the development and function of mammary epithelium. *Epithel Cell Biol* 2:79–89.
67. Foulds L (1969) *Neoplastic Development*. New York: Academic Press.
68. Cardiff RD (1984) Protoneoplasia: The molecular biology of murine mammary hyperplasia. *Adv Cancer Res* 42:167–190.
69. Schedin PJ, Strange R, Kaeck M, Singh M, Thompson HJ (1995) Treatment with chemopreventive agents DFMO and retinoic acid results in altered mammary mesenchyme and epithelial cell loss. *Carcinogenesis* 16:1787–1794.
70. Verma AK (1990) Inhibition of tumor promotion by DL-α-difuoromethyl-ornithine, a specific irreversible inhibitor of ornithine decarboxylase. *Basic Life Sci* 52:195–204.
71. Maiorana A, Gullino PM (1980) Effect of retinyl acetate on the incidence of mammary carcinomas and hepatomas in mice. *J Natl Cancer Inst* 64:655–663.
72. Guenette RS, Corbeil HB, Léger J, Wong K, Mézl V, Mooibroek M, Tenniswood M (1994) Induction of gene expression during involution of the lactating mammary gland of the rat. *J Mol Endocrinol* 12:47–60.
73. Chammas R, Taverna D, Cella N, Santos C, Hynes N (1994) Laminin and tenascin assembly and expression regulate HC11 mouse mammary cell differentiation. *J Cell Sci* 107:1031–1040.

2. Tissue reconstitution, or transgenic mammary gland, technique for modeling breast cancer development

Paul A.W. Edwards

Introduction

Breast cancer appears to develop as a result of clones of cells accumulating a series of mutations. To model this process, we [1–9] and others [10–13] have introduced tumor mutations into individual clones of cells in mouse mammary epithelium, in mice, by a transplantation approach known as *tissue reconstitution* or constructing a *transgenic mammary gland*. Introducing oncogenes and growth factor genes in this way has shown how the three-dimensional growth pattern of mammary epithelium is altered by such genes and allows us to address basic questions, such as: What does an individual oncogene do to three-dimensional growth control? Do related oncogenes have similar or different effects? How do the effects of oncogenes relate to their normal role in controlling the three-dimensional growth pattern? How do clones of cells that express an oncogene behave among neighboring normal cells in an epithelium? The method also allows sequential introduction of more than one oncogene to follow tumor development.

Tissue reconstitution method for expressing genes in mammary epithelium

The tissue reconstitution method for expressing genes in mammary epithelium is shown in Figure 1 [6]. Mammary epithelial cells from an adult female mouse are put into primary culture, and a gene of interest is introduced into a small proportion of the cells by infection with helper-free (i.e., nonreplicating) retrovirus [14]. The cells are then transplanted into a *cleared mammary fat pad*, a mammary fat pad from which the natural epithelium has been removed [15]. The cleared fat pad is made by removing the nipple end of the #4 fat pad 3 weeks after birth, at which stage the natural epithelium has only grown a short distance into the fat pad. The injected cells reform an epithelium by growing out from the site of injection. This epithelium seems entirely normal by all criteria, except that it is not connected to a nipple, so that milk secretion stops immediately after parturition. In this reconstituted epithelium, a small fraction of the cells expresses the introduced gene (unless retrovirus infection

R. Dickson and M. Lippman (eds.) MAMMARY TUMOR CELL CYCLE, DIFFERENTIATION AND METASTASIS. 1996. Kluwer Academic Publishers. ISBN 0-7923-3905-3. All rights reserved.

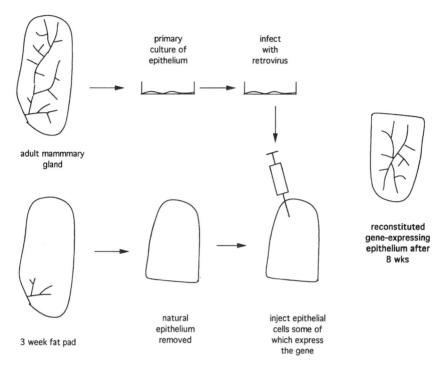

Figure 1. The tissue reconstitution method for introducing genes into mouse mammary epithelium in vivo. Mammary epithelial cells are prepared from an adult female gland by collagenase digestion and are put into primary culture. They are infected with helper-free retrovirus and then transplanted into a cleared mammary fat pad in vivo. The cleared fat pad is prepared in a 3-week-old female mouse. At this age the epithelium, represented in the diagram by lines, is a small cluster of ducts that has grown only a short way in from the nipple. It can be removed by cutting off the top of the fat pad. The genetically manipulated cells reform an epithelium that branches and fills the fat pad over about 10 weeks. The whole gland can then be whole mounted as shown in later figures. In our laboratory, cells are infected with retrovirus by subculturing the primary cells onto irradiated retrovirus-producing cells. The total time in culture is 4 days. For details see Edwards et al. [8].

conditions are modified to give a high proportion of infected cells [8]). An important feature of the method is that the primary epithelial cells are only kept in culture for a short time, 4 days in our protocol, so that they do not have time to adapt to culture or to acquire unknown mutations. Technical details have been reviewed elsewhere [8]. The tissue reconstitution approach has also been used to model neoplasia in other tissues, for example, in skin, prostate, and the hemopoietic system [5].

Comparison of the reconstituted mammary gland with transgenic models

There are currently three methods available for expressing genes in mammary epithelium: the tissue reconstitution method, direct introduction of genes, and mammary-specific expression in transgenic mice. In direct introduction, helper-free retroviruses are injected directly into the mammary gland through the nipple [16,17]. This approach works well in the rat and has been used to introduce the v-Ha-*ras* and *neu* oncogenes [16,17], but no studies in the mouse have yet been reported. It seems likely that the mouse gland, at least in the nonlactating animal, is too small to be manipulated this way. Mammary-specific expression of genes in transgenic mice is probably the most widely known of the methods. Here, genes are expressed in germ-line transgenic mice from mammary-specific promoters, for example, the promoters for whey acidic protein (WAP) [18] or mouse mammary tumor virus (MMTV) [19,20].

Tissue reconstitution and direct introduction have two major advantages over the transgenic mouse approach as models of the development of neoplasia. Firstly, they introduce genes into individual cell clones against a background of normal neighboring cells, as in natural tumor development (Figure 2c). In contrast, in transgenics all cells in the tissue express the introduced gene, causing a generalized hyperplasia, and it is not possible to see how

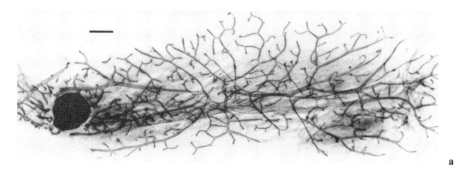

a

Figure 2. Examples of reconstituted mammary glands expressing oncogenes. Whole mounts of reconstituted glands expressing various genes. Whole glands were stained and then cleared by immersion in methyl salicylate. Except in b, they are stained with the nuclear stain carmine. Epithelium appears as dark treelike structures within clear adipose tissue. The oval dark body at the end of the fat pads is a lymph node. The magnification is the same in all the photographs, scale bar = 1 mm. **a.** Control transplant infected with a retrovirus that carries no oncogene. **b.** Reconstituted gland expressing the enzyme beta-galactosidase, stained histochemically for the enzyme. In this typical example, a small region of the epithelium expresses the gene and stains deep blue, which appears black in the photograph. The rest of the epithelium, unstained, is a faint yellow color and appears pale grey. Primary mouse mammary epithelial cells were infected with the retrovirus IRV-BAG, which expresses beta-galactosidase from a beta-actin promoter [41], and were transplanted as shown in Figure 1. After 10 weeks of growth of the transplant, the glands were stained as whole mounts for beta-galactosidase activity using X-gal as the substrate [41]. **c.** Lesion (marked by the arrow) caused by the expression of the activated *c-erbB-2* oncogene *neu,* as described previously [3,8,9]. Primary cells were infected with a retrovirus that expresses *neu* from a beta-actin promoter. **d.** Transplant expressing the *Wnt-1* oncogene, as described in Edwards et al. [7]. With this oncogene, unlike with *erbB-2,* the whole of the epithelium is hyperplastic. **e.** Hyperplasia induced by *v-myc,* as described in Edwards et al. [6]. As with *Wnt-1,* the abnormal growth pattern is often uniform throughout the transplant.

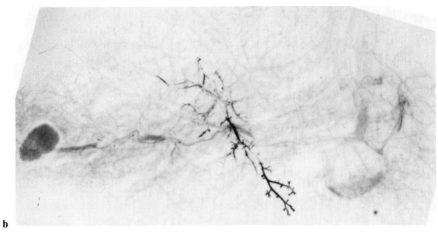

b

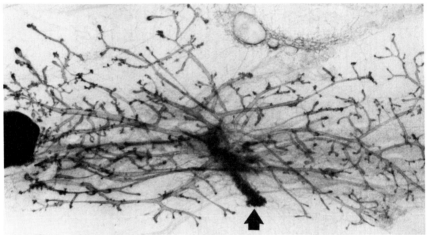

c

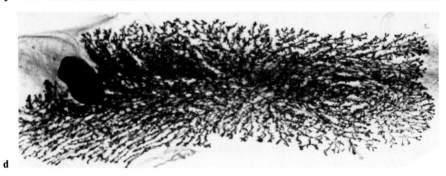

d

Figure 2 (continued)

26

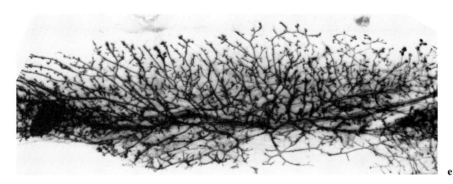

e

Figure 2 (continued)

focal, clonal lesions develop. Secondly, any promoter can be used to drive the expression of a gene in the reconstitution system. For example, we have used the beta-actin promoter, and, in the future, inducible promoters could be used if reliable ones become available. Transgenic experiments have to use the available mammary-specific promoters, which have limitations. They are not completely mammary specific, so that growth abnormalities can occur elsewhere and may even be lethal during development [21]. The WAP, BLG, and some forms of the MMTV promoters are essentially lactation specific [20], and are weak or inactive in the virgin (resting) gland, the state most relevant to modeling breast cancer.

The tissue reconstitution approach is probably also less expensive and quicker than making transgenic mice, especially because any individual transgenic line may show effects specific to the integration site of the transgene and at least two lines have to be compared. In transplants, many different sites of retrovirus integration are generated within one experiment, so integration-specific effects do not influence the overall picture. One technical limitation of the reconstitution approach is that there may be immune responses to the introduced gene product. For example, we have seen obvious lymphocyte infiltration around epithelium that expressed the MC29 *gag-myc* fusion protein [6] and SV40 large T [unpublished], both viral proteins that may be very immunogenic. Other oncogenes have not elicited a detectable response, notably OK10 *v-myc*. One solution is to use mouse genes; another may be to induce tolerance to the introduced protein.

What does an individual oncogene do to three-dimensional growth control?

Mammary epithelium is particularly suited to studying the steps in tumor development because the entire epithelium can be visualized in three dimensions by whole mounting. In this technique the whole mammary gland is stained and made transparent to display its three-dimensional structure

27

(Figure 2). This shows even small local changes in spatial organization caused by oncogenes (Figure 2). Several oncogenes and growth factors have now been expressed in mammary epithelium, and overall there is a striking diversity of effects; for example, altered branching of ducts, inappropriate alveolus formation, and changes in hormone responsiveness. The altered growth patterns produced are in most cases quite well ordered and stable, rarely, if at all, giving rise to tumors on the time scale of the experiments (usually 3–4 months). Work with the reconstitution system has concentrated on early, simple preneoplastic lesions that reveal the consequences of the introduced mutation acting alone, without subsequent unknown changes that occur in tumor development.

Pattern of expression of an introduced gene

To show where in the gland an introduced gene might be expressed, beta-galactosidase was introduced into transplanted epithelium, using a retrovirus that transduces beta-galactosidase, and whole glands were stained histochemically with X-gal to show where the enzyme was expressed (Figure 2b) [8]. Typically, expressing cells were scattered over part of a transplant — some cells alone, and others in clusters — in a manner that would be consistent with all of them deriving from one, two, or occasionally three clones per transplant, although we have not confirmed this interpretation. Figure 2b shows a typical transplant in which the distribution of stained cells looks as though they may be a single clone.

The beta-galactosidase staining clearly shows the position of retrovirus-infected cells in the whole mount, and in the future it would be an advantage to coexpress betagalactosidase with the oncogenes introduced so that changes in growth pattern can be related to the presence of genetically manipulated cells. We [8; C.L. Abram, M.J. Page, and P.A.W. Edwards, unpublished] have made a new retrovirus vector, pCA1, that directs the translation of both beta-galactosidase and a gene of interest from a single message, giving well-coordinated expression of the two genes. The translation of two reading frames from a single message is achieved using a picornavirus IRES sequence [22]. *neo* activity has also been incorporated by using *beta-geo*, a fusion protein combining beta-galactosidase and *neo* activity [23].

ErbB2: Focal development of a spectrum of lesions

ErbB2 is a growth factor receptor closely related to the EGF receptor, ErbB, and is normally expressed in the lactating mammary gland [24]. It is one of the best candidates for an oncogene of importance in human breast cancer, with around 20% of breast carcinomas, and a high proportion of carcinomas in situ, expressing high levels of the protein [25]. Several groups have shown that the overactive mutant form of rat *erbB2*, *neu*, is very effective at causing carcinoma in situ and frank carcinoma when expressed in mammary epithelium [3,17,26,27]. Wild-type *erbB2* was also reported to produce tumors when expressed in mammary epithelium in transgenic mice, but subsequently the introduced *erbB2* was found to have acquired activating mutations during tumor development [28].

When *neu* was introduced into reconstituted epithelium, focal lesions developed in the transplanted epithelium (Figure 2c) [3,8,9]. The focal distribution of abnormal growth was as expected from the experiments in which beta-galactosidase was expressed (Figure 2b). In whole mount the more obvious lesions were dense aggregates of cells, often of rather ill-defined shape, although some suggested the 'bunch-of-grapes' shape formed by clusters of alveoli in the lactating gland [3,8]. These lesions were classified by the standard criteria of human histopathology as hyperplasias with or without atypia, sclerosing adenosis, carcinoma in situ, and frank carcinoma [3].

To try to understand the development of these lesions, we have examined whole mounts and sections for mild lesions [8,9]. Many whole mounts showed clusters of alveoli on ducts in the virgin gland, apparently representing inappropriate development of alveoli in the virgin gland. They occurred either focally as distinct lesions or peripherally to more advanced lesions. Alveoli were also often prominent in glands that had been taken through lactation and involution [illustrated in 3,8]. In this case, they could have been present as inappropriate alveoli before lactation or they could have arisen normally in lactation but have been retained as a result of *erbB2/neu* expression. Antibody staining of sections through clusters of alveoli showed expression of ErbB2 [3]. Histologically, a continuum of morphologies was seen, from essentially normal clusters of alveoli through to more advanced lesions [3,9]. One interpretation is that ErbB2 is normally involved in initiating or maintaining alveoli in lactation, and that inappropriate activation of the receptor leads to inappropriate alveolus formation.

erbB2 *compared with* erbB: *Do related oncogenes have similar or different effects?*

ErbB and ErbB2 are closely related growth factor receptors, and yet constitutively active mutants of them alter the growth of transplanted epithelium in quite different ways. This is a clear illustration of the diversity of oncogene effects on growth, which would not be revealed by in vitro experiments. In contrast to the alveolar lesions produced by expressing *neu*, v-*erbB* produced enlarged ducts in which the luminal surface was fragmented and there were frequently loose epithelial cells in the lumen. There was little alteration to the surrounding stroma [1]. Thus two closely related oncogenes have different effects, although we do not yet know whether this is because ErbB and ErbB2 activate different signal transduction pathways or because the mode of activation of the oncogenes was different — v-*erbB* is chicken c-*erbB*, with both ends truncated, while *neu* is rat c-*erbB2*, with a point mutation in the transmembrane domain. This is currently under investigation.

myc *and* Wnt-1 — *clonal expansion?*

Examples of oncogenes that have a completely different kind of effect on the epithelium are *myc* and *Wnt-1* (originally known as *int-1*). They alter the pattern of duct branching in the gland (Figure 2d and 2e). The effect of expressing *myc*, both in the form v-*myc* [6] or c-*myc* [unpublished], is to produce a closer spacing of ducts (Figure 2e). *Wnt-1* produces an even more dramatic increase in the density of ducts (Figure 2d) [7], originally observed when *Wnt-1* was expressed in transgenic mice [29]. With both genes, rather than the growth pattern being disturbed focally, a large part or all of the transplant is abnormal. This is not what we would expect from the beta-galactosidase experiment (Figure 2b). The effect is very local, and not a systemic effect due to hormone release, since in both cases normal epithelium can be found only 100–200 µm away from the affected epithelium [6,7,30]. The most interesting interpretation of this result is that cells that express either of these oncogenes outgrow their normal neighbors and take over most or all of the tansplant, the kind of clonal expansion postulated to occur in neoplastic development. In support of this idea, the morphology of the transplants is usually rather uniform, particularly in the case of *Wnt-1*, but varies between transplants, suggesting that they are clonal. However, other explanations have not yet been ruled out. For example, the hyperplasias could be a mixture of oncogene-expressing cells and normal cells, the normal cells being influenced by their abnormal neighbors. This is certainly plausible for *Wnt-1*, as the Wnt-1 product is a secreted, growth-factor–like molecule. We have not been able to stain cells for the presence of these oncogenes — *myc* is expressed at too low a level, and there are no antisera suitable for immunocytochemistry of *Wnt-1* — so the resolution of this question awaits coexpression with a marker gene, as described earlier.

Is Wnt-1 *an oncogene because it mimics other* Wnts?

Wnt-1 was originally discovered as *int-1*, a gene whose expression is often activated in mammary tumors induced by MMTV [reviewed in 31]. The *Wnt-1* product is a secreted glycoprotein, and its close homology to the Wingless gene product of *Drosophila* suggests that it is involved in short-range signaling between cells. For some time its oncogenic activity was a puzzle: If it was not expressed in normal mammary gland, why should there be a receptor for it? However, more recently a large family of closely related glycoproteins, the Wnt family, has been discovered, and several of these are normally expressed in mammary gland in various stages of development [32,34]. Wnts seem to be involved in controlling a wide range of developmental processes [36]. Wnt-1 might therefore alter mammary growth pattern by mimicking one or more other Wnt glycoproteins that are normally involved in regulating mammary development.

We had also suggested that the hyperplastic epithelium induced by expressing Wnt-1 (Figure 2d) looked somewhat like a mid-pregnant epithelium. In early pregnancy new side branches develop on the duct framework laid down in the virgin animal. To show the resemblance, transplants of normal mammary epithelium were grown in a pregnant mouse, and their growth pattern was quite similar to the Wnt-1–expressing transplant in a virgin mouse [7].

It followed that one or more of the Wnt gene products might be responsible for directing side-branch growth in early pregnancy, so we expressed some of the likely Wnts in transplants. Wnt-4 seemed to fulfil the prediction [4]. In the normal mammary gland, it is expressed only weakly in the virgin, and expression increases early in pregnancy [32,34]. Reconstituted epithelium expressing Wnt-4, in the virgin gland, showed an overbranched pattern of growth close, but not identical, to that of early pregnancy [4]. Comparing the patterns of growth induced by Wnt-4 and Wnt-1, the Wnt-4 pattern was closer to that of early pregnancy. Although much more needs to be done, it seems likely that Wnt-4 plays a key role in pregnancy, changing the growth pattern of the epithelium, and that the oncogenic effect of Wnt-1 is at least in part through its ability to mimic Wnt-4. Wnt-1 may also mimic other Wnt proteins that are normally expressed in mammary gland, such as Wnt-6 and Wnt-7b [32,34]. Wnt-1, Wnt-6, and Wnt-7b transform fibroblasts, while Wnt-4 has little or no effect [35], suggesting that Wnt-1 is also a ligand for a receptor that binds Wnt-6 and Wnt-7b.

Hormone-independent growth of epithelium that expresses Wnt-1

Because the dependence of mammary growth on ovarian hormones is a major practical issue in breast cancer, any situations in which the growth of mammary epithelium is independent of ovarian hormones are of interest, even if the genes involved are probably not relevant to the human situation. When Tsukamoto et al. [29] expressed Wnt-1 in mammary epithelium in transgenic mice they found that the hyperplastic epithelium developed in male mice as well as in females, so its growth was independent of ovarian hormones. In the transgenic mice the effect could have been systemic. To show that it was local, Wnt-1–expressing epithelium and normal epithelium were transplanted into opposite ends of the same fat pad in normal mice [7,30]. The two epithelial outgrowths grew until they confronted each other in the fat pad, with a separation of about 100–200 µm. The morphology of the normal epithelium was completely unaffected, showing not only that the effect of Wnt-1 was not systemic, but also that it was of very limited range within the fat pad, as expected from the behavior of Wnts in other systems [31].

In normal mice, growth of epithelial tubes can be divided into two phases: growth of major ducts in the virgin animal, and growth of side branches in pregnancy. These two growth phases have different hormone/growth factor sensitivity; for example, they respond differently to transforming growth factor (TGF)-beta [37]. Growth of major ducts occurs at characteristic terminal endbud structures, but these are not found in side branch growth. Wnt-1–expressing epithelium has terminal endbuds when growing in intact females, but they are absent during growth in males or ovariectomized females, showing that Wnt-1 does not simply substitute for ovarian hormones. We suggested an alternative, if speculative, interpretation, based on our hypothesis that Wnt-1 caused the side branch growth that would normally occur in pregnancy (see earlier): Growth of the side-branch type might be independent of ovarian hormones and so Wnt-1–driven growth was also ovarian independent [7]. If this is correct, then estrogen-independent tumor growth might be driven by signals that would normally only be issued in pregnancy or lactation.

hst/FGF-4

hst/FGF-4 is a member of the fibroblast growth factor family, which seems occasionally to be expressed in MMTV-induced mouse mammary tumors, and is coamplified with *int-2* and *PRAD-1*, but apparently not expressed, in human tumors. It causes what seem to be alveoli to develop singly or in clusters, along major ducts [for illustrations see 5,8]. This is similar to the mildest effects of *FGF3/int-2* [38]. As in the case of ErbB2, this raises the possibility that an FGF is normally involved in controlling the growth of alveoli.

v-Ha-ras

v-Ha-*ras* has also been introduced both by retrovirus infection of primary cultures [2,10,13] and by calcium-phosphate transfection of plasmid DNA followed by mild selection [11]. Some of the resulting transplants showed irregular, dilated duct structures with enlarged, dense endbuds, increased alveolar budding, and multilayered epithelium [10,13]. Others developed tightly clustered groups of alveolar structures [2,11].

Sequential introduction of more than one oncogene to follow tumor development

The tissue reconstitution method permits an elegant reconstruction of the sequential development of a tumor [2,10]. One oncogene can be introduced to produce a preneoplastic growth pattern, and then a second oncogene can be added to some of the preneoplastic cells, creating clones of cells expressing both oncogenes against a background of cells expressing the first oncogene, as in the clonal development of neoplasia. This is done by making a transplant expressing the first oncogene, putting the resulting abnormal growth into primary culture, infecting with a retrovirus that carries the second oncogene, and making a second round of transplants. We made hyperplastic epithelium by introducing v-*myc* and then introduced v-Ha-*ras* as the second oncogene [2]. Tumors developed fairly rapidly at the site of transplantation, with no discernible intermediate between the *myc* hyperplasia and the tumor. Similarly, Aguilar-Cordova et al. [10] used the mammary epithelial cell line Comma-D, which gives mildly dysplastic growths on transplantation, as a preneoplastic state. They introduced v-Ha-*ras* and obtained tumors on transplantation. Incidentally, both these experiments demonstrated, as one might expect, that v-Ha-*ras* could act as a second mutation in tumor development. This is in contrast to its initiating role in the induction of mammary tumors by certain carcinogens [39].

Is this a valid way to model human breast cancer?

At a fundamental level, there is little doubt that experiments of this kind are invaluable. They show how tumor mutations alter the three-dimensional organization of tissue, and they illustrate how little we learn about the ultimate effects of tumor mutations from in vitro experiments. For example, who would have predicted that v-*myc* would alter mammary epithelial branching (Figure 2), or that it would antagonize the apoptosis that normally occurs after lactation during involution, causing the epithelium to retain the morphology of lactation [18; J.M. Bradbury and P.A.W. Edwards, unpublished]? Mouse mammary tumorigenesis was classically considered a poor model of the human disease, but the reason for this was in part that the tumor mutations caused by MMTV or chemical carcinogen treatment were not in general the mutations that occur in the human. This is no longer relevant, now that we can introduce tumor mutations of choice. In particular, the histology of lesions caused by mutant *erbB2* is close to that of human premalignant lesions [3]. On a more applied level, tissue reconstitution can also provide syngeneic preneoplastic lesions and tumors with defined oncogene expression for the testing of new therapies in vivo, a better target in some respects than the xenografted human tumor.

Future directions

To date the tissue reconstitution approach has been used to express oncogene and growth factor genes, while a complete model of tumor development clearly requires inactivation of tumor suppressor genes as well. There are various possible ways this might be achieved. Dominant negative mutants of some tumor suppressor genes may become available. Gene expression might be inhibited by retroviruses that express antisense or ribozyme constructs, but these methods remain to be generally proven. Deletion of genes may be more effective and might be achieved using the *lox-cre* system [40]. Transgenic mice would be engineered so that the gene to be deleted was flanked by *lox* sequences. The gene would then be deleted by expression of the *cre* recombinase, which catalyzes recombination between pairs of *lox* sites. This deletion step could be achieved in the reconstituted mammary gland using a retrovirus that expresses *cre* to give clones of mutant cells.

Conclusions

The tissue reconstitution method for expressing genes in mammary epithelium has proved to be a valuable method to find out what tumor mutations do to intact tissue and is arguably the method of choice. Its main limitation at present is that inhibition or deletion of genes, while probably feasible, has not yet been demonstrated.

What have we learned from expressing oncogenes and growth factors in mammary epithelium? That most oncogenes affect the growth pattern of mammary epithelium and the effects are very diverse. Even closely related oncogenes may give quite distinct effects. Some ideas have emerged about how the action of oncogenes may be related to their normal functions or the normal functions of related molecules. Experience with *erbB2*, in particular, encourages us to believe that this mouse model will be relevant to human disease.

Acknowledgments

I thank my coworkers, particularly Dr. Jane Bradbury. Our work was supported by the Agriculture and Food Research Council, the Breast Cancer Research Trust, Association for International Cancer Research and the Cancer Research Campaign.

References

1. Abram CL, Bradbury JM, Page MJ, Edwards PAW (1995) v-erbB induces abnormal patterns of growth in mammary epithelium. In *Intercellular Signalling in the Mammary Gland*. CJ Wilde, CH Knight, M Peaker (eds). New York: Plenum, pp 67–68.
2. Bradbury JM, Sykes H, Edwards PAW (1991) Induction of mouse mammary tumours in a transplantation system by sequential introduction of the myc and ras oncogenes. *Int J Cancer* 48:908–915.
3. Bradbury JM, Arno J, Edwards PAW (1993) Induction of epithelial abnormalities that resemble human breast lesions by the expression of the neu/erbB2 oncogene in reconstituted mouse mammary gland. *Oncogene* 8:1551–1558.
4. Bradbury JM, Edwards PAW, Niemeyer CC, Dale TC (1995) Wnt-4 expression induces a pregnancy-like growth pattern in reconstituted mammary glands in virgin mice. *Dev Biol* 170:553–563.
5. Edwards PAW (1993) Tissue reconstitution models of breast cancer. *Cancer Surv* 16:79–96.
6. Edwards PAW, Ward JL, Bradbury JM (1988) Alteration of morphogenesis by the v-myc oncogene in transplants of mouse mammary gland. *Oncogene* 2:407–412.
7. Edwards PAW, Hiby SE, Papkoff J, Bradbury JM (1992) Hyperplasia of mouse mammary epithelium induced by expression of the Wnt-1 (int-1) oncogene in reconstituted mammary gland. *Oncogene* 7:2041–2051.

34

8. Edwards PAW, Abram CL, Bradbury JM (1995) Genetic manipulation of mammary epithelium by transplantation. *J Mammary Gland Biology and Neoplasia* 1:75–90.
9. Edwards PAW, Abram CL, Hiby SE, Niemeyer C, Dale TC, Bradbury JM (1995) The role of erbB-family genes and Wnt genes in normal and preneoplastic mammary epithelium, studied by tissue reconstitution. In *Intercellular Signalling in the Mammary Gland*. CJ Wilde, CH Knight, M Peaker (eds). New York: Plenum, pp 57–66.
10. Aguilar-Cordova E, Strange R, Young LJT, Billy HT, Gumerlock PH, Cardiff RD (1991) Viral Ha-ras mediated mammary tumour progression. *Oncogene* 6:1601–1607.
11. Miyamoto S, Guzman RC, Shiurba RA, Firestone GL, Nandi S (1990) Transfection of activated Ha-ras protooncogenes causes mouse mammary hyperplasia. *Cancer Res* 50:6010–6014.
12. Smith GH, Gallaghan D, Zweibel JA, Freeman SM, Bassin RH, Callaghan R (1991) Long-term in vivo expression of genes introduced by retrovirus-mediated transfer into mammary epithelial cells. *J Virol* 65:6365–6370.
13. Strange R, Aguilar-Cordova E, Young LJT, Billy HT, Dandekar S, Cardiff RD (1989) Harvey-ras mediated neoplastic development in the mouse mammary gland. *Oncogene* 4:309–315.
14. Miller AD (1992) Retroviral vectors. *Curr Top Microbiol Immunol* 158:1–24.
15. DeOme KB, Faulkin LJ Jr, Bern HA, Blair PB (1959) Development of mammary tumors from hyperplastic alveolar nodules transplanted into gland-free mammary fat pads of female C3H mice. *Cancer Res* 19:515–520.
16. Wang B, Kennan WS, Yasukawa-Barnes J, Lindstrom MJ, Gould MN (1991) Carcinoma induction following direct in situ transfer of v-Ha-ras into rat mammary epithelial cells using replication-defective retrovirus vectors. *Cancer Res* 51:2642–2648.
17. Wang B, Kennan WS, Yasukawa-Barnes J, Lindstrom MJ, Gould MN (1991) Frequent induction of mammary carcinomas following neu oncogene transfer into in situ mammary epithelial cells of susceptible and resistant rat strains. *Cancer Res* 51:5649–5654.
18. Andres AC, van der Walk MA, Schonenberger CA, Fluckiger F, LeMeur M, Gerlinger P, Groner B (1988) Ha-ras and c-myc oncogene expression interferes with morphological and functional differentiation of mammary epithelial cells in single and double transgenic mice. *Genes Dev* 2:1486–1495.
19. DanKort DL, Muller WJ (1996) Transgenic models of breast cancer metastasis. In *Mammary Tumor Cell Cycle, Differentiation, and Metastasis*. RB Dickson, ME Lippman (eds). Boston: Kluwer.
20. Webster MA, Muller WJ (1994) Mammary tumorigenesis and metastasis in transgenic mice. *Semin Cancer Biol* 5:69–76.
21. Stocklin E, Botteri F, Groner B (1993) An activated allele of the c-erbB-2 oncogene impairs kidney and lung function and causes early death of transgenic mice. *J Cell Biol* 122:199–208.
22. Ghattas IR, Sanes JR, Majors JE (1991) The encephalomyocarditis virus internal ribosome entry site allows efficient coexpression of two genes from a recombinant provirus in cultured cells and in embryos. *Mol Cell Biol* 11:5848–5859.
23. Friedrich G, Soriano P (1991) Promoter traps in embryonic stem cells: A genetic screen to identify and mutate developmental genes in mice. *Genes Dev* 5:1513–1523.
24. Dati C, Antoniotti S, Taverna D, Perroteau I, De Bortoli M (1990) Inhibition of c-erbB-2 oncogene expression by estrogens in human breast cancer cells. *Oncogene* 5:1001–1006.
25. Varley JM, Walker RA (1993) The molecular pathology of human breast cancer. *Cancer Surv* 16:31–57.
26. Muller WJ, Sinn E, Pattengale PK, Wallace R, Leder P (1988) Single-step induction of mammary adenocarcinoma in transgenic mice bearing the activated c-neu oncogene. *Cell* 54:105–115.
27. Bouchard L, Lamarre L, Tremblay PJ, Jolicoeur P (1989) Stochastic appearance of mammary tumors in transgenic mice carrying the MMTV/c-*neu* oncogene. *Cell* 57:931–936.
28. Siegel PM, Dankort DL, Hardy WR, Muller WJ (1994) Novel activating mutations in the *neu* proto-oncogene involved in induction of mammary tumours. *Mol Cell Biol* 14:7068–7077.

29. Tsukamoto AS, Grosschedl R, Guzman RC, Parslow T, Varmus HE (1988) Expression of the int-1 gene in transgenic mice is associated with mammary gland hyperplasia and adenocarcinomas in male and female mice. *Cell* 55:619–625.
30. Lin T-P, Guzman RC, Osborn RC, Thordarson G, Nandi S (1992) Role of endocrine, autocrine and paracrine interactions in the development of mammary hyperplasia in Wnt-1 transgenic mice. *Cancer Res* 52:4413–4419.
31. Nusse R, Varmus HE (1992) Wnt genes. *Cell* 69:1073–1087.
32. Gavin BJ, McMahon AP (1992) Differential regulation of the Wnt gene family during pregnancy and lactation suggests a role in post natal development of the mammary gland. *Mol Cell Biol* 12:2418–2423.
34. Weber-Hall SJ, Phippard DJ, Niemeyer CC, Dale TC (1994) Developmental and hormonal regulation of Wnt gene expression in the mouse mammary gland. *Development* 57:205–214.
35. Bradbury JM, Niemeyer CC, Dale TC, Edwards PAW (1994) Alterations of the growth characteristics of the fibroblast cell line C3H10T1/2 by members of the Wnt gene family. *Oncogene* 9:2597–2603.
36. Parr BA, McMahon AP (1994) *Wnt* genes and vertebrate development. *Curr Opin Genetics Dev* 7:2181–2193.
37. Daniel CW, Silberstein GB, Van Horn K, Strickland P, Robinson S (1989) TGF-β1-induced inhibition of mouse mammary ductal growth: Developmental specificity and characterization. *Dev Biol* 135:20–30.
38. Ornitz DM, Moreadith W, Leder P (1991) Binary system for regulating transgene expression in mice: Targeting int-2 gene expression with yeast GAL4/UAS control elements. *Proc Natl Acad Sci USA* 88:698–702.
39. Sukumar S (1989) ras oncogenes in chemical carcinogenesis. *Curr Top Microbiol Immunol* 148:93–114.
40. Gu H, Marth JD, Orban PC, Mossmann H, Rajewsky K (1994) Deletion of a DNA polymerase β gene segment in T cells using cell type-specific gene targetting. *Science* 265:103–106.
41. Beddington RSP, Morgernstern J, Land H, Hogan A (1989) An in situ transgenic enzyme marker for the midgestation mouse embryo and the visualization of inner cell mass clones during early organogenesis. *Development* 106:37–46.

3. Preneoplasia in mammary tumorigenesis

Daniel Medina

Introduction

It is axiomatic that cancers in epithelial organs arise via multiple intermediate stages. This concept is termed *multistage carcinogenesis* and is based upon both clinical and experimental observations over the past 40 years in practically all major epithelial organs [1–3]. The intermediate stages have been labeled with various terms, the most common terms being *preneoplastic* or *premalignant*. Recently it has been recognized that the stage of preneoplasia itself represents a progression of several stages [4]. The past 10 years have witnessed the application of molecular biology approaches to examine basic questions in mammary carcinogenesis. These approaches, which include the development and characterization of transgenic mouse models and transgenic gland models; the successful development of cell culture systems to establish mammary epithelial cell lines of preneoplastic and neoplastic phenotypes; the identification and elucidation of oncogenes, tumor-suppressor genes, and growth factors; and recognition of the importance of the mammary stroma in mammary epithelial cell function, have provided new insights into the biological and molecular events that underlie the development of mammary carcinogenesis. In light of these new methodologies, the time is appropriate for a review of the preneoplastic state in mammary tumorigenesis. Although this review focuses on the mouse as a model, current results and ideas about rat and human preneoplastic or intermediate stage lesions are also discussed. It is hoped that this review will invite discussion and comments, stimulate new ideas, and attract new participants into this research area.

Preneoplastic phenotype as a model system

Mouse mammary preneoplasias

The biological properties of mouse mammary preneoplasias were extensively studied by DeOme and his coworkers [5] and have been reviewed extensively [3,5,6]. There are several different morphological forms of preneoplastic le-

R. Dickson and M. Lippman (eds.) MAMMARY TUMOR CELL CYCLE, DIFFERENTIATION AND METASTASIS. 1996. Kluwer Academic Publishers. ISBN 0-7923-3905-3. All rights reserved.

sions in the mouse mammary gland, which include hyperplastic alveolar nodules (HAN), ductal hyperplasias (DH), and keratinized nodules (KN). The most extensively characterized preneoplastic lesions are the HAN, which represent transformed cell populations histologically similar to the differentiated alveolar cells normally found in the normal pregnant mammary gland. The HAN are termed *preneoplastic* because they have been shown to exhibit a greater probability for tumor formation than their normal cell homologues, the alveolar cells found in pregnant mice.

Hyperplastic alveolar nodules have been induced by mammary tumor viruses (MMTV), both the exogenous and endogenous forms; chemical carcinogens such as 7,12-dimethylbenzanthracene (DMBA) and urethane; prolonged hormonal stimulation (prolactin plus estrogen plus progesterone); specific oncogenes (see discussion on transgenic glands and transgenic mice); and growth in cell culture [7,8]. Hyperplastic alveolar nodules were originally identified as persistent focal areas of alveolar hyperplasia in the ductal mammary glands of nonpregnant, nonlactating mice. Individual HAN transplanted into the mammary gland–free (cleared) fat pads of syngeneic virgin mice will grow and fill the fat pad with mammary alveolar cells, reminiscent of the normal pregnant mammary gland [5,9] (Figure 1A and 1B). These transplants are termed *hyperplastic outgrowth lines* and are abbreviated as HOG or HPO. The outgrowth lines can be perpetuated by serial transplantation into the cleared mammary fat pads at intervals of 8–12 weeks.

The hyperplastic outgrowth lines, like their progenitor primary HAN, have increased probabilities for tumor formation. The transplantation method allows the neoplastic potential of hyperplastic outgrowth lines to be tested directly. In the absence of additional exposure to MMTV, chemical carcinogens, exogenously administered hormones, or specific oncogenes, the HOG lines produce mammary tumors at a rate characteristic for each line. The tumor-producing capabilities, measured as the percent of transplants that produce tumors at 12 months after transplantation, or as the time (months) for 50% of the transplants to produce tumors (TE_{50}), extends over a wide range. For example, outgrowth lines like TM2L and TM3 have an extremely low tumorigenic potential (<3% and <1% at 12 months, respectively), others like TM2H and TM4 have a TE_{50} of 4–5 months, D2 has a TE_{50} of 7.5 months, and TM10 has a TE_{50} of 11 months. The tumor potential of an outgrowth line is relatively stable with serial transplantation; however, there are several well-documented cases of selection by transplantation of more tumorigenic variants within the outgrowth cell population. For example, outgrowth line D1 had a very low tumor potential of 4% when initially isolated, but at transplant generations 45–47, a variant was inadvertently selected with a much higher tumor potential.

The additional exposure of MMTV, chemical carcinogens, γ-irradiation, some hormones, and certain drugs increases the tumor potential of outgrowth lines significantly [10], whereas specific hormones or chemopreventive agents will decrease the tumor potential [11,12]. The response of the mammary

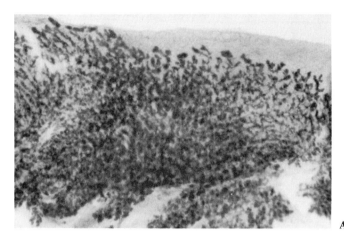

A

Figure 1. Whole mount preparations of BALB/c mammary outgrowths. The glands were placed in 10% formalin, defatted in acetone, processed as described in Medina [10], and stained with hematoxylin. **A:** TM2L HOG, which is a typical moderately dense alveolar outgrowth filling the entire mammary fat pad. ×10. **B:** Histological section of TM2L. The alveoli are arranged in small clusters. The large number of cytoplasmic lipid droplets is unusual in this outgrowth line as such droplets are seen infrequently in other BALB/c outgrowth lines. ×120. **C:** TM40D HOG, which contains a dense center of mammary cells and a periphery composed of apparent ductules. ×15. **D:** Histological section of TM40D showing the intraluminal epithelial proliferation that is seen both in the samples that are filling the fat pad and in those that have filled the fat pad. The cells are contained within the basement membrane until a neoplasm arises focally. ×120. **E:** EL12. An example of an immortalized ductal outgrowth. This outgrowth differs from EL11 in the presence of lateral alveolar buds along the ducts. Such alveoli can proliferate focally, and when transplanted they gave rise to the stable alveolar hyperplastic outgrowth line, TM12. ×12. **F:** A typical outgrowth from the cell line COMMA-1D. This cell line generates both ductal and alveolar outgrowths upon transplantation into the fat pad. The cells were transplanted in the center of the fat pad and segregated to give alveolar and ductal outgrowths. ×15. **G:** Hyperplastic alveolar outgrowths (line D2) transplanted into an intact mammary fat pad will extend into the available fatty stroma until their growth is inhibited by the host's growing mammary ducts. Note neither type of mammary epithelium (duct or alveoli) overlap into the other's territory. ×9. **H:** An exception to the general rule is shown in G. Here the outgrowth line TM2H (hyperplasia type III) is growing past the host's mammary ducts. The ducts had reached the spot marked by the arrow before encountering the transplanted hyperplasia. The hyperplasia does not apparently recognize the spatial-defining factors present in the gland. In this respect, this hyperplasia behaves like a neoplasia. ×18.

alveolar hyperplasias to chemical carcinogens is dissimilar to that of liver nodules. The later cell populations are postulated to be resistant to the subsequent effects of chemical carcinogens [2]. In a similar vein, the levels of phase 1 and phase 2 metabolic enzymes exhibit dissimilar patterns between mammary and liver preneoplastic cell populations [13].

A second common preneoplastic lesion found in mice is ductal hyperplasia (DH). These lesions are induced by chemical carcinogens [14], irradiation [15], and progestins [16] in vivo and by exposure to specific combinations of car-

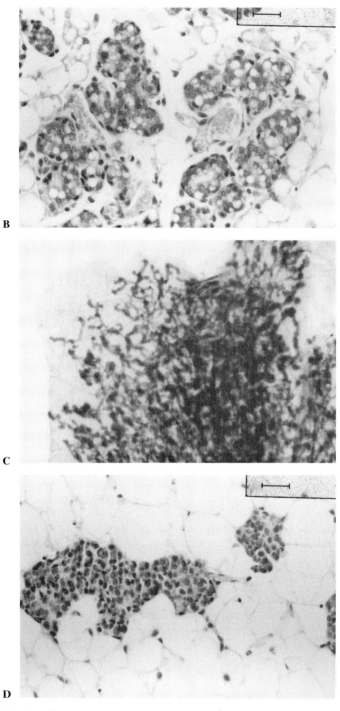

B

C

D

Figure 1 (continued)

40

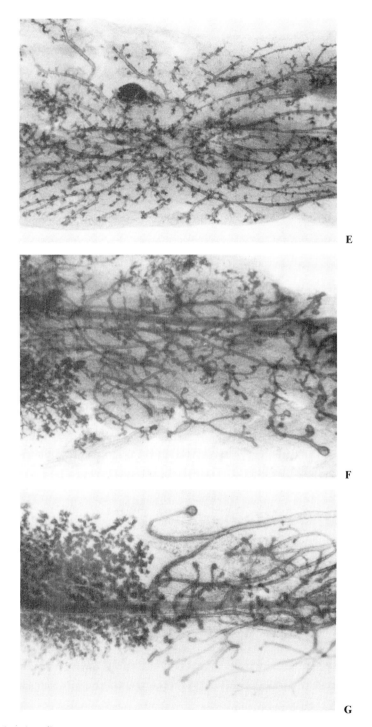

E

F

G

Figure 1 (continued)

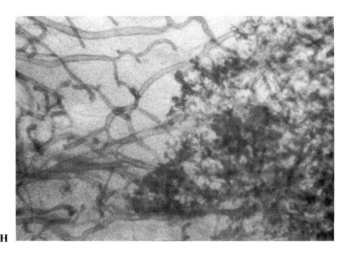

H

Figure 1 (continued)

cinogens and growth factors in vitro [17]. Ductal hyperplasias are a very heterogeneous group of lesions that are characterized by hyperplasia of the ducts and/or proliferation of duct epithelium intraluminally. In chemical carcinogen–treated mice, DH develop during the first 6–9 months after exposure, whereas HAN tend to develop later [14,18]. Ductal hyperplasias, like HAN, give rise to mammary adenocarcinomas upon transplantation into syngeneic mice. Ductal hyperplasias that exhibit intraductal epithelial proliferation progress through a phenotype very similar to human ductal carcinoma in situ (DCIS), in which the lumen becomes occluded with epithelial cells for long stretches of the duct. In a histological section, several ducts in one field are filled with epithelial cells (Figure 1C and 1D). Locally invasive carcinoma develops from these hyperplastic ducts. In contrast to HAN, it has been difficult to develop stable outgrowth lines of DH by serial transplantation because the transplants rapidly progress to carcinoma [19]. An exception may be a recently isolated outgrowth line, TM40D, which was derived from the cell line FSK4. This outgrowth line grows in the fat pad as an expansion of ductules whose lumina are filled to varying extents with epithelial cells. So far, after five transplant generations, tumors have not developed at up to 6 months. If the behavior of this line remains stable, it might be a model for DH/DCIS progression.

A second type of ductal lesion is represented by immortalized ducts that show little evidence of ductal hyperplasia (Figure 1E). These ducts are morphologically similar to normal ducts and are ovarian dependent for growth; however, they are immortalized cell populations [20]. Four outgrowth lines — DIM4, EL11, EL12, and HDH4 — have been studied. A curiosity of these lesions is their tendency to develop into mixed ductal-alveolar hyperplasias upon serial transplantation. With DIM4 and EL12, the morphological progression from ductal to alveolar hyperplasia was correlated with a change from low to high tumor potential and the gain of ovarian hormone independence [20,21]. The major difference between EL11 and EL12 cell populations was the ability of the latter to develop a limited extent of alveolar development and proliferation. The alveolar cell type had a higher rate of proliferation and therefore became the predominant cell type with transplantation and was very susceptible to the transforming effects of chemical carcinogens and hormones. Clearly, it is of interest to determine the molecular change(s) that distinguish EL11 from EL12 as such information will provide insight into the processes that regulate alveolar hyperplasia.

Preneoplastic stage in rat and human mammary glands

The emphasis on the viral etiology in mouse mammary cancer and the extensive characterization of the HAN as a model for preneoplasia has obscured the close parallel of chemical carcinogen–induced lesions in the mouse to those in the rat and human. Breast cancer arises in humans and in rodents exposed to chemical carcinogens from ductal cells altered in the terminal portions of the mammary tree [11,22]. The pathogenesis involves an initial intraductal epithelial hyperplasia, which progresses through cellular atypia and occlusion of the duct. The most extreme atypical hyperplasia is referred to as *neoplasia* in rodents and *DCIS* in humans. The sequence of events have been defined in human breast, and recently a cell line–xenograft model that mimics much of this progression has been described by Miller et al. [23]. The model uses Ha-*ras* transformed MCF10 cells transplanted subcutaneously into nude/beige mice. The successful development of this model should not only result in a careful molecular analysis of the essential changes involved in the intermediate stages of human breast carcinogenesis but also spur other investigators to develop additional xenograft models for human breast cancer.

The chemical carcinogen–treated rat mammary gland has been a favorite model for cancer research since its development by Huggins et al. in 1961 [24]. Although the terminal endbud is hypothesized to be a critical site for carcinogen-induced transformation, the development of models for intermediate stages has not been extensive and has been plagued with inconsistencies. Beuving et al. [25,26] presented transplantation experiments that suggested the HAN in carcinogen-treated rats was a preneoplastic lesion. Other investigators could not confirm these results [22,27,28]. Furthermore, the HAN and HAN outgrowths that arose from transplantation were ovarian hormone independent for maintenance, that is, they did not regress, whereas the vast majority of adenocarcinomas (>80%) arising in the carcinogen-treated rat are hormone dependent and regress in the absence of hormones. Russo et al. [29] presented the hypothesis that HAN have a low tumorigenic potential and develop primarily into adenomas and fibroadenomas. Transplantation experiments demonstrated that fibrous nodules, not HAN, develop into fibroadenomas in rats [26]. Russo et al. [29] also presented the hypothesis that the carcinogen-treated terminal endbud progresses into intraductal proliferations from which adenocarcinomas subsequently develop. Although the importance of DH [28] and the Russo hypothesis have been established for over 10 years, the ability to systematically model and study these intermediate changes in the rat mammary gland has only been recently developed by Thompson and Singh [30]. Rats that are given a single injection of nitrosomethylurea at 21 days of age developed hyperplastic lesions in the mammary gland similar to those observed in human breast. Some lesions were locally invasive into the lymph node. The quantification of these lesions and their transplantation behavior should provide an excellent basis for a model that allows dissection of the molecular changes associated with the early changes in breast carcinogenesis and might provide molecular probes applicable to the human disease.

Essential alterations in mouse mammary transformation

The biological properties of HAN outgrowth lines have been described in detail [7,10]. The examination of the growth properties of mammary outgrowth lines in vivo has provided important information on the regulation of their growth and tumorigenic potential. The early studies have defined four essential alterations in the regulation of growth that occur in hyperplasias and for the development of mammary tumors. The mammary hyperplastic outgrowth lines were shown to be immortal [31] and stably hyperplastic in morphology [5,10], to exhibit an enhanced tumorigenic potential [5,10], and still to be responsive to local environmental factors that regulated growth and spacing in the mammary fat pad [32]. Thus, unlike mammary tumors, HAN and HAN outgrowths, although immortal and preneoplastic, were not autonomous. However, many outgrowth lines have attained ovarian-hormone independence for growth and morphogenesis. These biological characteristics clearly place the HAN as an intermediate cell population on the path to development of neoplasia.

Immortalization was defined as the capacity for indefinite division potential. As initially demonstrated by Daniel [33], normal mammary cells, when serially transplanted in the mammary fat pad, exhibit a finite life span and are no longer transplantable after five to seven serial transplantations in vivo. The HAN outgrowth lines can be serially transplanted indefinitely. Some lines, like D1 and D2, have been serially transplanted for 30 years. It is of interest that immortality in vivo does not necessarily translate into immortality in vitro and vice versa. There is not a well-established in vitro assay for in vivo immortalization. For instance, preneoplastic immortalized cells are not more readily subculturable than normal cells, do not grow readily in anchorage-independent conditions, do not exhibit cytochalasin β–induced multinucleation, and do not exhibit altered $[Ca^{2+}]$ dependency [7].

Hyperplasia is initially represented as an increase in the number of alveolar cells maintained in the hormonal environment of the nonpregnant, non-lactating mouse. However, the histological and cytological architecture of the alveolar cells are similar to the normal alveolar cells found in the mammary glands of midpregnant mice [7]. Smith et al. [34] described experiments that suggested keratin 6 (K6) and keratin 14 (K14) expression was enhanced in preneoplastic alveolar cells and that these may represent a signature of the stem cell transformed in preneoplastic mammary cell populations. However, an extensive analysis of additional hyperplastic outgrowth lines could not confirm this conclusion but suggested that K6 and K14 coexpression was present in some outgrowth lines and not others. More importantly, there was no correlation between K6, K14 coexpression, and tumorigenic potential [35]. Despite the substantial amount of research attempting to define a set morphological, biochemical, cytological, or in vitro criteria unique to preneoplastic cells, the majority of experiments have reinforced the conclusion that the alveolar cell in mammary preneoplasias is astonishingly similar to the alveolar cell in the pregnant mammary gland [3,7,36].

Although preneoplastic mammary cells are immortal, they, like normal mammary cells, are dependent upon undefined local factors that regulate growth and spatial distribution. The best examples of this regulation are observed in the dependence of the preneoplastic cells upon the fat pad stroma for proliferation and tumor transformation [10] and the inability of preneoplastic cells to overgrow normal mammary ducts [32] (Figure 1G and 1H). Neoplastic cells have escaped this type of growth regulation. This property of autonomy represents the most fundamental biological difference observed between preneoplastic and neoplastic cells.

Many of the mammary preneoplasias (and neoplasias) seem to be ovarian hormone independent for growth yet retain hormone responsiveness for functional differentiation (these lesions are dependent upon prolactin for growth). Thus, the expression of hormone independence is probably a secondary or coincidental event, and not an essential characteristic of these preneoplasias. The relationship of the differentiated state of the preneoplasia to its altered growth potential is an intriguing question. The morphological phenotype of the preneoplastic HOG is alveolar, which represent the differentiated mammary cell expressed in the hormone-stimulated mouse. However, the HOG lines maintain the differentiated phenotype in the hormonal milieu of the virgin mouse. Indeed, the HOG lines are ovarian independent for morphogenesis and growth, but the cells remain hormonally responsive for casein and α-lactalbumin production, the milk proteins expressed by mammary differentiated cells. It is evident that the preneoplasias are not terminally differentiated, although they exhibit many but not all the hallmarks of the lactating cell. So far, the expression of whey acidic protein (WAP) has been difficult to detect in HOG transplants. One exception appears to be the C1D9 cell line, a derivative of the COMMA1-D cell line that produces both ductal and alveolar outgrowths in vivo. C1D9 cells grown on a matrigel substrate and in the presence of appropriate hormones will produce WAP [37].

The preneoplastic mammary cells seem to represent a cell state similar to that described by Scott and co-workers [38,39] in the 3T3-adipocyte system. In that system, 3T3 cells differentiate into two cell states: terminally differentiated cells and nonterminally differentiated cells. The latter cell state can re-enter the proliferation cycle. Both of the 3T3-cell states synthesize a full complement of products typical of differentiated adipocytes and cannot be distinguished cytologically or biochemically. Preneoplastic mammary cells seem to represent a nonterminally differentiated population. So far, the stimulation of casein and α-lactalbumin production in the majority of cells has not been sufficient to alter the tumorigenic potential of the population. The simplest interpretation of the relationship between the alveolar phenotype and preneoplasia would be that the HAN population represents transformation of an alveolar or an alveolar-progenitor cell. Alterations in ovarian dependence are not obligatory for a preneoplastic state. As suggested originally by DeOme et al. [40] and reasserted recently [36], the characteristics of ovarian hormone independence and tumorigenic potential are independently assortable properties.

Recent experiments have demonstrated that the properties of immortality, hyperplasia, and tumorigenicity are independent and assortable characteristics [4,20,35]. Early experiments that investigated the properties of HAN generally used well-defined HAN isolated from MMTV or chemical carcinogen–treated mice [5–7,10]. The primary HAN had generally progressed far along the developmental path to neoplasias, and therefore all exhibited the properties of immortalization, hyperplasia, and enhanced tumorigenicity. Recent experiments focused on growing normal mammary cells in short-term cell cultures, treating with chemical carcinogens, and transplanting the cells into the mammary fat pads of syngenic mice. The recipient mice then selected for any variants in growth potential that arose in the cell cultures [8]. Variant cell populations selected in this manner were of two classes: ductal outgrowths and alveolar outgrowths. The majority of ductal outgrowths were composed of cells with a limited proliferation potential and therefore could be serially transplanted only three to four times. Several independent populations could be transplanted repeatedly and therefore showed an extended proliferation potential [20]. Two of these populations, termed *EL11* and *EL12*, are now in transplant generation 25 (Figure 1E). Both lines are ductal outgrowths, ovarian hormone dependent, and nonhyperplastic but are immortal (Table 1). The presence of these lines clearly established that the immortalization phenotype could develop independently from the properties of morphological hyperplasia and enhanced tumorigenicity characteristic of previously described mammary preneoplastic lesions. Whereas the EL11 line is purely ductal and has never produced a mammary tumor unless exposed to DMBA, the EL12 line generates variable amounts of lateral alveolar budding, and these alveolar cells are ovarian hormone independent, progress to neoplasia, and can be transformed by very low doses of DMBA. Thus, with these two lines the early stages of the development of neoplasia are present, and, there-

Table 1. Biological properties of mouse mammary outgrowth lines

Outgrowth line	Morphological phenotype[a]	Immortal	Hormone dependence[b]	Tumor potential[c] (TE$_{50}$)	DMBA responsiveness[d]
Normal	Ductal	No	Yes	0	Nil
EL11	Ductal	Yes	Yes	0	Nil
EL12	Ductal-alveolar	Yes	Yes	9%	Moderate
TM3	Alveolar	Yes	Yes	<1%	Nil
TM2L	Alveolar	Yes	Partial	<3%	Strong
TM2H	Alveolar	Yes	No	>90% (4)	N.D.[e]
TM4	Alveolar	Yes	No	>90% (4)	N.D.
TM10	Alveolar	Yes	No	60% (11.5)	N.D.
TM12	Alveolar	Yes	No	66% (9.0)	Strong
TM40	Ductal	Yes	Partial	N.D.	N.D.
D1	Alveolar	Yes	No	11%	Strong
D2	Alveolar	Yes	No	70% (7.5)	Strong
C4	Alveolar	Yes	No	32%	Strong

[a] Determined in mature virgin BALB/c mice.
[b] Dependence on ovarian hormones for growth and norphogenesis.
[c] Percent tumors by 12 months after transplantation. The numbers in parentheses reflect the months after transplantation for 50% of the transplants to produce tumors.
[d] Tumorigenic response to a single dose of 1 mg DMBA at 10 months after treatment.
[e] N.D. = not determined.

fore, they provide excellent models to examine the molecular correlates of the biological phenotypes.

The second type of outgrowths selected from normal cells cultured for short time periods were alveolar outgrowths, designated *TM* for transformed mammary (Table 1). These outgrowths were morphologically similar to the typical preoplastic alveolar hyperplasias derived from in situ HAN. A study of their biological properties demonstrated that the two other phenotypes of preoplasias, those of hyperplasia and enhanced tumor potential, were independently assortable properties. The dissociation of these two properties was evident in outgrowth lines TM3 and TM2L. Both outgrowth lines are composed of alveolar cells and produce adenocarcinomas only sporadically.

TM3 is unusual in several respects. First, it grows very slowly, is absolutely ovarian hormone dependent for growth, and takes 7 months to fill 75% of the fat pad. Starting at 6–7 months, the alveolar cells regress so that by 11–12 months, a sparse skeleton of atrophied ducts populate the fat pad [35]. The cell and molecular factors that mediate this unusual behavior are unknown but are currently being examined. Second, TM3 in situ is absolutely resistant to the transforming effects of low doses of DMBA (1 mg). TM3 cells established as a cell line in culture also are resistant to the cytotoxic effects of 1 μg DMBA. In contrast, TM12 cells in culture are sensitive to DMBA-induced cytotoxity at 0.1 μg. However, TM3 cells are capable of forming adenocarcinomas if exposed to continuous hormone stimulation and 3 mg DMBA (Medina, unpublished) or if transfected with specific oncogenes (see Molecular alterations in mammary preneoplasias). TM3 seems to represent an immortalized, hyperplastic, but non-preoplastic cell population.

TM2L is similar to TM3 in its very poor tumorigenic potential and is partially ovarian hormone dependent in situ, but exhibits normal growth rates in situ, does not regress, and is sensitive to the transforming effects of low doses of DMBA. An unusual aspect of TM2L hyperplasia is the extensive cytoplasmic lipid formation, a feature generally observed in mammary cells of lactating mice but not pregnant mice. This might indicate that the cells populating TM2L hyperplasia are further along the differentiation pathway. It is likely that TM3 and TM2L hyperplasias are blocked in their tumorigenic progression by different mechanisms. An understanding of the molecular events that are responsible for the blocked progression would provide new targets for intervention or therapy.

In contrast, the majority of the outgrowth lines, such as D1, D2, C4, TM10, TM12, and TM4, fulfill the criteria for the mammary preneoplastic phenotype. They are immortal, alveolar, and have enhanced tumor potential. As discussed later, the TM2H outgrowth line seems to represent the extreme end in the spectrum of the preneoplastic phenotype. In summary, an examination of the biological properties of mammary preneoplasias has revealed that the three essential characteristics of immortalization, hyperplasia, and enhanced tumor potential are independent and assortable properties. The presence of in vivo outgrowth lines that can also grow in cell culture provides powerful tools to examine the molecular changes that underlie preneoplastic development.

The scheme (Figure 2) illustrated later for mouse mammary tumorigenesis has evolved to account for the new information on preneoplasias. The scheme emphasizes the individual events that occur as preneoplasias evolve and suggests that preneoplasia is a heterogeneous and dynamic state. In this scheme, hyperplasia I represents immortalized, hyperplastic, nontumorigenic cell populations such as TM3 and TM2L; hyperplasia II represents immortalized, hyperplastic cell populations with a weak to moderate tumorigenic potential, such as D1, C4, TM10, and TM12; and hyperplasia III represents immortalized, hyperplastic cell populations with a very high tumorigenic potential, such as TM2H and TM4. This latter class of hyperplasias consists of cell populations that are morphologically hyperplastic and do not grow subcutaneously but appear to contain subpopulations with the cell cycle dysregulation patterns that are characteristic of mammary neoplasms (see Summary and future directions). It is not necessary that each preneoplasia or tumor proceed through all the steps sequentially. Although there is evidence that immortal-

normal → immortalized → hyperplasia I → hyperplasia II → hyperplasia III → neoplasia

Figure 2. Scheme of mammary preneoplastic development.

ized cells do progress to hyperplasias (e.g., EL12 → TM12) and hyperplasias I can progress to hyperplasia II, it is clear that many primary HAN at the time of initial detection have the attributes of hyperplasia type II or type III. The scheme is intended to emphasize the multistage nature of preneoplastic development, just as the preneoplastic stage itself is just one stage of neoplastic development.

Molecular alterations in mammary preneoplasias

The development of specific cDNA probes to mammary tumor virus genes, to mammary tumor–related genes (*wnt*-1, *int*-2, *int*-3), and to proto-oncogenes has provided the means to analyze the relative importance of the expression of these genes in the development of preneoplasias and neoplasias.

MMTV-related genes

The experiments of Nusse et al. [41] and Peters et al. [42] demonstrated that exogenous MMTV integrates preferentially at specific regions of the cellular genome and activates the expression of adjacent genes. The genes (*wnt*-1, *int*-2) are found expressed in a great majority of tumors induced by the C3H and GR/RIII variants of the MMTV. Other integration sites have been documented for Czech II (*int*-3) [43], BALB/cf/Cd (*int*-41) [44], and C3H mice (*wnt*-3, Fgf4) [45,46]. Additionally, overexpressed genes have been described in mammary preneoplasias (*int*-5) [47]. The activated genes have different cellular functions, which include developmental genes (*wnt*-1) [49], fibroblast growth factors (*int*-2, *hst*-8) [49], aromatase (*int*-5) [50], and cell fate determination (*int*-3) [51]. Experiments have directly demonstrated that overexpression of these genes results in mammary hyperplasia and neoplasia. For example, the mammary glands of *wnt*-1 transgenic mice exhibit diffuse hyperplasia and develop mammary carcinomas in all females by 10 months of age [52]. Mammary tumor development is enhanced by coexpression of *int*-2 [53]. Moreover, overexpression of *wnt*-1 achieved by retroviral infection of the gland leads to diffuse alveolar hyperlasia, which is ovarian hormone independent [54].

Activation of *wnt/int* genes is not observed in all mammary tumors. Morris and Cardiff [55] showed that spontaneous tumors in BALB/c mice induced by GR and C3H viruses did not exhibit a high level of *wnt/int* gene activations (50%). Tumors arising from hyperplastic outgrowth lines of GR and C3H origin rarely exhibited *wnt/int* gene activation [55,56]. Similarly, mammary tumors in C3Hf/Ki mice did not exhibit *wnt*-1 or *int*-2 gene activation [57]. Finally, *int* gene activation was not detected in BALB/c tumors induced by DMBA [58], those arising spontaneously from the D1 HOG line [59], or those from the TM HOG lines [4]. Therefore, the importance of the activation of *wnt/int* genes in mammary tumors other than those induced by the exogenous

MMTV, and perhaps in the D2 HOG line, remains problematic. The results of Morris and Cardiff [55] and Schwartz et al. [56] are intriguing because they suggest that preneoplasias and tumors arising from them do not require *wnt/int* gene activation. Experiments that investigate the role of *wnt*-1 and *int*-2 utilizing transfection of normal or preneoplastic cells will provide important information regarding the functions of these genes in mammary transformation.

The role of endogenous MMTV in the generation of HAN and tumors has been neglected, except for the special case of the GR virus. There are several observations that suggest activation or insertion of endogenous MMTV might initiate mammary tumorigenesis. First, the BALB/cV strain was described as a BALB/c subline that arose after brother-sister mating of a single little from a female that developed a mammary tumor at 10 months [60]. Breeding females of the BALB/cV strain had a moderate incidence of mammary tumors (47%, mean latent period 10.2 months) and the MMTV was milk transmitted. Competition radioimmunoassays for the MMTV major core protein and restriction enzyme digestion patterns of proviral DNA suggested the MMTV was not of C3H or GR MMTV origin. Recently, nucleotide sequence analysis of the LTR ORF of the BALB/cV virus indicated it has extensive homologies to endogenous MMTV [61,62]. Furthermore, the pattern of deletion of the VB2 subset of T lymphocytes places the virus as distinct from C3H, GR, or RIII MMTV and identical to the MMTV active in C4 and D2 hyperplasias, both of which are lines that arose in the same BALB/c colony from which the BALB/cV line orginated [63].

Second, the levels of LTR ORF mRNA are elevated in lactating tissues and numerous hyperplastic outgrowth lines of BALB/c origin [4,59,64,65]. Several functions have been suggested for the ORF protein. It acts as a superantigen (sag) and plays a role in the life cycle of MMTV infection by stimulating T and B lymphocyte proliferation. One consequence of stimulation of specific subsets of T cells is the deletion of specific VB subsets [63,66]. Each MMTV variant deletes specific VB subsets. Additionally, pORF (sag) may act as an oncogene, as it has been isolated from transforming DNA [67] and overexpression of the LTR ORF cDNA in nontumorigenic TM3 outgrowth lines by transfection results in rapid formation of tumors [68].

Finally, in the same BALB/c strain from which the BALB/cV subline arose, a unique *int* gene, *int*-5, has been identified, sequenced, and functionally defined [47,50,69,70]. The gene activated in the *int*-5 locus is identical to aromatase, a cytochrome P450–related gene. The proliferation of D2 tumor cells in vitro is stimulated by androstenedione, a substrate for aromatase, and is blocked by an aromatase inhibitor and by the anti-estrogen 1C1 164384 [70]. These studies suggested that estrogen formed within the D2 cells acted as a mitogen. If *int*-5 activation can be demonstrated as one of the common mechanisms occurring in HAN induced by hormones or spontaneously, it would represent a novel but logical pathway for the initiation and/or progression of mammary alveolar hyperplasias.

Several investigators have examined the interaction of chemical carcinogens and endogenous MMTV. The majority of mouse strains have endogenous MMTV genes [71]. Only in rare instances does chemical carcinogen treatment lead to activation of expression of endogenous MMTV genes [58,72,73]. In a very rare instance, complete activation leading to virion production can occur [58]. In the BALB/c series of HOG lines, neither the preneoplasias nor tumors derived from them uniformly exhibit expression of the endogenous MMTV genes, except the LTR ORF. New proviruses can occur in preneoplasias and tumors, but these are not obligatory for transformation [53,58,74]. On occasions when new proviruses occurred, the expression of *int* genes was not thoroughly evaluated.

Until recently, the possible role of endogenous retroposons in mammary tumorigenesis had been relatively unexplored. The studies by Asch and co-workers [75,76] have demonstrated that the increased expressions of at least two classes of retrotransposons, MuLVs and intracisternal A particles (IAP), are common in BALB/c mammary preneoplasias and neoplasias. In one study [75], they demonstrated that the expression of IAPs was common in D2 and C4 HOG and tumors, as well as in tumors induced by C3H and BALB/cV MTVs and by DMBA. Expression of IAPs in virgin and pregnant glands was nil. In a second study, the expression of IAPs and/or MuLV sequences was increased 3–100×, whereas VL30 sequences were decreased 5–35× in a series of mammary cancers induced by MMTV, chemical carcinogen, or hormonal agents [76]. The overexpression of IAPs and/or MuLV sequences was also increased in the hyperplasias generating the tumors [Asch, personal communication]. The significance of increased expression lies in the increased probability of gene activation by transposition. Indeed, gene activation in mammary preneoplasias and neoplasias by retroposition has been reported by two research groups [77,78]. In one case, *int*-3 was activated and resulted in progression from preneoplasia to tumor [78].

In summary, it would seem appropriate to reinvestigate the involvement of the various *wnt* and *int* genes in the development of mouse mammary hyperplasias for both the alveolar and ductal types. It is striking that the gene most consistently overexpressed in mammary hyperplasias is *pORF* (*sag*), the function of which remains speculative yet intriguing.

Proto-oncogene expression

Several approaches have been used to examine the relative importance of proto-oncogene expression in preneoplastic and neoplastic mammary development. First, experiments have examined the levels of expression of proto-oncogenes in preneoplastic and neoplastic tissues relative to expression levels in normal mammary gland. Second, the effects of overexpression in transfected or retroviral infected cells have been evaluated in several immortalized cell lines in vivo and in vitro. Third, the presence and type of hyperplasias have been documented in transgenic mice.

ras expression. DMBA is a powerful carcinogen for both the rat and mouse normal mammary gland [14,79], and also for the conversion of mouse mammary preneoplasia to neoplasias [21]. DMBA activates the c-Ha-*ras* gene by mutation at codon 61 in both the rat and mouse mammary glands [79,80]. The original experiment in the mouse system utilized tumors arising from the DI/UCD HOG subline. Spontaneous tumors arose from this subline at a high frequency, but such tumors were negative for c-Ha-*ras* activation, in contrast to the same tumors induced by DMBA [80]. In a subsequent experiment, the low-tumor-incidence C4 HOG line was treated with DMBA. The rare spontaneous tumors and the untreated preneoplasias were negative for c-Ha-*ras* activation, while the DMBA-induced tumors exhibited a high frequency of c-Ha-*ras* activation by mutation at codon 61 [81]. Mutations included both the commonly observed A to T transversion and a novel A to G transition. It appeared that the DMBA-induced mutated Ha-*ras* oncogenes potentiated the conversion of hyperplastic outgrowths to carcinomas. The mutations were detected in only two of six fat pads containing hyperplastic outgrowths, which supported the concept that tumors arise from preneoplasias in a clonal fashion [82]. The demonstration of *ras* activation also provided an explanation of why DMBA-treated preneoplasias do not behave homogeneously in transplantation experiments [83]. Previous experiments have shown that subdivision of a DMBA-treated outgrowth into 40 pieces, followed by transplantation into cleared fat pads, resulted in very few tumors, whereas, if left untransplanted, each outgrowth eventually would produce a tumor. The frequency of transformed cells, as detected by the transplantation experiments, was directly proportional to the amount of DMBA exposure of the preneoplastic outgrowths [83]. Activation of Ha-*ras* is presumably a rare event, yet once activated, it results in the development of tumors from the preneoplasias.

Methylnitrosourea (MNU) induces rat mammary tumors characterized by mutated c-Ha-*ras* at codon 12 and mouse mammary tumors characterized by mutated c-Ki-*ras*. The mutation in c-Ki-*ras* was also detected in mammary preneoplasias, indicating the Ki-*ras* mutation is also a preneoplastic event [84]. Interestingly, the induction of Ki-*ras* mutations appears to be dependent on cell type and/or hormonal influences, because mammary ductal hyperplasias induced by MNU in the presence of EGF do not contain Ki-*ras* mutations [85] and alveolar hyperplasias induced in lithium-containing medium do not contain *ras* mutations [86]. The latter hyperplasias contain novel transforming genes [86].

The concept that *ras* activation is not sufficient for mammary tumorigenesis is supported by several experiments. First, the frequency and pattern of tumor development in transgenic mice carrying an MMTV-LTR– or a WAP-promoter–driven *ras* transgene suggests that more than one event is needed [87,88]. Second, experiments of normal mouse mammary cells transfected with activated *ras* in cell culture yielded hyperplastic outgrowths upon transplantation into fat pads of syngeneic mice; however, these outgrowths were not immortal upon serial transplantation [89]. However, immortalized preneoplastic mammary cells (COMMA1D) transfected with viral *ras* yielded adenocarcinomas [90].

Other experiments, both in vitro and in vivo, have demonstrated that the transformation of mammary cells by *ras* is strongly concentration dependent [91,92]. The level of activated *ras* expression affects cell morphology and cloning efficiency in vitro [91,93] as well as in vivo tumorigenicity. In some mammary cell lines, like EF43, v-*ras* abolishes epithelial differentiation resulting in anaplastic tumors [93].

Other proto-oncogenes. Normal mammary cells and established mammary cells have been transformed by v-*mil*, v-*myc*, *wnt*-1, and *wnt*-4 [54,91–93]. The transforming abilities are dependent, in part, upon the cell line as well as the level of expression of the oncogene. For instance, v-*mil* overexpression in cell line EF43 resulted in carcinomas that retain an epithelial morphology, unlike the same cells transformed with v-*ras* [93]. V-*myc* overexpression did not transform cell lines EF43 or COMMA-1D [93,94] but was transforming for normal mammary cells [95] and a BALB/c immortalized cell line designated MMEC [96]. In the COMMA-1D/CL14 cell line, v-*myc* increased casein mRNA and protein levels 50- to 60-fold [94].

Although numerous studies have demonstrated the transforming capabilities of several proto-oncogenes or oncogenes for mammary normal and hyperplastic cells, the quantitative analysis of proto-oncogene expression in preneoplastic cells has resulted in a less informative picture as to the possible involvement of specific genes. One study that examined the expression of a battery of proto-oncogenes in preneoplastic HOG line D1 and D1 tumors detected elevated expression (2–6×) of c-Ha-*ras* and c-Ki-*ras* RNA in tumors compared with the preneoplasias [59]. The levels of these RNAs in preneoplasias were not increased compared with that seen in normal pregnant mammary gland. In general, the levels of c-*fos*, c-*myc*, v-*sis*, v-*abl*, v-*fps*, v-*ros*, *wnt*-1, and *int*-2 were not consistently increased in tumors compared with preneoplasias, although elevated levels of v-*abl* and v-*fps* were seen in a few tumors. Amplification of *neu* DNA was not detected by Southern analysis. A second study examined the expression of proto-oncogenes in the TM series of hyperplasias and tumors [4]. In these outgrowth lines and tumors, altered mRNA expression was not detected for c-Has-*ras*, c-*myc*, retinoblastoma, c-*neu*, *wnt*-1, and *int*-2; however, MMTV-LTR ORF was elevated in the hyperplasias and tumors, and gelsolin was markedly decreased in tumors. In a third study, *wnt*-2, *wnt*-4, and *wnt*-5b mRNAs were not inappropriately expressed in the hyperplasias [97]. The cumulative data do not provide any support for the role of many of the more common oncogenes in the development of mouse mammary hyperplasias, except for a possible role of *ras* and MMTV-LTR ORF.

Tumor suppressor genes

The expression of the tumor suppressor gene p53 is altered in up to 40% of human breast carcinomas as well as the comedo variant of ductal carcinoma in situ [98]. Altered expression of p53 has been reported in a significant number of mouse mammary hyperplasias [99–101]. Aberrant p53 expression was detected frequently by nuclear and cytoplasmic immunohistochemical staining patterns (Table 2). Sequence analysis of the p53 gene revealed a variety of mechanisms yielding misexpression of p53. Outgrowth lines exhibited point mutations, leading to accumulation of p53 protein, point mutations resulting in a truncated message and no protein, insertions and deletions resulting in protein accumulation, as well as alterations in expression not due to p53 mutation. Although dysregulation of the p53 gene appears to be common in mouse mammary hyperplasias, dysregulation did not appear to correlate directly with tumorigenic potential, because outgrowth lines TM2L and TM3 infrequenty produce tumors yet contained dysregulation of p53. Furthermore, dysregulation is not apparently related to immortality because the immortalized ductal lines EL11 and EL12 express normal patterns of p53 expression [Medina, unpublished]. Finally, DMBA-induced BALB/c mammary tumors exhibited normal immunohistochemical staining patterns of p53. Sequence analysis of p53 gene in these tumors indicated a wild-type phenotype. The study of p53 gene expression in BALB/c mammary hyperplasias and neoplasias is just beginning, and it is likely that information on the functional significance of specific mutations and on the factors that regulate p53 stability, that is, mdm-2, will be necessary to integrate definitively the role of p53 in mouse mammary tumorigenesis. It is already clear that not all p53 mutations result in enhancement of mammary tumorigenesis [102].

Table 2. Analysis of p53 expression in mouse mammary hyperplasias

Outgrowth line	Immunohistochemical staining pattern[a]	Codon affected; result
TM2L	No	Exon 5; truncated message
TM2H	No	Exon 4; C→T stop 112
TM3	Yes, nuclear	Exon 7; insertion Ser 233–234
TM4	Yes, nuclear	Exon 5; deletion 123–129 Exon 5; C→G Trp 138
TM9	Yes, cytoplasmic	Exon 5; G→A, Met 170
TM10	No	Not analyzed
TM12	No	Not analyzed
TM40	Yes, nuclear	Not analyzed
D1	Yes, nuclear	Wild type
D2	Yes, nuclear	Wild type

[a] No = no protein detected; Yes = protein detected immunohistochemically.

Transgenic models

Transgenic mice. Transgenic mouse models of mammary tumorigenesis have been developed with activated *ras*, c-*myc*, activated *neu*, c-*neu*, *wnt*-1, *int*-2, *int*-3; and polyoma virus middle T, growth hormone, specific p53 mutations, cyclin D1, TGF-α, and TGF-β using the mammary specific promoters MMTV-LTR and WAP [103,104]. In general, mammary tumors developed focally and stochastically that supported the concept of multistage mammary carcinogenesis. The latency of mammary tumor formation varied with the oncogene and the promoter. In most transgenics, morphologically abnormal mammary gland has been noted; however, transplantation analysis was not performed to determine the biological behavior of the mammary gland lesions.

Of particular interest are the mammary glands from the *wnt*-1, *int*-2, cyclin D1, and TGF-α transgenic mice [52,105–110]. In each of these cases, the primary mammary phenotype was extensive epithelial hyperplasia, which persisted in nonpregnant, nonlactating mice. The mammary hyperplasias in *wnt*-1 transgenic mice were ovarian hormone independent and developed a high incidence of mammary tumors. The mammary hyperplasias in *int*-2, cyclin D1, and TGF-α transgenic mice produced very few tumors. Transplantations studies of the *wnt*-1, and *int*-2 hyperplasias into the fat pad of syngeneic mice suggested that both proto-oncogenes are acting as autocrine, not paracrine, growth factors [105,107]. The mammary hyperplasia in transgenic mice showed marked increased susceptibility for tumorigenic transformation as bitransgenics *wnt*-1 × *int*-2 [53], c-*myc* × TGF-α [111], *wnt*-1 × p53 null [112], and TGF-α mice exposed to DMBA [113] exhibited very high tumor incidences with very short latent periods. These experiments support the concept of multistage carcinogenesis and suggest that the mammary hyperplasias in transgenic mice are biologically similar to the HAN and HAN outgrowths that have been extensively characterized by other investigators [3,6,10].

Experiments utilizing TGF-β, p53 arg-leu, and *int*-3 as transgenes resulted in mammary hypoplasia [102,114–117]. Transplantation experiments suggested that TGF-β1 overexpression blocks the proliferation of alveolar progenitor cells, thus resulting in a alveolar hypoplastic gland that does not produce tumors [116]. Similarly, transplantation experiments of mammary epithelium with deregulated expression of *int*-3 suggested that *int*-3 alters the cell developmental pathways in normal morphogenesis and functional differentiation [118]. The result in this case was enhanced tumorigenesis; however, the reasons for enhanced tumorigenesis are not understood. It seems likely that *int*-3 expression results in a cell population with altered responsiveness to or expression of growth factors [Smith, personal communication]. It would be interesting to examine p53 expression in the *int*-3–expressing cells or their resulting tumors to determine the possible involvement of the p53 gene in this tumorigenic pathway. On the other hand, the overexpression of p53 arg-leu mutant results in increased apoptosis, blockage of mammary epithelial differentiation at the first week of pregnancy, and a total resistance to DMBA-induced mammary tumorigenesis [102]. The results of the TGF-α–DMBA, TGF-β, and the p53 arg-leu-DMBA experiments support the concept that alveolar progenitor (or alveolar) cells are the primary transformed cell in many mouse mammary tumor models [7,119,120], in contrast to the mammary duct progenitor cell or the mammary totipotent stem cell, which is the transformed cell in chemical carcinogen or irradiation-initiated mouse mammary tumors.

Transgenic glands. The development of transgenic mammary glands was pioneered by several investigators [90,95,121]. The methodology allows long-term in vivo expression of genes transferred into normal mammary epithelial cells. The system allows examination of the overexpression of specific genes in mammary cells growing in their normal microenvironment and macro-environment in a normal mouse. In this situation, the transformed cells are surrounded by normal mammary cells, which mimics the natural situation. The disadvantages are that the frequency of infection is low and the resulting outgrowth in the fat pad is heterogeneous. Experiments in which v-*ras*, c-*myc*, activated *neu*, *wnt*-1, and *wnt*-4 were overexpressed in normal mammary epithelial cells resulted in a hyperplastic phenotype [reviewed in 122]; however, the specific patterns of hyperplasia were subtly different. V-*myc* and *wnt*-1 glands exhibited a diffuse hyperplasia [54,95], v-*ras*/v-*myc* glands exhibited focal tumor development in a field of hyperplasia [123], and activated *neu* led to focal atypical hyperplasias and the comedo variant of DCIS [124]. The latter result is particularly intriguing, since this model would seem closely related to the human disease. The results demonstrate that transgenic mammary glands represent a powerful, sensitive, selective, and rapid approach to examine the molecular events initiated by specific gene expression during the early stages of mammary tumorigenesis, as well as examining the combined effects of genes during complete tumorigenesis.

Growth factors

The development of the normal mammary gland is regulated by the interactions of hormones, growth factors, and growth inhibitors [reviewed in 17]. These growth factors include EGF, TGF-α, TGF-β, IGF-I, IGF-II, PDGF, bFGF, and MDGI [reviewed in 17,125]. TGF-α is a more potent growth stimulatory factor than EGF in normal gland development [126]; in contrast, TGF-β inhibits normal ductal development [127]. The constitutive expression of several of these growth factors, such as TGF-α and related cognate receptors, occurs in mammary cancers [reviewed in 125]. In other cases, the levels of some of these factors are increased (i.e., TGF-α, IGFI, IGFII, PDGF, cathespin) or decreased (i.e., TGF-β, mammastatin) by estrogen [125]. The roles of most of these growth factors and growth inhibitors in the development of mammary hyperplasias have been less studied than in normal or neoplastic

Table 3. EGF dependency in vitro, in vivo hormone dependency and tumorigenic potential, and TGF-α protein expression in mouse mammary hyperplastic outgrowth lines

Outgrowth line	EGF dependency[a]	Hormone dependency[b]	TGF-α protein[c]	Tumorigenic potential, %
TM2L	N	P	ND	<3
TM2H	N	N	N	>90
TM3	Y	Y	N	<1
TM4	N	N	N	>90
TM9	N	N	N	25
TM10	N	N	N	60
TM12	Y	N	Y	66

[a] N = no requirement for growth in vitro; Y = absolute requirement.
[b] Refers to ovarian hormones required for growth of the epithelial cells line in the fat pad; N = no requirement as cells grew equally well in ovariectomized as in intact mice; P = partial requirement as cells grew slower in ovariectomized mice than in the intact mice; Y = absolute requirement as no growth was observed.
[c] Immunohistochemical staining on neutral-buffered, formalin-fixed, paraffin-embedded sections using the R9 polyclonal antibody. N = no reaction; Y = positive reaction; ND = not determined.

mammary gland. The paucity of information can be summarized in three conclusions.

First, transformation of immortalized nontumorigenic mammary cell lines of mouse (NOG8, HC11) and human origin by activated *ras* results in increased expression of TGF-α and changes in growth properties characteristic of neoplastic cells [125,128]. Some of the mouse cell lines also show a decreased responsiveness to the growth stimulatory effects of EGF [128]. In this context, it is interesting that the majority of in vitro epithelial cell lines established from in situ hyperplastic outgrowth lines (e.g., TM2H, TM4, TM9, TM10, TM40D) are independent of an EGF requirement for growth [4]. Some cell lines, as in TM3 and TM12, show a strong requirement for EGF in vitro. The EGF requirement is independent of tumorigenic potential or in vivo hormone dependency (Table 3). Of six outgrowth lines examined, only one line (TM12) showed evidence of TGF-α protein by immunohistochemical staining. An occasional TM2H tumor showed *cripto* protein expression immunohistochemically, and no tumor showed a positive immunohistochemical staining reaction for amphiregulin [Medina, unpublished]. The latter two proteins are often upregulated in human mammary tumors [129]. It is interesting that rat mammary tumor cell lines that are growth factor independent in vitro and produce neoplastic growths in vivo overexpress TGF-α and an EGF-related membrane receptor [130, 131]. It would be interesting to determine if the EGF-independent phenotype in mouse hyperplasias is correlated with enhanced expression of the EGF-related receptors Erbβ3 and Erbβ4 or synthesis of an FGF-related protein. Although the mouse hyperplasias discussed earlier do not show activation of the *int*-2 (FGF-3) gene, there is no information regarding activation of other FGF genes. It is known that the EGF-independent TM cell lines in vitro are responsive to the proliferative effects of bFGF (FGF2) in the absence of serum [4].

Second, the responsiveness of the alveolar hyperplastic outgrowths to TGF-β in vitro or in vivo has not been examined. Daniel and coworkers [132,133] reported that normal alveolar cells in pregnant mice in situ are unresponsive to the growth inhibitory effects of TGF-β1; however, it remains to be determined if this is true for hyperplastic alveolar outgrowths. It has been reported that estrogen decreases TGF-β1 mRNA expression in human breast cancer cell lines in vitro [125,134]. If TGF-β1 is hormonally regulated, this class of growth inhibitors may have little effect on the ovarian hormone–independent mouse hyperplastic outgrowth lines under in situ conditions.

Third, the expression patterns of a significant number of growth factors, such as IGF I and IGF II, FGFs, mammastatin, and their cognate receptors, have not been examined in mouse mammary hyperplasias. In summary, it would appear that this area is in need of careful and systematic examination.

Cell cycle control

The study of the factors involved in cell cycle control has produced dramatic new understanding of these processes in the past 5 years [135,136]. Cyclin-dependent kinases (CDK) control cell cycle progression and are highly conserved in all eukaryotic cells. The regulation of CDK kinase activity involves a complex, multitiered system that involves phosphorylation and dephosphorylation of specific amino acid residues, and physical association with positive regulatory proteins, termed *cyclins*, and negative regulatory proteins, termed *inhibitors of kinases* (INK). In higher eukaryotes, G1 and S phase functions are controlled by distinct structurally related kinases, cdk2, cdk4, and cdk6. Basic insight into the regulation and function of these cdks has come from studies in yeast and mammalian cells in vitro. The cdk2 and cdk4 kinase activities are high in breast tumor cells, which reflects their high proliferative state [137–139]. This has resulted in the hypothesis that the overexpression of cyclins may be an important rate-limiting step in breast cancer. Indeed, cyclins A, D, and E are often overexpressed in human breast cancers [138–140], and overexpression of cyclin D1 in transgenic mice results in mammary hyperplasia and a low incidence of mammary tumors [108]. Very little information on the regulation of cell cycle proteins in hyperplastic states has been published.

Table 4 summarizes the expression patterns of the cell cycle–related proteins in the TM series of mouse mammary hyperplasias [141–143]. As far as this author is aware, these data represent the first systematic description of the expression patterns of cdks and cyclins in hyperplastic and preneoplastic tissues of any organ. Briefly, the data indicate that elevated levels of cdk kinase activities (cdc2, cdk2, cdk4) occur only in neoplastic tissues that have also an

Table 4. Expression patterns of cell cycle–related proteins in mouse mammary hyperplasias and neoplasias

Protein or function	Stage of tumor development[a]			
	Hyperplasia I	Hyperplasia II	Hyperplasia III	Neoplasia
cdc2 K.A.[b]	1	1	4	11
cdk4 K.A.	1	1	2	4.5
cyclin D1 (cdk4)[c]	1	10	4	65
cyclin D2 (cdc4)[c]	47	85	7.5	1
cdk2 K.A.[b]	1	1	7	14
cyclin A (cdk2)	5	5	5	5
cyclin E (cdk2)	1.5	1.5	2.8	8.5
cdk5 K.A.	1	1	1	1
p34 tyrosine phosphorylation	21	27	8	7.5
PCNA L.I.[b]	1	1	1.6	3.3

[a] Fold increase compared with normal pregnant mammary gland, except where noted otherwise.
[b] Fold increase compared with TM2L hyperplasia since kinase activity could not be detected in normal mammary gland.
[c] Fold increase compared with neoplasias.

elevated proliferative index. The increases for the three kinases ranged from 4 to 14× compared with hyperplasia types I and II. However, the cellular amounts of the different cdk proteins are not necessarily increased during mammary tumor development. Evaluation of the regulatory cyclins showed different patterns. Cyclin-A protein levels (bound to cdk2) were elevated 5× in nontumorigenic hyperplasias (hyperplasia I) compared with normal and did not increase further. Cyclin D1 (bound to cdk4) levels started to increase in tumorigenic hyperplasias (at 10-fold) and jumped dramatically in tumors (>60-fold) compared with normal mammary cells. Interestingly, the cyclin D1 protein level in TM2L (hyperplasia I) was the same as in normal mammary cells. DNA amplification has not been examined yet. Cyclin E (bound to cdk2) increased only in the most deviated hyperplasias (hyperplasia III) and increased further in tumors (at eightfold). The increase in cyclin E protein in tumors was also accompanied by an increase in cyclin E protein isoforms, an observation also reported for human breast cancer [137]. In contrast, cyclin D2 bound to cdk4 was markedly elevated in hyperplasias types I and II, and then dropped precipitously in hyperplasia type III and tumors. This result suggests that cyclin D2 may actually prevent activation of cdk4, thereby acting to inhibit neoplastic development. This hypothesis is unique and so far similar results on cyclin D2 have not been reported in other organ systems in situ. However, some support for the hypothesis is provided by the observation that cyclin D2 mRNA levels were significantly lower in human breast cancer cell lines compared with normal breast epithelial cells in these same cancer cell lines; cyclin D1 mRNA levels were elevated compared with normal cells [139].

Another regulatory step, tyrosine phosphorylation, was decreased in hyperplasias III and tumors compared with earlier stage hyperplasias. The role of phosphatases, for example, cdc25, and inhibitory proteins, remains to be elucidated. The results, so far, present an intriguing picture of cell cycle regulation in mammary neoplastic development and stress the need for more information. Clearly, hyperplasia III, the most deviant hyperplasia, which morphologically appears hyperplastic yet contains a subpopulation of highly proliferative cells, reflects the cell cycle control pattern of an incipient neoplasia. It would be interesting to determine if DCIS in humans exhibits cdk kinase activities and cyclin patterns similar to hyperplasia type III.

Summary and future directions

Mouse mammary hyperplasias represent a model for the early developmental stages of mammary tumorigenesis. The evolution of the model has progressed on several fronts over the past 5 years. First, the biological properties of immortality, hyperplasia, and tumorigenicity have been demonstrated to be independent and assortable characteristics. Separate mammary outgrowth lines that grow in vivo and in vitro have been isolated that are characterized by one or more of these properties. These outgrowth lines provide a powerful tool to examine the molecular changes responsible for these biological properties. One method that might exploit the existence of these cell lines is RNA differential display. Preliminary experiments are identifying the presence of unique RNA expression associated with the acquisition of immortalization and tumorigenicity [144].

Second, the appliation of molecular biological methods to study mammary hyperplasia has demonstrated the possible roles of a variety of protooncogenes, tumor suppressor genes, and growth factors. The initiation and development of mammary cancer is very complex and can be influenced by viral, chemical carcinogen, hormone, and dietary factors. It is important to address not only what a particular oncogene can do in an established cell line, but also whether and how a gene is actually involved in mammary transformation. It is important to determine which genes are differentially expressed during mammary preneoplastic and neoplastic transformation in vivo and then to critially test the function of these genes on mammary transformation. In all cases, it is important to examine the functions of these genes under conditions in which the cells retain their morphogenic and functional properties. In this respect, the development of transgenic gland methodology is a powerful tool because it allows the introduction of a specific gene into normal or immortalized cells, the expression of these genes under defined in vivo conditions, and the interaction of genes and mammary cells in an organ microenvironment that allows for a valid assessment of the gene's effects on cell growth and differentiation. Furthermore, the ability to transplant mammary gland from transgenic animals into the mammary fat pads of syngeneic wild-type mice

60

provides a tool to dissect the possible functions and consequences of transgene expression at the cellular and tissue level.

Third, the role of growth factors and growth inhibitors has not been extensively studied in mammary hyperplastic development. It is evident that the alveolar hyperplasias are ovarian hormone independent. Several experiments demonstrate that overexpression of *wnt*-1 or *int*-2 generates a hyperplastic phenotype that is ovarian hormone independent. Since these two genes are preferentially activated by viral carcinogens, the results of the transgenic gland experiments are logical and offer an explanation for the hyperplastic phenotype. It is disappointing that neither of the *wnt/int* genes are generally activated in mammary hyperplasias generated under other etiological conditions. However, there is compelling evidence to suggest, however, that other members of the *wnt* family or FGF family may play an essential role in generating and maintaining hyperplasias. Both the *wnt* and Fgf families are composed of multiple genes. The *wnt* genes are differentially expressed during normal mammary gland development. Furthermore, the different *wnt* genes are highly conserved and play fundamental roles in pattern development in species from flies to mammals. The signal transduction pathways impacted by *wnt* genes include basic cellular components, such as the catenins, the latter being proteins whose function is disrupted in carcinogenesis. It will not be surprising if the elucidation of the *wnt* signal transduction pathway results in the explanation for alveolar hyperplasia. It is also likely that the Fgf family of genes will turn out to play essential roles in the acquisition of hyperplasia and tumorigenic potential. Therefore, the study of these two gene families would seem to merit a high priority in the study of mammary tumorigenesis. Likewise, the recent results of Friedman et al. [145], which document that homeobox genes are hormonally regulated in normal mammary gland development and are differentially expressed in neoplasias, provides another developmental gene family that is likely to play a fundamental role in mammary tumorigenesis.

Finally, the recent descriptions of a rat model and a human xenograft model in which hyperplastic and dysplastic lesions are reproducibly generated are exciting new developments that provide new models to study the pathogenesis, and cell and molecular biology of the early or preneoplastic stage of mammary tumorigenesis. Knowledge of the critical events that occur during the early stages of mammary tumorigenesis will provide not only new targets for detection and intervention, but also knowledge applicable to understanding the cancer problem in all epithelial organ systems.

Acknowledgments

Much of the work on the mammary hyperplasias carried out in the author's laboratory over the past 20 years that is partly summarized in this review could not have been attained without the expert and dedicated assistance of my senior research associate, Frances Kittrell. I am deeply indebted to her for her skill, loyalty, and expertise. Some of the unpublished results described herein are supported by research grants CA11944 and CA47112 from the National Cancer Institute.

References

1. Moolgavkar SH, Luebeck EG (1992) Multistage carcinogenesis: Population-based model for colon cancer. *J Natl Cancern Inst* 84:610–618.
2. Farber E, Cameron R (1980) The sequential analysis of cancer development. *Adv Cancer Res* 31:125–226.
3. Medina D (1988) The preneoplastic state in mouse mammary tumorigenesis. *Carcinogenesis* 9:113–119.
4. Medina D, Kittrell FS, Oborn CJ, Schwartz M (1993) Growth factor dependency and gene expression in preneoplastic mouse mammary epithelial cells. *Cancer Res* 53:668–674.
5. DeOme KB, Faulkin LJ Jr, Bern HA, Blair PE (1959) Development of mammary tumors from hyperplastic alveolar nodules transplanted into gland-free mammary fat pads of female C3H mice. *Cancer Res* 19:515–520.
6. Cardiff RD, Wellings SR, Faulkin, LJ Jr (1977) Biology of breast preneoplasia. *Cancer* 39:2734–2746.
7. Medina D (1982) Mammary tumors. In *The Mouse in Biomedical Research*, HL Foster, D Small, JG Fox (eds). Vol IV. New York: Academic Press, pp 373–396.
8. Kittrell FS, Oborn CJ, Medina D (1992) Development of mammary preoplasias in vivo from mouse mammary epithelial cells in vitro. *Cancer Res* 52:1924–1932.
9. Medina D (1996) The mammary gland: A unique organ for the study of development and turmorigenesis. *J Mammary Gland Biol Neoplasia* 1:5–19.
10. Medina D (1973) Preneoplastic lesions in mouse mammary tumorigenesis. *Methods Cancer Res* 7:3–53.
11. Medina D (1977) Tumor formation in preneoplastic mammary nodule lines in mice treated with nafoxidine, testosterone, and 2-bromo-α-ergocryptine. *J Natl Cancer Inst* 58:1107–1110.
12. Medina D, Lane HW (1983) Stage specificity of selenium-mediated inhibition of mouse mammary tumorigenesis. *Biol Trace Elem Res* 5:297–306.
13. Mekhail-Ishak K, Medina D, Batist G (1989) Biochemical characteristics of mouse mammary tissues, preneoplastic lesions and tumors. *Carcinogenesis* 10:2363–2366.
14. Medina D, Warner M (1976) Mammary tumorigenesis in chemical carcinogen-treated mice. IV. Induction of mammary ductal hyperplasia. *J Natl Cancer Inst* 57:331–337.
15. Ethier SP, Ullrich RL (1982) Detection of ductal dysplasia in mammary ontgrowths derived from carcinogen-treated virgin female BALB/C mice. *Cancer Res* 42:1753–1760.
16. Lanari C, Molinolo AA, Pasqualini CD (1986) Induction of mammary adenocarcinomas by medroxyprogesterone acetate in BALB/c female mice. *Cancer Lett* 32:215–223.
17. Imagawa W, Yang J, Guzman R, Nandi S (1994) Control of mammary gland development. In *The Physiology of Reproduction*. E Knobil, JD Neill (eds). 2nd (ed), Vol 2. New York: Raven Press, pp 1033–1065.
18. Medina D (1976) Mammary tumorigenesis in chemical carcinogen-treated mice. VI. Tumor-producing capabilities of mammary dysplasias in BALB/cCrgl mice. *J Natl Cancer Inst* 57:1185–1189.
19. Medina D (1979) Serial transplantation of chemical carcinogen-induced mouse mammary ductal dysplasias. *J Natl Cancer Inst* 62:397–405.
20. Medina D, Kittrell FS (1993) Immortalization phenotype dissociated from the preneoplastic phenotype in mouse mammary epithelial outgrowths in vivo. *Carcinogenesis* 14:25–28.
21. Medina D, Kittrell FS (1987) Enhancement of tumorigenicity with morphological progression in a BALB/c preneoplastic outgrowth line. *J Natl Cancer Inst* 79:569–576.

22. Russo J, Gusterson BA, Rogers AE, Russo IH, Wellings SR, Zwieten MJ (1990) Comparative study of human and rat mammary tumorigenesis. *Lab Invest* 62:244–278.
23. Miller FR, Soule HD, Tait L, Pauley RJ, Wolman SR, Dawson PJ, Heppner GH (1993) Xenograft model of progressive human proliferative breast disease. *J Natl Cancer Inst* 85:1725–1731.
24. Huggins C, Grand LC, Brillantes FP (1961) Mammary cancer induced by a single feeding of polynuclear hydrocarbons and its suppression. *Nature* 189:204–207.
25. Beuving LJ, Faulkin LJ Jr, DeOme KB, Bergs VV (1967) Hyperplastic lesions in the mammary glands of Sprague-Dawley rats after 7,12-dimethylbenz(α)anthracene treatment. *J Natl Cancer Inst* 39:423–429.
26. Beuving LJ (1968) Mammary tumor formation within outgrowths of transplanted hyperplastic models from carcinogen-treated rats. *J Natl Cancer Inst* 40:1287–1289.
27. Sinha D, Dao TL (1975) Brief communication: Site of origin of mammary tumors induced by 7,12-dimethylbenzanthracene in the rat. *J Natl Cancer Inst* 54:1007–1009.
28. Haslam SZ, Bern HA (1977) Histopathogenesis of 7,12-dimethylbenz(α)anthracene-induced rat mammary tumors. *Proc Natl Acad Sci USA* 74:4020–4024.
29. Russo J, Saby WM, Isenberg WM, Russo IH (1977) Pathogenesis of mammary carcinomas induced in rats by 7,12-dimethylbenz(α)anthracene. *J Natl Cancer Inst* 59:435–445.
30. Thompson HJ, Singh M (1995) Morphological identification of early stages of neoplasia in a rat model for human breast carcinogenesis. *Proc Am Assoc Cancer Res* 36:778.
31. Daniel CW, Aidells BD, Medina D, Faulkin LJ Jr (1975) Unlimited division potential of precancerous mouse mammary cells after spontaneous or carcinogene-induced transformation. *Fed Proc* 34:64–67.
32. Faulkin LJ Jr, DeOme KB (1960) Regulation of growth and spacing of gland elements in the mammary fat pad of the C3H mouse. *J Natl Cancer Inst* 24:953–969.
33. Daniel CW (1972) Aging of cells during serial propagation in vivo. *Adv Gerontol Res* 4:167–200.
34. Smith GH, Mehrel T, Roop DR (1990) Differential keratin gene expression in developing, differentiating, preneoplastic and neoplastic mouse mammary epithelium. *Cell Growth Differ* 1:161–170.
35. Medina D, Kittrell FS, Liu Y-J, Schwartz M (1993) Morphological and functional properties of TM preneoplastic mammary outgrowths. *Cancer Res* 53:663–667.
36. Medina D, Schwartz M, Taha M, Oborn CJ, Smith GH (1987) Expression of differentiation-specific proteins in preneoplastic mammary tissues in BALB/c mice. *Cancer Res* 47:4686–4693.
37. Roskelley CD, Desprez PY, Bissill MJ (1994) Extracellular matrix-dependent tissue-specific gene expression in mammary epithelial cells requires both physical and biochemical signal transduction. *Proc Nat Acad Sci USA* 91:12378–12382.
38. Wier ML, Scott RE (1985) Defective control of terminal differentiation and its role in carcinogenesis in the 3T3 T proadipocyte stem cell line. *Cancer Res* 45:3339–3346.
39. Sparks RL, Seibel-Ross EI, Wier ML, Scott E (1986) Differentiation, dedifferentiation, and transdifferentiation of BALB/c 3T3 T mesenchymal stem cell: Potential significance in metaplasia and neoplasia. *Cancer Res* 46:5312–5319.
40. DeOme KB, Blair PB, Faulkin LJ Jr (1961) Some characteristics of the preneoplastic hyperplastic nodules of C3H/Crgl mice. *Acta Unio Int Contra Cancer* 18:973–982.
41. Nusse R, van Ooyen A, Cox D, Fung YKT, Varmus H (1984) Mode of proviral activation of a putative mammary oncogene *int*-1 on mouse chromosome 15. *Nature* 307:131–136.
42. Peters G, Brookes S, Smith R, Dickson C (1983) Tumorigenesis by mouse mammary tumor virus: Evidence for a common region for provirus integration in mammary tumors. *Cell* 33:369–377.
43. Gallahan D, Callahan R (1987) Mammary tumorigenesis in feral mice: Identification of a new *int* locus in mouse mammary tumor virus (Czech II)-induced mammary tumors. *J Virol* 61:66–74.

44. Garcia M, Wellinger R, Vessaz A, Diggelmann H (1986) A new site of integration for mouse mammary tumor virus proviral DNA common to BALB/cfC3H mammary and kidney adenocarcinomas. *EMBO J* 5:127–136.

45. Roelink HE, Waganaar E, Lopes da Silva S, Nusse R (1990) Wnt-3, a gene activated by proviral insertion in mouse tumors, in homologous to int-1/Wnt-1 and is normally expressed mouse embryos and adult brain. *Proc Natl Acad Sci USA* 87:4519–4523.

46. Peters G, Brookes S, Smith R, Placzek M, Dickson C (1989) The mouse homolog of the hst/k-FGF gene is adjacent to int-2 and is activated by proviral insertin in some virally induced mammary tumors. *Proc Natl Acad Sci USA* 86:5678–5682.

47. Morris VL, Rao TR, Kozak CA, Gray DA, Lee-Chen ECM, Cornell TJ, Taylor CB, Jones RF, McGrath CM (1991) Characterization of *int-5*, a locus associated with early events in mammary carcinogenesis. *Oncogene Res* 6:53–63.

48. Gavin BJ, McMahon JA, McMahon AP (1990) Expression of multiple novel Wnt-1/int-1-related genes during fetal and adult mouse development. *Genes Dev* 4:2319–2332.

49. Smith R, Peters G, Dickson C (1988) Multiple RNAs expressed from the int-2 gene in mouse embryonal carcinoma cell lines encode a protein with homology to fibroblast growth factors. *EMBO J* 1:1013–1023.

50. Durgam VR, Tekmal RR (1994) The nature and expression of int-5, a novel MMTV integration locus gene in carcinogen-induced mammary tumors. *Cancer Lett* 87:179–186.

51. Robbins J, Blondel BJ, Gallahan D, Callahan R (1992) Mouse mammary tumor gene INT-3: A member of the Notch gene family transforms mammary epithelial cells. *J Virol* 66:2594–2599.

52. Tsukomoto AS, Grosschedl R, Guzman RC, Parslow T, Varmus HE (1988) Expression of the *int-1* gene in transgenic mice is associated with mammary gland hyperplasia and adenocarcinomas in male and female mice. *Cell* 55:619–625.

53. Kwan H, Pecenka V, Tsukamoto A, Parslow TG, Guzman RC, Lin T-P, Muller WJ, Lee FS, Leder P, Varmus HE (1992) Transgene expressing the *Wnt-1* and *int-2* proto-oncogenes cooperate during mammary carcinogenesis in doubly transgenic mice. *Mol Cell Biol* 12:147–154.

54. Edwards PAW, Hiby SE, Papkoff J, Bradbury JM (1992) Hyperplasia of mouse mammary epithelium induced by expression of the Wnt-1 (int-1) oncogene in reconstituted mammary gland. *Oncogene* 7:2041–2051.

55. Morris DW, Cardiff RD (1987) Multistep model of mouse mammary tumor development. *Adv Viral Oncol* 7:123–140.

56. Schwartz MS, Smith GH, Medina D (1992) The effect of parity, tumor latency and transplantation on the activation of *int* loci in MMTV-induced, transplanted C3H mammary preneoplasis and their tumors. *Int J Cancer* 51:805–811.

57. Popko BJ, Pauley RJ (1985) Mammary tumorigenesis in C3Hf/Ki mice: Examination of germinal mouse mammary tumor viruses and the *int-1* and *int-2* putative proto-oncogenes. *Virus Res* 2:231–243.

58. Knepper JE, Medina D, Butel JS (1987) Activation of endogenous MMTV provirus in murine mammary cancer induced by chemical carcinogens. *Int J Cancer* 40:414–422.

59. Knepper JE, Kittrell FS, Medina D, Butel JS (1989) Spontaneous progression of hyperplastic outgrowths of the D1 lineage to mammary tumors: Expression of mouse mammary tumor virus and cellular proto-oncogenes. *Mol Carcinog* 1:229–238.

60. Drohan W, Teramoto YA, Medina D, Schlom J (1981) Isolation and characterization of a new mouse mammary tumor virus variant from BALB/c mice. *Virology* 114:175–186.

61. Kang JJ, Schwegel T, Knepper JE (1993) Sequence similarity between the long terminal repeat coding regions of mammary tumorigenic BALB/cV and renal-tumorigenic C3H-K strains of mammary tumor virus. *Virology* 196:303–308.

62. Brandt-Carlson C, Butel JS, Wheeler D (1993) Phylogenetic and structural analyses of MMTV. LTR-ORF sequences of exogenous and endogenous origins. *Virology* 193:171–185.

63. Wei WZ, Ficsor-Jacobs R, Tsai SJ, Pauley R (1991) Elimination of V-beta 2 bearing T-cells

in BALB/c mice implanted with syngeneic preneoplastic and neoplastic mammary lesions. *Cancer Res* 51:3331–3333.

64. Knepper JE, Medina D, Butel JS (1986) Differential expression of endogenous mouse mammary tumor virus genes during development of the BALB/c mammary gland. *J Virol* 51:518–521.

65. Wheeler DA, Butel JS, Medina D, Cardiff RD, Hager GL (1983) Transcription of mouse mammary tumor virus: Identification of a candidate mRNA for the long terminal repeat gene product. *J Virol* 46:42–29.

66. Ocha-Orbea H, Shakhov AN, Scarpellino L, Kolb E, Muller V, Vessaz-Shaw A, Fucho R, Blochlinger K, Rollini P, Billotte J, Sarafidou M, MacDonald HR, Diggelmann H (1991) Clonal deletion of VB14-bearing T cells in mice transgenic for mammary tumor virus. *Nature* 350:207–211.

67. Van Klaveren P, Haaksma T, Dijk H, Bentvelzen P (1994) Plasmid rescue of an oncogenic sequence containing a mouse mammary tumor virus gene. *Anticancer Res* 14:597–602.

68. Mukhopadhyay R, Medina D, Butel J (1995) Expression of the mouse mammary tumor virus long terminal repeat open reading frame promotes tumorigeneic potential of hyperplastic mouse mammary epithelial cells. *Virology* 211:84–93.

69. Gray DA, McGrath CM, Jones RF, Morris VL (1986) A common mouse mammary tumor virus integration site in chemically induced precancerous mammary hyperplasia. *Virology* 80:360–368.

70. Tekmal RR, Durgam VR (1995) The overexpression of *int*-5/aromatose, a novel MMTV integration locus gene, is responsible for D2 mammary tumor cell proliferation. *Cancer Lett* 88:147–155.

71. Cohen JC, Varmus HE (1979) Endogenous mammary tumor virus DNA varies among wild mice and segregates during inbreeding. *Nature* 278:418–423.

72. Butel JS, Dusing-Swartz S, Socher SH, Medina D (1981) Partial expression of endogenous mouse mammary tumor virus in mammary tumors induced in BALB/c mice by chemical, hormonal and physical agents. *J Virol* 38:571–580.

73. Michalides R, Van Deemter L, Nusse R, Hageman P (1979) Induction of mouse mammary tumor virus RNA in mammary tumors of BALB/c mice treated with urethane, X-irradiation and hormones. *J Virol* 31:63–72.

74. Schwartz MS, Medina D (1987) Characterization of the DIM series of BALB/c preneoplasias for mouse mammary tumor virus-mediated oncogenesis. *Cancer Res* 47:5707–5714.

75. Asch BB, Asch HL (1990) Expression of the retrotransposons, intracisternal A-particles, during neoplastic progression of mouse mammary epithelium analyzed with a monoclonal antibody. *Cancer Res* 50:2404–2410.

76. Asch BB, Asch HL, Stoler DL, Anderson GR (1993) Deregulation of endogenous retrotransposons in mouse mammary carcinomes of diverse etiologies. *Int J Cancer* 54:813–819.

77. Asch BB, Natoli F, Asch HL (1994) DNA mutations involving endogenous murine leukemia virus-related elements in mouse carcinomas. *Proc Am Assoc Cancer Res* 35:3513.

78. Kordon E, Smith GH, Callahan R, Gallahan D (1994) *Int*-3, a cell fate gene, is activated by retroposon insertion during progression from preneoplasia to tumor. *Mol Cell Biol* 5:387A.

79. Zarbl H, Sukumar S, Arthur AV, Martin-Zanca D, Barbacid M (1985) Direct mutagenesis of Ha-*ras*-1 oncogenes by *N*-nitroso-*N*-methylurea during initiation of mammary carcinogenesis in rats. *Nature* 315:382–385.

80. Dandekar S, Sukumar S, Zarbl H, Young LJT, Cardiff RD (1986) Specific activation of the cellular Harvey-*ras* oncogene in dimethylbenz-anthracene-induced mouse mammary tumors. *Mol Cell Biol* 6:4104–4108.

81. Kumar R, Medina D, Sukumar S (1990) Activation of H-*ras* oncogenes in preneoplastic mouse mammary tissues. *Oncogene* 5:1271–1277.

82. Cardiff RD, Fanning TG, Morris DW, Ashley RL, Faulkin LJ (1981) Restriction endonuclease studies of hyperplastic outgrowth lines form BALB/cfC3HY mouse hyperplastic mammary nodules. *Cancer Res* 41:3024–3029.

65

83. Medina D (1978) Preneoplasia in breast cancer. In *Experimental Breast Cancer*, Vol II. WL McGuire (ed). New York: Plenum Press, pp 47–102.

84. Miyamoto S, Sukumar S, Guzman RC, Osborn R, Nandi S (1990) Transforming c-Ki-ras mutation is a preneoplastic event in mouse mammary carcinogenesis induced in vitro by N-methyl-N-nitrosourea. *Mol Cell Biol* 10:1593–1599.

85. Guzman RC, Osborn RC, Swanson SM, Sakthivel R, Hwang S-I, Miyamoto S, Nandi S (1992) Incidence of c-Ki-ras activation in N-methyl-N-nitrosourea-induced mammary carcinomas in pituitary-isografted mice. *Cancer Res* 52:5732–5737.

86. Bera TK, Guzman RC, Miyamoto S, Panda DK, Sasaki M, Hanyu K, Enami J, Nandi S (1994) Identification of a mammary transforming gene (MAT1) associated with mouse mammary carcinogenesis. *Proc Natl Acad Sci USA* 91:9789–9793.

87. Sinn E, Muller W, Pattengale P, Tepler J, Wallace R, Leder P (1987) Co-expression of MMTV/v-Ha-*ras* and MMTV/c-*myc* genes in transgenic mice: Synergistic action of oncogenes in vivo. *Cell* 49:465–475.

88. Andres A-C, Schonenberger C-A, Groner B, Hennighausen L, LeMeur M, Gerlinger P (1987) Ha-*ras* oncogene expression directed by milk protein gene promoter: Tissue specificity, hormonal regulation and tumor induction in transgenic mice. *Proc Natl Acad Sci USA* 84:1299–1303.

89. Miyamoto S, Guzman RC, Shiurba RA, Firestone GL, Nandi S (1990) Transfection of activated Ha-*ras* protooncogenes causes mouse mammary hyperplasia. *Cancer Res* 50:6010–6014.

90. Aguilar-Cordora E, Strange R, Young LJ, Billy HT, Gumerlock PH, Cardiff RD (1991) Viral Ha-*ras* mediated mammary tumor progression. *Oncogene* 6:1601–1607.

91. Redmond SMS, Reichmann E, Muller RG, Friis RR, Groner B, Hynes NE (1988) The transformation of primary and established mouse mammary epithelial cells by p21-*ras* is concentration dependent. *Oncogene* 2:259–265.

92. Andres A-C, Bchini O, Schubaur B, Dolder B, LeMeur M, Gerlinger P (1991) H-*ras* induced transformation of mammary epithelium is favored by increased oncogenes expression or by inhibition of mammary regression. *Oncogene* 6:771–779.

93. Gunzberg WH, Salmons B, Schlaeffli A, Moritz-Legrand S, Jones W, Sarkar NH, Ullrich R (1988) Expression of the oncogenes *mil* and *ras* abolishes the in vivo differentiation of mammary epithelial cells. *Carcinogenesis* 9:1849–1856.

94. Ball RK, Ziemiecki A, Schonenberger CA, Reichman E, Redmond SMS, Groner B (1988) V-*myc* alters the response of a cloned mouse mammary epithelial cell line to lactogenic hormones. *Mol Endocrinol* 2:133–142.

95. Edwards PAW, Ward JL, Bradbury JM (1988) Alteration of morphogenesis by the v-*myc* oncogene in transplants of mammary gland. *Oncogene* 2:407–412.

96. Telang NT, Osborne MP, Sweterlitsch LA, Narayanan R (1990) Neoplastic transformation of mouse mammary epithelial cells by deregulated *myc* expression. *Cell Regul* 1:863–872.

97. Medina D, White A, Said TK (1996) Hormones, growth factors and gene expression in preneoplasias of the mouse mammary gland. In *Hormonal Carcinogenesis*. JJ Li, S Li (eds). Raven Press, NY, pp 132–140.

98. Allred DG, O'Connell P, Fuqua SAW (1993) Biomarkers in early breast neoplasia. *J Cell Biochem* 17G:125–131.

99. Jerry DJ, Ozbun MA, Kittrell FS, Lane DP, Medina D, Butel JS (1993) Mutations in p53 are frequent in the preneoplastic stage of mouse mammary tumor development. *Cancer Res* 53:3374–3381.

100. Jerry DJ, Butel JS, Donehower LA, Paulson EJ, Cochran C, Wiseman RW, Medina D (1994) Infrequent p53 mutations occur infrequently in 7,12-dimethylberz anthracene-induced mammary tumors in BALB/c and p53 hemizygous mice. *Mol Carcinog* 9:175–183.

101. Ozbun MA, Jerry JD, Kittrell FS, Medina D, Butel JS (1993) p53 mutations selected in vivo when mouse mammary epithelial cells form hyperplastic outgrowths are not necessary for establishment of mammary cells in vitro. *Cancer Res* 53:1646–1652.

102. Li B, Greenberg N, Stephens LC, Meyn R, Medina D, Rosen JM (1994) Preferential overexpression of a 172 Arg-Leu mutant p53 in the mammary gland of transgenic mice results in altered lobuloalveolar development. *Cell Growth Differ* 5:711–721.

103. Cardiff RD, Muller WJ (1993) Transgenic mouse models of mammary tumorigenesis. *Cancer Surv* 16:97–113.

104. Cardiff RD (1996) The biology of mammary transgenes: Five rules. *J Mammary Gland Biol Neoplasia* 1:61–73.

105. Lin T-Z, Guzman RC, Osborn RC, Thordarson G, Nandi S (1992) Role of endocrine, autocrine and paracrine interactions in the development of mammary hyperplasia in Wnt-1 transgenic mice. *Cancer Res* 52:4413–3319.

106. Muller WJ, Lee FS, Dickson C, Peters G, Pattengale P, Leder P (1990) The *int-2* gene product acts as an epithelial growth factor in transgenic mice. *EMBO J* 9:907–913.

107. Ornitz DM, Cardiff RD, Kuo A, Leder P (1992) *Int-2*, an autocrine and/or ultra-short-range effector in transgenic mammary tissue transplants. *J Natl Cancer Inst* 84:887–892.

108. Wang TC, Cardiff RD, Zukerberg L, Lees A, Arnold A, Schmidt EV (1994) Mammary hyperplasia and carcinoma in MMTV-cyclin D1 transgenic mice. *Nature* 369:669–671.

109. Matsui Y, Halter SA, Holt JT, Hogan BLM, Coffey RJ (1990) Development of mammary hyperplasia and neoplasia in MMTV-TGFα transgenic mice. *Cell* 61:1147–1155.

110. Sandgren EP, Luetteke NC, Palmiter RD, Brinster RL, Lee DC (1990) Overexpression of TGFα in transgenic mice: Induction of epithelial hyperplasia, pancreatic metaplasia, and carcinoma of the breast. *Cell* 61:1121–1135.

111. Amundadottir LT, Johnson MD, Smith GH, Merlino G, Dickson RB (1995) Synergistic interaction of transforming growth factor α and c-*myc* in mouse mammary and salivary gland tumorigenesis. *Cell Growth Differ* 6:737–748.

112. Donehower LA, Godley LA, Aldaz CM, Pyle R, Yu-Ping S, Pinkel D, Gray J, Bradley A, Medina D, Varmus HE (1995) Deficiency of p53 accelerates mammary tumorigenesis in *wnt-1* transgenic mice and promotes chromosomal instability. *Genes Dev*, in press.

113. Coffey RJ Jr, Meise KS, Matsui Y, Hogan BLM, Dempsey PJ, Halter SA (1994) Acceleration of mammary neoplasia in transforming growth factor α transgenic mice by 7,12-dimethylbenzanthracene. *Cancer Res* 54:1678–1683.

114. Pierce DF, Johnson MD, Matsui Y, Robinson SD, Gold LI, Purchio AF, Daniel CW, Hogan BL, Moses HL (1993) Inhibition of mammary ductal development but not alveolar outgrowth during pregnancy in transgenic mice expression active TGFB1. *Genes Dev* 7:2308–2317.

115. Jhappan C, Geiser AG, Kordon EC, Bagheri D, Henninghausen L, Roberts AB, Smith GH, Merlino G (1993) Targeting expression of a TGFB1 transgene to the pregnant mammary gland inhibits alveolar development and lactation. *EMBO J* 12:1835–1845.

116. Kordon EC, McKnight R, Jhappan C, Henninghausen L, Merlino G, Smith GH (1995) Ectopic TGFB1 expression in the secretory mammary epithelium induces early senescence of the epithelial stem cell population. *Dev Biol* 168:47–61.

117. Jhappan C, Gallahan D, Stahle C, Chu E, Smith GH, Merlino G, Callahan R (1992) Expression of an activated *Notch*-related *int*-3 transgene interferes with cell differentiation and induces neoplastic transformation in mammary and salivary glands. *Genes Dev* 6:345–355.

118. Smith GH, Gallahan D, Diella F, Jhappan C, Merlino G, Callahan R (1995) Constitutive expression of a truncated *int*-3 gene in mouse mammary epithelium impairs differentiation and functional development. *Cell Growth Differ* 6:563–577.

119. Smith GH, Arthur LA, Medina D (1980) Evidence of separate pathways for viral and chemical carcinogenesis in C3H/StWi mouse mammary glands. *Int J Cancer* 26:373–379.

120. Medina D, Smith GH (1990) In search of mammary gland stem cells. *Protoplasma* 159:77–84.

121. Smith GH, Gallahan D, Zwiebel JA, Freeman SM, Bassin RH, Callahan R (1991) Long-term in vivo expression of genes introduced by retrovirus-mediated transfer into mammary epithelial cells. *J Virol* 65:6365–6370.

67

122. Edwards PAW, Abram CL, Bradbury JM (1996) Genetic manipulation of mammary epithelium by transplantation. *J Mammary Gland Biol Neoplasia* 1:75–89.
123. Bradbury JM, Sykes H, Edwards PAW (1991) Induction of mouse mammary tumors in a transplantation system by sequential introduction of the *myc* and *ras* oncogenes. *Int J Cancer* 48:908–915.
124. Bradbury JM, Arno J, Edwards PAW (1993) Induction of epithelial abnormalities that resemble human breast lesions by the expression of the *neu*/erbB2 oncogene in reconstituted mouse mammary gland. *Oncogene* 8:1551–1558.
125. Salomon DS, Dickson RB, Normanno N, Saeki T, Kim N, Kenney N, Ciardiello F (1992) Interaction of oncogenes and growth factors in colon and breast cancer. In *Current Perspectives on Molecular and Cellular Oncology*, Vol 1. DA Spandidos (ed). London: JAI Press, pp 211–260.
126. Vonderhaar BK (1987) Local effects of EGF, TGFα, and EGF-like growth factors on lobuloalvealar development of the mouse mammary gland in vivo. *J Cell Physiol* 132:581–584.
127. Silberstein GB, Daniel CW (1987) Reversible inhibition of mammary gland growth by TGFβ. *Science* 237:291–293.
128. Salomon DS, Perroteau I, Kidwell WR, Tam J, Derynck R (1987) Loss of growth responsiveness to epidermal growth factor and enhanced production of TGFα in *ras*-transformed mouse mammary epithelial cells. *J Cell Physiol* 130:397–409.
129. Normanno N, Ciardello F, Brandt R, Salomon DS (1994) Epidermal growth factor-related peptides in the pathogenesis of human breast cancer. *Breast Cancer Res Treat* 29:11–27.
130. Ethier SP, Moorthy R (1991) Multiple growth factor independence in rat mammary carcinoma cells. *Breast Cancer Res Treat* 18:73–82.
131. Ethier SP, Moorthy R, Dilts CA (1991) Secretion of an epidermal growth factor-like growth factor by epidermal growth factor-independent rat mammary carcinoma cells. *Cell Growth Differ* 2:593–602.
132. Daniel CW, Silberstein GB, Van Horn K, Strickland P, Robinson SD (1989) TGFβ1-induced inhibition of mouse ductal growth: Developmental specificity and characterization. *Dev Biol* 135:20–30.
133. Robinson SD, Silberstein GB, Roberts AB, Flanders KC, Daniel CW (1991) Regulated expression and growth inhibitory effects of transforming growth factor-β isoforms in mouse mammary gland development. *Development* 113:867–878.
134. Knabbe C, Wakefield L, Flanders K, Kasid A, Derynck R, Lyppman ME, Dickson RB (1987) Evidence that TGFβ is hormonally regulated negative growth factor in human breast cancer. *Cell* 48:417–428.
135. Norbury C, Nurse P (1992) Animal cell cycles and their control. *Annu Rev Biochem* 61:441–470.
136. Hartwell LH, Kastan MB (1994) Cell cycle control and cancer. *Science* 266:1821–1828.
137. Keyomarsi K, O'Leary N, Molnar G, Leas E, Howard JF, Pardee AB (1994) Cyclin E, a potential prognostic marker for breast cancer. *Cancer Res* 54:380–385.
138. Keyomarsi K, Pardee AB (1993) Redundant cyclin overexpression and gene amplification in breast cancer cells. *Proc Natl Acad Sci USA* 90:1112–1116.
139. Buckely MF, Sweeney KE, Hamilton JA, Sini RL, Manning DL, Nicholson RI, deFazio A, Watts CKW, Musgrove EA, Sutherland RL (1993) Expression and amplification of cyclin genes in human breast cancer. *Oncogene* 8:2127–2133.
140. Gillett C, Fanth V, Smith R, Fisher C, Bartek J, Dickson C, Barnes D, Peters G (1994) Amplification and overexpression of cyclin D1 in breast cancer detected by immunohistochemical staining. *Cancer Res* 54:1812–1817.
141. Said TK, Medina D (1995) Tyrosine phosphorylation in mouse mammary hyperplasias. *Carcinogenesis* 16:923–930.
142. Said TK, Medina D (1995) Cell cyclins and cyclin-dependent kinase activities in mouse mammary tumor development. *Carcinogenesis* 16:823–830.

143. Said TK, Luo L, Medina D (1995) Mouse mammary hyperplasies and neoplasies exhibited different patterns of cyclins D1 and D2 binding to cdK4. *Carcinogenesis* 16:2507–2513.
144. Zhang L, Medina D (1993) Gene expression screening for specific genes associated with mouse mammary tumor development. *Mol Carcinog* 8:123–126.
145. Friedmann Y, Daniel CA, Strickland P, Daniel CW (1994) *Hox* genes in normal and neoplastic mouse mammary gland. *Cancer Res* 54:5981–5985.

4. Transgenic models of breast cancer metastasis

David L. Dankort and William J. Muller

Introduction

Traditionally it has been difficult to genetically define the events that lead to the formation of metastatic mammary tumors. While a number of gene products have been implicated in the development of mammary carcinomas, few have been demonstrated to play causative roles in mammary tumor formation. With the advent of transgenic mouse technology, the basic researcher can now target the expression of a gene product to a particular tissue. This has provided scientists with the ability to create mouse models of human diseases. Of particular interest is the generation of transgenic mice carrying genes thought to play important roles in the initiation/progression of mammary carcinomas. From these model systems have emerged murine tumors that not only mimic human pathologies but have the propensity to metastasize to the lung, mirroring one of the major sites of human metastases. Here we review transgenic models of mammary tumorigenesis, with particular emphasis on those that develop metastatic mammary carcinomas.

Genetic changes occur in the development of mammary carcinomas

There are several lines of evidence to suggest that there is an increased risk of subsequent breast cancer development amongst women with proliferative disorders of increasing severity (atypical hyperplasias to in situ carcinomas) compared with those with proliferative disorders lacking atypia or those with normal epithelium [1]. These observations suggest that the occurrence of metastatic breast cancer requires multiple genetic events. While data linking these morphological changes to genetic alterations are lacking, it appears that distinct cytological abnormalities do exist. These consist of gene amplification of proto-oncogenes and conversely the loss of heterozygosity (LOH) at putative tumor suppressor loci. In fact, specific LOHs have been observed in human breast cancer samples on at least six chromosomes.

Interestingly, subsets of LOH mutations correlate with increased aggressiveness of the tumors [2]. While the identity of the genes affected in these

R. Dickson and M. Lippman (eds.) MAMMARY TUMOR CELL CYCLE, DIFFERENTIATION AND METASTASIS. 1996. Kluwer Academic Publishers. ISBN 0-7923-3905-3. All rights reserved.

deletions is unclear, there appears to be a requirement to remove several genes that likely negatively regulate cell growth. In addition to gross deletions involving these putative tumor suppressors, specific tumor suppressor genes, such as p53, appear to be frequently mutated [3]. Several genes are amplified and/or overexpressed in mammary tumors. These include growth factor receptor molecules (EGFR [4,5] c-ErbB2 [6]), growth factor–like molecules (int-2 [7,8]), transcription factors (c-myc [9]), and cell cycle regulators (cyclin D1/PRAD-1 [10,11]). Again, there appears to be a correlation between the amplification of specific genes and specific LOHs with tumorigenesis [12], but to date there have been no systematic studies linking these genetic alterations with the morphology of breast lesions.

While there is an increasing effort to identify prognostically valuable genes, correlative studies are limited to identifying genes that may in some way be involved in the production of carcinomas. However, these studies do not provide insight into the functional roles these genes play in tumor formation and progression. For this reason, researchers have chosen to employ transgenic mouse technologies as a powerful tool in directly assessing the transforming potential of proto-oncogenes known to be involved in mammary tumorigenesis [13,14]. Transgenic mouse models expressing a number of proto-oncogenes in the mammary epithelium have provided important insight into the complex in vivo requirements for aspects of malignant tumor formation, such as tumor initiation, angiogenesis, and metastasis.

Mammary targeted expression of transgenes

Mammary specific expression of oncogenes in transgenic mice has been achieved by fusing oncogenes to either the mouse mammary tumor virus (MMTV) long terminal repeat (LTR) or the whey acidic protein (WAP) promoter/enhancer. While these promoter/enhancer elements confer high levels of transcription to the mammary epithelium, their activities differ both temporally and spatially. Specifically, the WAP promoter/enhancer is transcriptionally active exclusively in the mid-pregnant mammary gland [15–17], whereas the MMTV-LTR directs transcription throughout all stages of mammary gland development [18]. Additionally, the MMTV LTR is transcriptionally active in epithelial cells derived from the seminal vesicles, epididymis, and the salivary, Harderian, and prostate glands. Table 1 lists the sites of transgene expression observed in a number of well-characterized transgenic mice bearing either WAP or MMTV linked oncogenes.

Mammary hyperproliferative disorders in transgenic mice

Several transgenic strains have been made that express gene products found to be overexpressed in human breast cancers (Table 1). As previously noted,

Table 1. Comparison of MMTV and WAP oncogene transgenic strains

Construct	Pathology	Mammary tumor occurrence	Onset[a]	Metastases[b]	References
MMTV/c-*myc*	M. gl. tumors, B and T cell lymphomas	Stochastic	325 days (50)	N.P.	28–30
MMTV/v-Ha-*ras*	M. gl. and Sal. gl. adenocarcinoma, Har. gl. hyperplasia, liver and lung met., lymphomas	Stochastic	168 days (52)	Infrequent lung and liver met.	29
MMTV/c-*myc*/v-Ha-*ras*	M. gl. and Sal. gl. adenocarcinoma, Har. gl. hyperplasia, lymphomas	Stochastic	46 days (9)	N.A.	29
WAP/c-*myc*	M. gl. adenocarcinomas	Stochastic	N.D.	N.P.	17
WAP/v-Ha-*ras*	M. gl. and Sal. gl. adenocarcinoma, lung met.[c]	Stochastic	N.D.	Lung met.[c]	15,92
WAP/c-*myc*/v-Ha-*ras*	M. gl. hyperplasia, dysplasia and adenocarcinoma	Stochastic	3–4 months	N.A.	16
MMTV/cyclin D1	M. gl. hyperplasia and adenocarcinoma, testicular or uterine sarcomas, liver met.[d]	Stochastic	18 months (17)	Liver met.[d]	24
MMTV/*int*-2	M.gl. hyperplasia and tumors	Stochastic	>18 months	N.P.	22
MMTV/*Wnt*-1	M. gl. hyperplasia and adenocarcinomas, lymph node met., Sal. gl. adenocarcinoma	Stochastic	4–6 months (43)	Infrequent lymph node met.	37,39
MMTV/*neu*[NT]	M. gl. adenocarcinoma, Sal. gl. and Epid. hyperplasia, pulmonary met.	Rapid progression	89 days	Pulmonary met.	54
MMTV/*neu*[NT]	M. gl. adenocarcinoma, Epid. and Har. hyperplasia, lung and pulmonary met.	Stochastic	7–10 months (29,69)	Lung (3/5) and pulmonary (1/5) met.	55
MMTV/*neu*	M. gl. hyperplasia and adenocarcinoma, lung met.[c]	Stochastic	205, 261 days (57,21)	Lung met.[c] (29/41)	56
MMTV/PyV mT	M. gl. adenocarcinoma, lung met.[c]	Rapid progression	34, 94 days (35,20)	Lung met.[c] (33/35,18/20)	68
MMTV/PyV mT src[−/−]	M. gl. hyperplasia and rare adenocarcinoma	Stochastic	>200 days (24)	N.P.	83
MMTV/PyV mT yes[−/−]	M. gl. adenocarcinoma, lung met.	Rapid progression	80 days (31)	Lung met.	83

M. gl. = mammary gland; Sal. gl. = salivary gland; Har. gl. = Harderian gland; Epid. = epididymis; met. = metastases.

[a] Refers to mammary tumor onset of 50% of female carriers. Number in parentheses represents number of mice observed. Where there are two numbers, the numbers refer to the number of mice analyzed from each strain that correspond to the latencies. N.D. = not determined.

[b] N.P. = metastases not present; N.A. = data not available. The number of mice with metastases of those examined are given in parentheses.

[c] The majority of lung metastases were of salivary origin.

[d] The liver metastases were derived from testicular or uterine sarcomas.

cyclin D1 and *int*-2 genes are often found amplified and/or overexpressed in these tumors. Interestingly, these genes reside on an amplicon that also includes the c-Src substrate cortactin, which is also frequently overexpressed in human breast cancers [19–21]. The generation of transgenic mice that individually express elevated levels of either *int*-2 or cyclin D1 in the mammary epithelium has provided important insight into the relative contribution of these molecules to mammary tumorigenesis. In both sets of MMTV transgenic mice, expression of the cyclin D1 or the *int*-2 transgene led to widespread mammary epithelial hyperplasias [22–24]. The hyperplasia associated with both the MMTV/cyclin D1 and MMTV/*int*-2 transgenic mice did give rise to focal mammary tumors, but did so with protracted latencies (Table 1). Together, these data suggest a high mitotic rate alone exhibited by these hyperplasias is insufficient for rapid progression to an in situ carcinoma.

Mammary tumorigenesis is a multistep process in transgenic mice

As previously indicated, human breast cancer appears to arise as a consequence of multiple genetic perturbations. Early work with primary embryo fibroblasts suggested that transformation of primary mammalian cells could be effected by the coexpression of a cytoplasmic oncogene, such as v-Ha-*ras*, and a nuclear proto-oncogene, such as c-*myc* [25,26]. Moreover, it appeared that a cytoplasmic oncogene could transform immortalized cell lines but not primary cells without the help of a nuclear 'immortalizing' gene product [27].

Although these studies provided important information of the genetic requirements for the transformation of cells cultivated in vitro, whether this was also true in the context of the living organism was unclear. To test whether this was also the case in vivo, separate strains of transgenic mice bearing either c-*myc* or v-Ha-*ras* under the control of the MMTV-LTR were established and subsequently interbred [28–30]. As expected, female animals from either strain overexpressed the respective transgene in the mammary gland and developed focal mammary adenocarcinomas [28–30]. The average onset of tumor formation was approximately 168 and 325 days for v-Ha-*ras* and multiparous c-*myc* transgenic females, respectively (Table 1). While both strains developed mammary tumors, the pathological features of the c-*myc* and v-Ha-*ras* mammary tumors were distinct. MMTV/c-*myc* tumors appeared as moderately well differentiated, locally invasive adenocarcinomas comprising large basophilic cells, that is, cells containing enlarged nuclei [14]. By contrast to these c-*myc* tumors, the MMTV/v-Ha-*ras*–derived lesions were adenosquamoid carcinomas comprised of small eosinophilic cells juxtaposed to normal epithelium [18].

While both tumors were locally, albeit infrequently, invasive, only the MMTV/v-Ha-*ras*–derived tumors metastasized beyond the mammary fat pad into the lung and/or liver [29,31; W.J. Muller, unpublished results]. To assess whether coexpression of v-Ha-*ras* and c-*myc* in the mammary epithelium were sufficient for rapid tumorigenesis, bitransgenic mice carrying both transgenes were generated [29]. Although bitransgenic mice coexpressing c-*myc* and v-Ha-*ras* in the mammary epithelium resulted in a dramatic acceleration in the development of mammary tumors, these tumors arose adjacent to morphologically normal mammary epithelium that also coexpressed elevated levels of c-*myc* and v-Ha-*ras* [29]. These observations argued that, although c-*myc* and v-Ha-*ras* could cooperate in mammary tumorigenesis, their expression was not sufficient for tumorigenesis. Rather, these results suggested that further genetic events were required for the conversion of mammary epithelial cells to a malignant phenotype. As with the parental MMTV/v-Ha-*ras* and MMTV/c-*myc* strains, distant metastases in tumor bearing bitransgenic mice were rare. This observation may suggest that activation of the c-*myc* and v-Ha-*ras* oncogenes is insufficient to facilitate metastatic progression.

Collaboration of oncogenes has also been observed in transgenic mice coexpressing *int*-2 and *Wnt*-1 growth factors in the mammary gland. Int-2 is a member of the fibroblast growth factor family [32], whereas *Wnt*-1 (previously termed *int*-1) is a member of a family of secreted growth factors [33]. Both genes were initially identified as being preferential MMTV integration sites within MMTV-induced murine mammary tumors [34–36]. The MMTV/*Wnt*-1 transgenic animals from a single line develop mammary hyperplasias prior to pregnancy [37]. From these hyperplasias emerge adenocarcinomas that are phenotypically indistinguishable from those arising from MMTV infection [38]. Interbreeding of these strains produced *int*-2/*Wnt*-1 bitransgenics and resulted in a dramatic acceleration of tumor formation [39]. However, like the c-*myc*/v-Ha-*ras* bitransgenics, coexpression of the *int*-2 and *wnt*-1 was not sufficient for global transformation of the murine mammary gland. Interestingly, in MMTV induced mammary tumorigenesis, insertional activation of both *int*-2 and *Wnt*-1 is frequently observed. Taken together, these transgenic and retroviral experiments illustrate that, like the *myc*/*ras* bitransgenics, there is cooperativity amongst different subsets of proto-oncogenes in mammary carcinogenesis.

Role of the c-*ErbB*-2/*neu* oncogene in mammary tumorigenesis and metastasis

The *neu* oncogene was initially isolated [40] and cloned [41] from chemically induced rat neuroglioblastomas. Sequence analyses revealed that *neu*, and its human homolog, c-*ErbB*-2, were structurally related to the epidermal growth factor receptor (EGFR) [41–43]. Upon sequence comparison with the cloned wild-type cellular gene, it was found to differ by a single nucleotide [44], resulting in a nonconservative amino acid change within the transmembrane domain. This conferred upon the receptor a constitutive ligand-independent kinase activity [45]. For the purpose of clarity, the oncogenic form is referred to as *activated neu* or *neu^{NT}*, whereas the wild-type rat and human genes are termed *neu* and c-*ErbB*-2, respectively.

The results of numerous studies demonstrate overexpression of c-*ErbB*-2 is detected in a large proportion of human breast and ovarian cancers and their derived cell lines [6,46–50]. Moreover, the overexpression of c-*ErbB*-2 in these cancers can be further correlated with poor prognosis [49–52] as well as poor clinical outcome [53]. Because poor clinical outcome is reflective of the occurrence of metastatic disease, these studies suggested that mammary tumor cells expressing elevated levels of c-*ErbB*-2 had the propensity to metastasize.

To directly test the oncogenic potential of the *neu* oncogene in the mammary epithelium, transgenic mice expressing a constitutively activated version of *neu*, termed *neu^{NT}* [42,43], under the transcriptional control of the MMTV promoter were established [52,53]. In several of these strains, mammary epithelial expression of the *neu^{NT}* oncogene resulted in the development of multifocal mammary tumors in 100% of both male and female transgenic mice [52]. Histological examination of virgin females revealed multiple dysplastic nodules arising synchronously in the mammary epithelium. Interestingly, within 3 months all female carriers had developed multiple mammary carcinomas involving the entire mammary epithelium. Furthermore, these tumors histologically resembled the human comedo-carcinomas that are also known to express elevated levels of Neu [3,14]. Therefore these transgenic mouse models may be direct models of the human disease.

Although these strains of transgenic mice possessed a much shortened life span, pulmonary metastasis was observed in several instances [52,53]. Notably, the observed metastases were intravascular at the time of autopsy, suggesting that these tumors could not readily traverse the pulmonary vein endothelium. Taken together, these observations provided direct evidence that expression of activated Neu in the mammary epithelium resulted in the induction of metastatic disease.

Although transgenics expressing *neu^{NT}* in the mammary epithelium did provide direct evidence of this tyrosine kinase's oncogenic potential in mammary tumorigenesis, the phenotype, one-step progression, did not mirror the epidemiological data of human breast cancer development. Moreover, examination of human breast cancer samples failed to reveal a comparable activating mutation. Thus, on the basis of these observations it appeared that overexpression of the wild-type c-*ErbB*-2 was the primary mechanism by which c-*ErbB*-2 induced mammary tumors in humans. To test if overexpression of wild-type *neu* was capable of inducing mammary carcinoma, transgenic mice carrying MMTV/*neu* were established [55,56]. Female transgenic mice derived from several independent lines developed focal mammary adenocarcinomas juxtaposed to hyperplastic epithelium after a long latency period (Table 1). Like the *neu^{NT}* tumors, these tumors resembled the human comedo-carcinomas that express elevated levels of c-*ErbB*-2 [3].

Transgene expression was detected in all tumors examined at both the level of RNA and protein. In a proportion of the samples examined, *neu* transgene RNA and protein were detected in the surrounding hyperplastic epithelium [56]. Interestingly, Neu derived from tumor lysates displayed elevated tyrosine kinase activity compared with that of hyperplasia-derived lysates within the same MMTV/*neu* animal. In many cases, the differences in kinase activities could not be attributed to the amount of Neu present [56]. These observations argued that the increased specific activity of Neu in tumors was directly correlated with tumorigenesis. Because, *neu* is known to be activated by somatic mutations, one possible explanation for this observation is that activation of Neu in these tumors occurs through somatic mutations in the transgene itself. To explore this possibility, RNA derived from tumor and adjacent normal epithelium was examined for the presence of altered transcripts using either RT/PCR or RNAse protection analyses [57].

The results of these analyses revealed multiple in-frame deletions occurred within the transgenes of MMTV/*neu* derived from tumors but not the adjacent hyperplastic epithelium. Notably, within the same animal different deletions were detected, each being restricted to a single tumor and not found in the adjacent epithelium, suggesting that each tumor had arisen from a clonal antecedent. These deletions, ranging in size from 5 to 12 amino acids, occurred in the extracellular domain proximal to the transmembrane region [57; P.M. Siegel and W.J. Muller, unpublished]. RNAse protection analysis suggested 65% of the MMTV/*neu*-derived tumors express aberrant *neu* transcripts. Introduction of these deletions into the *neu* proto-oncogene resulted in its oncogenic activation in in-vitro transformation assays.

Furthermore, these mutant receptor molecules appear to have elevated kinase activities, as assessed by phosphotyrosine immunoblot analysis. Together, these data suggest that the majority of MMTV/*neu* tumors arise through somatic mutations of the transgene resulting in constitutive activation of Neu. Moreover, these data would predict MMTV-directed expression of these *neu* deletion mutants (*NDL*) in the transgenic animal would lead to accelerated mammary adenocarcinomas compared with that of MMTV/*neu* mice.

Another important feature of the MMTV/*neu* tumors is that they frequently metastasized. In fact, over 70% of the tumor-bearing animals eventually develop metastases to the lung, albeit only after long onset. These tumors were likely derived from the mammary epithelium because they expressed mammary differentiation markers [56]. The penetrance of this metastatic phenotype contrasts with the relatively infrequent occurrence of pulmonary metastases observed in transgenic strains expressing *neu*[NT]. One possible explanation for this apparent discrepancy is that MMTV/*neu*[NT], with its high tumor burden, possess a shortened life span compared with MMTV/*neu* (Table 1).

Multiple pathways are required for rapid progression

Another tyrosine kinase that has been associated with the induction of mammary cancers is that associated with the polyomavirus (PyV) middle T (mT) antigen. However, unlike Neu, PyV middle T does not possess an intrinsic biochemical activity [58] but rather exerts its oncogenic effects through its association with the c-Src family of tyrosine kinases and other signaling molecules (Figure 1b). The first indication that PyV mT may be involved in the induction of mammary carcinoma stems from the observation that infection of newborn or *nu/nu* mice with PyV frequently results in the induction of mammary tumors [59]. A functional mT antigen is required for PyV-induced tumor formation [60] and is sufficient to transform established cells in tissue culture [61]. Furthermore, genetic analysis has demonstrated that mT mutants that are deficient in Src, PI3′K, or SHC associations are invariably transformation incompetent [62–67]. Taken together, these data suggest that mT antigen mediates transformation through activation of several cellular signaling pathways.

To directly test the oncogenic potential of middle T in the mammary epithelium, transgenic mice carrying a MMTV/PyV middle T fusion gene were established. Like MMTV/*neu*^{NT} mice, all transgenic mice expressing the PyV mT antigen in the mammary epithelium synchronously developed multifocal tumors with a short latency [68]. Remarkably, the presence of multifocal mammary adenocarcinomas could be detected by whole-mount analysis as early 3 weeks of age in female mice. Because transformation of the mammary epithelium is concurrent with detectable transgene expression, it appears that expression of PyV middle T is sufficient for mammary tumorigenesis.

Of particular relevance to this review, a striking phenotype exhibited by the MMTV/PyV middle T mice is the frequent occurrence of pulmonary

---

Figure 1. Schematic representation of signal transduction from the *Neu/Erb*B-2 receptor tyrosine kinase and the polyomavirus middle T antigen. **A:** Proteins that bind *Neu/Erb*B-2 directly or indirectly as determined by coimmunoprecipitation assays. Proteins that bind directly to the receptor by 'far-western' blot analyses include Src and Yes tyrosine kinases [79; S.K. Muthuswamy and W.J. Muller, unpublished], GRB7 [93], and GRB2 [93]. The latter protein is depicted as binding the receptor through tyrosine phosphorylated SHC, although it can bind directly. Those proteins identified by coimmunoprecipitation analyses include phospholipase Cγ1 (PLCγ1) [94], SHC [93,95], phosphoinositol 3′kinase (PI3′kinase) [96–98], and protein tyrosine phosphatases (PTP) 1D and 1C [99]. Ras GTPase activating protein (ras-GAP) has been shown to interact with *neu*^{NT} in in-vitro association assyas [S.K. Muthuswamy, D.L. Dankort, and W.J. Muller, unpublished]. The GRB2-Sos (mammalian son of sevenless) complex is pre-existing in quiescent cells [100–102]. The Sos protein is a Ras-specific GTP exchange factor that has been shown to activate Ras [103]. **B:** Middle T antigen associated proteins are indicated. Depicted are PI3′kinase [104,105], SHC proteins [65,66], src family tyrosine kinases (Src [78,106], Yes [107], and Fyn [108,109]), and protein phosphatase 2A (PP2A) subunits [110,111]. Also indicated is a simplified signal transduction kinase cascade eminating from Ras [112–114], culminating in the modulation of transcription factor activity [115,116].

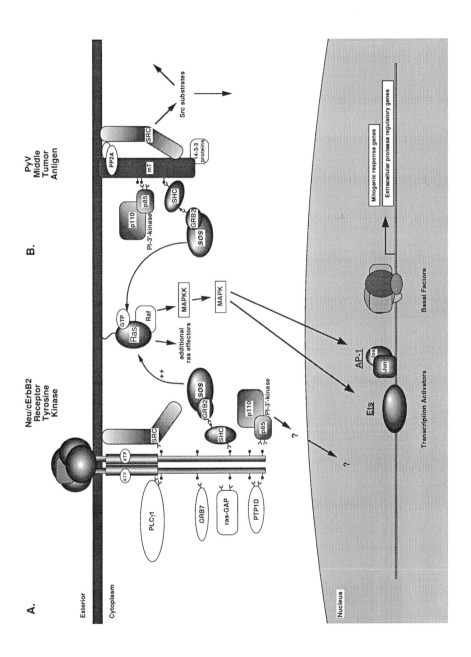

79

metastases. In fact, by 3 months of age approximately 95% of MMTV/PyV middle T females have developed pulmonary metastases. Given that these lung metastases express differentiated mammary epithelial markers, it is likely that they originated from the primary mammary tumors [68]. Consistent with this view, both transplantation of these mammary tumors into the mammary fat pads or injection of mT-tumor derived cell lines into the tail veins of syngeneic mice resulted in lung metastases [Cardiff and Muller, unpublished observations]. Interestingly, the majority of these lesions appeared to be intra-alveolar rather than intravascular. This contrasts with observations made with the metastatic lesions exhibited in the MMTV/*neu* strains, which appeared to lack the ability to traverse the pulmonary vascular endothelium and remained lodged within pulmonary vessels [56]. The molecular basis, however, for this difference has not been determined.

These transgenic studies suggest that expression of PyV mT antigen or activated forms of Neu were capable of predisposing the mammary epithelial cell to metastasize. In vivo studies placing tumors in hypovascularized positions have demonstrated that, in the absence of neovascularization, tumors grow at a linear rate and upon vascularization a rapid exponential growth ensues [69]. In both human breast carcinomas and skin melanomas, the appearance of neovascularization is prognostic for a poor clinical outcome [70,71], presumably due to metastasis from the primary tumor. Angiogenesis may play two roles in allowing metastasis. First, it allows for tumor expansion beyond a critical volume [72,73]. Secondly, newly formed vasculature often contains basement membrane defects that likely facilitate metastatic cell invasion of these vessels [74]. Interestingly, PyV mT antigen–induced tumors appear to possess the ability to promote angiogenesis. For example, both PyV middle T induced hemanginomas and MMTV/mT–derived mammary tumors have the capacity to induce angiogenesis [75,76; L.J.T. Young and R.D. Cardiff, unpublished]. Moreover, in the case of the MMTV/mT–derived mammary tumors, approximately 50% of these transplants appear to metastasize to the lung. While it is not yet clear which factors mediate this angiogenesis, this system should prove invaluable in evaluating inhibitors of this process in the context of the living animal.

The ability of PyV mT antigen to induce mammary metastasis may also reflect its capacity to alter the balance of extracellular protease activities. In the PyV mT-induced hemanginomas, expression of mT appears to upregulate the levels of the urokinase-type plasminogen activator (uPA) and to downregulate its cognate inhibitor, PAI-1. The uPA protein is a key regulatory enzyme that activates a proteolytic cascade important in tissue remodeling, cell migration, and tumor cell invasiveness. Thus the occurrence of highly invasive hemanginomas in mice expressing mT antigen in the endothelial compartment appears to correlate with induction of a proteolytic imbalance [77]. Although it is unclear whether a similar situation is responsible for the metastatic behavior of the PyV middle T mammary tumor cells, elevated proteolytic activity has also been observed in these tumor cells [C.T. Guy and W.J. Muller, unpublished].

Molecular basis for the metastatic behavior of the PyV middle T– and Neu-induced mammary tumors

While the generation of transgenic mice has demonstrated the role of many genes in tumor initiation, metastatic mammary tumors arise infrequently and do so with a poor penetrance in most strains (see Table 1). As mentioned previously, lung metastases were observed infrequently in the MMTV/v-Ha-ras and MMTV/neu^NT strains and occurred with a high penetrance in the MMTV/neu and MMTV/mT strains [29,54–56,68]. These observations raise the intriguing possibility that the frequent induction of metastases occurs via a common mechanism. In fact, although both Neu and PyV middle T oncogenes bear little sequence homology, they appear to activate common sets of signaling pathways. For example, both PyV middle T and Neu activate members of the c-Src tyrosine kinase family by forming physical complexes [78–80]. In addition, both molecules can activate pathways involving PI-3′ kinase and SHC proteins.

The importance of c-Src in mT-induced mammary tumorigenesis and metastasis derives from the results of interbreeding the MMTV/mT strains with c-Src– or c-Yes–deficient mice [81,82]. The results of these analyses revealed that a functional c-Src gene was required for the efficient induction of mammary tumors by PyV middle T [83]. While *src* appears to be required for mT-induced mammary tumorigenesis, it is dispensable for mT-induced endothelial or fibroblast transformation [84,85]. This suggests Src may play a tissue-specific role in mT-mediated tumorigenesis. This notion is supported by the observation that the *yes* gene product appears to be dispensable for MMTV/mT-induced carcinogenesis [83]. Whether c-Src is also required for Neu-induced tumorigenesis awaits future experimentation. Taken together, these data would argue that the mammary epithelium is exquisitely sensitive to the actions of activated Src in mediating transformation.

Although these observations suggest that c-Src appears important in Neu- and PyV mT–induced mammary tumorigenesis, recent studies have demonstrated that expression of a constitutively activated c-Src in the mammary epithelium is not sufficient for mammary tumorigenesis and metastasis [M.A.Webster, Muller, and Cardiff, unpublished]. Thus middle T antigen and likely Neu must activate additional pathways that contribute to these phenotypes. Middle T mutants exist that are deficient in binding the PI3′kinase p85 subunit or SHC proteins yet still retain Src association capacities. In tissue transformation assays, these mT mutants are severely impaired in their transformation abilities [65–67], suggesting a requirement for the simultaneous activation of the PI3′kinase and SHC (and thus presumably Ras) pathways.

These mutants, when expressed in the mammary gland, are debilitated in their capacity to induce mammary carcinoma while being capable of activating endogenous Src molecules [M.A. Webster, R.A. Cardiff, and W.J. Muller, unpublished]. Taken together, these data demonstrate a need for the simultaneous activation of several cellular signaling pathways in order to attain rapid transformation in this system. Both Neu and mT antigen (Figure 1) have the ability to activate similar pathways. Perhaps the recruitment and activation of several of these pathways is required to possess the potent transforming abilities these molecules display. Neu mutants now exist that should prove useful in dissecting the pathways required for mammary tumorigenesis.

Another common feature of the PyV mT– and Neu-induced mammary tumors is that they both express elevated levels of the Ets-related transcription factor PEA-3 [86,87]. Interestingly, the promoter regions of several extracellular proteases, and their cognate inhibitors contain PEA-3 binding sites. Furthermore, it has been demonstrated that expression of non-nuclear oncogenes such as PyV mT antigen and v-src can activate the transcription of the stromelysin 1 promoter through these PEA-3 motifs [88,89]. Interestingly, EGF has been shown to stimulate activity from this promoter, perhaps indicting that EGFR family members can transcriptionally activate these proteases as well [90]. Conversely, these same PEA-3 elements appear to downregulate the expression of protease inhibitors such as TIMP-1 [91]. Thus the activation of Ets-related transcription factors through the action of tyrosine kinases, such as Neu- and the PyV middle T–associated c-Src kinase, may have influence metastasis by altering proteolytic balance. Future genetic dissection of these pathways will hopefully provide important insight into the roles each of these pathways play in mammary tumorigenesis and metastasis.

Acknowledgment

The authors thank Peter M. Siegel and Jennifer E. LeCouter for their critical reviews of this manuscript.

References

1. Dupont WD, Page DL (1985) Risk factors for breast cancer in women with proliferative breast disease. N Engl J Med 312:146–151.
2. Sato T, Tanigami A, Yamakawa K, Akiyama F, Kasumi F, Sakamoto G, Nakamura Y (1990) Allelotype of breast cancer: Cumulative allele losses promote tumor progression in primary breast cancer. Cancer Res 50:7184–7189.
3. Morrison BW (1994) The genetics of breast cancer. Hemotol Oncol Clin North Am 8:15–27.
4. Gasparini G, Bevilacqua, Pozza F, Meli S, Boracchi P, Marubini E, Sainsbury JRC (1992) Value of epidermal growth factor receptor status compared with growth fraction and other factors for prognosis in early breast cancer. Br J Cancer 66:970–976.
5. Sainsbury JRC, Nicholson S, Angus B, Farndon JR, Malcolm AJ, Harris AL (1988)

Eidermal growth factor receptor status of histological sub-types of breast cancer. *Br J Cancer* 58:458–460.

6. Slamon DJ, Godolphin W, Jones LA, Holt JA, Wong SG, Keith DE, Levin WJ, Stuart SG, Udove J, Ullrich A, Press MF (1989) Studies of the HER-2/neu proto-oncogene in human breast and ovarian cancer. *Science* 244:707–712.

7. Zhou DJ, Casey G, Cline MJ (1988) Amplification of human int-2 in breast cancers and squamous carcinomas. *Oncogene* 2:279–282.

8. Schuuring E, Verhoeven E, van Tinteren H, Peterse JL, Nunnink B, Thunnissen FBJM, Devilee P, Cornelisse CJ, van der Vijver MJ, Mooi WJ (1992) Amplification of genes within the chromosome 11q13 region is indicative of poor prognosis in patients with operable breast cancer. *Cancer Res* 52:5229–5234.

9. Berns EMJJ, Klijn JGM, van Putten WLJ, van Staveren IL, Portengen H, Foekens JA (1992) c-myc amplification is a better prognostic factor than HER2/neu amplification in primary breast cancer. *Cancer Res* 52:1107–1113.

10. Buckley MF, Sweeney KJE, Hamilton JA, Sini RL, Manning DL, Nicholson RI, deFazio A, Watts CKW, Musgrove EA, Sutherland RL (1993) Expression and amplification of cyclin genes in human breast cancer. *Oncogene* 8:2127–2133.

11. Bartkova J, Lukas J, Muller H, Lutzhoft D, Strauss M, Bartek J (1994) Cyclin D1 protein expression and function in human breast cancer. *Int J Cancer* 57:353–361.

12. Ben Cheickh M, Rouanet P, Louason G, Jeanteur P, Theillet C (1992) An attempt to define sets of cooperating genetic alterations in human breast cancer. *Int J Cancer* 51:542–547.

13. Webster MA, Muller WJ (1994) Mammary tumorigenesis and metastasis in transgenic mice. *Semin Cancer Biol* 5:69–76.

14. Cardiff RD, Muller WJ (1993) Transgenic mouse models of mammary tumorigenesis. *Cancer Surv* 16:97–113.

15. Andres A-C, Schonenberger C-A, Groner B, Henninghausen L, LeMeur M, Gerlinger P (1987) Ha-ras oncogene expression directed by a milk gene promoter; tissue specificity, hormonal regulation, and tumor induction in transgenic mice. *Proc Natl Acad Sci USA* 84:1299–1303.

16. Andres A-C, van der Valk MA, Schonenberger C-A, Fluckiger F, LeMeur M, Gerlinger P, Groner B (1988) Ha-ras and c-myc oncogene expression interferes with morphological and functional differentiation of mammary epithelial cells in single and double transgenic mice. *Genes Dev* 2:1486–1495.

17. Schoonenberger C-A, Andres A-C, Groner B, van der Aalk M, LeMeur M, Gerlinger P (1988) Targeted c-myc expression in mammary glands of transgenic mice induces mammary tumors with constitutive milk protein gene transcription. *EMBO J* 7:169–175.

18. Pattengale PK, Stewart TA, Leder A, Sinn E, Muller W, Tepler I, Schmidt E, Leder P (1989) Animal models of human disease: Pathology and molecular biology of spontaneous neoplasms occurring in transgenic carrying and expressing activated cellular oncogenes. *Am J Pathol* 135:39–61.

19. Casey G, Smith R, McGillivray D, Peters G, Dickson C (1986) Characterization and chromosome assignment of the human homolog of int-2, a potential proto-oncogene. *Mol Cell Biol* 6:502–510.

20. Lammie GA, Peters G (1991) Chromosome 11q13 abnormalities in human cancer. *Cancer Cells* 3:413–420.

21. Schuuring E, Verhoeven E, Litvinov S, Michalides RJAM (1993) The product of the EMS1 gene, amplified and overexpressed in human carcinomas, is homologous to a v-src substrate and is located in cell-substratum contact sites. *Mol Cell Biol* 13:2891–2898.

22. Muller WJ, Lee FS, Dickson C, Peters G, Pattengale P, Leder P (1990) The int-2 gene product acts as an epithelial growth factor in transgenic mice. *EMBO J* 9:907–913.

23. Ornitz DM, Moreadith RW, Leder P (1991) Binary system for regulating transgene expression in mice: Targeting int-2 expression with yeast GAL4/UAS control elements. *Proc Natl Acad Sci USA* 88:698–702.

83

24. Wang TC, Cardiff RD, Zukerberg L, Lees E, Arnold A, Schmidt EV (1994) Mammary hyperplasia and carcinoma in MMTV/cyclin D1 transgenic mice. *Nature* 369:669–671.
25. Land H, Parada LF, Weinberg RA (1983) Tumorigenic conversion of primary embryo fibroblasts requires at least two cooperating oncogenes. *Nature* 304:596–602.
26. Weinberg RA (1985) The action of oncogenes in the cytoplasm and the nucleus. *Science* 230:770–776.
27. Weinberg RA (1989) Oncogenes and multistep carcinogenesis. In *Oncogenes and the Molecular Origins of Cancer*. RA Weinberg (ed). Cold Spring Harbor, NY: Cold Spring Harbor Laboratory, pp 307–326.
28. Stewart TA, Pattengale PK, Leder P (1984) Spontaneous mammary adenocarcinomas in transgenic mice that carry and express MTV/myc fusion genes. *Cell* 38:627–637.
29. Sinn E, Muller W, Pattengale P, Tepler I, Wallace R, Leder P (1987) Coexpression of MMTV/v-Ha-ras and MMTV-c-myc genes in transgenic mice: Synergistc action of oncogenes in vivo. *Cell* 49:465–475.
30. Leder A, Pattengale PK, Kuo A, Stewart TA, Leder P (1986) Consequences of widespread deregulation of the c-myc gene in transgenic mice: Multiple neoplasms and normal development. *Cell* 45:485–495.
31. Tremblay PJ, Pothier F, Hoang T, Trembley G, Brownstein S, Liszaur A, Jolicoeur P (1989) Transgenic mice carrying the mouse mammary tumor virus ras fusion gene: Distinct effects in various tissues. *Mol Cell Biol* 9:854–859.
32. Yoshida T, Miyagawa K, Odagiri H, Sakamoto H, Little PFR, Terada M, Sugimura T (1987) Genomic sequences of hst, a transforming gene encoding a protein homologous to fibroblast growth factors and the int-2-encoded protein. *Proc Natl Acad Sci USA* 84:7305–7309.
33. Nusse R, Varmus HE (1992) Wnt genes. *Cell* 69:1073–1088.
34. Pathak VK, Strange R, Young LJT, Morris DW, Cardiff RD (1987) Survey of int region DNA rearrangements in 3 and BALB/cfCH3 mouse mammary tumor system. *J Natl Cancer Inst* 78:327–331.
35. Gray DA, Jackson DP, Percy DH, Morris VL (1986) Activation of int-1 and int-2 loci in GRf mammary tumors. *Virology* 154:271–278.
36. Peters G, Lee AE, Dickson C (1989) Concerted activation of two potential proto-oncogenes in carcinomas induced by mouse mammary tumour virus. *Nature* 320:628–631.
37. Tsukamoto AS, Grosschedi R, Guzman RC, Parslow T, Varmus HE (1988) Expression of the int-1 gene in transgenic mice is associated with mammary gland hyperplasia and adenocarcinomas in male and female mice. *Cell* 55:619–625.
38. Medina D (1982) Mammary tumors. In *The Mouse in Biomedical Research*. HL Foster, JD Small, JG Fox (eds). New York: Academic Press, pp 373–396.
39. Kwan H, Pecenka V, Tsukamoto A, Parslow TG, Guzman R, Lin T-P, Muller WJ, Lee FS, Leder P, Varmus HE (1992) Transgenes expressing the WntI-1 and int-2 proto-oncogenes cooperate during mammary carcinogenesis in doubly transgenic mice. *Mol Cell Biol* 12:147–154.
40. Padhy LC, Shih C, Cowing D, Finkelstein R, Weinberg RA (1982) Identification of a phosphoprotein specifically induced by the transforming DNA of rat neuroblastomas. *Cell* 28:865–871.
41. Bargmann CI, Hung M-C, Weinberg RA (1986) The neu oncogene encodes an epidermal growth factor receptor-related protein. *Nature* 319:226–230.
42. Coussens L, Yang-Feng TL, Liao Y-C, Chen E, Gray A, McGrath J, Seeburg PH, Libermann TA, Schlessinger J, Francke U, Levinson A, Ullrich A (1985) Tyrosine kinase receptor with extensive homology to EGF receptor shares chromosome location with neu oncogene. *Science* 230:1132–1139.
43. Yamamoto T, Ikawa S, Akiyama T, Semba K, Nomura N, Miyajima N, Saito T, Toyoshima K (1986) Similarity of protein encoded by the human c-erb-B-2 gene to the epidermal growth factor receptor. *Nature* 319:230–234.
44. Bargmann CI, Hung M-C, Weinberg RA (1986) Multiple independent activations of the neu oncogene by a point mutation altering the transmembrane domain of p185. *Cell* 45:649–657.

84

45. Bargmann CI, Weinberg RA (1988) Increased tyrosine kinase activity associated with the protein encoded by the activated neu oncogene. *Proc Natl Acad Sci USA* 85:5394–5398.

46. Slamon DJ, Clark GM, Wong SG, Levin WJ, Ullrich A, McGuire WL (1987) Human breast cancer: Correlation of relapse and survival with the amplification of the HER-2/neu oncogene. *Science* 235:177–182.

47. van de Vijver MJ, Peterse JL, Mooi WJ, Wisman P, Lomans J, Dalesio O, Nusse R (1988) Neu overexpression in breast cancer. *N Engl J Med* 319:1239–1245.

48. King C, Kraus MH, Aaronson SA (1985) Amplification of a novel v-erbB-related gene in a human mammary carcinoma. *Science* 229:974–976.

49. Mansour EG, Ravdin PM, Dressler L (1994) Prognostic factors in early breast carcinoma. *Cancer* 74:381–400.

50. Hynes NE, Stern DF (1994) The biology of erbB-2/neu/HER-2 and its role in cancer. *Biochim Biophys Acta* 1198:165–184.

51. Gullick WJ, Love SB, Wright C, Barnes DM, Gusterson B, Harris AL, Altman DG (1991) C-erbB-2 protein overexpression in breast cancer is a risk factor in patients with involved and uninvolved lymph nodes. *Br J Cancer* 63:434–438.

52. Patterson MC, Dietrich KD, Danyluk J, Paterson AH, Lees AW, Jamil N, Hanson J, Jenkins H, Krause BE, McBlain WA, Slamon DJ, Fourney RM (1991) Correlation between c-erbB2 amplification and risk of recurrent disease in node-negative breast cancer. *Cancer Res* 51:556–567.

53. Tripathy D, Benz C (1994) Growth factors and their receptors. *Hematol Oncol Clin North Am* 8:29–50.

54. Muller WJ, Sinn E, Pattengale PK, Wallace R, Leder P (1988) Single-step induction of mammary adenocarcinoma in transgenic mice bearing the activated c-neu oncogene. *Cell* 54:105–115.

55. Bouchard L, Lamarre L, Trembley PJ, Jolicoeur P (1989) Stochastic appearance of mammary tumors in transgenic mice carrying the c-neu oncogene. *Cell* 57:931–936.

56. Guy CT, Webster MA, Schaller M, Parsons TJ, Cardiff RA, Muller WJ (1992) Expression of the neu protooncogene in the mammary epithlium of transgenic mice induces metastatic disease. *Proc Natl Acad Sci USA* 89:10578–10582.

57. Siegel PM, Dankort DL, Hardy WR, Muller WJ (1994) Novel activating mutations in the neu proto-oncogene involved in induction of mammary tumors. *Mol Cell Biol* 14:7068–7077.

58. Kaplan DR, Pallas DC, Morgan B, Schaffhausen B, Roberts TM (1988) Mechanisms of transformation by polyoma middle T antigen. *Biochim Biophys Acta* 948:345–364.

59. Berebbi M, Martin PM, Berthois Y, Bernard AM, Blangy D (1990) Estradiol dependence of the specific mammary tissue targetting of polyoma virus oncogenicity in nude mice. *Oncogene* 5:505–509.

60. Israel MA, Chan HW, Hourihan SA, Rowe WP, Martin MA (1979) Biological activity of polyoma viral DNA in mice and hamsters. *J Virol* 29:990–996.

61. Treisman R, Novak U, Favaloro J, Kamen R (1981) Transformation of rat cells by an altered polyoma virus genome expressing only the middle T protein. *Nature* 292:595–600.

62. Charmichel G, Schaffhausen BS, Mandel G, Liang TJ, Benjamin TL (1984) Transformation by polyoma virus is drastically reduced substitution of phenylalanine for tyrosine at residue 315 of middle-sized tumor antigen. *Proc Natl Acad Sci USA* 81:679–683.

63. Markland W, Oostra BA, Harvey R, Markham AF, Colledge WH, Smith AE (1986) Site directed mutagenesis of polyomavirus middle-T antigen sequence encoding tyrosine 315 and tyrosine 250. *J Virol* 59:384–391.

64. Druker BJ, Sibert L, Roberts TM (1992) Polyomavirus middle T-antigen NPTY mutants. *J Virol* 66:5770–5776.

65. Campbell KS, Ogris E, Burke B, Su W, Auger KR, Druker BJ, Schaffhausen BS, Roberts TM, Pallas DC (1994) Polyoma middle tumor antigen interacts with SHC protein via the NPTY (Ans-Pro-Thr-Tyr) motif in middle tumor antigen. *Proc Natl Acad Sci USA* 91:6344–6348.

66. Dilworth SM, Brewster CEP, Jones MD, Lanfrancone L, Pelicci G, Pelicci PG (1994)

Transformation by polyoma middle T-antigen involves the binding and tyrosine phosphorylation of Shc. *Nature* 367:87–90.

67. Markland W, Smith AE (1987) Mutants of polyomavirus middle-T antigen. *Biochim Biophys Acta* 907:299–321.

68. Guy CT, Cardiff RA, Muller WJ (1992) Induction of mammary tumors by expression of polyomavirus middle T oncogene: A transgenic mouse model for metastatic disease. *Mol Cell Biol* 12:954–961.

69. Folkman J (1992) The role of angiogenesis in tumor growth. *Semin Cancer Biol* 3:65–71.

70. Srivastava A, Laidler P, Davies RP, Horgan K, Hughes LE (1988) The prognostic significance of tumor vascularity in intermediate-thickness (0.76–4.0 mm thick) skin melanoma. *Am J Pathol* 133:419–423.

71. Weidner N, Semple JP, Welch WR, Folkman J (1991) Tumor angiogenesis and metastasis — correlation in invasive breast carcinoma. *N Engl J Med* 324:1–8.

72. Folkman J, Watson K, Ingber D, Hanahan D (1989) Induction of angiogenesis during the transition from hyperplasia to neoplasia. *Nature* 339:58–61.

73. Folkman J, Klagsbrun M (1987) Angiogenic factors. *Science* 235:442–447.

74. Aznavoorian S, Murphy AN, Stetler-Stevenson WG, Liotta LA (1993) Molecular aspects of tumor cell invasion and metastasis. *Cancer* 71:1368–1382.

75. Williams RL, Courtneidge SA, Wagner EF (1988) Embryonic lethalities and endothelial tumors in chimeric mice expressing the polyoma virus middle T oncogene. *Cell* 52:121–131.

76. Williams RL, Risau W, Zerwes H-G, Drexler H, Aguzzi A, Wagner EF (1989) Endothelioma cells expressing the polyoma middle T oncogene induce hemangiomas by host cell recruitment. *Cell* 57:1053–1063.

77. Montesano R, Pepper MS, Mohle-Steinlein U, Risau W, Wagner EF, Orci L (1990) Increased proteolytic activity is responsible for abberant behaviour of endothelial cells expressing the middle T oncogene. *Cell* 62:436–445.

78. Courtneidge SA, Smith AE (1983) Polyoma transforming protein associates with the product of the c-src cellular gene. *Nature* 303:435–439.

79. Muthuswamy SK, Siegel PS, Dankort DL, Webster MA, Muller WJ (1994) Mammary tumors expressing the neu proto-oncogene possess elevated c-Src tyrosine kinase activity. *Mol Cell Biol* 14:735–743.

80. Lutrell DK, Lee A, Lansing TJ, Crosby RM, Jung KD, Willard D, Luther M, Rodriguez M, Berman J, Gilmer TM (1994) Involvement of pp60c-src with two major signaling pathways in human breast cancer. *Proc Natl Acad Sci USA* 91:83–97.

81. Soriano P, Montgomery C, Geske R, Bradley A (1991) Targeted disruption of the c-src proto-oncogene leads to osteopetrosis in mice. *Cell* 64:693–702.

82. Stein PL, Vogel H, Soriano P (1994) Combined deficiences of Src, Fyn and Yes tyrosine kinases in mutant mice. *Genes Dev* 8:1999–2007.

83. Guy CT, Muthuswamy SK, Cardiff RA, Sariano P, Muller WJ (1994) Activation of the c-Src tyrosine kinase is required for the induction of mammary tumors in transgenic mice. *Genes Dev* 8:23–32.

84. Thomas JE, A. A, Soriano P, Wagner EF, Brugge J (1993) Induction of tumor formation and cell transformation by polyoma middle T antigen in the absence of src. *Oncogene* 8:2521–2526.

85. Kiefer F, Anhauser I, Soriano P, Aguzzi A, Courtneidge, Wagner EF (1994) Endothelial cell transformation by polyomavirus middle T antigen in mice lacking Src-related kinases. *Curr Biol* 4:100–109.

86. Xin JH, Cowie A, Lachance P, Hassell JA (1992) Molecular cloning and characterization of PEA3, a new member of the Ets oncogene family that is differentially expressed in mouse embryonic cells. *Genes Dev* 6:481–496.

87. Trimble MS, Xin J-H, Guy CT, Muller WJ, Hassell JA (1993) PEA3 is overexpressed in mouse metastatic mammary adenocarcinomas. *Oncogene* 8:3037–3042.

88. Wasylyk C, Flores P, Gutman A, Wasylyk B (1989) PEA3 is a nuclear target for transcription activation by non-nuclear oncogenes. *EMBO J* 8:3371–3378.

89. Wasylyk C, Gutman A, Nicholson R, Wasylyk B (1991) The c-Ets oncoprotein activates the stromelysin promoter through the same elements as several non-nuclear oncoproteins. *EMBO J* 10:1127–1134.
90. McDonnell SE, Kerr LD, Matrisian LM (1990) Epidermal growth factor stimulation of stromelysin mRNA in rat fibroblasts requires induction of proto-oncogene c-fos and c-jun and activation of protein kinase C. *Mol Cell Biol* 10:4284–4293.
91. Edwards DR, Rocheleau H, Sharma RR, Wills AJ, Cowie A, Hassell JA, Heath JK (1992) Involvement of AP1 and PEA3 binding sites in the regulation of murine tissue inhibitor of metalloproteinases-1 (TIMP-1) transcription. *Biochim Biophys Acta* 1171:41–55.
92. Nielsen LL, Discafani CM, Gurnani M, Tyler RD (1991) Histopathology of salivary and mammary gland tumors in transgenic mice expressing a human Ha-ras oncogene. *Cancer Res* 51:3762–3767.
93. Stein D, Wu J, Fuqua SA, Roonprapunt C, Yajnik V, D'Eustachio P, Moskow JJ, Buchberg AM, Osborne CK, Margolis B (1994) The SH2 domain protein GRB7 is co-amplified, overexpressed and in a tight complex with HER2 in breast cancer. *EMBO J* 13:1331–1340.
94. Peles E, Ben Levy R, Or E, Ullrich A, Yarden Y (1991) Oncogenic forms of the neu/HER2 tyrosine kinase are permanently coupled to phospholipase Cg. *EMBO J* 10:2077–2086.
95. Segatto O, Pelicci G, Giuli S, Digeiesi G, Di Fiore PP, McGlade J, Pawson T, Pelicci PG (1993) Shc products are substrates of erbB-2 kinase. *Oncogene* 8:2105–2112.
96. Scott GK, Dodson JM, Montgomery PA, Johnson RM, Sarup JC, Wong WL, Ullrich A, Shepard HM, Benz CC (1991) p185HER2 signal transduction in breast cancer cells. *J Biol Chem* 266:14300–14305.
97. Peles E, Lamprecht R, Ben-Levy R, Tzahar E, Yarden Y (1992) Regulated coupling or the Neu receptor to phosphoinositol 3'-kinase and its release by oncogenic activation. *J Biol Chem* 267:12266–12274.
98. Ojan X, Dougall WC, Fei Z, Greene MI (1995) Intermolecular association and transphosphorylation of different neu-kinase forms permit SH2-dependent signaling and oncogenic transformation. *Oncogene* 10:211–219.
99. Vogel W, Lammers R, Huang J, Ullrich A (1993) Activation of a phosphotyrosine phosphatase by tyrosine phosphorylation. *Science* 259:1611–1614.
100. Li N, Batzer A, Daly R, Yajnik V, Skolnik E, Chardin P, Bar-Sagi D, Margolis B, Schlessinger J (1993) Guanine-nucleotide-releasing factor hSOS1 binds to GRB2 and links receptor tyrosine kinases to ras signalling. *Nature* 363:85–88.
101. Rozakis-Adcock M, Fernley R, Wade J, Pawson T, Bowtell D (1993) The SH2 and SH3 domains of mammalian GRB2 couple the EGF receptor to the ras activator mSOS1. *Nature* 363:83–85.
102. Egan SE, Giddings BW, Brooks MW, Buday L, Sizeland AM, Weinberg RA (1993) Association of SOS ras exchange protein with GRB2 is implicated in tyrosine kinase signal transduction and transformation. *Nature* 360:45–51.
103. Buday L, Downward J (1993) Epidermal growth factor regulates p21ras through the formation of a complex of receptor, Grb2 adapter protein, and SOS nucleotide exchange factor. *Cell* 73:611–620.
104. Courtneidge SA, Hebner A (1987) An 81 kDa protein complexed with middle T antigen and pp60c-src: A possible phosphatidylinositol kinase. *Cell* 50:1031–1037.
105. Whitman M, Kaplan DR, Schaffhausen B, Cantley LT, Roberts TM (1985) Association of phosphatidylinositol kinase activity with polyoma middle T competent for transformation. *Nature* 315:239–242.
106. Bolen JB, Theile CJ, Israel MA, Yonemoto W, Lipsich LA, Brugge JS (1988) Enhancement of cellular src gene product-associated tyrosine kinase activity following polyomavirus infection and transformation. *Cell* 38:767–777.
107. Kornbluth S, Sueul M, Hanafusa H (1986) Association of the polyomavirus middle T antigen with the c-yes protein. *Nature* 325:171–173.
108. Kypta RM, Hemming A, Courtneidge SA (1988) Identification and characterization of p59

fyn (a Src like protein kinase) in normal and polyomavirus transformed cells. *EMBO J* 7:3837–3844.

109. Cheng SH, Harvey R, Espino PC, Semba K, Yamanota T, Toyoshima K, Smith AE (1988) Peptide antibodies to the human pp59 c-fyn are capable of complex formation with the middle-T antigen of polyomavirus. *EMBO J* 7:3845–3855.

110. Pallas DC, Shahtik LK, Martin BL, Jasper S, Miller TB, Brautigan DL, Roberts TM (1990) Polyoma small and middle T antigens and SV40 small t antigen form stable complexes with protein phosphatase 2A. *Cell* 60:167–176.

111. Walter GRR, Slaughter C, Mumby M (1990) Association of protein phosphatase 2A with polyoma virus medium tumor antigen. *Proc Natl Acad Sci USA* 87:2521–2521.

112. Moodie SA, Wolfman A (1994) The 3Rs of life: ras, raf, and growth regulation. *Trends Biol Sci* 10:44–48.

113. Marshall CJ (1994) MAP kinase kinase kinase, MAP kinase kinase, and MAP kinase. *Curr Opin Gen Dev* 4:82–89.

114. Daum G, Eisenmann-Tappe I, Fries H-W, Troppmair J, Rapp UR (1994) The ins and outs of raf kinases. *Trends Biol Sci* 19:474–480.

115. Karin M (1994) Signal transduction from the cell surface to the nucleus through the phosphorylation of transcription factors. *Curr Opin Cell Biol* 6:415–424.

116. Hill CS, Treisman R (1995) Transcriptional regulation by extracellular signals: Mechanisms and specificity. *Cell* 80:199–211.

B

Human breast cancer: Receptors, signaling, and the cell cycle

5. Protein kinase C and breast cancer

Nancy E. Davidson and M. John Kennedy

Introduction

Protein kinase C (PKC) was first described by Nishizuka's laboratory in 1977 as a proteolytically activated kinase [1–3]. Subsequent work has established the importance of PKC activity in a multitude of cell functions that regulate growth and differentiation in a variety of cell types [4,5]. More recently, molecular cloning approaches have established that PKC is actually a family of closely related isoenzymes [6,7]. These include the calcium-dependent isoenzymes α, β_I, β_{II}, and γ; the calcium-independent isoenzymes δ, ϵ, η, θ, and μ; and the atypical isoenzymes, ζ and i(λ) (Table 1). These enzymes are the products of distinct genes, with the exception of PKC β_I and β_{II}, which are derived from alternative splicing of a single gene. The PKC enzymes are structurally quite similar. They are composed of a single polypeptide chain with a regulatory domain at the amino terminus and a catalytic domain at the carboxyl terminus. The isoenzymes can be divided into four regions that are conserved across isoenzymes (C1–C4) and five regions that vary between isoenzymes but are conserved within the isoenzyme across species (V1–V5) [9,10].

Many excellent reviews of the general properties and regulation of PKC have been published [4–8], as has a summary of the role of PKC in cancer biology [11]. This chapter focuses specifically on the role of PKC family members in the growth and behavior of breast cancer.

PKC activity in human breast tumors

The potential importance of PKC activity in mammary carcinogenesis is supported by the finding that PKC activity is elevated in primary breast cancers compared with adjacent normal breast tissue. O'Brian et al. [12] showed that PKC activity was higher in 8 of 9 breast tumors (8 invasive cancers and 1 cystosarcoma phylloides) than in normal breast tissue from the same individual. The mean PKC specific activity was 166 ± 63 pmol ^{32}P/min/mg in the histologically normal breast tissue and 460 ± 182 pmol ^{32}P/min/mg in the breast neoplasms. A single specimen of atypical ductal and lobular hyperplasia from

R. Dickson and M. Lippman (eds.) MAMMARY TUMOR CELL CYCLE, DIFFERENTIATION AND METASTASIS. 1996. Kluwer Academic Publishers. ISBN 0-7923-3905-3. All rights reserved.

Table 1. Some isoforms of protein kinase C

Calcium dependent	α
	β$_I$
	β$_{II}$
	γ
Calcium independent	δ
	ε
	η
	θ
	μ
Atypical	ζ
	i (λ)

a woman with a family history of breast cancer had a specific activity of 346 ± 63 pmol ^{32}P/min/mg. Thus, in this small study the net level of PKC activity was higher in breast tumor tissue than normal breast tissue, a finding that suggests a role for PKC in human breast carcinogenesis.

Further, Wyss et al. [13] have demonstrated a relationship between PKC activity and steroid hormone receptor status in primary tumors. In a study of 238 primary breast cancer specimens, total PKC, as determined by binding of [^{3}H] 4-β-phorbol-12,13-dibutyrate, was found to correlate inversely with progesterone receptor (PR) levels ($p < 0.005$) but not with estrogen receptor (ER) levels. However, if ER+/PR− tumors were excluded (i.e., those with a presumably nonfunctional ER), there was a significant inverse correlation between PKC and ER as well. No relationship between epidermal growth factor receptor (EGFR) and total PKC activity was observed, although the presence of EGFR was inversely correlated with ER or PR. Since increased EGFR and absence of ER expression in clinical breast cancer specimens is associated with loss of differentiation and poorer clinical outcome in many studies, these data suggest that increased PKC activity may be linked to a more aggressive tumor type.

Attempts to link a particular pattern of isozyme expression with malignant versus normal breast tissue or recognized clinical parameters for breast cancers have not been revealing thus far. Imber et al. [14] isolated primary cultures from 25 normal and malignant human mammary tissues. Cytosol and membrane fractions of each individual culture were prepared before and after the addition of the protein kinase C activator, 12-0-tetradecanoylphorbol-13-acetate (TPA), and Western blot analysis for PKC isoforms α, β, γ, δ, ε, and ζ was performed. No PKC-β nor PKC-γ was detected in any of the cultures. The level of ζ PKC was similar across cultures and did not translocate or downregulate upon the addition of TPA in any culture. Up to fivefold differences in the expression of PKC-α, -δ, and -ε were found, but levels of these isoforms were not correlated within individual cultures. TPA caused efficient translocation and downregulation of PKC-α, but PKC-ε was only partially translocated to membrane and was slowly downregulated. High levels of expression of α, δ, and ε isoforms occurred equally frequently in both normal and malignant epithelial cultures. No relationship between PKC isoform expression and age, tumor size, nodal status, or steroid receptor status was noted, although the sample size is extremely small. It is possible that the establishment of primary cell lines masked any differences in PKC isoform expression that may exist in vivo, and studies of PKC isoform expression in situ would be required to address this possibility. In addition, a larger sample size would be critical to draw definitive conclusions about the relationship between PKC isoform expression and clinical parameters in a disease as heterogeneous as breast cancer.

PKC activity in human breast cancer cell lines

Because of the difficulty of performing mechanistic studies in vivo, most studies of PKC function in breast cancer have used established human breast cancer cell lines as model systems. Early studies documented that ER-negative human breast cancer cell lines have significantly higher cytosolic PKC activity [15] and immunoreactive protein [16] than ER-positive human breast cancer cell lines. In contrast, there is a positive correlation between the number of EGFR and the level of PKC activity within the same cell lines. Thus, the findings in cell lines generally parallel those in primary cancer specimens, validating the use of cell lines as a model system for the study of PKC action in breast cancer cells.

Effects of phorbol esters on human breast cancer cell lines

The tumor-promoting phorbol esters have been useful tools to dissect the effects of PKC activity on human breast cancer cells in vitro (Table 2). PKC is

Table 2. Phorbol ester effects on MCF-7 cells

Inhibition of cell number and thymidine incorporation
Block in G_1 phase of cell cycle
Characteristic morphological changes
Decreased estrogen receptor mRNA half-life
Decreased EGF binding
Increased EGFR gene transcription
Decreased prolactin receptor gene transcription
Increased TFG-β activity and TFG-$β_1$ mRNA
Increased cell invasiveness and motility
Increased adherence to fibronectin, laminin, and Matrigel

---

the major intracellular receptor for phorbol esters [9,17]. Under physiological conditions, diacylglycerol (DAG), a product of the phosphatidylinositol cycle, transiently activates PKC. Phorbol esters can substitute for DAG as PKC activators but act in a more prolonged fashion than DAG because of their metabolic stability [18]. Thus, treatment with phorbol esters results in activation and translocation of PKC from cytosol to membrane with subsequent downregulation. Therefore, effects of phorbol esters may be related to either prolonged activation of PKC or subsequent downregulation of PKC or both.

Growth effects of TPA

The growth modulatory effects of phorbol esters in human breast cancer cell lines have been well documented [19–26]. Treatment with 10 ng/ml TPA for 6 days inhibited MCF-7 cell proliferation and DNA content by more than 50% [19]. Subsequent studies showed a correlation between the relative potency of various phorbol esters as inhibitors of binding of phorbol 12,13-dibutyrate and cell proliferation, suggesting that phorbol esters induced growth arrest of MCF-7 cells through a PKC-mediated pathway [21].

In MCF-7 cells, a TPA-dependent translocation of cytosolic PKC activity to membranes was observed within 30 minutes of TPA exposure. Removal of TPA at that time resulted in a slow increase in cytosolic PKC activity and a slow decrease in membrane-associated PKC activity, with full recovery only after many hours. Prolonged TPA exposure resulted in loss of PKC activity after 12 hours, and PKC activity increased and regained its usual pattern of subcellular localization after several days of incubation in TPA-free medium. This corresponded with a return to normal growth rates [26]. Darbon et al. demonstrated through direct studies that TPA induces subcellular translocation and subsequent downregulation of both phorbol binding and protein kinase C activity in MCF-7 cells, thus linking phorbol ester binding and PKC activity [27].

Although MCF-7 cells are the best studied of the human breast cancer cell lines, TPA also brought about similar growth responses in a variety of other human breast cancer cell lines. Treatment of MDA-MB-468, Hs578t, and MDA-MB-231 cells with TPA for 5 days led to a dose-dependent inhibition of growth by >50% at concentrations of >10 nM [24]. TPA had little effect on the growth of T47D or ZR-75 cells, perhaps because of variable effect on PKC activity, as discussed later [20,24,25].

Flow cytometry studies in MCF-7 cells showed that TPA treatment disrupts the cell cycle, resulting in a G1 block and delayed passage through G2 [22]. These effects were seen within 6–12 hours after TPA addition and were maximal by 24 hours. They are reversible in that removal of TPA from the medium resulted in restoration of MCF-7 cell proliferation within 3–4 days. In most studies this coincided with a gradual upregulation of PKC.

Morphological changes

TPA treatment also elicited very characteristic morphological changes in MCF-7 cells [19,22,24]. After 24–28 hours, cells became markedly enlarged and flattened, and striking vacuolization was seen by light microscopy. Electron microscopy showed extensive granular endoplasmic reticulum and an appearance of secretory granules and microvilli suggestive of a more differentiated state. These changes were reversible over time with removal of TPA from the medium.

Effects on expression of steroid, epidermal growth factor, and prolactin receptors, and transforming growth factor β_1

As noted earlier, PKC activity in human breast cancer cells is inversely related to ER expression. Thus, the effects of phorbol esters on ER regulation have been examined [28–30]. Treatment of MCF-7 cells with 100 nM TPA resulted in an 80% decrease in the level of ER mRNA within 6 hours. Nuclear run-on assays showed that this did not result from a change in ER gene transcription. Rather mRNA half-life studies showed that the decrease was a consequence of post-transcriptional effects of TPA on the stability of the ER mRNA as TPA decreased ER mRNA half-life from 4 hours to 40 minutes. That this effect was related to PKC is supported by the finding that the inactive phorbol, 4α-phorbol, had no effect. Also the PKC inhibitor, H7, blocked TPA modulation of ER mRNA. Interestingly, TPA effects were biphasic in that low concentrations of TPA (10^{-11} to 10^{-10} M) actually increased ER mRNA by about twofold.

Similar results were obtained for ER protein as determined by enzyme immunoassay or ligand binding assay. Maximum loss was observed after 24 hours of TPA treatment. Measurement of PKC activity in parallel flasks suggests that activation of PKC by TPA, rather than its subsequent loss, was responsible for the decrease in ER [29].

Washout experiments showed that these effects were reversible after 48 hours in the study of Saceda et al. [29]. However, Ree et al. [28] noted continuing depression of ER mRNA and protein despite similar washout procedures. Finally, TPA did not universally lead to a decrease in ER protein in ER-positive breast cancer cell lines. TPA at the same concentration of 100 nM had no effect on ER expression in T47D or ZR-75 cells [29], two cell lines that manifest little change in growth upon TPA exposure [24]. It is of note that T47D cells particularly have relatively low endogenous PKC activity and TPA elicited little evidence of PKC translocation in these cells [24,26].

The effects of TPA on EGFR mRNA have also been examined [29,30]. Treatment of MCF-7 cells with 100 nM TPA led to a 14-fold increase in EGFR mRNA within 24 hours. Nuclear run-on studies showed that this was associated with a fourfold increase in EGFR gene transcription by 6 hours. Again, the inactive 4-α-phorbol had no demonstrable effect, attesting to the involvement of PKC. These mRNA changes occur in parallel with an acute decrease in EGF binding affinity, which is felt to result from phosphorylation of the EGFR as a consequence of TPA activation of PKC [19,20,30]. Together, these studies are notable in that the pattern of ER and EGFR mRNA expression after PKC activation by TPA mirrored the relationship between PKC activity and ER and EGFR in primary tumors — high PKC activity in conjunction with high EGFR and low ER. They also provided evidence for involvement of PKC in the regulation of expression of two critical receptors in breast cancer cells.

TPA treatment was also associated with decreased expression of prolactin receptor in all five breast cancer cell lines examined [31]. In MCF-7 cells, 10 nM TPA caused a 70% loss of prolactin receptor mRNA within 12 hours, with a subsequent decrease in prolactin receptor at the cell surface. Molecular studies showed that this was due to a reduction in prolactin receptor gene transcription without any effect on mRNA stability. Thus TPA has pleiotropic effects on receptor expression, leading to diminished expression of ER and prolactin receptor but increased expression of EGFR, suggesting variable effects of PKC on the regulation of these receptor types.

Multiple studies suggest that transforming growth factor β (TGF-β) inhibits growth of MCF-7 cells. Increased TGF-β activity in conditioned medium as well as increased TGF-β_1 mRNA levels are also a consequence of TPA treatment of MCF-7 cells [25,32]. Treatment with TPA resulted in rapid induction of TGF-β_1 mRNA between 6 and 12 hours. This effect was dose dependent, first seen at 0.8 nM and maximal at concentrations $\geq$10 nM. This is no doubt in part a consequence of the interaction of TPA with a phorbol ester–responsive element in the promoter region of the TGF-β_1 gene. The potential importance of this finding is that increased TGF-β activity could contribute to the growth inhibitory effects of TPA on MCF-7 cells via an autocrine loop.

Metastasis formation and PKC in breast cancer

The ability to metastasize is a key property of the cancer cell. Formation of metastasis depends on a series of discrete steps, including attachment of tumor cells to the basement membrane, proteolysis of the basement membrane, and migration of tumor cells through the membrane. A relationship between PKC activity, cell motility, and metastatic capacity has been previously reported in a variety of model systems. Several lines of experimental evidence in those systems suggest that downregulation of PKC activity abrogates the invasive and metastatic phenotype [33,34].

The role of PKC in breast cancer metastasis has been studied using TPA-treated MCF-7 cells [35]. MCF-7 cells are poorly metastatic in nude mouse models. In a Boyden chamber assay, TPA effected an 18-fold increase in invasiveness of MCF-7 cells. This was associated with a 14-fold increase in cell motility. TPA also increased the ability of MCF-7 cells to adhere to fibronectin, laminin, and Matrigel, an important observation in that the metastatic process is also dependent on the ability of the cell to bind to substratum such as basement membrane. Finally, TPA increased the expression of certain matrix metalloproteinases (MMP-1 and MMP-9) by up to 100-fold, suggesting that TPA treatment could enhance the ability of MCF-7 cells to degrade extracellular matrix. Together these findings highlight the possibility that PKC might act as a critical mediator in the regulation of invasion and metastasis of human breast cancer cells.

Multidrug resistance and PKC in breast cancer cells

Cancer cells frequently manifest de novo or acquired resistance to antineoplastic drugs. One phenotype of resistance, multidrug resistance (*mdr*), is associated with the presence of a membrance glycoprotein, the p170 glycoprotein, which functions as an efflux pump for a variety of chemotherapeutic agents derived from natural products. A number of features of the *mdr* phenotype suggested a role for calcium-dependent processes, but a role for PKC specifically was first suggested by the work of Fine et al. [36]. In these studies, PKC activity was sevenfold higher in a multidrug-resistant cancer cell line, MCF-7/ADR, than in the sensitive parental MCF-7 line. Exposure of the sensitive parent line to phorbol-12,13-dibutyrate increased PKC activity and induced resistance to doxorubicin and vincristine (agents included in the *mdr* phenotype) but not melphalan (an alkylating agent). This increased resistance was at least partially reversed by a calcium channel blocker, verapamil.

Imunohistochemical and subcellular fractionation studies of MCF-7/ADR cells suggested that these cells had four- to eightfold higher nuclear PKC activity, a three- to fivefold higher cytosolic activity, and a less than twofold higher membrane activity than parental MCF-7 cells [37]. Studies with isotype-specific antisera showed that nuclei from MCF-7/ADR cells contained high levels of an altered form of PKC-α. These results have been confirmed by Blobe et al. [38], who found that MCF-7/ADR cells have a 10-fold increase in calcium-dependent PKC activity and a 10-fold decrease in calcium-independent PKC activity. These changes are associated with increased PKC-α expression and decreased expression of PKC-δ and PKC-ϵ. Finally, MCF-7 cells transfected with the human *mdr1* gene (BC-19 cells) exhibited greater multidrug resistance when stably transfected with PKC-α as well [39]. However, BC-19 cells transfected with PKC-γ show no demonstrable change in their drug resistance phenotype, although they had increased PKC activity (all accounted for by PKC-γ) [40]. Taken together, these findings underscore the possibility that PKC-α may play a role in the *mdr* phenotype in breast cancer cells.

Overexpression of PKC-α in MCF-7 cells

The isolation and cloning of specific PKC isoforms have made it possible to examine the effects of sustained overexpression of a single PKC isoform. Ways et al. [41] studied the effects of stable overexpression of PKC-α in MCF-7 cells using standard transfection and selection techniques (Table 3). A pool of MCF-7–PKC-α clones was derived, as was a pool of vector clones; MCF-7–PKC-α cells demonstrated 5- to 16-fold greater PKC activity using a variety of substrates than MCF-7–vector cells. This was associated with a three- to fivefold increase in PKC-α expression. Western blot analysis of endogenous expression of other PKC isoforms showed that MCF-7–PKC-α cells expressed higher levels of PKC-α and -β isoforms, and decreased levels of γ and η compared with MCF-7-vector or parental MCF-7 cells, while levels of PKC-ε and -ζ were unchanged. The mRNA transcripts for PKC-α, -β, -γ, and -η paralleled protein expression.

MCF-7–PKC-α cells proliferated more rapidly and had a higher S-phase fraction than parental cells (MCF-7 23%, MCF-7–PKC-α 39%). Soft agar cloning showed that MCF-7–PKC-α cells grew readily in anchorage-independent conditions, while parental cells grew poorly. MCF-7–PKC-α cells also demonstrated marked alterations in morphology. Whereas parental and MCF-7–vector cells displayed an epithelial appearance and grew attached to the plastic substratum, MCF-7–PKC-α cells were more spherical, formed giant cells, and detached from the plastic surface to grow in suspension. Electron microscopy showed increased expression of secondary lysosomal granules and intermediate filaments. Northern analysis showed an increase in mRNA transcripts for vimentin, an intermediate filament not normally expressed in MCF-7 cells.

Given the inverse relationship between ER and PKC activity and the observation that TPA downregulates ER mRNA transcripts, the ER status of the MCF-7–PKC-α cells was examined. In contrast to parental MCF-7 or MCF-7-vector cells, MCF-7–PKC-α cells lacked ER mRNA; had decreased mRNA

Table 3. Characteristics of MCF-7 cells overexpressing PKC-α

Increased proliferation and S-phase fraction
Anchorage-independent growth
Morphological changes
Increased vimentin mRNA
Loss of ER and estrogen-mediated responses
Tumorigenic and metastatic in nude mice
Increased PKC-α and -β protein, and mRNA
Decreased PKC-γ and -η protein, and mRNA
Stable PKC-ε and -ζ protein

Adapted from Ways et al. [41], with permission.

expression of two estrogen-responsive genes, pS2 and cathepsin D; and activated an estrogen-responsive vit-tk-CAT reporter construct only minimally. Finally, MCF-7–PKC-α cells were uniformly tumorigenic in female nude mice, and microscopic metastases to lung, perinephric fat, and lymph nodes was documented in about one third of the animals. Parental MCF-7 cells formed microscopic tumors at the inoculation site in 2 of 10 animals without evidence of metastases. Thus, these studies suggest that MCF-7–PKC-α cells display a more undifferentiated phenotype, characterized by increased proliferation, anchorage-independent growth, loss of ER expression, and increased tumorigenicity and metastatic potential in nude mice. Whether these changes were a direct consequence of PKC-α overexpression or an indirect result of modulation of the activity of other PKC isoforms such as PKC-β remains to be determined.

PKC as a therapeutic target in breast cancer

Given the role of PKC in a number of fundamental cellular mechanisms in breast cancer cells, the possibility that PKC might be a therapeutic target in breast cancer is worthy of exploration. Several agents that might act via PKC pathways are at various stages of clinical development. These include tamoxifen, UCN-01, and bryostatin 1.

Tamoxifen

Tamoxifen, a synthetic, nonsteroidal antiestrogen, is a mainstay of hormonal therapy for breast cancer. Its primary mechanism of action is via competition with estrogen for binding to the ER. However, nonreceptor activities have also been proposed. One possible target is PKC. O'Brian et al. [42] showed that tamoxifen inhibited rat brain PKC in vitro with an IC_{50} of about $100\,\mu M$. It also inhibited binding of [^{3}H] phorbol dibutyrate to high-affinity membrane receptors or C3H10T½ cells with an IC_{50} of $5\,\mu M$. Related triphenethylene compounds, including clomiphene, 4-hydroxytamoxifen, and N-desmethyltamoxifen, were also PKC inhibitors, with IC_{50}s in the micromolar range [43]. The inhibitory potencies of these drugs against PKC were correlated with their estrogen-irreversible cytotoxic effects against MCF-7 cells.

In vitro studies further showed that the triphenylethylenes do not interact with the active site of PKC. Rather, there is evidence that these agents may inhibit PKC via specific interactions with other undefined domain(s) of the PKC enzyme as well as nonspecific interaction between antiestrogen and lipid cofactors [44]. Bignon et al. [45] extended these studies to show that two triphenylethylene derivatives inhibited PKC activity in ER-negative BT-20 cells in a concentration-dependent manner with an IC_{50} of 3–$7\,\mu M$. Fractionation studies showed that PKC isoforms α and β were both reduced. These findings raise the possibility that specific PKC antagonists could be developed from this class of agents and suggest that PKC may be an alternate target through which tamoxifen exerts its effects. Also, given tamoxifen's ability to inhibit PKC, especially PKC-α, the possibility that it might reverse the *mdr* phenotype is under investigation [46].

UCN-01

UCN-01 or 7-hydroxystaurosporine was isolated from the culture broth of *Streptomyces* species. Although developed as a potentially selective inhibitor of PKC, it can inhibit a number of tyrosine and serine-threonine kinases. In vitro studies showed that UCN-01 inhibited the growth of MCF-7, MDA–MB-453, SK–BR-3, MDA–MB-468, and Hs578t cells with a 50% inhibitory concentration range of 30–100 nM after 6 days of exposure. Washout studies suggested that a 24 hour exposure to UCN-01 irreversibly inhibited cell growth in MCF-7 and MDA–MB-453 cells but that continuous treatment was necessary for maximal growth-inhibitory effects in other cell lines. Detailed studies in MDA-MB-468 cells showed that UCN-01 inhibited the progression from G1 to S phase at low concentrations and progression within S phase at higher concentrations [47]. Clinical trials with this agent are slated to begin shortly.

Bryostatin 1

Bryostatin 1, a macrocyclic lactone isolated from the marine bryozoan, *Bugula neritina*, is a potent modulator of PKC in many systems [48]. It has been found to have effects both agonistic and antagonistic to those of TPA [49]. Like TPA, it can substitute for DAG through its ability to bind to PKC and to elicit its subsequent subcellular translocational activation [50]. From a chemotherapeutic perspective, it is an attractive compound as it stimulates the proliferation of normal human hematopoietic progenitors [51], has significant antineoplastic activity against leukemias [52], and lacks the tumor-promoting activities of TPA [53]. A phase I trial has been completed in the United Kingdom and other trials are in progress in the United States [54,55].

Initial studies of bryostatin 1 showed that it inhibited growth of human breast cancer cells relatively poorly when compared with TPA [24,25,56]. However, it completely antagonized the growth inhibition and morphological changes induced by TPA in MCF-7 cells [24]. It was therefore postulated that the differences between TPA and bryostatin in their effects on cell growth may be associated with differential effects on PKC isoform activity. Kennedy et al. [24] reported that 100 nM TPA induced rapid translocation of the PKC-α isoform and PKC activity from the cytosolic to membrane fraction in MCF-7 cells. In contrast, 100 nM bryostatin 1 treatment resulted in loss of PKC activity and PKC-α isozyme from both cytosol and membrane compartments within minutes.

In combination assays, the bryostatin 1 effect was dominant over the TPA effect. These disparate effects of TPA and bryostatin 1 were seen in MCF-7 and MDA–MB-468 cells, both cell lines whose growth was inhibited by TPA but only minimally affected by bryostatin 1. Interestingly, T47D cells, whose growth is only slightly affected by TPA or bryostatin 1, showed no transloca-tion of PKC-α isozyme or PKC activity in response to TPA. But bryostatin 1 still caused rapid loss of PKC activity and PKC-α isozyme from both cytosolic and membrane-associated fractions in T47D cells. These results are compat-ible with the hypothesis that distinct effects of bryostatin 1 and TPA in human breast cancer cells may be explained by their different effects on the expres-sion and activity of the PKC-α isoform, although involvement of other targets certainly cannot be excluded.

Stanwell et al. [56] also showed that TPA had similar effects on PKC-α in MCF-7 cells with redistribution of the α isoform to the membrane and nuclear fractions in a concentration-dependent manner. However, in this study bryostatin 1 had little effect except at a concentration of 1 μM, at which translocation of PKC-α isozyme to the membrane fraction was evident. Mod-est redistribution of PKC-ζ from the cytosol to membrane (bryostatin) or the membrane and nucleus (TPA) was seen and was also not concentration depen-dent. Finally, PKC-ε was also translocated to the membrane and nucleus by both drugs. Effects of TPA or bryostatin 1 on total PKC activity were not examined. Differences in cell culture conditions or use of variable MCF-7 sublines may account for some of these differences. In any case, these studies point out the complexities of studies designed to tease apart the effects of various PKC isoforms.

Although bryostatin 1 does not inhibit the growth of human breast cancer cell lines in vitro, its potential ability to induce the rapid loss of PKC activity from the cytosolic fraction of treated human breast cancer cells may have significant biological and clinical implications. As noted earlier, there is a large body of evidence that downregulation of PKC may reduce the metastatic capacity of tumor cells; thus, the ability of bryostatin 1 to act as an antimetastatic agent should be further explored. Indeed, Johnson et al. [35] have shown that bryostatin 1 blocked TPA-induced increases in MCF-7 cell invasiveness and motility. In addition, the fact that bryostatin 1 may be a potent downregulator of PKC-α raises the possibility that it may be useful in the management of malignancies with the *mdr* phenotype because overexpression of PKC-α particularly was observed in MCF-7/ADR cells.

Finally, multiple studies in a variety of experimental models support a role for PKC as a mediator of programmed cell death. In these systems, activation of PKC is associated with a block of programmed cell death, while PKC inhibition is associated with potentiation of programmed cell death. Thus, treatment of human breast cancer cells with bryostatin 1, which appears to downregulate PKC, could render cells more sensitive to the apoptotic effects of commonly used chemotherapeutic agents. Studies of Grant et al. [57] have confirmed the feasibility of this approach in other cell systems.

Conclusions

Systemic therapy for breast cancer has reached a plateau, suggesting that new approaches based on an improved understanding of basic breast cancer biology are necessary. Ample evidence from studies using both human tissues and established breast cancer cell lines suggests a pivotal role for PKC in breast cancer. Its involvement in cell growth and differentiation, metastatic capability, and drug resistance is only now beginning to be understood. It is hoped that enhanced knowledge about regulation of PKC and its isoforms will permit the development of new approaches to breast cancer treatment and prevention.

Acknowledgment

This work was supported by grant U01 CA66084 from the National Cancer Institute.

References

1. Takai Y, Kishimoto A, Inove M, Nishizuka Y (1977) Studies on a cyclic nucleotide-independent protein kinase and its proenzyme in mammalian tissues and purification and characterization of an active enzyme from bovine cerebellum. *J Biol Chem* 252:7603–7609.
2. Takai Y, Kishimoto A, Iwasa Y, et al. (1979) Calcium-dependent activation of a multifunctional protein kinase by membrane phospholipids. *J Biol Chem* 254:3692–3695.
3. Kishimoto A, Takai Y, Mori T, Kikkawa V, Nishizuka Y (1980) Activation of calcium and phospholipid-dependent protein kinase by diacylglycerol, its possible relation to phosphatidylinositol turnover. *J Biol Chem* 255:2273–2276.
4. Nishizuka Y (1986) Studies and perspectives of protein kinase C. *Science* 233:305–312.
5. Nishizuka Y (1989) Studies and perspectives of the protein kinase C family for cellular regulation. *Cancer* 63:1892–1903.
6. Nishizuka Y (1988) The molecular heterogeneity of protein kinase C and its implications for cellular regulation. *Nature* 334:661–665.
7. Hug H, Sarre TF (1993) Protein kinase C isoenzymes: Divergence in signal transduction? *Biochem J* 291:329–343.
8. Dekker K, Parker P (1994) Protein kinase C — a question of specificity. *Trends Biochem Sci* 19:73–77.
9. Parker PJ, Coussens L, Totty N, et al. (1986) The complete primary structure of protein kinase C — the major phorbol ester receptor. *Science* 233:853–859.
10. Coussens L, Parker PJ, Rhee L, et al. (1986) Multiple, distinct forms of bovine and human protein kinase C suggest diversity in cellular signaling pathways. *Science* 233:859–866.
11. Blobe GC, Obeid LM, Hannun YA (1994) Regulation of protein kinase C and role in cancer biology. *Cancer Metastasis Rev* 14:411–421.
12. O'Brian CA, Vogel VG, Singletary SE, Ward NE (1989) Elevated protein kinase C expression in human breast tumor biopsies relative to normal breast tissue. *Cancer Res* 49:3215–3217.
13. Wyss R, Fabbro D, Regazzi R, Borner C, et al. (1987) Phorbol ester and epidermal growth factor receptors in human breast cancer. *Anticancer Res* 7:721–728.
14. Imber R, Haberthür F, Meier F, Filipuzzi I, Almendral AC (1994) No tumor-specific expres-

sion levels of protein kinase C isoenzymes and of c-fos in human breast cancer cell cultures. *Carcinogenesis (Lond)* 15:359–363.

15. Fabbro D, Küng W, Roos W, Regazzi R, Eppenberger U (1986) Epidermal growth factor binding and protein kinase C activities in human breast cancer cell lines: Possible quantitative relationship. *Cancer Res* 46:2720–2725.

16. Borner C, Wyss R, Regazzi R, Eppenberger U, Fabbro D (1987) Immunological quantitation of phospholipid/Ca^{2+}-dependent protein kinase of human mammary carcinoma cells: Inverse relationship to estrogen receptors. *Int J Cancer* 40:344–348.

17. Neidel JE, Kohn LJ, Vandenbark GR (1983) Phorbol diester receptor copurifies with protein kinase C. *Proc Natl Acad Sci USA* 80:36–40.

18. Castagna M, Takai Y, Kaibuchi K, et al. (1982) Direct activation of calcium-activated, phospholipid-dependent protein kinase by tumor-promoting phorbol esters. *J Biol Chem* 257:7874–7851.

19. Osborne CK, Hamilton B, Nover M, Ziegler J (1981) Antagonism between epidermal growth factor and phorbol ester tumor promoters in human breast cancer cells. *J Clin Invest* 67:943–951.

20. Roos W, Fabbro D, Küng W, Costa SD, Eppenberger U (1986) Correlation between hormone dependency and the regulation of epidermal growth factor receptor by tumor promoters in human mammary carcinoma cells. *Proc Natl Acad Sci USA* 83:991–995.

21. Darbon J-M, Valette A, Bayard F (1986) Phorbol esters inhibit the proliferation of MCF-7 cells. *Biochem Pharmacol* 35:2683–2686.

22. Valette A, Gas N, Jozan S, et al. (1987) Influence of 12-0-tetradecanoylphorbol-13-acetate on proliferation and maturation of human breast carcinoma cells (MCF-7): Relationship to cell cycle events. *Cancer Res* 47:1615–1620.

23. Issandou M, Bayard F, Darbon J-M (1988) Inhibition of MCF-7 cell growth by 12-0-tetradecanoylphorbol-13-acetate and 1,2-dioctanoyl-sn-glycerol: Distinct effects on protein kinase C activity. *Cancer Res* 48:6943–6950.

24. Kennedy MJ, Prestigiacomo L, Tyler G, May WS, Davidson N (1992) Differential effects of bryostatin-1 and phorbol ester on human breast cancer cells. *Cancer Res* 52:1278–1283.

25. Nutt JE, Harris AL, Lunec J (1991) Phorbol ester and bryostatin effects on growth and the expression of oestrogen responsive and TGF-β1 genes in breast tumour cells. *Br J Cancer* 4:671–676.

26. Fabbro D, Regazzi R, Costa SD, Borner C, Eppenberger U (1986) Protein kinase C desensitization by phorbol esters and its impact on growth of human breast cancer cells. *Biochem Biophys Res Commun* 135:65–73.

27. Darbon J-M, Oury F, Clamens S, Bayard F (1987) TPA induces subcellular translocation and subsequent down-regulation of both phorbol ester binding and protein kinase C activities in MCF-7 cells. *Biochem Biophy Res Commun* 146:537–546.

28. Ree AH, Landmark BF, Walaas SI, et al. (1991) Down-regulation of messenger ribonucleic acid and protein levels for estrogen receptors by phorbol ester and calcium in MCF-7 cells. *Endocrinology* 129:339–344.

29. Saceda M, Knabbe C, Dickson RB, et al. (1991) Post-transcriptional destabilization of estrogen receptor mRNA in MCF-7 cells by 12-0-tetradecanoylphorbol-12-acetate. *J Biol Chem* 25:17809–17812.

30. Lee CSL, Koga M, Sutherland RL (1989) Modulation of estrogen receptor and epidermal growth factor receptor mRNAs by phorbol ester in MCF-7 breast cancer cells. *Biochem Biophys Res Commun* 162:415–421.

31. Ormandy CJ, Lee CSL, Kelly PA, Sutherland RL (1993) Regulation of prolactin receptor expression by the tumor promoting phorbol ester 12-0-tetradeccanoylphorbol-13-acetate in human breast cancer cells. *J Cell Biochem* 52:47–56.

32. Guerin M, Prats H, Mazars P, Valette A (1992) Antiproliferation effect of phorbol esters on MCF-7 human breast adenocarcinoma cells: Relationship with enhanced expression of transforming growth factor-β1. *Biochim Biophys Acta* 1137:116–120.

33. Schwartz GK, Redwood SM, Ohunma T, et al. (1990) Inhibition of invasion of invasive human

bladder carcinoma cells by protein kinase C inhibitor staurosporine. *J Natl Cancer Inst* 82:1753–1756.

34. Dumont JA, Jones WD, Bitonti AJ (1992) Inhibition of experimental metastasis and cell adhesion of B16F1 melanoma cells by inhibitors of protein kinase C. *Cancer Res* 52:1195–1200.

35. Johnson MD, Torri JT, Lippman ME, Dickson RB (1994) Regulation of the invasiveness of the human breast cancer cell line MCF-7 by agents that act through protein kinase C (abstr). *J Cell Biochem* 18D(Suppl):243.

36. Fine RL, Patel J, Chabner BA (1988) Phorbol esters induce multidrug resistance in human breast cancer cells. *Proc Natl Acad Sci USA* 85:582–586.

37. Lee SA, Karaszkiewicz JW, Anderson WB (1992). Elevated level of nuclear protein kinase C in multidrug-resistant MCF-7 human breast carcinoma cells. *Cancer Res* 52:3750–3759.

38. Blobe GC, Sachs CW, Khan WA, et al. (1993) Selective regulation of expression of protein kinase C (PKC) isoenzymes in multidrug-resistant MCF-7 cells. *J Biol Chem* 268:658–664.

39. Yu G, Ahmad A, Aquino C, et al. (1991) Transfection with protein kinase C α confers increased multidrug resistance to MCF-7 cells expressing P-glycoprotein. *Cancer Commun* 3:181–189.

40. Ahmad S, Trepel JB, Ohno S, et al. (1992) Role of protein kinase C in the modulation of multidrug resistance: Expression of the atypical γ isoform of protein kinase C does not confer increased resistance to doxorubicin. *Mol Pharmacol* 42:1004–1009.

41. Ways DK, Kukoly CA, deVente J, et al. (1995) MCF-7 breast cancer cells transfected with protein kinase C-α exhibit altered expression of other protein kinase C isoforms and display a more aggressive neoplastic phenotype. *J Clin Invest* 95:1–10.

42. O'Brian CA, Liskamp RM, Solomon DH, Weinstein IB (1985) Inhibition of protein kinase C by tamoxifen. *Cancer Res* 45:2462–2465.

43. O'Brian CA, Liskamp RM, Solomon DH, Weinstein IB (1986) Triphenylethylenes: A new class of protein kinase C inhibitors. *J Natl Cancer Inst* 76:1243–1247.

44. O'Brian CA, Housey GM, Weinstein IB (1988) Specific and direct binding of protein kinase C to an immobilized tamoxifen analogue. *Cancer Res* 48:3626–3629.

45. Bignon E, Ogita K, Kishimoto A, Nishizuka Y (1990) Protein kinase C subspecies in estrogen receptor-positive and -negative human breast cancer cell lines. *Biochem Biophys Res Commun* 171:1071–1078.

46. Trump DL, Smith DC, Ellis PG, et al. (1992) High-dose oral tamoxifen, a potential multidrug-resistance-reversal agent: Phase I trial in combination with vinblastine. *J Natl Cancer Inst* 84:1811–1816.

47. Seynaeve CM, Stetler-Stevenson M, Sebers S, et al. (1993) Cell cycle arrest and growth inhibition by the protein kinase antagonist UCN-01 in human breast carcinoma cells. *Cancer Res* 53:2081–2086.

48. Berkow RL, Kraft AS (1985) Bryostatin, a non-phorbol macrocyclic lactone, activates intact human polymorphonucler leukocytes and binds to the phorbol ester receptor. *Biochem Biophys Res Commun* 131:1109–1115.

49. Gschwendt M, Fürstenberger G, Rose-John S, et al. (1988) Bryostatin 1, an activator of protein kinase C, mimics as well as inhibits biological effects of the phorbol ester TPA in vivo and in vitro. *Carcinogenesis (Lond)* 9:555–562.

50. Kraft AS, Baker VV, May WS (1987) Bryostatin induces changes in protein kinase C location and activity without altering c-*myc* gene expression in human promyelocytic leukemia cells (HL-60). *Oncogene* 1:111–118.

51. May WS, Sharkis SJ, Esa A, et al. (1987) Antineoplastic bryostatins are multipotential stimulators of human hematopoietic progenitor cells. *Proc Natl Acad Sci USA* 84:8483–8487.

52. Pettit GR, Dey JF, Hartwell JL, Wood HB (1970) Antineoplastic components of marine animals. *Nature* 227:962–963.

53. Hennings H, Blumberg PM, Pettit GR, et al. (1987) Bryostatin 1, an activator of protein kinase C, inhibits tumor promotion by phorbol esters in SENCAR mouse skin. *Carcinogenesis (Lond)* 8:1343–1346.

54. Prendiville J, Crowther D, Thatcher N, et al. (1993) A phase I study of intravenous bryostatin 1 in patients with advanced cancer. *Br J Cancer* 68:418–425.
55. Philip PA, Rea D, Thavasu P, et al. (1993) Phase I study of bryostatin 1: Assessment of interleukin 6 and tumor necrosis factor α induction in vivo. *J Natl Cancer Inst* 85:1812–1818.
56. Stanwell C, Gescher A, Bradshaw TD, Pettit GR (1994) The role of protein kinase C isoenzymes in the growth inhibition caused by bryostatin 1 in human A549 lung and MCF-7 breast carcinoma cells. *Int J Cancer* 56:585–592.
57. Grant S, Jarvis WD, Swerdlow PS, et al. (1992) Potentiation of the activity of 1-β-D-arabinofuranosyl-cytosine by the protein kinase C activator bryostatin 1 in HL-60 cells: Association with enhanced fragmentation of mature DNA. *Cancer Res* 52:6270–6278.

6. Protein tyrosine phosphatases:
Cellular regulators of human breast cancer?

Yi-Fan Zhai, Julie J. Wirth, Clifford W. Welsch, and Walter J. Esselman

Introduction

Protein tyrosine phosphorylation and dephosphorylation are believed to be key regulatory mechanisms in the control of signal transduction, cell proliferation, differentiation, and neoplastic transformation [1–4]. The net cellular level of tyrosine phosphorylation is maintained dynamically by the opposing actions of protein tyrosine kinases (PTKs) and protein tyrosine phosphatases (PTPases). While the involvement of PTKs in these cellular processes has been examined extensively, an investigation of the concomitant role of PTPases has only just begun.

PTPases have been identified in many different eukaryotic cell types. The diverse family contains both transmembrane glycoproteins and cytosolic proteins [2,3]. The transmembrane receptor-type PTPases contain distinct extracellular domains, a single hydrophobic transmembrane region and two tandem repeated conserved cytoplasmic PTPase domains. The cytoplasmic PTPases generally contain one PTPase domain and regulatory segments containing diverse elements [3]. Examples of primary structures of the PTPases relevant to this communication are shown in Figure 1.

In the studies reported in this communication, we have examined the receptor-type PTPases, LAR-PTPase and CD45, and two cytoplasmic PTPases, PTP1B and TCPTP. PTP1B and TCPTP, although initially isolated from human placenta and a human T-cell library, respectively [5,6], are widely distributed in many tissue types. CD45 is expressed primarily in nucleated hematopoietic cells [7]. LAR-PTPase (leukocyte-common antigen related) is expressed on endothelial and epithelial cells of a broad range of tissue and cell types, including breast, kidney, thymus, brain, intestine, muscle, and different tumor cell lines [3,8,9]. The objective of our studies has been to define the role of PTPases in human breast carcinoma development and/or growth, in particular in those breast carcinomas that have a high expression of PTK activity. More specifically, our objectives in this communication are to examine the expression levels of specific PTPases in human breast carcinoma cells that have a high expression level of PTK and to assess the influence of increased PTPase expression, via transfection of PTPase cDNA, on in vitro growth of

R. Dickson and M. Lippman (eds.) MAMMARY TUMOR CELL CYCLE, DIFFERENTIATION AND METASTASIS. 1996. Kluwer Academic Publishers. ISBN 0-7923-3905-3. All rights reserved.

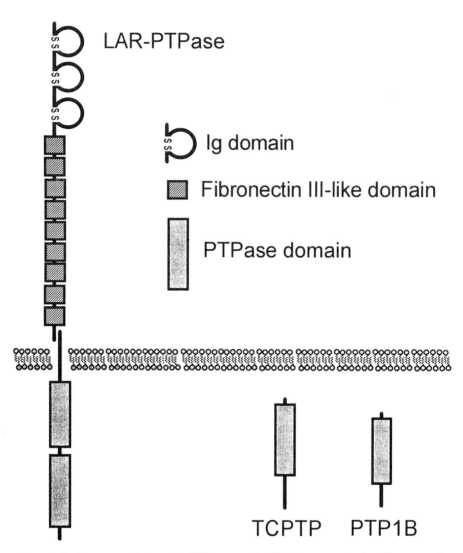

Figure 1. Basic structure of the major PTPases examined in this communication. Shown are the receptor-type PTPase, LAR-PTPase, and the cytoplasmic-type PTPases, PTP1B and TCPTP. The homologous PTPase domains are shown and, for LAR-PTPase, the domains homologous to Ig and fibronectin III are shown.

human breast carcinoma cells and in vivo tumorigenicity of these cells in athymic nude mice. We intend to test the hypothesis that the elevation in expression of certain PTPases, if expressed in sufficient quantities, would alter or suppress the neoplastic transforming and tumorigenic effects of aberrant hyperphosphorylation caused by PTK oncogenes.

Materials and methods

Cell lines

A benzopyrene-induced, immortalized, but nontumorigenic human breast epithelial cell line, 184B5, was obtained from Dr. M. Stampfer (Livermore Laboratory, Berkeley, CA). 18-Rn1, 18-Rn2, and 18-Hn1 cell lines and 184B5 cells were grown in MCDB170, prepared by mixing equal amounts of minimum essential medium (MEM; Gibco, Grand Island, NY) and keratinocyte basal medium, that is, modified MCDB153 (Clonetics, San Diego, CA), supplemented with EGF (10 ng/ml), insulin (10 μg/ml), transferrin (10 μg/ml) (Collaborative Research, Bedford, MA), hydrocortisone (0.5 μg/ml, Sigma Chemical, St. Louis, MO), and gentamicin (5 μg/ml, Gibco). MCF-7 and SK-BR-3 human breast carcinoma cell lines were obtained from the American Type Culture Collection (Bethesda, MD). MCF-7 and SK-BR-3 cell lines were grown in Dulbecco's modified Eagle's medium (DMEM) with 10% fetal calf serum (Gibco). All cells were incubated at 37°C in 5% CO_2.

Animals

Female athymic nude mice (nu/nu) were obtained from Harlan Sprague-Dawley (Indianapolis, IN). The mice were maintained in our pathogen-free barrier facility (germ-free laminar airflow), and the drinking water, feed, bedding, and cages were sterilized before use. The animals were housed in a temperature (24°C) and light (14 hr/day) controlled room. The mice were fed Wayne Autoclave Rodent Blox (8658) (Dyets, Bethelehem, PA).

neu *transfection*

18-Rn1 cells were derived by infecting 184B5 cells with a mutationally activated replication-defective amphotropic retrovirus vector, JR-*neu* (rat), containing a single amino acid substitution (Val[664] to Glu[664]) in the transmembrane region. 18-Rn2 cells (obtained from Dr. C. Aylsworth, Michigan State University, E. Lansing, MI) were derived by infecting 184B5 cells with mutationally activated rat *neu* oncogene (identical to that described earlier). The 18-Hn1 cell line was derived by transfecting 184B5 cells with a mutationally activated human *neu* (*erbB*-2) oncogene and was a gift from Dr. J. Pierce (National Cancer Institute, Bethesda, MD).

Oligonucleotide primers

All oligonucleotide primers were synthesized in the Macromolecular Synthesis Facility, Michigan State University. The primers (including position in cDNA and the size of amplified fragment in bp) were as follows: 1. GAPDH,

human CCATGGCACCGTCAAGGCTGAGAACG (228–253), CAAT-
GCCAGCCCCAGCGTCAAAGGT (964–939) 738 bp; 2. LAR, human
TCGAGCGCCTCAAAGCCAACG (4362–4382), GGCAGGCACCTCTG-
TGTGGCCG (5191–5170), 831 bp, 3. PTP1B, human CGGCCATTTACC-
AGGATATCCGACA (130–154), TCAGCCCCATCCGAAACTTCCTC
(839–817) 711 bp; 4. TCPTP, human GCTGGCAGCCGCTGTACTTG-
GAAAT (110–134), ACTACAGTGGATCACCGCAGGCCCA (687–663)
579 bp; 5. *neu*, rat TGCCCCATCAACTGCACCCACTCCTGT (1907–1933),
TCCAGGTAGCTCATCCCCTTGGCAATC (2541–2515), 636 bp; primers
for human *neu* were identical to those previously reported [10].

RT-PCR analysis

Total RNA was isolated from cultured cells before confluence and RT-PCR
was performed. Radioactive labeling was performed by addition of 1 μCi of (α-
^{32}p)dCTP (Dupont/NEN Research Products, Wilmington, DE) to each polymerase chain reaction (PCR) reaction mixture. At the end of every five PCR
cycles, one reaction was stopped and the amplified products were analyzed by
8% native polyacrylamide gels and autoradiography. The amount of incorporated radioactivity of each gel band was determined by using a Betascope 603
blot analyzer (Betagen, Waltham, MA).

Immunofluorescence analysis

Cells were seeded at 1×10^4 cells per chamber (eight chamber slides; Nunc,
Naperville, IL), incubated for 48 hours, then fixed with 100% methanol at
−20°C. Anti-human c-*erbB*-2 monoclonal antibody was obtained from
Oncogene Science (Uniondale, NY), and anti-human LAR mAb 11:1A and
anti PTP1B-mAb AE4-2J were generous gifts from Dr. M. Streuli (Dana-
Farber Cancer Institute, Boston, MA) and Dr. D. Hill (Applied Biotechnology, Cambridge, MA), respectively. The second antibody for c-*erbB*-2, LAR,
and PTP1B was FITC-conjugated goat anti-mouse IgG (Sigma Chemical
Company). The amount of p185^{neu}, LAR, and PTP1B proteins was quantitated
by measuring the fluorescence intensities of the samples on a single-cell basis
using an ACAS 570 interactive laser cytometer (Meridian Instruments,
Okemos, MI).

Northern blot analysis

RNA was isolated using guanidine thiocyanate, and poly-A mRNA was isolated using a PolyATract mRNA Isolation System (Promega, Madison, WI).
mRNA was separated on a 1% MOPS-formaldehyde agarose gel and transferred to a nylon membrane (Gene Screen, Dupont/NEN Research Products).
GAPDH (738 bp) and *neu* (622 bp) probes were prepared by PCR of cDNA of
18-Hn1 cells. The LAR (1306 bp) and PTP1B (1273 bp) probes were prepared

A. LAR cDNA (pSP6.DL-LAR)

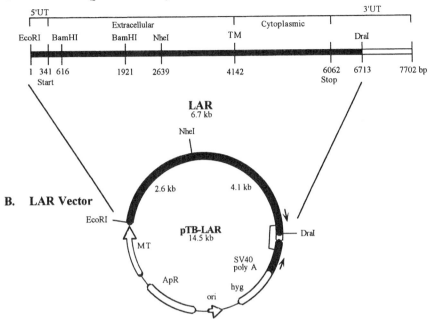

Figure 2. LAR-PTPase cDNA expression vector. **A:** The pSP6.DL-LAR plasmid region containing the full-length coding sequence of LAR-PTPase. The positions of the start and stop codons are
indicated, as well as the restriction enzyme sites used in the construction. The regions coding the
extracellular, cytoplasmic, and transmembrane (TM) domains of LAR-PTPase are indicated. **B:**
The plasmid, pTB-LAR (14.5 kb) contains the MT-1 heavy metal inducible metallothionein
promoter (MT), the LAR-PTPase coding sequence (solid, 6.7 kb from the *Eco*RI to *Dra*I sites), an
SV-40 polyadenylation signal (shaded), and a hygromycin-resistance gene as a selection marker.
The arrows indicate the position of the PCR primers, and the bracket indicates the position of the
segment spliced out of the PCR product.

by *Bam*HI or *Hind*III digestion, respectively, of cDNA. Probes were labeled
with $\alpha(^{32}P)dCTP$ (Dupont/NEN Research Products) using a random primer
labeling kit (United States Biochemical, Cleveland, OH).

LAR-PTPase expression vector

The vector containing human LAR-PTPase cDNA was constructed as follows
(Figure 2). The pSP6.DL-LAR plasmid (Figure 2A), containing the human
LAR-PTPase cDNA (a gift from Dr. M. Streuli), was digested with *Eco*RI +
*Nhe*I to yield 2.6 kb and 4.1 kb fragments, respectively. Then the 2.6 kb
pSP6.DL-LAR fragment was ligated to *Nru*I + *Nhe*I digested pTB-hyg (a gift
from Dr. J. McCormick, Michigan State University East Lansing, MI), generating a 10.5 kb intermediate plasmid pTG-LAR$_{EN}$. The 4.1 kb pSP6.DL-LAR

111

fragment was ligated into pTB-hyg after *Nhe*I + *Nae*I digestion, giving a second intermediate plasmid pTB-LAR$_{ND}$ (11.8 kb). The final plasmid pTB-LAR, constructed by ligating the 4.7 kb *Not*I + *Nhe*I fragment from pTB-LAR$_{EN}$ into pTB-LAR$_{ND}$ (after *Not*I + *Nhe*I digestion), contained the full-length coding sequence of LAR-PTPase (Figure 2B). The orientation and structure of the insertion were analyzed by restriction digestion. The pTB-LAR plasmid contained the human LAR-PTPase cDNA, the MT-1 heavy metal (zinc or cadmium) inducible metallothionein promoter, and a hygromycin resistance gene (*hyg*).

LAR-PTPase transfections

18-Hn1 cells were transfected with pTB-LAR or with control plasmid DNA (pTB-hyg alone) using lipofectin (Gibco) as described by the supplier with minor modifications. Cells were seeded at 5×10^5 per tissue culture dish (100 mm) in serum-containing growth medium. After 24 hours, 4 ml of medium with lipofectin reagent-DNA complex (30 µg of plasmid DNA and 30 µl of lipofectin reagent) were added to each dish and incubated overnight at 37°C. The DNA-containing medium was replaced with growth medium containing serum and was incubated for 48 hours before the addition of hygromycin (75 µg/ml).

LAR-PTPase expression

After hygromycin selection, LAR-transfected 18-Hn1 cell lines (18-Hn1-LAR) were cultured in Dulbecco's modified Eagle's medium (DMEM) containing 10% fetal bovine serum (GIBCO) and 10^{-3} M dexamethasone (Sigma Chemical). RT-PCR analysis (35 cycles) of LAR-PTPase transfected 18-Hn1 cells was performed using a sense primer in LAR-PTPase (5'-CGTCCAGCCCTCCTACGCAGA-3'; positioned just 3' to the LAR-PTPase termination codon) and an antisense primer 5' to the SV40 polyadenylation signal in the vector (5'-ATTTTATGTTTCASGGTTCA-GGGGGA-3'; see arrows, Figure 2B).

For analysis of LAR-PTPase protein expression, cells were grown in DMEM-containing serum with hygromycin B (150 mg/ml). When confluent, cells were washed twice in PBS and surface-labeled with N-hydroxysuccinimidobiotin (Sigma Chemical). Following labeling, cells were lysed with NP-40 cell lysis buffer (20 mM TRIS-HCl, pH 8.0, 1% NP-40; Pierce Chemical Co., Rockford, IL), 0.9% NaCl, 5 mM EDTA, 0.23 U/ml aprotinin, 2 mM PMSF, 1 µM pepstatin A, 1 µM leupeptin, 50 µg/ml RNAase A, and 50 µg/ml DNAase I (reagents from Sigma Chemical or Boehringer Manneheim, Indianapolis, IN). The protein concentration of the lysates was determined by the Bradford protein assay. Lysates (2 mg) from each LAR-PTPase clone were precleared twice by addition of 10 µg 104.21 mAb (anti-CD45) for 1 hour and 40 µl protein G agarose beads (Boehringer Manneheim) for 1 hour. Immunoprecipitation was performed by incubation with 5 μg anti-LAR-PTPase mAb 11.1A for 1 hour followed by 40 μl protein G-agarose beads for 1 hour. Immunoprecipitates were washed twice in PBS (pH 7.4), once in 0.5 M LiCl, and twice in 20 mM TRIS (pH 8.0), and were separated by SDS-PAGE (4–15% gradient). After electrophoresis, the proteins on the SDS-PAGE gel were transferred onto a 0.2 micron PVDF membrane (BioRad Laboratories, Melville, NY), blocked with 10% skim milk (w/v), 20 mM TRIS (pH 8), 0.137 M saline containing 0.1% Tween-20 (v/v) for 1 hour, and incubated with 1:5000 streptavidin-horseradish peroxidase conjugate (Immunopure, Pierce). Lastly, the blot was developed with a chemiluminescent detection system (ECL; Amersham, Arlington Heights, IL) and Hyperfilm (Amersham).

Cell proliferation rates in vitro

For comparison of cell proliferation rates, cells were seeded at 1×10^5 cells per 35 mm well in 6 well Costar culture cluster dishes in serum-free MCDB170 medium. At the indicated times, triplicate wells of each cell line were washed twice with PBS, trypsinized (0.05% trypsin, 0.53 mM EDTA), centrifuged, and resuspended in PBS, and the cells were counted individually using a Coulter Counter (Coulter Electronics, Hialeah, FL). For flow cytometric DNA analysis, bivariate flow cytometric measurement of BrdUrd incorporation was performed. Fluorescence intensity was determined with an Ortho cytofluorograph (Ortho Diagnostic Systems, Westwood, MA). Statistical analysis was performed by one-way analysis of variance and the Neuman-Keuls multiple comparison test.

Tumorigenicity assay

Tumorigenicity of cell lines was determined by the ability of cells to form tumors in mature female athymic nude mice. A total of 5×10^6 cells of each cell line were inoculated subcutaneously into athymic nude mice. Mice were observed at weekly intervals, and tumor diameters were obtained by using a vernier caliper. The tumor volumes were calculated based on the formula $V = 4/3\pi([A + B]/4)^3$, in which A and B are two perpendicular diameters obtained from each tumor. Tumor weights were obtained when the experiments were terminated 5 weeks after cell inoculation. Statistical analysis was performed by Student's t test and by one-way analysis of variance and the Neuman-Keuls multiple comparison test.

Results

Effect of neu *introduction on 184B5 cell proliferation in vitro*

The activated rat *neu* oncogene cDNA was introduced into the immortalized human breast epithelial cell line, 184B5. More than 1000 G418 resistant colonies were observed on each 100 mm plate following a single exposure to 1 ml of JR-*neu* virus at 2×10^4 colony-forming units (CFU)/ml. These colonies were pooled and designated as the cell line 18-Rn1. As a consequence of *neu* introduction, 18-Rn1 and a second *neu* transfected 184B5 cell line, 18-Hn1, were found to proliferate significantly more rapidly compared with parental 184B5 cells. The population doubling times for 184B5, 18-Rn1, and 18-Hn1 were 28, 24, and 19 hours, respectively. The *neu* transfection resulted in BrdUrd uptake of 30.3% and 38.9% in 18-Rn1 and 18-Hn1 cells, respectively, compared with 11.7% for 184B5 cells. These data provide evidence that increased *neu* expression resulted in a substantial elevation of DNA synthesis and cell proliferation.

Effect of neu *introduction on tumorigenicity of 184B5 cells in athymic nude mice*

As a direct test of the transforming potential of the *neu* oncogene, the capability of *neu* transfected 184B5 cells (18-Hn1 and 18-Rn1) to form tumors in athymic nude mice was determined. Both 18-Rn1 and 18-Hn1 cells readily formed palpable tumors after subcutaneous inoculation (Figure 3). 18-Rn1 cells formed tumors that initially grew progressively, followed by a period of slow growth; a number of these tumors ultimately regressed. 18-Hn1 cells formed rapidly growing progressive tumors; no evidence of regression was observed in these tumors. Histological analysis revealed that all 18-Rn1 tumors exhibited many characteristics of human breast carcinomas, including a high degree of nuclear polymorphism, central necrosis, and cysts. Histological characteristics of 18-Hn1 tumors were similar to 18-Rn1 tumors but lacked substantial cystic formation. No tumor development was observed from the parental 184B5 cell line.

Expression of neu *and PTPases in 184B5 cells and in* neu-*transformed 184B5 cells*

The PTPases studied by RT-PCR were LAR-PTPase, PTP1B, and TCPTP. Labeling of PCR products with (α-^{32}P)dCTP was used to determine the RT-PCR amplification efficiency and to semiquantitatively compare amplified PCR products. The amount of radioactive amplified product produced for each PTPase, GAPDH, and *neu* was measured every five PCR cycles. Since amplification was found to reach a plateau range at more than 25 cycles, the data used for comparative analysis were at 25 cycles of amplification. Thus, it was possible to obtain a semiquantitative comparison of the initial amounts of mRNA template by comparing the amounts of amplified PCR products. The expression of *neu* and PTPases in 18-Rn1, 18-Hn1, and 18-Rn2 cells and the parental 184B5 cells were compared using GAPDH as an internal control. By use of this method, *neu* elevation was estimated at from 5- to 22-fold in the three independently transformed 184B5 cell lines (18-Rn1, 18-Hn1, and 18-

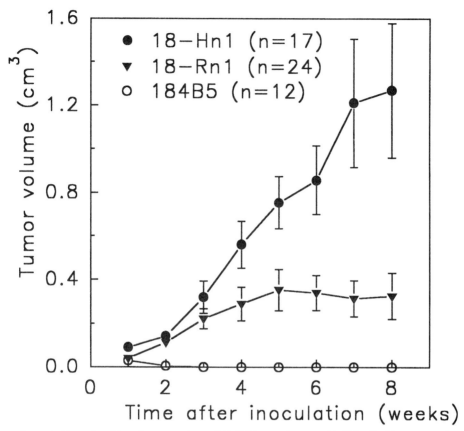

Figure 3. Tumorigenicity of *neu*-transformed 184B5 human breast epithelial cells. Tumor growth of *neu*-transformed 18-Hn1 (-●-) and 18-Rn1 (-▼-) cells, and parental 184B5 (-○-) cells was measured after subcutaneous inoculation of these cells into athymic nude mice. The number in parentheses is the number of inoculation sites for 184B5 cells, or the number of tumors resulting from inoculation of 18-Hn1 and 18-Rn1 cells. Data points are the mean tumor volume ± SEM.

Rn2). Of the PTPases examined, LAR-PTPase and PTP1B expression increased substantially over the very low levels found in 184B5 cells. TCPTP expression was also observed to increase, albeit slightly. Substantial expression of PTPases was not observed in SK-BR-3 and MCF-7 cell lines. Northern blot analysis was also performed and, although the PTPase mRNAs were present in extremely low amounts, the results were consistent with our RT-PCR data.

The expression levels of p185^{neu}, LAR-PTPase, and PTP1B were further confirmed by analysis of fluorescent-antibody labeled cells. Using respective primary antibodies and FITC second antibodies, the relative amounts of P185^{neu}, LAR-PTPase, and PTP1B proteins were estimated in individual cells as fluorescent units by using quantitative laser cytometry. The results indicated

Table 1. Expression of p185^{neu}, LAR-PTPase, and PTP1B proteins *neu*-transformed 185B5 human breast epithelial cells and in SK-BR-3 and MCF-7 human breast carcinoma cell lines determined by immunofluorescence analysis

Cells	Fluorescent units $\times$ 10^{-2}/cell (mean $\pm$ SEM)		
	P185^{neu}	LAR-PTPase	PTP1B
184B5	195 $\pm$ 3 (170)	489 $\pm$ 29 (114)	166 $\pm$ 1 (210)
18-Rn1	2943 $\pm$ 59 (235)	4641 $\pm$ 54 (181)	425 $\pm$ 6 (163)
18-Hn1	43,985 $\pm$ 376 (119)	5947 $\pm$ 252 (114)	1414 $\pm$ 20 (118)
SK-BR-3	6469 $\pm$ 4 (73)	464 $\pm$ 4 (86)	296 $\pm$ 10 (73)
MCF-7	344 $\pm$ 7 (125)	354 $\pm$ 1 (65)	163 $\pm$ 8 (83)

Numbers in parentheses represent the number of cells analyzed.

that p185^{neu} protein was expressed at elevated levels in 18-Rn1 and 18-Hn1 cell ($\sim$15- and $\sim$225-fold, respectively), compared with 184B5 cells (Table 1). LAR-PTPase was also expressed at elevated levels in 18-Rn1 and 18-Hn1 cells ($\sim$9- and $\sim$12-fold, respectively) compared with 184B5 cells. PTP1B was also expressed at elevated levels in 18-Rn1 and 18-Hn1 cells ($\sim$3- and $\sim$8-fold, respectively) compared with 184B5 cells. Of the two human breast carcinoma cell lines, SK-BR-3 expressed high levels of p185^{neu} protein, whereas MCF-7 cells expressed low levels of p185^{neu}, results that are in accord with literature reports. SK-BR-3, MCF-7, and 184B5 cells expressed LAR-PTPase and PTP1B proteins at low levels. We conclude from these data that LAR-PTPase and PTP1B expression were elevated in the *neu*-transfected 184B5 cells.

Transfection of LAR-PTPase cDNA into neu-*transformed 184B5 cells*

In the above-described study the levels of LAR-PTPase and PTP1B expression in *neu*-transformed cells were found to be increased above very low background levels in 184B5 cells. However, the observed levels of LAR-PTPase and PTP1B expression were still somewhat low in the *neu*-transformed cells. In order to test the hypothesis that the overexpression of LAR-PTPase would alter the transformed phenotype and tumorigenicity, we transfected *neu*-transformed 184B5 cells with an expression vector containing LAR-PTPase cDNA. A vector (pTB-LAR) was prepared incorporating full-length LAR cDNA and a metallothionine promoter Figure 2. The pTB-LAR vector was introduced into *neu*-transformed, 184B5 human breast epithelial cells using lipofectin. Selection using hygromycin resistance resulted in 25 clonal cell lines from which four independent clones (designated 18-Hn1-LAR5, LAR7, LAR10, and LAR13) were selected on the basis of elevated constitutive LAR-PTPase expression. Neither of these 4 cell lines, which were selected for further study, nor the other 21 cell lines, were found to be significantly inducible for LAR-PTPase expression with either zinc or cadmium treatments. However, the constitutive expression of the exogenous LAR-

PTPase gene in the cell lines selected was determined to be sufficient to perform the following experiments.

Expression of LAR-PTPase in LAR-PTPase–transfected neu-*transformed 184B5 cells*

RT-PCR was performed on 18-Hn1-LAR5, -LAR7, -LAR10, and -LAR13 cell lines using a LAR-PTPase sense primer and an antisense primer in the SV40 vector sequence. The expression of the introduced LAR-PTPase gene was confirmed by the presence of RT-PCR products of about 650 and 750 bp in each of the cell lines (confirmed by DNA sequencing). Expression of LAR-PTPase protein was determined using whole cell lysates from surface biotinylated 18-Hn1 and 18-Hn1-LAR5, -LAR7, -LAR10, and -LAR13 cells. Labeled cells were subjected to immunoprecipitation using monoclonal anti-human LAR-PTPase mAb 11.1A, SDS-PAGE separation, electrotransfer to PVDF membrane, and ECL chemiluminescence detection. Such analysis of 18-Hn1-LAR cells indicated that LAR-PTPase was overexpressed in each of the 18-Hn1-LAR cell lines compared with 18-Hn1-C cells transfected with the control plasmid (Figure 4).

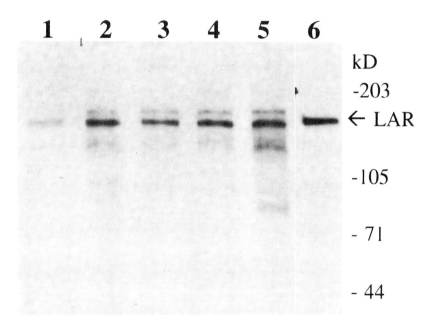

Figure 4. Immunoprecipitation of LAR-PTPase from 18-Hn1 and 18-Hn1-LAR cells. Cells were surface labeled with biotin, immunoprecipitation was performed with monoclonal anti-LAR-PTPase (11.1A), and detection was performed by chemiluminescence. Lane 1, 18-Hn1-C cells (transfected with pTB-hyg only); lane 2, 18-Hn1-LAR5 cells; lane 3, 18-Hn1-LAR7 cells; lane 4, 18-Hn1-LAR10 cells; lane 5, 18-Hn1-LAR13 cells; lane 6, HeLa cells (positive control). The scale is in kilodaltons, and the position of LAR-PTPase is indicated by the arrow at 150 kD.

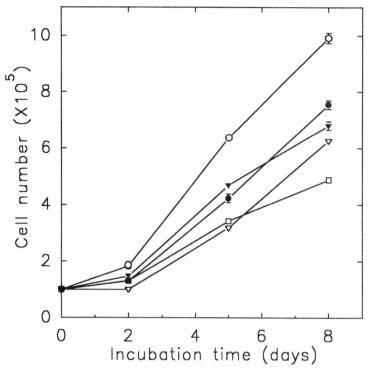

Figure 5. In vitro proliferation of 18-Hn1 and 18-Hn1-LAR cells. Cells were seeded at 1×10^5 cells per well and were cultured in serum-free medium. Triplicate wells of each cell line were collected and counted individually at the indicated times. (○), 18-Hn1 cells; (●), 18-Hn1-LAR5 cells; (▼), 18-Hn1-LAR10 cells; (▽), 18-Hn1-LAR7 cells; (□), 18-Hn1-LAR13 cells. The values represent the means ± SD. At certain time points the SD of the means were so small as to be nondiscernible in this figure. Mean numbers of cells/well, 18-Hn1 versus 18-Hn1-LAR5, 7, 10, or 13, $p < 0.01$.

Cell proliferation of LAR-PTPase–transfected neu-*transformed 184B5 cells*

Slight alterations in morphological appearance were observed in the 18-Hn1-LAR cell lines compared with 18-Hn1 and 18-Hn1 cells containing the control vector alone, that is, an increase in cell size, an increase in number of perinuclear granules or vesicles, and an increased proportion of large cells. The in vitro proliferation rate of 18-Hn1 cells containing the control vector was compared with those of the 18-Hn1-LAR cells in serum-free media (Figure 5). Each of the 18-Hn1-LAR cell lines proliferated significantly more slowly than the 18-Hn1 cells containing the control vector alone, a reduction in the rate of proliferation of approximately 23–50%. The reduction in growth rate was most apparent when the cells became confluent, between days 5 and

118

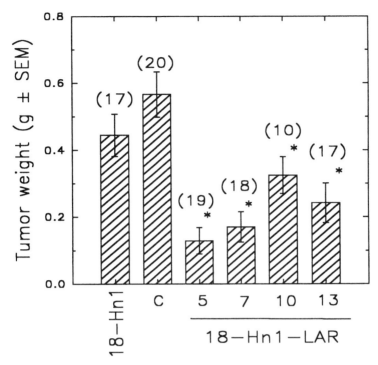

Figure 6. Tumorigenicity of 18-Hn1 cells, 18-Hn1 cells transfected with the control vector (C), and 18-Hn1-LAR cells in athymic nude mice. Tumor weight is shown 5 weeks after subcutaneous inoculation of 5×10^6 cells. Significant ($p < 0.05$) mean differences (indicated by *) were observed when comparing 18-Hn1 cells or 18-Hn1-C cells (18-Hn1 transfected with pTB-hyg) with 18-Hn1-LAR cells 5, 7, 10, and 13. The parentheses indicate the number of tumors measured, and error bars represent the standard error of the means.

7 of growth. These studies were performed three times with virtually identical results.

Tumorigenicity of LAR-PTPase–transfected neu-*transformed 184B5 cells*

The tumorigenic potential of 18-Hn1-LAR cell lines was compared with 18-Hn1 cells and 18-Hn1 cells transfected with the control vector following subcutaneous injection into athymic nude mice (Figure 6). Each cell line examined formed palpable tumors. Importantly, however, mean tumor weights were significantly smaller in each of 18-Hn1-LAR cell lines than those observed in 18-Hn1 cells or in 18-Hn1 cells containing the control plasmid alone (C). This tumorigenicity study was repeated two times with virtually identical results. Histopathological examination revealed that all the tumors were carcinomas with varying degrees of cystic necrosis. No unique histopathological distinction was apparent between tumors arising from 18-Hn1 and 18-Hn1-LAR cells.

Discussion

A positive association of *neu* expression with human breast carcinoma development was supported by our finding that transfection of activated *neu* oncogene cDNA into an immortalized nontumorigenic human breast epithelial cell line (184B5) resulted in (a) an increase in p185^{neu} expression and (b) the formation of progressively growing carcinomas after such cells were inoculated into athymic nude mice. Expression levels of *neu* were substantially higher in the faster growing, more progressive tumors (18-Hn1) than in the slower growing tumors (18-Rn1). An examination of the effect of *neu* overexpression on PTPase levels in these tumors indicated a significantly increased expression of specific PTPases, that is, LAR-PTPase and PTP1B. Although elevated, the expression level of these PTPases in 18-Hn1 and 18-Rn1 cells was still relatively low and could only be detected without difficulty by immunofluorescence and by RT-PCR (techniques such as immunoblotting or Northern analysis were only partly successful). To test the hypothesis that expression of LAR-PTPase at high levels would alter or suppress the transformed and tumorigenic phenotype, we undertook experiments to introduce LAR-PTPase into *neu*-transformed 184B5 cells (18-Hn1 cells). Transfection of LAR-PTPase cDNA into 18-Hn1 cells resulted in cells with an elevated expression level of this PTPase. Four clones exhibiting constitutive, elevated expression of LAR-PTPase had significantly reduced rates of proliferation in vitro and significantly reduced tumorigenicity after inoculation into athymic nude mice. These results provide evidence that specific PTPases (e.g., LAR-PTPase) may play a key suppressive regulatory role in the tumorigenicity of human breast carcinoma cells that overexpress p185^{neu} PTK.

The human *neu* proto-oncogene (also known as c-*erb*B-2 or HER-2) encodes a 185 kD transmembrane glycoportein (p185^{neu}) that shows extensive structural similarity with the epidermal growth factor receptor (EGFR), a 170 kD transmembrane protein. Like EGFR, p185^{neu} protein possesses a hydrophobic transmembrane spanning sequence, a cytoplasmic portion with PTK activity, and an extracellular portion containing two cysteine-rich clusters [10]. p185^{neu} specific ligands have been identified [11–14]. Point mutations containing a substitution of Glu for Val at position 664 in the transmembrane region of p185^{neu} result in constitutive receptor oligomerization, leading to an activation of the PTK, which is important for the neoplastic transforming activity of *neu* [15]. The transforming activity of the *neu* oncogene is manifested via multiple genetic mechanisms, all resulting in constitutive elevation of *neu* PTK activity.

As a receptor tyrosine kinase in the growth factor receptor family, p185^{neu} has been proposed to transduce signals in the cell via at least four pathways associated with the binding of SH2 domain-containing proteins to p185^{neu} autophosphorylation sites. Among the major signaling components implicated in early post-receptor events are phospholipase Cγ (PLCγ), p21^{ras} guanosine triphosphate-activating protein (GAP), phosphatidylinositol-3′ kinase (PI′3K,

120

p110/p85), and SHC [16,17]. These proteins are phosphorylated by the PTK activity of the receptor, and some serve as binding sites for additional 'adaptor' molecules containing SH2 domains (e.g., Grb2). A positive correlation between PLCγ1 expression and the expression of EGFR or p185^{neu} has been reported for human breast carcinomas [18], and both PLCγ and GAP have been reported to be phosphorylated by, and to coprecipitate with, p185^{neu} [19–21]. Furthermore, a variety of other tyrosine phosphorylated proteins are associated in a cytosolic complex with PLCγ and GAP [21]. In addition, PI'3K has also been identified as a substrate of activated p185^{neu} (chimeric protein) and forms a complex with p185^{neu} upon ligand binding [22]. SHC is also phosphorylated upon stimulation with growth factor receptor tyrosine kinases [23].

The human *neu* proto-oncogene has been found to be amplified and/or overexpressed in approximately 30% of primary human breast carcinomas [24–27]. The incidence and level of *neu* amplification has been found to remain consistent in matched primary and metastatic breast carcinomas from the same patient, suggesting that amplification is an early and possibly initiating event in human breast carcinomas [28]. In human breast carcinomas, *neu* proto-oncogene amplification and overexpression have been found to be highly correlated with poor prognostic factors [29]. These factors include large tumor size, lymph node positivity, a higher number of involved nodes, advanced stage, steroid receptor negativity, aberrant DNA content, and higher rate of cell proliferation. However, until recently the effects of induced *neu* overexpression in cultured human breast epithelial cells and the effects of such overexpression on the pathogenesis of these cells have remained unknown. Pierce et al. [30] first reported that overexpression of p185^{neu} alone was sufficient for neoplastic transformation of immortalized human breast epithelial cells. Our results, as reported in this communication, confirm and extend those of Pierce et al. [30]. These findings strongly suggest that amplification and/or overexpression of the *neu* proto-oncogene and the consequent continued overphosphorylation of tyrosine residues in cellular proteins are important and critical factors in the initiation, growth, and/or progression of human breast carcinomas.

LAR-PTPase is a transmembrane molecule composed of a 1234 amino acid extracellular, receptor-like region, a 24-amino acid transmembrane segment, and a 623 amino acid cytoplasmic region containing two tandem repeated PTPase domains (only the first PTPase domain is believed to be active) (Figure 2). LAR-PTPase has been found to be expressed on endothelial and epithelial cells of a broad range of tissue and cell types [3,8,9]. Streuli et al. [8] have demonstrated that the LAR-PTPase protein is proteolytically cleaved within the cell to produce a mature structure containing two subunits, termed the *LAR-P subunit* (PTPase) and the *LAR-E subunit* (LAR extracellular subunit), which can be released from the cell surface. The extracellular region of LAR-PTPase is composed of three immunoglobulin (Ig)–like domains and eight fibronectin type III (FN-III) domains, and resembles neural cell adhesion molecules (N-CAM) [8]. N-CAM facilitates cell adhesion by homotypic cell–cell interaction among Ig domains [31,32]. Hence, LAR-PTPase may also be a cell adhesion molecule. It was reported that the PTPase, RPTPμ, a receptor-type PTPase with both Ig and Fn-III domains, mediates homotypic cell aggregation [33]. Thus, the physiological function of LAR-PTPase may not only involve the regulation of cellular tyrosine phosphorylation of proteins but may also mediate cell–cell or cell–matrix recognition and interaction, the loss of which could lead to unreastrained cell proliferation and neoplastic transformation [2,3]. Supporting this hypothesis is the finding that the product of a colorectal tumor suppressor gene, DCC (deleted in colorectal cancer), which was shown to be frequently deleted in human colorectal carcinomas, is structurally similar to the extracellular region of LAR-PTPase [34,35]. In addition, Streuli et al. [8] have demonstrated that the LAR-PTPase gene is located on human chromosome 1p32–33, a chromosome that contains several candidate tumor suppressor genes. Altogether, the position of the LAR-PTPase gene and the results of our studies showing consistent and significant suppression of tumorigenicity in LAR-PTPase transfected human breast carcinoma cells raises the possibility that this gene may act, at least in part, as a tumor suppressor gene.

It is well established that protein tyrosine phosphorylation is a fundamental mechanism for regulating diverse cellular processes, including signal transduction, cell proliferation, and neoplastic transformation. The constitutive activation of certain PTKs causes unregulated cell proliferation, which is a very important component of oncogenesis. About one third of all known oncogenes are PTKs. Therefore, it is certainly reasonable that certain genes of the PTPase family may act as tumor suppressor genes [2,34,36]. Conceptually, hyperphosphorylation of a key signal transduction protein, driving tumorigenic processes, can occur either by overexpression of PTK activity or by the loss of PTPase activity. Therefore, one would predict that overexpression of a PTPase gene could counteract certain oncogenic PTKs, either by conferring resistance to neoplastic transformation or by reversing the neoplastically transformed phenotype. Conversely, loss or inactivation of one or both copies of a PTPase gene could result in constitutively increased tyrosine phosphorylation of particular cellular proteins, thus leading to the malignant phenotype.

In support of the concept that certain PTPases may function as tumor suppressor gene products is a report demonstrating the loss of one allele of the human RPTPγ-PTPase gene in approximately one half of the human tumor samples examined [37]. The gene for PTP1B may also qualify as a candidate tumor suppressor gene. Brown-Shimer et al. [38] have demonstrated that PTP1B, when transfected into NIH 3T3 cells, was capable of suppressing transformation by *neu*. In addition, Woodford-Thomas et al. [39] reported that overexpression of the PTPase, PTP1, in v-*src* transformed NIH 3T3 cells caused a 75% reduction in the ability of these cells to form colonies in soft agar, such cells reverted to a morphology characteristic of the parental cells.

Histochemically, PTPases have been reported to be increased in primary benign and malignant human breast disease [40,41], while a specific PTPase, that is, PTP1B, has been reported to be expressed in primary human breast carcinomas, an expression that is positively associated with the expression of *neu* [42].

Breast carcinoma continues to be one of the most common cancers in women throughout the western world. In the United States, the incidence of this disease has been steadily increasing; currently 1 in 9 women can expect to develop this disease in their lifetime. Despite this continued increase in breast carcinoma incidence and mortality, there has been a tremendous increase in the past 5–10 years in our understanding of this tumorigenic process at the cellular level. Most prominent has been the realization that certain proto-oncogenes have a critical role in this disease process. Of these, *neu* has generated much excitement. Like many other proto-oncogenes, activated p185^{neu} oncoprotein is a potent PTK. Continuous and/or increased activities of this enzyme system, leading to enhanced protein (tyrosine) phosphorylation, is clearly an important component of the induction of tumorigenic processes. Our understanding of the role of specific cellular PTPases as gene products that can potentially effectively modify PTK activities could lead to gene transfection strategies effective in the prevention of human breast neoplastic transformation and/or in the development of new therapies to modify the balance of tyrosine phosphorylation in the human breast carcinoma cell.

Acknowledgments

This work was supported by NIH research grants GM35774 (W.J.E.), CA50430 (C.W.W.), and CA64393 (W.J.E. & C.W.W.), and by a research grant from the Elsa U. Pardee Foundation (W.J.E. & C.W.W.). A portion of the studies described in this communication have been previously reported (Zhai et al., *Cancer Res* 53:2272–2278, 1993 and Zhai et al., *Mol Carcinogen*, 14:103–110, 1995).

References

1. Ullrich A, Schlessinger J (1990) Signal transduction by receptors with tyrosine kinase activity. *Cell* 61:203–212.
2. Fischer EH, Charbonneau H, Tonks NK (1991) Protein tyrosine phosphatases: A diverse family of intracellular and transmembrane enzymes. *Science* 253:401–406.
3. Saito H (1993) Structural diversity of eukaryotic protein tyrosine phosphatases: Functional and evolutionary implications. *Semin Cell Biol* 4:379–387.
4. Cool DE, Fischer EH (1993) Protein tyrosine phosphatases in cell transformation. *Semin Cell Biol* 4:443–453.
5. Tonks NK, Dlitz CD, Fischer EH (1988). Purification of the major protein-tyrosine-phosphatases of human placenta. *J Biol Chem* 263:6722–6730.
6. Cool DE, Tonks NK, Charbonneau H, Walsh KA, Fischer EH, Krebs EG (1989) cDNA

isolated from a human T-cell library encodes a member of the protein-tyrosine-phosphatase family. *Proc Natl Acad Sci USA* 86:5257–5261.

7. Trowbridge IS (1991) CD45. A prototype for transemembrane protein tyrosine phosphatases. *J Biol Chem* 266:23517–23522.

8. Streuli M, Krueger NX, Ariniello PD, Tang M, Munro JM, Blattler WA, Adler DA, Disteche CM, Saito H (1992) Expression of the receptor-linked protein tyrosine phosphatase LAR: Proteolytic cleavage and shedding of the CAM-like extracellular region. *EMBO J* 11:897–907.

9. Streuli M, Krueger NX, Hall LR, Schlossman SF, Saito H (1988) A new member of the immunoglobulin superfamily that has a cytoplasmic region homologous to the leukocyte common antigen. *J Exp Med* 168:1523–1530.

10. Saya H, Ara S, Lee PSY, Ro J, Hung M-C (1990) Direct sequencing analysis of transmembrane region of human *neu* gene by polymerase chain reaction. *Mol Carcinog* 3:198–201.

11. Lupu R, Colomer R, Zugmaier G, Sarup J, Shepard M, Slamon D, Lippman ME (1990) Direct interaction of a ligand for the *erb*B2 oncogene product with the EGF receptor and p185[erbB2]. *Science* 249:1552–1555.

12. Holmes WE, Sliwkowski MX, Akita RW, Henzel WJ, Lee J, Park JW, Yansura D, Abadi N, Raab H, Lewis GE, et al. (1992) Identification of heregulin, a specific activator of p185[erbB2]. *Science* 256:1205–1210.

13. Peles E, Bacus SS, Koski RA, Lu HS, Wen D, Ogden SG, Levy RB, Yarden Y (1992) Isolation of the *neu*/HER-2 stimulatory ligand: A 44kd glycoprotein that induces differentiation of mammary tumor cells. *Cell* 69:205–216.

14. Yarden Y, Peles E (1991) Biochemical analysis of the ligand for the *neu* oncogenic receptor. *Biochemistry* 30:3543–3550.

15. Weiner DB, Liu J, Cohen JA, Williams WV, Greene MI (1989) A point mutation in the *neu* oncogene mimics ligand induction of receptor aggregation. *Nature* 339:230–231.

16. Brugge JS (1993) New intracellular targets for therapeutic drug design. *Science* 260:918–919.

17. Cantley LC, Auger KR, Carpenter C, Duckworth B, Graziani A, Kapeller R, Soltoff S (1991) Oncogenes and signal transduction. *Cell* 64:281–302.

18. Arteaga CL, Johnson MD, Todderud G, Coffey RJ, Carpenter G, Page DL (1991) Elevated content of the tyrosine kinase substrate phospholipase C-gamma 1 in primary human breast carcinomas. *Proc Natl Acad Sci USA* 88:10435–10439.

19. Peles E, Levy RB, Or E, Ullrich A, Yarden Y (1991) Oncogenic forms of the *neu*/HER2 tyrosine kinase are permanently coupled to phospholipase C gamma. *EMBO J* 10:2077–2086.

20. Segatto O, Lonardo F, Helin K, Wexler D, Fazioli F, Rhee SG, Di-Fiore PP (1992) ErbB-2 autophosphorylation is required for mitogenic action and high-affinity substrate coupling. *Oncogene* 7:1339–1346.

21. Jallal B, Schlessinger J, Ullrich A (1992) Tyrosine phosphatase inhibition permits analysis of signal transduction complexes in p185[HER2/neu]-overexpressing human tumor cells. *J Biol Chem* 267:4357–4364.

22. Peles E, Lamprecht R, Ben-Levy R, Tzahar E, Yarden Y (1992) Regulated coupling of the Neu receptor to phosphatidylinositol 3'-kinase and its release by oncogenic activation. *J Biol Chem* 267:12266–12274.

23. Rozakis-Adcock M, McGlade J, Mbamalu G, Pelicci G, Daly R, Li W, Batzer A, Thomas S, Brugge J, Pelicci PG, et al. (1992) Association of the Shc and Brb2/Sem5 SH2-containing proteins is implicated in activation of the Ras pathway by tyrosine kinases. *Nature* 360:689–692.

24. Kraus MH, Popescu NC, Amsbaugh SC, King CR (1987) Overexpression of the EGF receptor-related proto-oncogene *erb*B-2 in human mammary tumor cell lines by different molecular mechanisms. *EMBO J* 6:605–610.

25. Slamon DJ, Clark GM, Wong SG, Levin WJ, Ullrich A, McQuire WL (1987) Human breast cancer: Correlation of relapse and survival with amplification of the HER-2 oncogene. *Science* 235:177–182.

26. Van de Vijver M, Van de Bersselaar R, De vilee P, Cornelisse C, Peterse J, Nusse R (1987) Amplification of the *neu* (c-*erb*B2) oncogene in mammary tumors is relatively frequent and is

often accompanied by amplification of the linked c-*erb*A oncogene. *Mol Cell Biol* 7:2019–2023.

27. Clark GM, McGuire WL (1991) Follow-up study of HER-2/*neu* amplification in primary breast cancer. *Cancer Res* 51:944–948.

28. Lacroix H, Iglehart JD, Skinner MA, Kraus MH (1989) Overexpression of *erb*B-2 or EGF receptor proteins present in early stage mammary carcinoma is detected simultaneously in matched primary tumors and regional metastases. *Oncogene* 4:145–151.

29. Van de Vijver M, Nusse R (1991) The molecular biology of breast cancer. *Biochim Biophys Acta* 1072:33–50.

30. Pierce JH, Arnstein P, DiMarco E, Artrip J, Kraus MH, Lonardo F, Di-Fiore PP, Aaronson SA (1991) Oncogenic potential of *erb*B-2 in human mammary epithelial cells. *Oncogene* 6:1189–1194.

31. Edelman GM (1985) Cell adhesion and the molecular processes of morphogenesis. *Annu Rev Biochem* 54:135–169.

32. Owens GC, Edelman GM, Cunningham BA (1987) Organization of the neural cell adhesion molecule (N-CAM) gene: Alternative exon usage as the basis for different membrane-associated domains. *Proc Natl Acad Sci USA* 84:294–298.

33. Gebbink MF, Zondag GC, Wubbolts RW, Beijersbergen RL, Van EI, Moolenaar WH (1993) Cell-cell adhesion mediated by a receptor-like protein tyrosine phosphatase. *J Biol Chem* 268:16101–16104.

34. Stanbridge EJ (1990) Human tumor suppressor genes. *Annu Rev Genet* 24:615–657.

35. Fearon ER, Cho KR, Nigro JM, Kern SE, Simons JW, Ruppert JM, Hamilton SR, Preisinger AC, Thomas G, Kinzler KW, et al. (1990) Identification of a chromosome 18q gene that is altered in colorectal cancers. *Science* 247:49–56.

36. Sager R (1989) Tumor suppressor genes: The puzzle and the promise. *Science* 256:1406–1412.

37. LaForgia S, Morse B, Levy J, Barnea G, Cannizzaro LA, Li F, Nowell PC, Boghosian-Sell L, Glick J, Weston A, et al. (1991) Receptor protein-tyrosine phosphatase gamma is a candidate tumor suppressor gene at human chromosome region 3p21. *Proc Natl Acad Sci USA* 88:5036–5040.

38. Brown-Shimer S, Johnson KA, Hill DE, Bruskin AM (1992) Effect of protein tyrosine phosphatase 1B expression on transformation by human *neu* oncogene. *Cancer Res* 52:478–482.

39. Woodford-Thomas TA, Rhodes JD, Dixon JE (1992) Expression of a protein tyrosine phosphatase in normal and v-*src*-transformed mouse 3T3 fibroblasts. *J Cell Biol* 117:401–414.

40. Partanen S, Pekonen F (1989) Histochemically demonstratable phosphotyrosyl-protein phosphatase in normal breast, benign breast diseases and in breast cancer. *Anticancer Res* 9:667–672.

41. Kidd KR, Kerns BJ, Dodge RK, Wiener JR (1992) Histochemical staining of protein-tyrosine phosphatase activity in primary human mammary carcinoma: Relationship with established prognostic indicators. *J Histochem Cytochem* 40:729–735.

42. Wiener JD, Kerns BM, Harvey EL, Conaway MR, Iglehart JD, Berchuck A, Bast RC (1994) Overexpression of the protein tyrosine phosphatase PTP1B in human breast cancer: Association with p185[c-erbB-2] protein expression. *J Natl Cancer Inst* 86:372–378.

7. Role of the nuclear matrix in breast cancer

Tracy S. Replogle and Kenneth J. Pienta

Introduction

The mammalian nucleus contains approximately 2 cm of DNA packed into a nucleus that is 10 microns in diameter. The packaging of DNA into the nucleus is organized by the nuclear matrix, the RNA-protein skeleton of the matrix. The nuclear matrix is the scaffold that organizes DNA at a structural as well as a functional level [1]. By organizing DNA in both structural and functional manners, the nuclear matrix plays a critical role in normal cellular function. Several reports have now demonstrated that the nuclear matrix is altered in cancer cells and is intimately involved in the function of several oncogenes. Defining how the nuclear matrix is involved in the process of cell transformation has implications not only for understanding malignancy, but also for the development of new biomarkers for diagnosis and prognosis.

The concept of a residual nuclear structure, composed predominantly of protein, was proposed in 1942 by Mayer and Gulick when it was noticed that high concentrations of sodium chloride used to extract nuclei resulted in insoluble protein [2]. In 1963, Smetana et al. reported the presence of a ribonucleoprotein network of fibers in nuclei after a series of extractions of soluble proteins and deoxyribonucleoproteins from Walker tumor and rat liver cells [3]. Eleven years later, the identification of a nuclear protein matrix was reported by Berezney and Coffey, who utilized a variety of extractions of rat liver nuclei to remove the major components of the nucleus. Figure 1 diagrams the steps necessary to isolate the nuclear matrix from intact cells. The procedure uses detergents and salt extractions to successively remove lipids, soluble proteins, intermediate filaments, DNA, and most of the RNA. The extractions revealed a nonchromatin framework that extended throughout the nucleus. Upon chemical analysis it was found that the nuclear matrix contained 98.2% protein, 0.1% DNA, 0.5% phospholipid, and 1.2% RNA [4]. A later report from the same laboratory stated that the structural components of the isolated matrix bear remarkable resemblance to well-defined structures of intact nuclei, suggesting that the nuclear matrix network is not a result of the extractions and enzyme treatments. Berezney and Coffey went on to suggest

R. Dickson and M. Lippman (eds.) MAMMARY TUMOR CELL CYCLE, DIFFERENTIATION AND METASTASIS. 1996. Kluwer Academic Publishers. ISBN 0-7923-3905-3. All rights reserved.

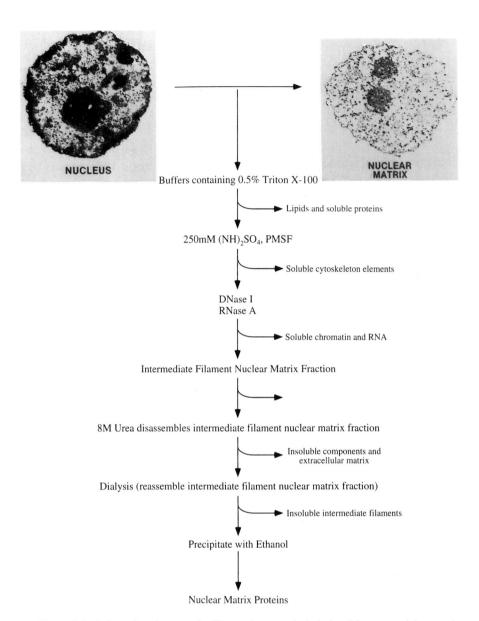

Figure 1. Isolation of nuclear matrix. The nuclear matrix is isolated by sequential extractions using non-ionic detergent, DNase I digestion, and a hypertonic salt buffer. These extractions remove over 98% of the DNA, 70% of the RNA, and 90% of the protein, resulting in the residual structure, which is essentially devoid of histones and lipids.

Table 1. Nuclear matrix is the dynamic structural subcomponent of the nucleus that directs the functional organization of DNA into loop domains and provides organizational sites for many of the functions involving DNA

Reported functions of the nuclear matrix

Nuclear morphology: The nuclear matrix contains structural elements of the pore complexes, lamina, internal network, and nucleoli, which give the nucleus its overall three-dimensional organization and shape.

DNA organization: DNA loop domains are attached to nuclear matrix at their bases, and this organization is maintained during both interphase and metaphase. Nuclear matrix shares some proteins with the chromosome scaffold, including topoisomerase II, an enzyme that modulates DNA topology.

DNA replication: The nuclear matrix has fixed sites for DNA replication and contains the replisome complex for DNA replication.

RNA synthesis: Actively transcribed genes are associated with the nuclear matrix. The nuclear matrix contains transcriptional complexes, newly synthesized heterogeneous nuclear RNA, and small nuclear RNA. RNA processing intermediates are bound to the nuclear matrix.

Nuclear regulation: The nuclear matrix has specific sites for steroid hormone receptor binding. DNA viruses are synthesized in association with the matrix. The nuclear matrix is a cellular target for transformation proteins, some retrovirus products such as the large T antigen, and E1A protein. Many of the nuclear matrix proteins are phosphorylated at specific times in the cell cycle.

that the nuclear matrix is a dynamically changing structure and therefore may play important roles in nuclear functions [5].

The nuclear matrix is defined as the RNA-protein skeleton of the nucleus that contributes to the structural and functional organization of DNA. In the last several decades, there has been a great deal of insight into the importance of the nuclear matrix, especially in the area of cancer. Five of the general functions of the nuclear matrix are listed in Table 1. They include nuclear morphology and regulation, DNA organization and replication, RNA synthesis and transport, and nuclear regulation.

A cellular hallmark of the transformed phenotype is abnormal nuclear shape and the presence of abnormal nucleoli. Nuclear structural alterations are so prevalent in cancer cells that they are commonly used as a pathological marker for transformation for many types of cancer. Nuclear shape is thought to reflect the internal nuclear structure and processes, and is determined, at least in part, by the nuclear matrix. The nuclear matrix contains structural elements of the pore complexes, lamina, internal network, and nucleoli that give the nucleus its overall three-dimensional organization and shape. The lamina forms the periphery of the matrix, while the nuclear matrix extends inward from the lamina [6]. The nucleolus, which is composed of RNA and proteins, is responsible for RNA synthesis and processing of pre-ribosomal RNA within the cell as well as assembly of ribosomal proteins [7]. The lamins comprise a structure that lies between the membrane and the peripheral chromatin. The predominant polypeptides are termed *lamins A, B,* and *C*; have a molecular weight (MW) range of 60,000–80,000; and have been found to be associated with the chromatin of cells [6]. It is now known that chromosomes are not free floating in the nucleus but must instead have a specific three-dimensional spatial organization, hence, much emphasis turned to the role of the nuclear matrix in DNA organization.

Vogelstein et al. were the first to visualize DNA loop structures attached to the nuclear matrix by releasing the supercoiled loops in the presence of a low concentration of ethidium bromide [8]. Using fluorescence microscopy, 3T3 nuclei devoid of soluble proteins and histones were placed in various concentrations of ethidium bromide and viewed. A halo, representing DNA intercalated with ethidium bromide, was seen surrounding the nuclear matrix skeleton. Intercalation of ethidium bromide into DNA caused positive supercoiling (i.e., unwinding of loops), which was experimentally represented as the enlargement of the halo. At higher concentrations of ethidium bromide, the DNA overwinds, causing positive supercoiling, represented by a decrease in halo size. Nicking the DNA resulted in uniform halos regardless of the ethidium bromide concentration used. The results of this study implicated DNA loop domains as an important level of DNA organization.

DNA is organized into loop domains of approximately 60 kilobases that are attached at their bases to the nuclear matrix. The points of attachments of DNA sequences to the matrix have been studied and have been termed *matrix attachment regions* (MARs) or *scaffold attachment regions* (SARs) [9]. The MARs generally contain AT-rich DNA sequences as well as sequences that are similar to topoisomerase II consensus sequences [10]. To date, no conserved consensus sequences are known for MARs; however, MARs have been found to be closely associated with actively transcribed genes and thus may control their expression. Romig et al. identified four novel DNA binding proteins that specifically bound to SARs, one of which (SAF-A) was found to specifically bind to several SAR elements from different species [11]. Other MARs have been purified and functionally characterized that bind lamins A and C [10]. Dickinson et al. cloned a DNA-binding protein that binds MARs called *SATB1*. SATB1 appears to recognize a particular type of AT-rich sequences, and binding occurs in the minor groove of DNA [12]. Most recently, Durfee et al. have isolated a 84-kD nuclear matrix protein (p84) that localizes to an area in the nucleus associated with RNA processing. In particular, p84 was found to specifically interact with the amino-terminal region of the retinoblastoma susceptibility gene [13].

The nuclear matrix has also been implicated in the replication of DNA. Vogelstein et al. demonstrated the rate of movement of newly synthesized DNA by autoradiography using ^{3}H-thymidine [8]. Using pulse-chase experiments, Pardoll et al. provided further evidence that the nuclear matrix provides fixed sites for the attachment of replication complexes [14]. These investigators demonstrated that after short pulse times with ^{3}H-thymidine given to rats, the matrix DNA had a very high specific activity when compared with the total DNA. This indicated that newly synthesized DNA is associated with the nuclear matrix, which had been shown by other investigators [15].

Berezney and Coffey also reported DNA that was labeled rapidly during DNA synthesis appeared to be associated with the nuclear matrix [16]. These replication sites that contain the enzymes needed to duplicate DNA have been named *replicases* by Reddy and Pardee [17]. Earnshaw and Heck demonstrated that topoisomerase II, an enzyme known to regulate DNA topology, is also a component of the DNA loops in mitotic chromosomes [18].

Berezney and Buchholtz provided further evidence to support the role of the nuclear matrix in eukaryotic DNA replication [19]. The replication of DNA occurs discontinuously in subunits on the long chromosomal DNA, called *replicons*. They proposed that DNA replication complexes remain bound to the nuclear matrix while DNA is reeled through during replication. Further evidence came from Valenzuela et al., when HeLa nuclei were shown to have an enrichment of replication forks (i.e., branched DNA) associated with the nuclear matrix [19]. Tubo et al. demonstrated that nuclear matrix prepared from labeled nuclei were enriched in DNA synthesized by the nuclei compared with the total nuclear DNA [21]. Younghusband observed that the nuclear matrix is the site of adenovirus DNA replication in infected HeLa cells [22]. Smith and Berezney reported a significant portion of DNA polymerase α bound to isolated nuclear matrices during active replication in regenerating liver [23].

The nuclear matrix has also been implicated in transcription. The nuclear matrix consists not only of protein, but also RNA, which has been shown to be an essential component [24]. Herlan et al. found that labeled RNAs associated tightly with the nuclear matrix and that the majority of the RNA included in the RNA–protein matrix consisted of pre-rRNA [25]. Small nuclear RNA complexed with proteins (snRNP) have also been localized to the nuclear matrix [26]. Heterogeneous nuclear RNA (hnRNA), which is the precursor to messenger RNA, has been shown to be associated with the nuclear skeleton after the removal of most of the chromatin, suggesting that the hnRNA is associated with nonchromatin structures within the nucleus [27]. This association was shown to be specific when labeled hnRNA was added to isolated nuclei, and very little hnRNA became associated with the nuclear structure of both intact and chromatin-depleted nuclei [27,28].

Van Eekelen and van Venrooij reported a specific set of proteins that were associated with the hnRNA and nuclear matrix complex, and concluded that proteins are involved in the binding of hnRNA to the nuclear matrix [29]. This association of hnRNA with the nuclear matrix led to the idea that the nuclear matrix may also play a role in transcription. In one study, all precursors of RNA were found to be exclusively associated with chick oviduct nuclear matrix, supporting the notion that the nuclear matrix may be the structural site for RNA processing [30]. In a series of experiments using HeLa nuclei, Jackson et al. demonstrated that RNA is synthesized at the nuclear cage (i.e., nuclear matrix) [31]. They observed, along with prior investigators, that RNA is attached in a specific manner to the nuclear matrix. In addition, transcribed sequences were found to be closely associated with the nuclear cage. This latter observation has been demonstrated in active viral genes using nine cell lines transformed with viral sequences of polyoma and/or avian sarcoma virus. The transcriptionally active genes were shown to be in close proximity to the nuclear cage [32].

Buckler-White et al. isolated nuclear matrix from mouse 3T3 cells infected with polyoma virus and showed that there is a fixed number of sites for T antigen on the matrix, implicating that the nuclear matrix does play a role in transcription. Additional evidence of the interaction of the nuclear matrix and transcriptionally active genes came from studies involving the thick oviduct [33,34], SV40-infected cells [35], chicken liver [36], and chicken erythrocytes [37]. Bidwell et al. examined nuclear matrix DNA-binding proteins that interacted with the osteocalcin gene promoter [38]. Their results were consistent with the involvement of the nuclear matrix in gene transcription.

The nuclear matrix has also been suggested to play a role in RNA processing. Using HeLa cells infected with adenovirus type 2, Mariman et al. provided evidence that adenoviral-specific nuclear matrix RNA contains precursors, intermediates, and products of RNA processing [39]. Other investigators have reported similar results [40–42]. Smith et al., using a previously isolated rat liver nuclear matrix protein and its corresponding antibody, provided evidence that the nuclear matrix does play a role in RNA splicing in vitro [43].

From the above-mentioned studies, it is easy to see why it has been proposed that the nuclear matrix is involved in gene regulation and expression. Gene expression can best be demonstrated by steroid hormones, which are thought to be involved in the transcriptional control of some genes. Barrack and Coffey used the induction of vitellogenin synthesis, which is a well-characterized model used in studying the regulation of specific gene expression by steroid hormones [44]. They found that nuclear matrix of an estrogen-responsive tissue (chicken liver) and of an androgen target tissue (rat ventral prostate) contained specific binding sites for both estradiol and dihydroxytestosterone, respectively. In addition, the levels of these matrix-associated steroid binding sites alter in response to changes of the hormonal status of the animal. In a later study, Barrack demonstrated the presence of specific acceptors for the androgen receptor in nuclear matrix of the prostate [45]. In addition, the majority of these acceptors were found in the internal network components of the matrix, while only 17% were found to be in the peripheral lamina. Kumara-Siri et al. reported that the T_3-nuclear receptor is associated with GC cells, suggesting that this association may help to regulate thyroid hormone action [46]. Ki-67, a mouse monoclonal antibody that recognizes a nuclear antigen expressed only in proliferating cells, also binds to the nuclear matrix and is now being introduced more into routine pathology [47]. It has also been observed that many of the nuclear matrix proteins are phosphorylated at specific times in the cell cycle. Phosphorylation is one common mechanism used by the cell to control gene expression. Henry and Hodge observed that there are changes in the phosphorylation pattern of several matrix proteins during the cell cycle [48].

Since the nuclear matrix plays crucial roles in the cell, it seems obvious to conclude that the nuclear matrix may play some role(s) in the development of cancer, perhaps as the result of protein alterations during transformation. Getzenberg et al. compared the nuclear matrix protein patterns from normal rat prostate and rat prostate tumors. Using two-dimensional gel electrophoresis, the complex mixture of nuclear matrix proteins was resolved. It was found that the protein pattern between prostate tumor nuclear matrix and normal nuclear matrix was different. In addition, the nuclear matrix proteins in several rat Dunning prostate adenocarcinoma lines were compared with the nuclear matrix composition of the dorsal prostate, the original tissue from which this tumor was derived. The nuclear matrix protein composition between the transformed cell lines contains a large number of common proteins, as well as nuclear matrix proteins that differed significantly from their tissue of origin [49]. These differences in the nuclear matrix protein composition could represent cell alterations during the tumor development. Pienta and Lehr went on to look at the protein composition of human prostate tumors as well as human prostate cell lines [50]. It was found that normal prostate cell transformation is accompanied by specific changes in nuclear matrix composition. Differences in nuclear matrix composition have also been reported in human hepatoma cells versus normal liver cells [51], human breast cancer tissue versus normal breast tissue [52], and in human laryngeal squamous cell carcinoma versus normal laryngeal epithelium [53].

Our laboratory has recently studied nuclear matrix protein composition of cancerous and normal breast tissue from 10 patients with infiltrating ductal carcinoma as well as the MCF-10 breast cell lines [52]. Using two-dimensional electrophoresis, it was found that the normal human breast tissue and tumor tissue possess a common set of nuclear matrix proteins as well as demonstrate specific protein protein changes. The two-dimensional patterns of nuclear matrix isolated from breast cancer tissue and normal breast tissue are shown in Figure 2A and 2B. A schematic representation illustrating the positions of proteins common to both normal and cancerous breast tissue, as well as proteins specific to each type of tissue, is given in Figure 3, and the molecular weights and the isoelectric points of several of these nuclear matrix proteins are listed in Table 2. We estimated that there were approximately 50–70 common proteins and arbitrarily identified 10 proteins that were common to all of the normal and malignant tissue samples and designated these *n*uclear *m*atrix *b*reast (NMB) 1–10. Four proteins were identified that were found only in the cancer specimens were identified as *n*uclear *m*atrix *b*reast *c*ancer (NMBC) W, X, Y, and Z (designated by arrows in Figure 2A). Two proteins were identified that were found only in normal tissue and not in the cancer specimens, and were designated *n*uclear *m*atrix *n*ormal *b*reast (NMNB) A and B (designated by arrows in Figure 2B).

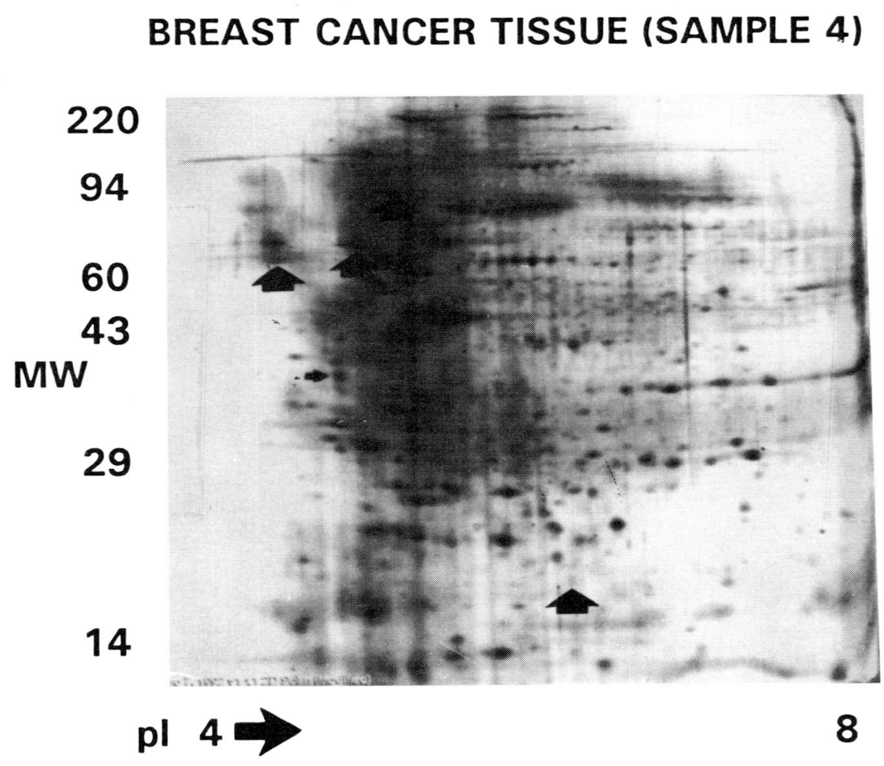

Figure 2. High-resolution, two-dimensional gel electrophoresis of nuclear matrix proteins. **A:** Infiltrating ductal carcinoma tissue, revealing four nuclear matrix proteins specific for breast cancer. **B:** Normal tissue from the same patient, revealing two nuclear matrix proteins specific for normal tissue as well as the absence of the four cancer-specific proteins.

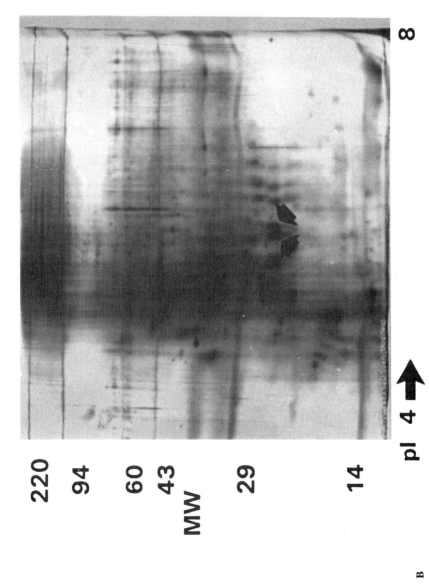

NORMAL BREAST TISSUE

220
94
60
43
MW
29

14

pl 4 → 8

B

Figure 2 (continued)

135

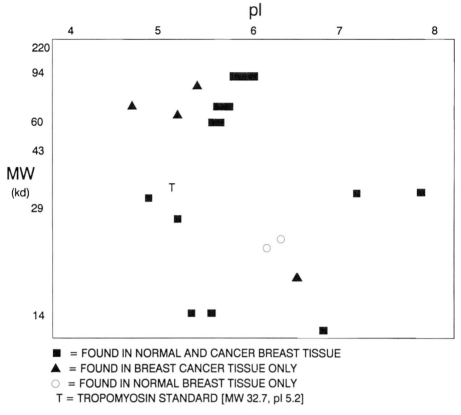

■ = FOUND IN NORMAL AND CANCER BREAST TISSUE
▲ = FOUND IN BREAST CANCER TISSUE ONLY
○ = FOUND IN NORMAL BREAST TISSUE ONLY
T = TROPOMYOSIN STANDARD [MW 32.7, pl 5.2]

Figure 3. Composite schematic representation of high-resolution gel electrophoresis shown in Figure 2A and 2B. Proteins common to all tissue are numbered 1–10. Cancer-specific proteins are labeled W, X, Y, and Z. Normal tissue specific proteins are labeled A and B.

These alterations in nuclear matrix protein composition found between the different tissue specimens could represent stromal or epithelial cell component changes. To help determine whether these changes were epithelial in origin, we investigated the nuclear matrix composition of the MCF-10 cell lines. The MCF-10 mortal line, the spontaneously immortalized MCF-10A, and the transfected variants of the immortalized line, H-RAS-MCF 10A and C-NEU-MCF10A, were all investigated. The MCF-10 cell line and its derivatives demonstrated a nuclear matrix phenotype that contained the proteins found in both normal and breast cancer tissue. These data suggest that these cell lines, which do not form tumors in athymic mice, may represent intermediate steps in the breast cancer transformation pathway. The nuclear matrix proteins that are lost and gained between normal and tumor tissues may be useful as intermediate endpoints or biomarkers if further characterization identifies them as mediators of transformation.

Table 2. Nuclear matrix proteins

Designation	M_2	Isoelectric point
NMB1[a]	12,000	6.8
NMB2	14,000	5.6
NMB3	14,000	5.7
NMB4	27,000	5.4
NMB5	30,000	4.9
NMB6	31,000	7.2
NMB7	31,000	7.8
NMB8	64,000	5.6–5.7
NMB9	76,000	5.7–5.9
NMB10	92,000	5.9–6.1
NMBC-W[b]	18,000	6.5
NMBC-X	62,000	5.3
NMBC-Y	64,000	4.7
NMBC-Z	80,000	5.5
NMNB-A[c]	24	6.2
NMNB-B	26	6.4

[a] NMB = nuclear matrix breast; NMB1-NMB10 are common nuclear matrix proteins found in both normal and cancerous breast.

[b] NMBC = nuclear matrix breast cancer; NMBC-W-NMBC-Z are nuclear proteins found in tumor samples but not in normal breast tissue.

[c] NMNB = nuclear matrix normal breast tissue; NMNB-A and NMNB-B are nuclear matrix proteins found in only normal breast tissue.

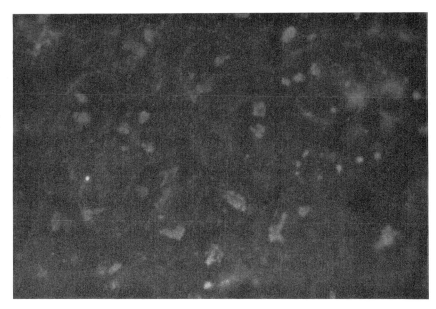

Figure 4. Expression of breast cancer-specific protein W. Immunohistochemistry utilizing a monoclonal antibody generated against protein W in the MCF10-A cell line. Protein W appears to localize to nucleoar regions, suggesting a possible role in transcription.

The determination of a function for a particular nuclear matrix protein is a tedious process. We have isolated NMBC-W by running multiple preparative gels of MCF-10A cells. After running approximately 400 mg of nuclear matrix protein on multiple gels, we cut the NMBC-W and produced a monoclonal antibody to spot W. In immunohistochemical experiments, this antibody targets nucleolar regions in the MCF10-A cells, suggesting that it may NMBC-W may have a role in transcription (Figure 4). This antibody will be utilized to screen cDNA libraries to elucidate the function of NMBC-W. By this method, our laboratory is currently isolating several nuclear matrix proteins. It is our belief that this approach will lead to a better understanding of the role of the nuclear matrix in cancer transformation, as well as identify potential intermediate biomarkers for breast cancer.

References

1. Pienta KJ, Murphy BC, Getzenberg RH, Coffey DS (1993) The tissue matrix and the regulation of gene expression in cancer cells. *Adv Mol Cell Biol* 7:131–156.
2. Mayer DT, Gulick A (1942) The nature of the proteins of cellular nuclei. *J Biol Chem* 146:433–440.
3. Smetana K, Steele WJ, Busch H (1963) A nuclear ribonucleoprotein network. *Exp Cell Res* 31:198–201.
4. Berezney R, Coffey DS (1974) Identification of a nuclear protein matrix. *Biochem Biophys Res Commun* 60:1410–1417.
5. Berezney R, Coffey DS (1977) Nuclear matrix: Isolation and characterization of a framework structure from rat liver nuclei. *J Cell Biol* 73:616–637.
6. Hancock R, Boulikas T (1982) Functional organization in the nucleus. *Int Rev Cytol* 79:165–214.
7. Verheijen R, Van Venrooij W, Ramaekers F (1988) The nuclear matrix: Structure and composition. 90:11–36.
8. Vogelstein B, Pardoll D, Coffey DS (1980) Supercoiled loops and eukaryotic DNA replication. *J Cell Science Cell* 22:79–85.
9. Ludérus MEE, de Graaf A, Mattia E, den Balen JL, Grande MA, de Jong L, Van Driel R (1992) Binding of matrix attachment regions to lamin B_1. *Cell* 70:949–959.
10. Hakes DJ, Berezney R (1991) DNA binding properties of the nuclear matrix and individual nuclear matrix proteins. *J Biol Chem* 266:11131–11140.
11. Romig H, Fackelmayer F, Renz A, Ramsperger U, Richter A (1992) Characterization of SAF-A, a novel nuclear DNA binding protein from HeLa cells with high affinity for nuclear matrix/scaffold attachment DNA elements. *EMBO J* 11:3431–3440.
12. Dickinson LA, Joh T, Kohwi Y, Kohwi-Shigematsu T (1992) A tissue-specific MAR/SAR DNA-binding protein with unusual binding site recognition. *Cell* 70:631–645.
13. Durfee T, Mancini MA, Jones D, Elledge SJ, Lew WH (1994) The amino-terminal region of the retinoblastoma gene product binds a novel nuclear matrix protein that colocalizes to centers for RNA processing. *J Cell Biol* 127:609–622.
14. Pardoll DM, Vogelstein B, Coffey DS (1980) A fixed site of DNA replication in eukaryotic cells. *Cell* 19:527–536.
15. Van der Velden HMU, Van Willigen G, Wetzels RHW, Wanka F (1984) Attachment of origin of replication to the nuclear matrix and the chromosome scaffold. *FEBS Lett* 171:13–16.
16. Berezney R, Coffey DS (1975) Nuclear protein matrix: Association with newly synthesized DNA. *Science* 189:291–292.

17. Reddy GPV, Pardee AB (1980) Multienzyme complex for metabolic channeling in mammalian DNA replication. *Proc Natl Acad Sci USA* 77:3312–3316.
18. Earnshaw WC, Heck MM (1985) Localization of topoisomerase I in mitotic chromosomes. *J Cell Biol* 100:1716–1725.
19. Berezney R, Buchholtz LA (1981) Dynamic association of replicating DNA fragments with the nuclear matrix of regenerating liver. *Exp Cell Res* 132:1–13.
20. Valenzuela MS, Mueller GC, Dasgupta S (1983) Nuclear matrix-DNA complex resulting from EcoRI digestion of HeLa nucleoids is enriched for DNA replicating forks. *Nucleic Acids Res* 11:2155–2164.
21. Tubo RA, Smith HC, Berezney R (1985) The nuclear matrix continues DNA synthesis at in vivo replicational forks. *Biochem Biophys Acta* 825:326–334.
22. Younghusband HB (1985) An association between replicating adenovirus DNA and the nuclear matrix of infected HeLa cells. *Can J Biochem Cell Biol* 63:654–660.
23. Smith HC, Berezney R (1980) DNA polymerase α is tightly bound to the nuclear matrix of actively replicating liver. *Biochem Biophys Res Commun* 97:1541–1547.
24. Nickerson JA, Krochmalnic G, Wan KM, Penman S (1989) Chromatin architecture and nuclear RNA. *Proc Natl Acad Sci USA* 86:177–181.
25. Herlan G, Eckert WA, Kaffenberger W, Wunderlich F (1979) Isolation and characterization of a RNA-containing nuclear matrix from *Tetrahymena* macronuclei. *Biochemistry* 18:1782–1788.
26. Nakayasu H, Mori H, Ueda K (1982) Association of small nuclear RNA-protein complex with the nuclear matrix from bovine lymphocytes. *Cell Struct Funct* 7:253–262.
27. Herman R, Weymouth L, Penman S (1978) Heterogenous nuclear RNA-protein fibers in chromatin-depleted nuclei. *J Cell Biol* 78:663–674.
28. Miller TE, Huang CY, Pogo AO (1978) Rat liver nuclei skeleton and ribonucleoprotein complexes containing hnRNA. *J Cell Biol* 76:675–691.
29. Van Eekelen CAG, van Venrooij WJ (1981) hnRNA and its attachment to a nuclear protein matrix. *J Cell Biol* 88:554–563.
30. Ciejek EM, Nordstrom JL, Tsai MJ, O'Malley BW (1982) Ribonucleic acid precursors are associated with the chick oviduct nuclear matrix. *Biochemistry* 21:4945–4953.
31. Jackson DA, McCready SJ, Cook PR (1981) RNA is synthesized at the nuclear cage. *Nature* 292:552–555.
32. Cook PR, Lang J, Hayday A, Lania L, Fried M, Chiswell DJ, Wyke JA (1982) Active viral genes in transformed cells lie close to the nuclear cage. *EMBO J* 1:447–452.
33. Robinson SI, Small D, Idzerda R, McKnight GS, Vogelstein B (1983) The association of transcriptionally active genes with the nuclear matrix of the chick oviduct. *Nucleic Acids Res* 11:5113–5130.
34. Ciejek EM, Tsai MJ, O'Malley BW (1983) Actively transcribed genes are associated with the nuclear matrix. *Nature* 306:607–609.
35. Abulafia R, Ben-Zeev A, Hay N, Aloni Y (1984) Control of late simian virus 40 transcription by the attenuation mechanism and transcriptionally active ternary complexes are associated with the nuclear matrix. *J Mol Biol* 172:467–487.
36. Jost JP, Seldran M (1984) Association of transcriptionally active vitellogenin II gene with the nuclear matrix of chicken liver. *EMBO J* 3:2005–2008.
37. Hentzen PC, Rho JH, Bekhor I (1984) Nuclear matrix DNA from chicken erythrocytes contains B-globin gene sequences. *Proc Natl Acad Sci USA* 81:304–307.
38. Bidwell JP, Van Wijen AJ, Fey EG, Dworetzky S, Penman S, Stein JL, Lian JB, Stein GS (1993) Osteocalcin gene promoter-binding factors are tissue-specific nuclear matrix components. *Proc Natl Acad Sci USA* 90:3162–3166.
39. Mariman ECM, Van Eekelen CAG, Reinders RJ, Berns AJM, Van Venrooij WJ (1982) Adenoviral heterogenous nuclear RNA is associated with the host nuclear matrix during splicing. *J Mol Biol* 154:103–119.
40. Long BH, Ochs RL (1983) Nuclear matrix, hnRNA, and snRNA in Friend erythroleukemia nuclei depleted of chromatin by low ionic strength EDTA. *Biol Cell* 48:89–98.

41. Long BH, Schrier WH (1983) Isolation from Friend erythroleukemia cells of an RNase-sensitive nuclear matrix fibril fraction containing hnRNA and snRNA. *Biol Cell* 48:99–108.
42. Ben-Zeev A, Aloni Y (1983) Processing of SV40 RNA is associated with the nuclear matrix and is not followed by the accumulation of low-molecular-weight RNA products. *Virology* 125:475–479.
43. Smith HC, Harris SG, Zillman M, Berget SM (1989) Evidence that a nuclear matrix protein participates in premessenger RNA splicing. *Exp Cell Res* 182:521–533.
44. Barrack ER, Coffey DS (1980) The specific binding of estrogens and androgens to the nuclear matrix of sex hormone responsive tissues. *J Biol Chem* 255:7265–7275.
45. Barrack ER (1983) The nuclear matrix of the prostate contains acceptor sites for androgen receptors. *Endocrinology* 113:430–432.
46. Kumara-Siri MH, Shapiro LE, Surks MI (1986) Association of the 3, 5, 3'-triiodo-L-thyronine nuclear receptor with the nuclear matrix of cultured growth hormone-producing rat pituitary tumor cells (GC cells). *J Biol Chem* 271:2844–2852.
47. Verheijen R, Kuijpers HJH, Schlingemann RO, Boehmer ALM, Van Driel R, Brakenhoff GJ, Ramaekers FCS (1989) Ki-67 detects a nuclear matrix-associated proliferation-related antigen. I. Intracellular localization during interphase. *J Cell Sci* 92:123–130.
48. Henry SM, Hodge LD (1983) Nuclear matrix: A cell-cycle-dependent site of increased intranuclear protein phsophorylation. *Eur J Biochem* 133:23–29.
49. Getzenberg RH, Pienta KJ, Huang EY, Coffey DS (1991) Identification of nuclear matrix proteins in the cancer and normal rat prostate. *Cancer Res* 51:6514–6520.
50. Pienta KJ, Lehr JE (1993) A common set of nuclear matrix proteins in prostate cancer cells. *Prostate* 23:61–67.
51. Berezney R, Basler J, Hughes BB, Kaplan SC (1979) Isolation and characterization of the nuclear matrix from *Zajdela ascites* hepatoma cells. *Cancer Res* 39:3031–3039.
52. Khanuja PS, Lehr JE, Soule HD, Gehani SK, Noto AC, Choudhury S, Chen R, Pienta KJ (1993) Nuclear matrix proteins in normal and breast cancer cells. *Cancer Res* 53:3394–3398.
53. Donat TL, Sakr W, Lehr JE, Pienta KJ (1996) Nuclear matrix protein alteration in intermediate biomarkers in squamous cell carcinoma of the head and neck. *Otolaryngol Head Neck Surge.*

8. Cyclins and breast cancer

Kimberley J.E. Sweeney, Elizabeth A. Musgrove, Colin K.W. Watts,
and Robert L. Sutherland

Introduction

There is unequivocal evidence that cancer is a disease resulting from abnormal
gene function [1]. In the past 20 years, up to 100 positively acting oncogenes [2]
have been identified, along with a dozen negatively acting tumor suppressor
genes [3]. The proteins encoded by the majority of these genes are components
of growth regulatory pathways, that is, they are growth factor receptors, signaling molecules, transcription factors, and proteins involved in entry into,
progression through, and exit from the cell cycle. It is not surprising, therefore,
that the cyclins, a family of molecules that play a central role in regulating
progression through the cell cycle, have been implicated in oncogenesis.

In eukaryotic cells, specific classes of cyclin regulatory subunits form complexes with cyclin dependent kinase (CDK) molecules to form active holoen-
zymes that are responsible for controlling cell cycle transitions during different
phases of the cell cycle. Although the mechanistic basis for control of cell cycle
progression during G_1, S phase, and mitosis has largely been defined in studies
using nonmammalian species, particularly yeast [4], a clear pattern of sequential cyclin induction and CDK activation in mammalian cells is now emerging
and is summarized in Figure 1.

The A and B type cyclins, which were the first to be identified, are partners
for Cdk2 and Cdc2, and are active in the S and G_2/M phases of the cell cycle.
These cyclins must be destroyed for the cells to exit mitosis, and hence in
normal cells overexpression of these genes leads to cell cycle arrest rather than
unbridled cell cycle progression [5]. Cyclin E/Cdk2 and cyclin D/Cdk4 or
cyclin D/Cdk6 complexes are active during the G_1 phase of the cell cycle and
are induced in response to growth factor stimulation. Activation of these
complexes allows cells to pass through G_1 and become committed to DNA
synthesis and cell division. These processes do not require the complete
destruction of the G_1 cyclins. Thus, of the cyclins, G_1 cyclins are the most likely
to act as oncogenes through overexpression or activating mutations. It is
conceivable, however, that the perturbation of any of the cyclin complexes
could lead to deregulation of all other checkpoints in the cell cycle, since
interconnections between the various cyclins, such as common negative regu-

*R. Dickson and M. Lippman (eds.) MAMMARY TUMOR CELL CYCLE, DIFFERENTIATION AND
METASTASIS. 1996. Kluwer Academic Publishers. ISBN 0-7923-3905-3. All rights reserved.*

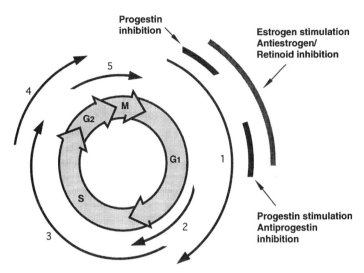

Figure 1. Points of action of cyclins, CDKs, and steroids during the cell cycle. The mammalian cell cycle consists of four distinct phases, designated G_1, DNA synthesis or S phase, G_2, and mitosis, as illustrated. The proposed points of action of estrogens and progestins, and their antagonists and retinoic acid, are shown. The sequence of cyclin–CDK complex formation throughout the cell cycle and their times of maximal activity are also shown schematically. After stimulation of breast cancer cells by mitogens or estrogens, progression through the cell cycle is accompanied by cyclin D/Cdk4 kinase activity (1), followed by cyclin E/Cdk2 activity at the G_1/S phase boundary (2), and cyclin A/Cdk2 activity upon entry into the S phase (3). During late S phase, cyclin A associates with Cdc2 to perform its functions during the G_2/M phase of the cell cycle (4) and cyclin B/Cdc2 complexes are formed in late G_2 to become activated during mitosis (5).

lators, exist. There is also the possibility that overexpression of one cyclin is able to usurp the role of other cyclin/CDK complexes. Additionally, several reports describe relationships between cyclin/CDK complexes and known oncoproteins and tumor suppressors, for example, Myc, Ras, Rb, and p53. A key question in determining a role for cyclins in oncogenesis is whether cyclins themselves have oncogenic potential or if oncogenic proteins exert their effects by binding or activating cyclin/CDK complexes to deregulate ordered progression through the cell cycle.

This chapter reviews the roles of cyclins in mammalian cell cycle progression, illustrating how these molecules can become dysregulated and in so doing potentially contribute to the initiation and progression of breast cancer. This includes discussion of the documented aberrant expression of various cyclins and related molecules in human breast cancer cells and the likely implications of these changes, based on an emerging understanding of the role of these genes in mediating the growth stimulatory effects of steroid and growth factor mitogens and the growth inhibitory effects of steroid antagonists and differentiation agents.

Role of cyclins, cyclin dependent kinases, and associated proteins in cell cycle control

The contemporary model of the mammalian cell cycle is an increasingly complex system of checks and balances with a currency of phosphates. Progression through the cell cycle is controlled by the sequential formation, activation, and inactivation of cyclin/CDK complexes. Each CDK phosphorylates specific substrates, many of which remain to be identified, orchestrating the appropriate changes necessary for progression through that checkpoint in the cell cycle [6]. The cyclin/CDK complexes are subject to several levels of control [7]. First, most cyclins are only available at the appropriate time in the cell cycle due to precise control of their abundance. Secondly, the CDKs are regulated post-transcriptionally by reversible phosphorylation by phosphatases and CDK activating kinases (CAK, itself a cyclin/CDK complex regulated by phosphorylation, e.g., cyclin H/Cdk7 is the CAK that phosphorylates Cdc2). Finally, the cyclin/CDK complexes have to contend with small protein molecules that inhibit their kinase activity (CDK inhibitors), including p15, p16, p21, and p27.

Roles in S and G_2/M phase

The cyclin B protein, which is predominantly involved in control in G_2 and at mitosis, is synthesized during the S and G_2 phases of the cell cycle, where it binds to the Cdc2 molecule. The Cdc2-cyclin B complex was initially called the *maturation promoting factor* (MPF), based on it first being identified as a critical component for oocyte maturation, and promotes G_2/M transition in all eukaryotes that have been studied [4]. Ectopic expression of cyclin B in rat fibroblasts results in increased Cdc2 kinase activity, but there is no change in the rate of cell cycle progression [8]. Conversely, early studies involving microinjection of Cdc2 into mammalian fibroblasts resulted in events that mimic those occurring during the early phases of mitosis, including the rounding up of cells, loss of the cell-substratum interaction, reduction of interphase microtubules, actin microfilament redistribution, and premature chromatin condensation. These cells did not pass further into division; nonetheless, these experiments provided evidence that Cdc2 activation plays a key role in the rearrangement of cellular structures associated with mammalian cell mitosis [9].

The primary function of cyclin A is to control progression through S phase and, as with cyclin B, this property is common to all eukaryotes. The promoter of cyclin A is repressed during the early and mid G_1 phase of the cell cycle and is activated at the beginning of S phase [10]. Microinjection of cyclin A antibody inhibits both DNA synthesis and entry into mitosis [11]. Cyclin A, therefore, is recognized as having two roles in the cell cycle: one in G_2 with Cdc2 as the partner and the other in S phase with the formation of cyclin A/Cdk2 complexes. Likely S phase substrates for cyclin A/Cdk2 include the single-stranded DNA-binding replication protein A [12,13], indicating a role in DNA replication itself.

In both NRK and NIH3T3 fibroblasts, the appearance of cyclin A mRNA and protein in late G_1 is dependent on cell adhesion. Transfection of NRK cells with a cyclin A cDNA resulted in adhesion-independent accumulation of cyclin A protein and cyclin A–associated kinase activity, allowing these cells to enter the S phase and to complete multiple rounds of cell division in the absence of cellular adhesion. Thus, the cyclin A promoter is also the target of the adhesion-dependent signals that control cell proliferation [14]. This loss of cell adhesion is a common trait of transformed cells.

Roles of cyclins in G_1 phase

In budding yeast the G_1 to S phase transition is accompanied by the accumulation of a novel family of G_1 cyclins (Clns), distinct from the cyclins that are required for progression through G_2 and M phases [15]. G_1 cyclins with analogous functions exist in mammalian cells and include cyclin E, cyclin C, and the D-type cyclin family, cyclins D1, D2, and D3. In mammalian cells, the G_1 phase of the cell cycle is the primary point of action for growth regulating factors, and therefore studying the cyclins involved in the regulation of this phase of the cell cycle is pertinent to the loss of normal growth control in cancer. Figure 2 illustrates the intricate network of regulatory pathways, both proven and hypothesized to exist, in the G_1 phase of the cell cycle. The presence of seemingly redundant checks and balances may reflect the importance of G_1 cyclins in reacting appropriately to outside stimuli and either initiating the cell cycle, directing the cell into the quiescent G_0 phase, or initiating a pathway of terminal differentiation.

It is now clear that cyclin E has a major role in controlling G_1/S phase transition. Cyclin E gene expression is increased in mid to late G_1 phase, and levels of cyclin E protein are maximal during late G_1 [16,17]. Cyclin E-associated kinase activity, which is maximal in late G_1, is regulated by both phosphorylation of the Cdk2 subunit and accumulation of cyclin E protein. Ectopic expression of cyclin E in fibroblasts and HeLa cells causes a shortening of the G_1 phase, often accompanied by diminished cell size [8,18,19]. Although overexpression of cyclin E diminished the serum requirement of some cells, they did not become serum independent. Indeed, rat fibroblasts overexpressing cyclin E retain the ability to quiesce under serum-free conditions [8].

The three D-type cyclins — D1, D2, and D3 — are differentially expressed in various cell types; for example, cyclin D2 rather than cyclin D1 is expressed in hemopoietic cells. In contrast to the other cyclins, the abundance of D-type cyclins does not oscillate dramatically throughout the cell cycle, although immunohistochemical studies demonstrate that cyclin D1 protein is predominantly nuclear during G_1 phase but cytoplasmic in S phase [20].

144

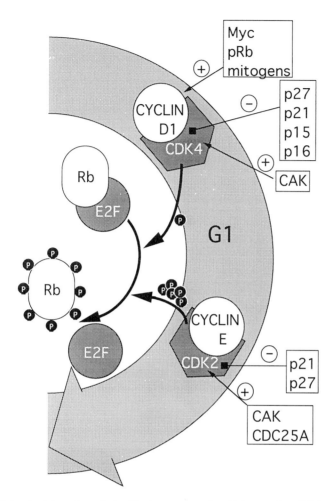

Figure 2. Molecular interactions during G_1 phase progression. D-type cyclins, Cdk4 and Cdk6, are induced as part of the delayed early response to mitogens in cells entering the G_1 phase. Myc and pRb may also stimulate cyclin D1 expression. pRb is initially present in its inhibitory hypophosphorylated form, sequestering transcription factors such as E2F. Cyclin D-bound Cdk4 or Cdk6 must be phosphorylated by CAK to become enzymatically active. The kinase activity of this cyclin/CDK complex is negatively regulated by the CDK inhibitors, p15, p16, p21, and p27. Cyclin E is expressed later in G_1 phase, binds to CDK2, and the associated kinase activity is regulated in a similar manner to cyclin D/CDK4 by CAK, CDC25A, and the p21 and p27 CDK inhibitors. The activation of the G_1 CDK complexes results in the accumulation of inactive hyperphosphorylated pRb and consequently the release of the E2F transcription factor.

The effect of ectopic expression of either cyclin D2 or D3 depends on the cell type studied. NIH3T3 cells engineered to express both cyclin D3 and its partner Cdk4 did not undergo significant phenotypic changes despite supraphysiological levels of kinase activity [21]. These cells do not ordinarily express cyclin D3. In contrast, overexpression of cyclin D2 or D3 in hemopoietic 32Dc13 cells, which normally express both proteins, resulted in an increased number of cells in S phase, apparently related to a shortening of G_1. Unlike stimulation with cyclin E, this was not accompanied by a change in cell size, nor was it associated with a change in cell viability, the rate of cell proliferation, or dependence on exogenous mitogens [22]. The constitutive expression of cyclin D2 in these cells was not accompanied by an increase in the cyclin D2–associated pRb kinase activity [23], suggesting that cyclin D2 may be altering the distribution of cells through the cell cycle in a manner independent of CDK-associated activity. Quelle et al. also observed an acceleration from G_0 to S phase in rodent fibroblasts engineered to overexpress cyclin D2 [24].

Of all the G_1 cyclins, cyclin D1 has been studied in most detail. Several methods have been employed for the ectopic expression of cyclin D1 in a variety of fibroblast cells, all with the same general conclusion: Overexpression of cyclin D1 causes a shortening of G_1 phase but the cells remain serum dependent [8,24,25]. The assembly of the holoenzyme cyclin D1/Cdk4 was rate limiting for progression through G_1 in quiescent cells stimulated to progress into the S phase, and the kinase activity lagged behind the appearance of cyclin D1 protein, paralleling the appearance of Cdk4 [21]. The rate-limiting event was the activation of Cdk4 by CAK, which was present in proliferating cells but present and inactive in cells emerging from quiescence [26]. Evidence that cyclin D1 is necessary for cell cycle progression is provided by studies that showed microinjection of a cyclin D1 antibody prevented cells from entering S phase [27].

Two independent studies have examined the role of cyclin D1 in the G_1 to S transition in cancer cells. Expression of cyclin D1 under the control of an inducible promoter and microinjection of cyclin D1 antibodies demonstrated that the protein is rate limiting for G_1 transit and is necessary for progression into S phase [28,29]. The dependence of cell cycle progression on cyclin D1 does, however, require functional pRb [20]. In T-47D breast cancer cells, induction of cyclin D1 was sufficient for growth arrested cells to complete a round of cell division in the complete absence of exogenous growth factors [28]. Thus cyclin D1 was both necessary and sufficient for cell cycle progression, in marked contrast to normal fibroblasts, in which cyclin D1 regulated the rate of G_1 progression but could not replace the requirement for serum to stimulate proliferation.

Roles in differentiation and senescence

Although investigations of cyclin/CDK function and regulation have concentrated on their roles in the control of proliferation, there is accumulating evidence for cyclin/CDK involvement in differentiation and senescence. Differentiation of myeloid cells can be blocked by altering the expression of cyclin D genes. These cells normally express cyclins D2 and D3 but not cyclin D1.

146

Upon differentiation these cyclins cease to be expressed, although the levels of their kinase partners Cdk4 and Cdk2 are sustained. Constitutive expression of cyclin D2 or D3, but not D1, stopped the cells from differentiating.

Changes in cyclin gene expression during terminal differentiation are cell type specific and include induction of expression, an unexpected finding in view of the cell cycle arrest accompanying differentiation, but understandable when one notes that induction of the CDK inhibitor, p21, is a common feature of differentiated cells [30]. L6 skeletal muscle precursors, for example, exhibit little change in the levels of cyclins D1 and D2 upon differentiation but undergo a significant increase in the amount of cyclin D3, although the D3 protein was not part of an active complex [31]. There are no published data from breast epithelial cells, although treatment of some breast cancer cell lines with differentiation agents is associated with decreased expression of cyclin D1, elevated levels of cyclin D3 and E, and increased expression of the CDK inhibitor, p21 [deFazio et al., unpublished data].

Senescence is a state of irreversible cell cycle arrest when cells reach the end of their life span and fail to enter DNA synthesis, even when serum stimulated. In senescent human fibroblasts, cyclin A and Cdc2 are downregulated, and constitutive expression of active cyclin A and Cdc2 does not prevent senescence [32]. Independent studies have reported both modestly reduced expression and overexpression of cyclins D1 and E, respectively, in senescent cells [32,33]. The latter report noted that the accumulated cyclin E/Cdk2 complexes in senescent cells harbored very little kinase activity, and an unexpected finding was that the majority of the Cdk2 was associated with cyclin D1 in an inactive complex. Again, this may be due to the increased expression of the CDK inhibitor p21 in senescent cells [34].

Interaction of the G_1 cyclins and the tumor suppressor pRb

Cyclins and CDKs interact with cellular proteins, in addition to those that directly regulate the activity of the complex. These include the product of the retinoblastoma susceptibility gene, pRb. In its hypophosphorylated state, pRb binds and thus inhibits a number of transcription factors, for example, E2F. Hyperphosphorylation and concomitant inactivation of the pRb protein, resulting in the release of bound transcription factors, occurs in late G_1 phase and is necessary for cell cycle progression. Cyclin D/Cdk4 and cyclin D/Cdk6 complexes are pRb kinases in vitro [21]. These cyclin D–associated kinases, together with cyclin E/Cdk2, are also believed to be the important Rb kinases in vivo [35].

D-type cyclins bind directly to the pRb protein, suggesting that these cyclins both regulate CDK activity and direct the kinase to the pRb substrate [36]. Several transfection studies in Saos cells, which do not express pRb, have demonstrated that expression of pRb causes cell cycle arrest. Coexpression of cyclin D1 and pRb results in the cells being rescued from their arrest, but this does not coincide with the expected hyperphosphorylation of pRb [37]. This suggests that cyclin D1 is not solely bound to pRb in order to phosphorylate the molecule but may have as yet undefined functions in cell cycle progression. There is, however, a codependent relationship between cyclin D1 and pRb. Cells that do not express functional pRb and express only very low levels of cyclin D1 mRNA and protein fail to form cyclin D1/Cdk4 or cyclin D1/Cdk6 complexes [38,39]. Consequently, these cells have been relieved of the necessity for cyclin D1 function in the G_1 phase of the cell cycle, as shown by lack of cell cycle arrest following microinjection of cyclin D1 antibodies into such cells [29]. Furthermore, cells lacking endogenous pRb take on an absolute need for cyclin D1 upon reintroduction of pRb, and microinjection of cyclin D1 antibodies under these circumstances causes cells to arrest in G_1 [29].

The relationship between cyclin D1 and pRb is regulatory as well as functional, since cyclin D1 promoter activity is stimulated, either directly or indirectly, by the pRb protein, suggesting cyclin D1 is also an object of pRb regulation [40]. This implies the existence of an autoregulatory loop in G_1 in which hypophosphorylated pRb binds to transcription factors and inhibits cell cycle progression while stimulating the expression of pRb. Upon formation and activation of the cyclin D1/Cdk4 complex phosphorylation, and hence inactivation, of the pRb protein is initiated, thus unleashing pRb-bound transcription factors but at the same time relieving stimulation of the cyclin D1 promoter [41]. A further degree of complexity in this association has arisen with data demonstrating that coexpression of wild-type cyclin D1 with a mutated form of cyclin D1 unable to bind pRb results in an increased percentage of cells rescued from a pRb-induced block [42]. Clearly, the interaction between cyclin D1 and pRb is not a simple enzyme/substrate interaction, and the many facets of this relationship have yet to be assimilated.

In summary, a model of cell cycle progression in G_1 phase involves transcriptional activation of D type cyclin gene expression followed by assembly and activation of cyclin D/Cdk4 or /Cdk6 complexes, which independently or together with cyclin E/Cdk2 phosphorylate pRb and relieve its inhibitory role by releasing E2F and other transcription factors essential for progression through S phase. While this is clearly an oversimplification, as evidence by the data cited earlier, it provides a framework for interpretation of the likely consequences of aberrant cyclin gene expression in breast cancer.

Expression and regulation of cyclins in breast cancer cells

Early studies on cell cycle control in hormone-responsive breast cancer cell lines showed that these cells are responsive to growth factors, steroids, and steroid agonists during the G_1 phase of the cell cycle [43] (see Figure 1). At that time, the target genes mediating the growth factor and steroid effects were largely unknown. However, the emerging role for G_1 cyclins in the control of G_1 progression indicated that these genes were likely targets for the mitogenic and inhibitory effects of steroids and their antagonists. The potential actions of such factors on cyclin function could be manifest at several levels, including direct transcriptional control, post-transcriptional regulation, regulation of CDK inhibitors and complex formation, changes in protein degradation machinery, or possibly alterations in spatiotemporal distributions.

Expression of cyclins in breast epithelial cells

The differential expression of various cyclin genes has been investigated in both normal and neoplastic breast epithelial cell lines [44,45]. These cells represent a variety of phenotypes, ranging from more differentiated cell lines that are estrogen receptor–positive and hormone responsive, to estrogen receptor–negative, hormone-independent cell lines that represent more aggressive, less differentiated tumors. Evidence of aberrant cyclin expression in breast cancer has been obtained. Cyclin A mRNA levels are increased in two lines, MDA-MB-157 and BT-549, while increased mRNA expression of cyclin B1 was also observed in BT-549 cells. Cyclin E mRNA was overexpressed in one cell line, MDA-MB-157, at a level which was estimated to be some 64-fold increase compared with normal cells and resulted in marked overproduction of the cyclin E protein. There was little variability in cyclin D3 mRNA expression between the cell lines examined, although Tam et al. found this protein was overexpressed in MCF-7 cells [46]. Cyclin D2 mRNA, however, was abundant in normal breast epithelial cells but was expressed at very low levels or was absent in most breast cancer cell lines [44]. This has been confirmed at the protein level [46] and raises the interesting possibility that loss of expression of cyclin D2 is in some way associated with transformation and oncogenesis.

   Cyclin D1 mRNA was highly expressed in MDA–MB-134, -175, -330, -453, and MCF-7M compared with the levels observed in other breast cancer lines and two normal breast epithelial lines. Other researchers observed elevated cyclin D1 mRNA expression in T-47D cells [47] as well as ZR-75 and CAMA cells [48]. Very low levels of cyclin D1 mRNA expression were noted in two breast cancer cell lines (DU-4475 and BT-549) and in HBL-100, a cell line derived from normal breast epithelial cells but containing SV40 sequences. Cyclin D1 protein expression is generally consistent with these observations of cyclin D1 mRNA [39,46]. The very low expression of cyclin D1 in two cell lines and reduced expression in some others is likely to be associated with deletion or inactivation of pRb [46,49]. The mRNA expression of G1 cyclins, p16, and the state of the pRb protein for several cell lines are compared in Table 1.

Cyclin gene amplification in breast cancer cell lines

To determine if the increased expression of certain cyclin genes observed in these breast cancer cell lines was due to gene amplification, gene copy number

Table 1. Relationship between G1 cyclin mRNA expression, p16 mRNA (*INK* 4) expression, and Rb mutation

Cell line	Cyclin				*INK 4*	RB inactivation
	D1	D2	D3	E		
Normal breast Cells	+ +	+ + + +	+ +	+ +	+	nd
MCF-7M	+ + + +	+	nd	+ +	−	−
MCF-7	+ + + +	−	+ + + +	+ +	−	−
ZR-75-T	+ + + +	nd	+ + + +	+ +	nd	nd
ZR-75-1	+ +	−	nd	+ +	+	−
BT-474	+ +	−	nd	+ +	+	−
BT-483	+ +	−	nd	+ +	+	−
BT-20	+ +	−	+ +	+ +	−	−
BT-549	+	−	nd	+ +	+ + + +	+
MDA-MB-134	+ + + +	+ +	nd	+ +	+	−
MDA-MB-361	+ +	−	nd	+ +	+	−
MDA-MB-157	+/+ +	−	+ + + +	+ + + +	+ + + +	−
MDA-MB-175	+ + + +	−	nd	+ +	+	−
MDA-MB-330	+ + + +	−	nd	+ +	−	−
MDA-MB-453	+ + + +	−	nd	+ +	+	−
MDA-MB-231	+ +	−	+ + + +	+ +	−	−
MDA-MB-436	+ +/+	−	+ +	+ +	+ + + +	+
MDA-MB-468	+ +/+	−	nd	+ +	+ + + +	+
T-47D	+ +	−	+ +	+ +	+	−
DU-4475	+	−	nd	+ +	+	+
Hs-578T	+ +	−	+ + + +	+ +	−	−
SK-BR-3	+ +	−	+ +	+ +	+	−
HBL-100	+	−	+ +	+ +	+ + + +	+

p16 mRNA (INK 4) expression; −, not expressed; +, normal level expression; + + + +, overexpression; nd, not determined (ref. 49).

Cyclin mRNA expression: −, undetectable expression; +, weak expression; + +, moderate expression, + + + +, overexpression; + +/+, differing reports from independent studies; nd, not determined. Cyclin data collated from references 39, 44–48.

RB: +, mutation present; nd, not determined; −, normal gene present. Rb data from references 39, 142–144.

was determined by Southern blot analysis. In MDA–MB-157 cells, an eight-fold amplification of the cyclin E gene accompanied increased expression [44,50]. Cyclin D1 gene amplification was detected in six cell lines, but amplification was not a prerequisite for increased cyclin D1 expression. No gross rearrangements were noted for any of the genes examined, although a subsequent study identified a truncation of the cyclin D1 gene in the MDA–MB-453 cell line [51]. Thus aberrant expression of cyclins typically involves deregulated expression of a normal protein rather than expression of a mutated protein.

150

Cyclin dependent kinase expression in breast epithelial cell lines

Protein expression of Cdc2 or Cdk2 does not vary dramatically between breast cancer cell lines and normal breast epithelial cells (unpublished data); this result is consistent with a study of 12 breast cancer cell lines that revealed only moderate variations in the expression of Cdc2 protein [52]. These data are in marked contrast to the study of Keyomarsi and Pardee in which Cdc2 was overexpressed at both the mRNA and protein level in 9 of 10 breast cancer cell lines when compared with normal breast epithelial cells [45].

Tam et al. examined the protein expression of the two G_1 CDKs, Cdk4 and Cdk6 [46]. Cdk6 protein was undetectable in any of the cell lines examined, although we have observed strong mRNA expression in normal breast epithelial cells and in MDA–MB-157 and DU-4475 breast cancer cells. Cdk4 was expressed in all cell lines investigated at levels that varied widely when compared with the expression of the other CDKs. Two cell lines that lacked cyclin D1 protein had exceptionally high levels of Cdk4 protein (HBL-100 and BT-549). Conversely, the cell line with the highest level of cyclin D1 protein (MDA–MB-134) also exhibited high levels of Cdk4. Whether this is translated into increased activity of cyclin D1/Cdk4 complexes in this cell line is yet to be established. Thus there is evidence for aberrant expression of selected CDK molecules in some breast cancer cell lines, although the functional consequences of these changes have yet to be defined. Furthermore, there are no published data on tumor samples to determine if similar lesions occur in clinical breast cancer, and if so at what frequency.

Cell cycle oscillations of cyclin expression in breast cancer cells

The expression of cyclin genes at various stages of the cell cycle and following mitogen stimulation has been examined in normal breast epithelial cells and in several breast cancer cell lines [45,53–55]. These studies involved monitoring cyclin gene expression following release from a block in cell cycle progression [45] or growth factor stimulation of growth arrested cells [53]. Serum-starved T-47D cells stimulated to re-enter the cell cycle with insulin [54] showed the sequential induction of cyclin expression depicted in Figure 3. The sequence and timing of increased expression of cyclin D1 in early to mid G_1, cyclin D3 later in G_1, cyclin E in late G_1, cyclin A in S phase, and cyclin B1 during G_2/M was common to growth factor stimulation of both normal breast epithelial cells and breast cancer cells [45,53,54]. Indeed, mRNA changes for cyclins A, E, and B and kinases Cdc2 and Cdk2 were generally consistent with results obtained using mitogen-stimulated fibroblasts and HeLa cells [56,57], supporting the view that these are critical events conserved in mammalian cell cycle progression.

Studies comparing synchronized normal breast and breast cancer cells suggested that the basal levels of cyclins A and B in G_1 phase in tumor cells were significantly higher than the negligible levels detected in normal cells. It was

151

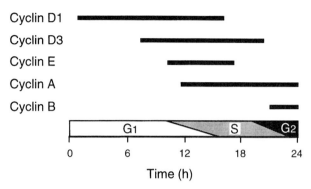

Figure 3. Sequential induction of cyclin mRNA in T-47D cells. Sequential induction of cyclin mRNA following growth factor stimulation of T-47D breast cancer cells. Bars indicate approximate times of maximum expression of individual cyclins after growth factor stimulation of growth-arrested cells at 0 hours.

proposed the untimely appearance of these cyclins in G_1 may contribute to loss of normal growth control in breast cancer [45]. Although high basal expression may be a consequence of the synchronization methods employed, two-parameter flow cytometry to examine cyclin expression in different phases of the cell cycle has confirmed that in some breast cancer cell lines, cyclins E and B are expressed during phases of the cell cycle when their expression was expected to be negligible [58,59]. Whether this cell cycle phase–independent expression is associated with inappropriately timed kinase activity remains to be determined. Nevertheless, the various cyclins reached peak abundance in the same sequence in normal and neoplastic cells.

These studies also demonstrated that in normal breast epithelial cells cyclin D1 mRNA expression was rapidly downregulated in late G_1 so as to be barely detectable in S phase, while in T-47D cells treated with insulin, cyclin D1 expression did not begin to decline until the start of S phase and declined slowly, returning to control levels as the cells entered G_2 phase [45,54,60]. This may merely reflect the duration of action of the mitogenic stimulus but could be of functional significance, given that microinjection of cyclin D1 in late G_1 can inhibit progression into S phase in human fibroblasts [61] but does not inhibit the progression of T-47D cells into S phase. A concentration-dependent increase of cyclins D1, D3, and E was observed with increasing concentrations of mitogen in T-47D cells, and this was concomitant with an increase in the number of cells that subsequently entered S phase. Further experiments demonstrated similar patterns of cyclin expression for other mitogens (IGF-1, bFGF, and FCS), suggesting that the induction of cyclin genes was a common response to mitogenic stimulation by peptide growth factors in these cells. This relationship suggests that sequential induction of cyclins D1,

D3, and E is involved in the commitment to DNA synthesis in breast cancer cells, as has been documented in other cell systems [20].

This question was specifically addressed by engineering T-47D cells for inducible cyclin D1 expression. Induction of cyclin D1 expression shortened the length of G_1 phase, and in serum-starved cells the induction of cyclin D1 alone was sufficient to initiate a round of cell division. This study demonstrated that cyclin D1 was indeed rate limiting for progress through the G_1 phase in the T-47D breast cancer cell line and provided a model to further define the consequences of cyclin D1 expression [28]. Induction of cyclin D1 mRNA and protein resulted in the accumulation of cyclin D1/Cdk4 complexes that support pRb-associated kinase activity in vitro, and this was followed by an increase in cyclin E/Cdk2 associated kinase activity and pRb phosphorylation in vivo [62]. In other cellular systems, specifically quiescent fibroblasts, the ectopic expression of a G_1 cyclin, such as cyclin D1, in the absence of serum is insufficient to induce kinase activity; therefore, there may be other factors that are rate limiting in these systems, such as downregulation of inhibitor action, CDK activation by CAK phosphorylation, or phosphatase activity [27]. It is possible that the differences observed between fibroblasts and breast cancer cells are due to the former cells being arrested in G_0 as opposed to early G_1 following serum deprivation.

Estrogen and antiestrogen action on cyclins

It is well established that estrogen is essential for both the initiation and progression of breast cancer, and several well-studied breast cancer cell lines have an absolute dependence on estrogens for tumor formation and growth in nude mice [63]. Dissection of the cell cycle effects of estrogens in a breast cancer cell model showed that cells were sensitive to estrogen in early G_1 phase, immediately following mitosis [64,65]. Similarly, antiestrogens inhibit proliferation of breast cancer cells, and their action is restricted to the same window within early G_1 phase [66]. Since this point of action within the cell cycle coincides with mitogenic induction of G_1 cyclins, particularly cyclin D1, we investigated whether the same regulatory genes that are involved in growth factor regulation of breast cancer cells might also be responsible for steroidal regulation of cell growth.

The possible involvement of cyclins in antiestrogen action was tested in T-47D and MCF-7 cells [54,67]. The antiestrogen ICI 164384 inhibits the insulin-stimulated growth of T-47D cells, and examination of cyclin expression showed decreases in the level of cyclin D1 and cyclin E but not cyclin D3 [54]. In MCF-7 cells decreases in cyclin D1 mRNA were detected in response to both steroidal (ICI 164384) and nonsteroidal (4-hydroxytamoxifen) antiestrogens and preceded any changes in %S phase by several hours. These effects were concentration dependent and reversible with the simultaneous addition of estrogen. A more recent study has revealed that decreased pRb phosphorylation is an early response to antiestrogen treatment. Within 6 hours

153

of treatment with ICI 182780, hypophosphorylated pRb was evident, and this preceded the beginning of the decline in the %S phase cells by at least 2 hours. This led to the hypothesis that a primary mechanism of growth arrest by antiestrogens is the decreased ability of Cdk4 to phosphorylate pRb [63]. Whether the decrease in Cdk4 activity can be accounted for by decreased cyclin D1 expression alone or involves effects of antiestrogen on CAK or CDK inhibitor expression and function is under study.

The ability of estrogen to reverse the decrease in cyclin D1 mRNA induced by antiestrogens suggests that cyclin D1 is in fact an estrogen-regulated gene [67]. This has been confirmed in T-47D cells in which in serum-free medium containing insulin, estrogen had a similar effect as other mitogens in inducing cyclin D1 mRNA expression [Musgrove et al., unpublished data]. It remains to be determined whether these effects on cyclin D1 gene expression by estrogens and antiestrogens are directly transcriptionally mediated or whether they involve immediate early genes such as c-myc. No classical estrogen response elements are evident within the published sequence for the cyclin D1 promoter, suggesting that direct transcriptional control by the estrogen receptor is unlikely. There are, however, data suggesting that c-myc, an estrogen-regulated protein, regulates expression of the cyclin D1 gene [68,69].

These results have implications for an improved understanding of the major problem in antiestrogen therapy: the development of resistance. Since rapid downregulation of cyclin D1 expression appears to be an early event following antiestrogen treatment of breast cancer cells, it is possible that overexpression of this gene is a potential mechanism for antiestrogen resistance. Our demonstration that inducible expression of cyclin D1 can reinitiate cell cycle progression in antiestrogen-arrested cells provides further support for this view.

Progestin and antiprogestin action on cyclins

T-47D and MCF-7 breast cancer cells exhibit a biphasic response to progestin treatment. There is an initial transient increase in cell cycle progression, followed by cell cycle arrest and long-term growth inhibition [70]. Both actions are mediated during the G_1 phase.

Addition of the synthetic progestin ORG 2058 to T-47D cells proliferating exponentially in insulin-supplemented serum-free medium results in a transient increase in cyclin D1 expression, which precedes the increase in cell cycle progression [54]. Experiments conducted in the presence of cycloheximide showed that the response of cyclin D1 to progestin treatment depends in part on the synthesis of new protein. Ectopic expression of cyclin D1 leads to effects similar to the stimulatory effect of progestins, that is, acceleration of G_1 phase progression [28,70], strongly implicating progestin induction of cyclin D1 as the mechanism underlying this response. Growth arrest following ORG 2058 treatment is accompanied by decreased expression of both cyclin D1 and c-myc, and by reduced pRb phosphorylation. Preliminary data suggest that both Cdk2 and cyclin D1/Cdk4 activity also decrease.

The synthetic antiprogestin RU486 also induces growth inhibition in T-47D cells but acts through a different inhibitory pathway than progestin, as evidenced by the temporal displacement of these two effects and differential effects on cyclin gene expression [71]. In contrast to both progestin and antiestrogen, following RU486 treatment cyclin D1 mRNA expression was not reduced but cyclin D3 expression was clearly decreased, concomitant with a decrease in %S phase [54]. Rb phosphorylation also decreased, but the changes in CDK activity responsible for this remain to be determined.

Retinoid effects on cyclins

Retinoids exert antiproliferative effects on breast cancer cells in culture and exhibit anticarcinogenic effects in rodent models of mammary carcinoma [72]. The hypothesis that retinoids have antiestrogenic properties in breast cancer cells [73] led to a comparison of the effects of retinoids and antiestrogens on breast cancer cell cycle progression and cyclin gene expression [74]. The inhibitory effects of retinoids on T-47D cell cycle progression are delayed by at least 16 hours compared with antiestrogen effects, suggesting that they may act via different mechanisms. Differential effects on cyclin gene expression support this view. Retinoid treatment does not significantly alter the expression of cyclins D1, D3, E, nor the Cdk2 and Cdk4 kinase partners, but the hypophosphorylated, cell cycle inhibitory form of pRb is markedly increased, providing a potential mechanism by which retinoids exert their inhibitory effects on the cell cycle. Although there is no change in the abundance of cyclin D1 and Cdk4, cyclin D1/Cdk4 kinase activity is decreased in retinoid-treated cells [74].

It is clear from these experiments that the mechanisms by which progestins, antiestrogens, progestin antagonists, and retinoids cause growth inhibition are not identical. Although decreased phosphorylation of pRb appears to be a universal feature, the effects on cyclin/CDK complex abundance and activity are specific for each class (Table 2). It is also clear that while regulation of cyclin gene expression is an important component of the mechanisms for proliferation control by steroids, steroid antagonists, and retinoids, other elements, including CDK inhibitors and CAK activity, are likely to contribute to these responses.

Cyclins as oncogenes

Over the past 5 years there has been fragmented evidence linking cyclins to cancer [75,76]. There is as yet no undisputed, formal proof for intrinsic oncogenic activity for any of the cyclins, although it has been frequently reported that cyclins are involved in chromosomal translocations associated with neoplasia, are located adjacent to viral integration sites, and cooperate

Table 2. Summary of effects of steroids, steroid antagonists, and retinoids on cell cycle regulatory genes in breast cancer cells[a]

		Cyclins[b]				
	c-*myc*[b]	D1	D3	E	pRb[c]	p21
Estrogen	↑	↑	ND	↑	↑	↓
Antiestrogen	↓	↓	NS	↓	↓	↑
Progestin[d]	↑	↑	ND	ND	↑	↓
Progestin[e]	↓	↓	ND	ND	↓	ND
Antiprogestin	↓	NS	↓	↓	↓	ND
Retinoic acid	NS	NS	NS	NS	↓	NS

[a] Determined under serum-free conditions, except for retinoic acid and estrogen.
[b] mRNA.
[c] Degree of protein phosphorylation.
[d] Changes associated with progestin stimulation of cell cycle progression.
[e] Changes associated with progestin inhibition of cell cycle progression.
ND = not determined; NS = no significant change.

Table 3. Cyclins as oncogenes

Cyclin	Link to oncogenesis	Ref.
Cyclin A	Site of hepatitis B virus integration in hepatocellular carcinoma	145,146
	Target of the human adenovirus oncoprotein E1A	147–150
Cyclin D1	Inversion in chromosome 11 in parathyroid adenomas places cyclin D1 under the control of the parathyroid hormone promoter	82,151, 152
	t(11;14)(q13;q32) in B-cell lymphoma places cyclin D1 under control of IgG heavy chain enhancer	96
	Cooperates with Myc to induce B-cell neoplasms in transgenic mice	98,101
	Confers transformed properties on established fibroblasts when overexpressed	25
	Induces mammary hyperplasia and carcinoma in transgenic mice	100
Cyclin D2	Part of the fusion protein resulting from the 5′ portion of the AML1 gene fusing with the 3′ portion of a chromosome 8 t(8;21) gene in acute myelogenous leukemia	153
	vin-1 gene, a provirus integration site in retrovirus induced rodent T-cell leukemia	154

with known oncogenes to promote tumorigenesis. A summary of the involvement of cyclins in various forms of human cancer is outlined in Table 3.

Cyclin D1 and breast cancer

Amplification of the q13 region of chromosome 11 has been reported in squamous cell carcinomas of the head and neck, esophagus, and lung; in carcinoma of the breast and bladder; and in a single case of melanoma and hepatoma [77], supporting the view that genes within this region harbor oncogenic activity. The amplified region is up to 15 million base pairs long and consists of somewhere between 15 and 150 genes. Among these genes, the potential proto-oncogenes identified include INT-2 (FGF3), HST-1 (FGF4), EMS-1, and BCL-1. INT-2 and HST-1 are rarely expressed in normal human breast tissue or breast cancer [78,79], and since it is more likely that the gene providing the selective advantage for 11q13 amplification is expressed in normal tissue, these two genes are unlikely to play a role in the pathogenesis of breast cancer. EMS-1 is consistently overexpressed in some breast cancer cell lines and breast carcinomas. EMS-1 is a cytoskeletal protein that is a substrate for Src kinase, suggesting it may have a role in cell motility and invasion [47,80]. BCL-1 has undoubtedly received the most attention. This is not a cellular gene but identifies the breakpoint for the well-documented t(11;14) chromosomal translocation in B-cell lymphomas. The cyclin D1 gene (PRAD1, CCND1, D11S287E) is now the favored BCL-1 candidate oncogene [81,82]. It was originally thought that all these genes were amplified together as a single amplicon [83], but more recently evidence has been presented for independent amplification, suggesting that as many as four amplification units exist around 11q13 [80,84–86]. The most commonly amplified region of 11q13 in breast cancer includes cyclin D1.

11q13 amplification has been examined in breast cancer in a number of studies [77,78]. Of the 2000 breast tumor samples examined, 13% showed amplification at the 11q13 locus. Following demonstration of discordance between cyclin D1 gene amplification and expression in breast cancer cell lines, a series of 124 breast tumor samples and 16 normal breast tissue controls was examined for overexpression of cyclin D1 mRNA. Forty-five percent of tumor samples expressed cyclin D1 to a greater extent than the normal tissue samples [44]. In a similar study, 5 of 10 tumor samples had a two- to eightfold increased expression of cyclin D1 mRNA [87]. Two laboratories employing immunohistochemical detection of cyclin D1 in approximately 350 breast tumor samples found that 43–55% had increased cyclin D1 staining [39,88,89]. The latter study reveals that overexpression of cyclin D1 protein is a relatively early event in breast cancer in that it was apparent in samples of ductal carcinoma in situ [39,89]. These studies exemplify the fact that overexpression and amplification of cyclin D1 can occur independently since the frequency of overexpression is greater. The mechanisms responsible for elevated expression have yet to be defined, but mutations in the promoter region, altered expression of negative regulators, or extended half-lives could all contribute to the accumulation of cyclin D1 in breast tumors.

There are a number of reports correlating 11q13 amplification and selected clinicopathological parameters in breast cancer, but there is little consensus on these relationships. In patients with operable breast cancer, amplification of the 11q13 locus, including the cyclin D1 gene, has been weakly associated with the presence of lymph node metastases, tumor size, early presentation, and poor prognosis, as judged by relapse-free and overall survival [47,80,90–95]. A stronger relationship exists between 11q13 amplification and steroid hormone receptor positivity, although even this relationship has not been universally demonstrated [83]. The possibility of 11q13 amplification or expression acting as a useful prognostic marker remains unresolved. Since the frequency of overexpression of the cyclin D1 mRNA and protein is greater than amplification of this gene, correlating expression with clinicopathological parameters may be more relevant and indeed may allay the discrepancies in the current literature.

The functional consequences of cyclin D1 expression in breast tumors remains unclear. Overexpression of cyclin D1 in B cell neoplasms is powerful enough to subvert control of G_1 phase and, despite its absence in normal B cells, cyclin D1 becomes essential for the cell cycle progression in these transformed cells [20]. Parathyroid adenomas that express high levels of cyclin D1 exhibit rapid growth, but since they are noninvasive, overexpression of the cyclin D1 gene is considered to be a purely proliferative lesion [96]. It is possible that overexpression of the cyclin D1 gene in breast tumors may promote premature S phase entry, as has been described for breast cell lines in culture [28]. It is highly probable that any oncogenic potential of the cyclin D1 protein would involve its interaction with the tumor suppressor gene pRb.

Cyclin D1 alone may not be sufficient to transform primary breast cells but may cooperate with other oncogenes. Although this has not been studied in normal breast epithelial cells, there is evidence of cyclin D1 cooperating in transformation with Ha-Ras in primary rat kidney cells or rat embryo fibroblasts and Myc in B cell lymphomas [97–99]. Furthermore, overexpression of cyclin D1 alone confers transformed properties on established fibroblasts [25]. Perhaps the most convincing evidence supporting the view that cyclin D1 can act as an oncogene in breast cancer comes from studies in transgenic mice, in which overexpression of cyclin D1 resulted in mammary hyperplasia and carcinoma, albeit after a long latency period [100]. To date this study stands alone but anticipates a link between tumorigenic potential and the expression of cyclin D1 in breast tissue, perhaps in association with other oncogenes, such as c-*myc*, as has been demonstrated in the lymphoid system [98,101].

Other cyclins and breast cancer

Cyclin D2 appears to be important in the development of certain leukemias (Table 3); these cells normally express cyclin D2 but not cyclin D1. Cyclin D2 functions in these cells in a manner analogous to cyclin D1 in other cell types. Overexpression of both cyclin D2 and cyclin D3 disables the differentiation pathway in lymphocytes, perhaps sentencing them to continuous proliferation [102]. There is, however, no apparent involvement of either gene in breast cancer, although it is curious that cyclin D2 expression is abundant in normal

158

breast epithelial cell lines but not in most breast cancer cell lines examined [44,46].

A role for cyclin E in breast cancer has been suggested based on a sample of nine breast tumors in which both qualitative and quantitative changes in cyclin E protein were observed independent of the S phase fraction. Increased expression correlated with increased tumor stage and grade, indicating that cyclin E may be a prognostic indicator [45]. This interesting observation remains to be confirmed in a larger series of tumors. There are no published reports examining cyclin A and B in clinical breast cancer, although the infrequent abnormalities noted in breast cancer cell lines suggest that aberrations in either of these cyclins are likely to be rare.

Inhibitors of cyclin dependent kinases as tumor suppressor genes

Arguably the most important recent advance in cell cycle research is the discovery of CDK inhibitors. Independent lines of research have converged on the identification of small proteins that inhibit the kinase activity of all CDKs (p21 and p27) or solely inhibit the partners of the D-type cyclins, Cdk4 and Cdk6 (p15, p16, p18). These proteins are putative tumor suppressor genes, providing a link between the negative control of cell cycle progression and cancer. Inactivation of these inhibitory molecules might be expected to have consequences similar to cyclin overexpression.

p21

The cyclin-dependent kinase inhibitor p21 was discovered independently as a protein induced by the tumor suppressor p53 (WAF1), as a CDK kinase inhibitor (CIP1), and as a protein (SDI1) induced as cells senesce [34,103,104]. The induction of p21 alone is sufficient to arrest the cell cycle of normal fibroblasts, and under these circumstances the protein is associated with cyclin A/Cdk2, cyclin E/Cdk2, and cyclin D1/Cdk4 complexes [34,103,104]. p21 mRNA expression is high at the G_0/G_1 boundary but decreases as cells reach S phase in both human fibroblasts and human breast carcinoma cells [105,106]. The p21-containing cyclin/CDK complexes exist in both active and inactive forms, with inhibition of kinase activity occurring abruptly with saturating levels of p21 [107,108].

p21 can be induced independently of p53 [109], and this is often concomitant with initiation of terminal differentiation [30,110–112]. This inhibitor is induced in human breast carcinoma cells following treatment with etoposide, the differentiation agent sodium butyrate [deFazio et al., unpublished data], or in response to serum starvation [106]. In addition to inhibiting CDK activity, p21 blocks polymerase δ-dependent DNA replication [113,114]; these separate functions are mediated by different domains within the molecule [115]. p21 does not, however, hinder damage-responsive DNA repair [105].

The common mutation of p53 in human cancers strengthens the likelihood that aberrations in its targets might also occur. Deletions or dysfunctional mutations of the p21 gene, however, have not been described, although non-functional polymorphisms have been reported in one breast epithelial cell line and in 2 of 45 colorectal cancers [116,117]. There is no direct evidence linking p21 to tumorigenesis, although there is evidence for subunit rearrangements of the normal cyclin/CDK/p21/PCNA quaternary complex following transformation [107]. This may be a way in which oncogenic proteins can alter the action of p21 in the absence of inactivating mutations. These observations are limited to virally transformed and p53 'null' fibroblasts, and it remains to be determined whether such alterations in subunit configuration also occur in carcinoma, including breast carcinoma.

A study of CDK inhibitors in breast cancer cells has shown that, unlike p16, deletions of p21 alleles are not observed in breast cancer cell lines. There are, however, wide variations in p21 gene expression associated with the presence or absence of p53 mutations: Cell lines harboring mutations in p53 have markedly reduced p21 mRNA. Furthermore, in addition to regulation by differentiation agents, p21 gene expression was regulated by the growth states of the cells and by several steroids and their antagonists [49]. Whether or not changes in p21 are causal or a consequence of growth regulation by these agents remains to be elucidated.

p16 and p15

The p16 protein was originally identified in Cdk4 and Cdk6 complexes lacking cyclin in some transformed cells [118], and was later cloned and identified as a specific Cdk4/Cdk6 inhibitor [119]. An inverse association between p16 and pRb has been observed, with p16 mRNA expression increased in cells lacking functional pRb (Table 1), consistent with data documenting repression of p16 mRNA by pRb [120]. p15 was identified as a Cdk4/Cdk6 inhibitor and is transcriptionally regulated by TGF-β [121]. The p15 and p16 genes are adjacent on chromosome 9p21, and this region became the focus of widespread attention when it was discovered that the p16 gene alone or with p15 was deleted in a substantial number of tumor cell lines, including breast cancer cells [122–124]. Controversy emerged when it was suggested that the rate of p16 deletions reported in cell lines was an artifact of cell culture since the frequency of deletions was significantly less in related primary tumors [125,126]. Further detailed studies have found that p16 is frequently mutated or deleted in pancreatic adenocarcinoma and in 19% of bladder carcinomas [126,127]. Additionally, p16 mutations segregate with the disease in some but not all familial melanoma families [128,129]. Although p16 is a strong candidate for a tumor suppressor gene in some cancers, particularly familial melanoma, current mutation analysis techniques are inadequate to unequivocally confirm this. In primary breast carcinoma, the limited data currently available

160

do not support a major role for p16, despite the frequent deletion of this gene in breast cancer cell lines [49,130].

Evidence for a tumor suppressor function for p16 comes from studies in rat embryo fibroblasts in which cells stimulated by oncogenic Ha-Ras and Myc were blocked from entering S phase by ectopic expression of p16; this block was overcome by expression of Cdk4. Moreover, p16 suppressed cellular transformation of rat embryo fibroblasts by Ha-Ras and Myc, and these effects were not seen in cells that lacked pRb [119]. Furthermore, transfection of p16 cDNA into carcinoma cells appears to inhibit their colony-forming efficiency, since p16 expressing cells are selected against with continued passage in vitro [49,123]. These data are consistent with the hypothesis that p16 has tumor suppressor activity that may be important in the genesis of some cancers, but its involvement appears to be less widespread than was first suggested [124].

Another low molecular weight inhibitor p18, which is structurally and functionally similar to p16 and p15, has recently been identified. p18 is primarily a Cdk6 inhibitor and, like p16, its ability to suppress growth is reliant on functional pRb [131].

p27

Another CDK inhibitor, p27^{KIP1}, has been characterized and has been shown to have a role in growth arrest mediated by cell–cell contact, or treatment with TGF-β or cAMP [132–137]. This molecule shares sequence homology with p21 in a region of the molecule with known CDK inhibitor activity. In vitro p27 inhibits the ability of cyclin E/Cdk2, cyclin A/Cdk2, and cyclin D1/Cdk4 complexes to phosphorylate pRb [135]. In vivo p27 associates with cyclin E/Cdk2 complexes, preventing their activation. However, in the presence of increasing levels of cyclin D, the inhibitor is sequestered by cyclin D complexes, allowing activation of cyclin E/Cdk2. The role of p27, therefore, in the cell cycle appears to be to establish an order of activation for cyclin D1 and cyclin E [132,134,137].

There is emerging evidence that p27 is intimately involved in growth control by physiological and pharmacological agents, for example, cAMP is proposed to induce G_1 arrest in murine macrophages by raising the threshold of p27, preventing activation of the cyclin D1/Cdk4 complex by CAK [132]. More detailed studies on transforming growth factor (TGF-β) suggest that it arrests cells by inhibiting Cdk4 expression, which prevents free p27 binding to cyclin D1/Cdk4 complexes, thus allowing p27 to bind and inactivate the cyclin E/Cdk2 complex [135,137,138]. One of these studies employed normal human breast epithelial cells, providing a potential mechanism for the well-documented inhibitory effect of TGF-β in breast epithelial cell proliferation [137]. Since TGF-β has been implicated in mediating the growth inhibitory effects of antiestrogens [139], the synthetic progestin, gestodene [140], and retinoids [141], a description of the effects of these agents on p27 inhibitor function in normal breast epithelium and breast cancer cells is eagerly awaited. Given that the role of TGF-β in mediating the growth regulatory activity of steroids and steroid antagonists is controversial, and that transcriptional activation of p15 is an alternative pathway of TGF-β action, the regulation of CDK inhibitor function by factors known to control breast epithelial cell proliferation and differentiation is a priority for ongoing research.

Conclusions

An increased understanding of mammalian cell cycle control has identified new families of molecules with potential oncogene (cyclins and CDKs) and tumor suppressor gene function (CDK inhibitors). Accumulating evidence in diverse cancers supports such roles for a number of cyclins, particularly cyclin D1 and D2, and for p16, which specifically inhibits the G^1 active kinases, Cdk4 and Cdk6. Further evidence on the roles of cyclins, CDKs, and their inhibitors in the control of proliferation and differentiation by growth factors, steroids, steroid antagonists, and diverse differentiation factors in breast epithelial cells identify a central role for these molecules, specifically cyclin D1, in responding to extracellular stimuli.

Although our understanding of these mechanisms is far from complete, it is already apparent how aberrant expression of molecules controlling G_1 progression could subvert normal growth control mechanisms, including the need for extracellular stimuli to sustain cell proliferation. The overexpression of cyclin D1 in a significant proportion of breast carcinomas, including in situ cancers, and its oncogenic potential in the mammary gland of transgenic mice provide strong evidence for a role for cyclin D1 in the pathogenesis of breast cancer. If this is substantiated by further research, cyclin D1 will potentially provide a new marker of therapeutic responsiveness and prognosis, and a target for novel therapeutic intervention in breast cancer.

Acknowledgments

We thank all members of the Cancer Biology Division who contributed to the work described in this review, particularly Nicholas Wilcken, for advice during the drafting of this manuscript. Research work in this laboratory is supported by the National Health and Medical Research Council of Australia, the New South Wales State Cancer Council, the St. Vincent's Hospital Research Fund, and the Leo and Jenny Leukemia and Cancer Foundation.

References

1. Bishop JM (1991) Molecular themes in oncogenesis. *Cell* 64:235–248.
2. Varmus H (1989) An historical overview of oncogenes. In *Oncogenes and the Molecular*

Origins of Cancer. RA Weinberg (ed). Cold Spring Harbor, NY: Cold Spring Harbor Laboratory Press, pp 3–44.

3. Knudson AG (1993) Antioncogenes and human cancer. *Proc Natl Acad Sci USA* 90:10914–10921.
4. Norbury C, Nurse P (1992) Animal cell cycles and their control. *Annu Rev Biochem* 61:441–470.
5. Murray AW, Solomon MJ, Kirschner MW (1989) The role of cyclin synthesis and degradation in the control of maturation promoting factor activity. *Nature* 339:280–286.
6. Nigg EA (1993) Targets of cyclin-dependent protein kinases. *Curr Opin Cell Biol* 5:187–193.
7. Morgan DO (1995) Principles of CDK regulation. *Nature* 374:131–134.
8. Resnitzky D, Gossen M, Bujard H, Reed SI (1994) Acceleration of the G_1/S phase transition by expression of cyclins D1 and E with an inducible system. *Mol Cell Biol* 14:1669–1679.
9. Lamb NJ, Cavadore JC, Labbe JC, Maurer RA, Fernandez A (1991) Inhibition of cAMP-dependent protein kinase plays a key role in the induction of mitosis and nuclear envelope breakdown in mammalian cells. *EMBO J* 10:1523–1533.
10. Henglein B, Chenivesse X, Wang J, Eick D, Bréchot C (1994) Structure and cell cycle-regulated transcription of the human cyclin A gene. *Proc Natl Acad Sci USA* 91:5490–5494.
11. Pagano M, Pepperkok R, Verde F, Ansorge W, Draetta G (1992) Cyclin A is required at two points in the human cell cycle. *EMBO J* 11:961–971.
12. Dutta A, Stillman B (1992) Cdc2 family kinases phosphorylate a human cell DNA replication factor, RPA, and activate DNA replication. *EMBO J* 11:2189–2199.
13. Fotedar R, Roberts JM (1992) Cell cycle regulated phosphorylation of RPA-32 occurs within the replication initiation complex. *EMBO J* 11:2177–2187.
14. Guadagno TM, Ohtsubo M, Roberts JM, Assoian RK (1993) A link between cyclin A expression and adhesion-dependent cell cycle progression. *Science* 262:1572–1575.
15. Reed SI (1991) G1-specific cyclins: In search of an S-phase-promoting factor. *Trends Genet* 7:95–99.
16. Koff A, Giordano A, Desai D, Yamashita K, Harper JW, Elledge S, Nishimoto T, Morgan DO, Franza BR, Roberts JM (1992) Formation and activation of a cyclin E-cdk2 complex during the G_1 phase of the human cell cycle. *Science* 257:1689–1694.
17. Dulic V, Lees E, Reed SI (1992) Association of human cyclin E with a periodic G_1-S phase protein kinase. *Science* 257:1958–1961.
18. Ohtsubo M, Roberts JM (1993) Cyclin-dependent regulation of G_1 in mammalian fibroblasts. *Science* 259:1908–1912.
19. Wimmel A, Lucibello FC, Sewing A, Adolph S, Müller R (1994) Inducible acceleration of G_1 progression through tetracycline-regulated expression of human cyclin E. *Oncogene* 9:995–997.
20. Lukas J, Pagano M, Staskova Z, Draetta G, Bartek J (1994) Cyclin D1 protein oscillates and is essential for cell cycle progression in human tumour cell lines. *Oncogene* 9:707–718.
21. Matsushime H, Quelle DE, Shurtleff SA, Shibuya M, Sherr CJ, Kato J-Y (1994) D-type cyclin-dependent kinase activity in mammalian cells. *Mol Cell Biol* 14:2066–2076.
22. Ando K, Ajchenbaum-Cymbalista F, Griffin JD (1993) Regulation of G_1/S transition by cyclins D2 and D3 in hematopoietic cells. *Proc Natl Acad Sci USA* 90:9571–9575.
23. Ando K, Griffin JD (1995) Cdk4 integrates growth stimulatory and inhibitory signals during G1 phase of haematopoietic cells. *Oncogene* 10:751–755.
24. Quelle DE, Ashmun RA, Shurtleff SA, Kato J-Y, Bar-Sagi D, Roussel MF, Sherr CJ (1993) Overexpression of mouse D-type cyclins accelerates G_1 phase in rodent fibroblasts. *Genes Dev* 7:1559–1571.
25. Jiang W, Kahn SM, Zhou P, Zhang Y-J, Cacace AM, Infante AS, Doi S, Santella RM, Weinstein IB (1993) Overexpression of cyclin D1 in rat fibroblasts causes abnormalities in growth control, cell cycle progression and gene expression. *Oncogene* 8:3447–3457.
26. Kato J-Y, Matsuoka M, Strom DK, Sherr CJ (1994) Regulation of cyclin D-dependent kinase 4 (Cdk4) by Cdk4-activating kinase. *Mol Cell Biol* 14:2713–2721.

27. Baldin V, Lukas J, Marcote MJ, Pagano M, Draetta G (1993) Cyclin D1 is a nuclear protein required for cell cycle progression in G_1. *Genes Dev* 7:812–821.
28. Musgrove EA, Lee CSL, Buckley MF, Sutherland RL (1994) Cyclin D1 induction in breast cancer cells shortens G_1 and is sufficient for cells arrested in G_1 to complete the cell cycle. *Proc Natl Acad Sci USA* 91:8022–8026.
29. Lukas J, Jadayel D, Bartkova J, Nacheva E, Dyer MJ, Strauss M, Bartek J (1994) BCL-1/cyclin D1 oncoprotein oscillates and subverts the G1 phase control in B-cell neoplasms carrying the t(11;14) translocation. *Oncogene* 9:2159–2167.
30. Halevy O, Novitch BG, Spicer D, Skapek SX, Rhee J, Hannon GJ, Beach D, Lassar AB (1995) Correlation of terminal cell cycle arrest of skeletal muscle with the induction of p21 by MyoD. *Science* 267:1018–1021.
31. Kiess M, Montgomery GR, Hamel PA (1995) Expression of the positive regulator of cell cycle progression, cyclin D3, is induced during differentiation of myoblasts into quiescent myotubes. *Oncogene* 10:159–166.
32. Afshari CA, Vojta PJ, Annab LA, Futreal PA, Willard TB, Barrett JC (1993) Investigation of the role of G_1/S cell cycle mediators in cellular senescence. *Exp Cell Res* 209:231–237.
33. Dulic V, Drullinger LF, Lees E, Reed SI, Stein GH (1993) Altered regulation of G_1 cyclins in senescent human diploid fibroblasts: Accumulation of inactive cyclin E-Cdk2 and cyclin D1-Cdk2 complexes. *Proc Natl Acad Sci USA* 90:11034–11038.
34. Noda A, Ning Y, Venable SF, Pereira-Smith OM, Smith JR (1994) Cloning of senescent cell-derived inhibitors of DNA synthesis using an expression screen. *Exp Cell Res* 211:90–98.
35. Sherr CJ (1993) Mammalian G_1 cyclins. *Cell* 73:1059–1065.
36. Kato J-Y, Matsushime H, Hiebert SW, Ewen ME, Sherr CJ (1993) Direct binding of cyclin D to the retinoblastoma gene product (pRb) and pRb phosphorylation by the cyclin D-dependent kinase Cdk4. *Genes Dev* 7:331–342.
37. Hinds PW, Mittnacht S, Dulic V, Arnold A, Reed SI, and Weinberg RA (1992) Regulation of retinoblastoma protein functions by ectopic expression of human cyclins. *Cell* 70:993–1006.
38. Bates S, Bonetta L, MacAllan D, Parry D, Holder A, Dickson C, Peters G (1994) Cdk6 (PLSTIRE) and Cdk4 (PSK-J3) are a distinct subset of the cyclin-dependent kinases that associate with cyclin D1. *Oncogene* 9:71–79.
39. Bartkova J, Lukas J, Müller H, Lützhøft D, Strauss M, Bartek J (1994) Cyclin D1 protein expression and function in human breast cancer. *Int J Cancer* 57:353–361.
40. Muller H, Lukas J, Schneider A, Warthoe P, Bartek J, Eilers M, Strauss M (1994) Cyclin D1 expression is regulated by the retinoblastoma protein. *Proc Natl Acad Sci USA* 91:2945–2949.
41. Hinds PW, Weinberg RA (1994) Tumor suppressor genes. *Curr Opin Gen Dev* 4:135–141.
42. Dowdy SF, Hinds PW, Louie K, Reed SI, Arnold A, Weinberg RA (1993) Physical interaction of the retinoblastoma protein with human D cyclins. *Cell* 73:499–511.
43. Sutherland RL, Lee CSL, Feldman RS, Musgrove EA (1992) Regulation of breast cancer cell cycle progression by growth factors, steroids and steroid antagonists. *J Steroid Biochem Mol Biol* 41:315–321.
44. Buckley MF, Sweeney KJE, Hamilton JA, Sini RL, Manning DL, Nicholson RI, deFazio A, Watts CKW, Musgrove EA, Sutherland RL (1993) Expression and amplification of cyclin genes in human breast cancer. *Oncogene* 8:2127–2133.
45. Keyomarsi K, Pardee AB (1993) Redundant cyclin overexpression and gene amplification in breast cancer cells. *Proc Natl Acad Sci USA* 90:1112–1116.
46. Tam SW, Shay JW, Pagano M (1994) Differential expression and cell cycle regulation of the cyclin-dependent kinase 4 inhibitor p16[INK4]. *Cancer Res* 54:5816–5820.
47. Schuuring E, Verhoeven E, van Tinteren H, Peterse JL, Nunnink B, Thunnissen FBJM, Devilee P, Cornelisse CJ, van de Vijver MJ, Mooi WJ, Michalides RJAM (1992) Amplification of genes within the chromosome 11q13 region is indicative of poor prognosis in patients with operable breast cancer. *Cancer Res* 52:5229–5234.

164

48. Lammie GA, Peters G (1991) Chromosome 11q13 abnormalities in human cancer. *Cancer Cells* 3:413–420.
49. Musgrove EA, Lilischkis R, Cornish AL, Lee CSL, Seshadri R, Sutherland RL (1995) Expression and regulation of the cyclin-dependent kinase inhibitors p16[INK4], p15[INK4B] and p21[WAFI/CIPI] in human breast cancer cell lines. *Int J Cancer* 63:584–591.
50. Keyomarsi K, O'Leary N, Molnar G, Lees E, Fingert HJ, Pardee AB (1994) Cyclin E, a potential prognostic marker for breast cancer. *Cancer Res* 54:380–385.
51. Lebwohl DE, Muise-Helmericks R, Sepp-Lorenzino L, Serve S, Timaul M, Bol R, Borgen P, Rosen N (1994) A truncated cyclin D1 gene encodes a stable mRNA in a human breast cancer cell line. *Oncogene* 9:1925–1929.
52. Bartek J, Staskova Z, Draetta G, Lukas J (1993) Molecular pathology of the cell cycle in human cancer cells. *Stem Cells* 1:51–58.
53. Musgrove EA, Buckley MF, deFazio A, Watts CKW, Sutherland RL (1994) Expression and regulation of cyclin genes in breast cancer cells. In *The Cell Cycle: Regulators, Targets and Clinical Applications.* V Hu (ed). New York: Plenum Press, pp 323–329.
54. Musgrove EA, Hamilton JA, Lee CSL, Sweeney KJE, Watts CKW, Sutherland RL (1993) Growth factor, steroid and steroid antagonist regulation of cyclin gene expression associated with changes in T-47D human breast cancer cell cycle progression. *Mol Cell Biol* 13:3577–3587.
55. Arnold A, Kim HG, Gaz RD, Eddy RL, Fukushima Y, Byers MG, Shows TB, Kronenberg HM (1989) Molecular cloning and chromosomal mapping of DNA rearranged with the parathyroid hormone gene in a parathyroid adenoma. *J Clin Invest* 83:2034–2040.
56. Elledge SJ, Richman R, Hall FL, Williams RT, Lodgson N, Harper JW (1992) *CDK2* encodes a 33-kDa cyclin A-associated protein kinase and is expressed before *CDC2* in the cell cycle. *Proc Natl Acad Sci USA* 89:2907–2911.
57. Ninomiya-Tsuji J, Nomoto S, Yasuda H, Reed SI, Matsumoto K (1991) Cloning of a human cDNA encoding a Cdc2-related kinase by complementation of a budding yeast *cdc28* mutation. *Proc Natl Acad Sci USA* 88:9006–9010.
58. Gong J, Traganos F, Darzynkiewicz Z (1993) Simultaneous analysis of cell cycle kinetics at two different DNA ploidy levels based on DNA content and cyclin B measurements. *Cancer Res* 53:5096–5099.
59. Gong J, Ardelt B, Traganos F, Darzynkiewicz Z (1994) Unscheduled expression of cyclin B1 and cyclin E in several leukemic and solid tumor cell lines. *Cancer Res* 54:4285–4288.
60. Motokura T, Keyomarsi K, Kronenberg HM, Arnold A (1992) Cloning and characterization of human cyclin D3, a cDNA closely related in sequence to the PRAD1/cyclin D1 proto-oncogene. *J Biol Chem* 267:20412–20415.
61. Pagano M, Theodoras AM, Tam SW, Draetta GF (1994) Cyclin D1-mediated inhibition of repair and replicative DNA synthesis in human fibroblasts. *Genes Dev* 8:1627–1639.
62. Musgrove EA, Sarcevic B, Sutherland RL (1996) Inducible expression of cyclin D1 in T-47D human breast cancer cells is sufficient for CDK2 activation and pRB hyperphosphorylation. *J Cell Biochem*, in press.
63. Watts CKW, Wilcken NRC, Hamilton JA, Sweeney KJE, Musgrove EA, Sutherland RL (1995) Mechanisms of antiestrogen, progestin/antiprogestin and retinoid inhibition of cell cycle progression in breast cancer cells. In *Hormone Dependent Cancers. Molecular and Cellular Endocrinology.* JP Pasqualini, BS Katzenellenbogen (eds). New York: Marcel Dekker, pp 119–140.
64. Leung BS, Potter AH (1987) Mode of estrogen action on cell proliferation in CAMA-1 cell: II. Sensitivity of G_1 phase population. *J Cell Biochem* 34:213–225.
65. Sutherland RL, Hall RE, Taylor IW (1983) Cell proliferation kinetics of MCF-7 human mammary carcinoma cells in culture and effects of tamoxifen on exponentially growing and plateau-phase cells. *Cancer Res* 43:3998–4006.
66. Musgrove EA, Wakeling AE, Sutherland RL (1989) Points of action of estrogen antagonists and a calmodulin antagonist within the MCF-7 human breast cancer cell cycle. *Cancer Res* 49:2398–2404.

67. Watts CKW, Sweeney KJE, Warlters A, Musgrove EA, Sutherland RL (1994) Antiestrogen regulation of cell cycle progression and cyclin D1 gene expression in MCF-7 human breast cancer cells. *Breast Cancer Res Treat* 31:95–105.

68. Daksis JI, Lu RY, Facchini LM, Marhin WW, Penn LJ (1994) Myc induces cyclin D1 expression in the absence of de novo protein synthesis and links mitogen-stimulated signal transduction to the cell cycle. *Oncogene* 9:3635–3645.

69. Philipp A, Schneider A, Vasrik I, Finke K, Xiong Y, Beach D, Alitalo K, Eilers M (1994) Repression of cyclin D1: A novel function of MYC. *Mol Cell Biol* 14:4032–4043.

70. Musgrove EA, Lee CSL, Sutherland RL (1991) Progestins both stimulate and inhibit breast cancer cell cycle progression while increasing expression of transforming growth factor α, epidermal growth factor receptor, c-*fos* and c-*myc* genes. *Mol Cell Biol* 11:5032–5043.

71. Musgrove EA, Sutherland RL (1994) Cell cycle control by steroid hormones. In *Seminars in Cancer Biology*. MG Parker (ed). London: Academic Press, pp 5:381–389.

72. Moon RC, Pritchard JF, Mehta RG, Nomides CT, Thomas CF, Dinger NM (1989) Suppression of the rat mammary cancer development by N-(4-hydroxy-phenyl) retinamide (4-HPR) following surgical removal of first palpable tumour. *Carcinogenesis* 10:1645–1649.

73. Fontana JA (1987) Interaction of retinoids and tamoxifen on the inhibition of human mammary carcinoma cell proliferation. *Exp Cell Biol* 55:136–144.

74. Wilcken NRC, Sarcevic B, Musgrove EA, Sutherland RL (1996) Differential effects of retinoids and antiestrogens on cell cycle progression and cell cycle regulatory genes in human breast cancer cells. *Cell Growth and Diff* 7:65–74.

75. Hunter T, Pines J (1991) Cyclins and cancer. *Cell* 66:1071–1074.

76. Hunter T, Pines J (1994) Cyclins and cancer II: Cyclin D and CDK inhibitors come of age. *Cell* 79:573–582.

77. Peters G, Fantl V, Smith R, Brookes S, Dickson C (1995) Chromosome 11q13 markers and D-type cyclins in breast cancer. *Breast Cancer Res Treat* 33:125–135.

78. Fantl V, Smith R, Brookes S, Dickson C, Peters G (1993) Chromosome 11q13 abnormalities in human breast cancer. *Cancer Surv* 18:77–93.

79. Faust JB, Meeker TC (1992) Amplification and expression of the *bcl*-1 gene in human solid tumor cell lines. *Cancer Res* 52:2460–2463.

80. Schuuring E, Verhoeven E, Mooi WJ, Michalides RJAM (1992) Identification and cloning of two overexpressed genes, U21B31/*PRAD1* and *EMS1*, within the amplified chromosome 11q13 region in human carcinomas. *Oncogene* 7:355–361.

81. Withers DA, Harvey RC, Faust JB, Melnyk O, Carey K, Meeker TC (1991) Characterization of a candidate *bcl*-1 gene. *Mol Cell Biol* 11:4846–4853.

82. Rosenberg CL, Wong E, Petty EM, Bale AE, Tsujimoto Y, Harris NL, Arnold A (1991) *PRAD1*, a candidate *BCL1* oncogene: Mapping and expression in centrocytic lymphoma. *Proc Natl Acad Sci USA* 88:9638–9642.

83. Gaffey MJ, Frierson H Jr, Williams, ME (1993) Chromosome 11q13, c-erbB-2, and c-myc amplification in invasive breast carcinoma: Clinicopathologic correlations. *Mod Path* 6:654–659.

84. Karlseder J, Zeillinger R, Schneeberger C, Czerwenka K, Speiser P, Kubista E, Birnbaum D, Gaudray P, Theillet C (1994) Patterns of DNA amplification at band q13 of chromosome 11 in human breast cancer. *Genes Chromosom Cancer* 9:42–48.

85. Szepetowski P, Simon MP, Grosgeorge J, Huebner K, Bastard C, Evans GA, Tsujimoto Y, Birnbaum D, Theillet C, Gaudray P (1992) Localization of 11q13 loci with respect to regional chromosomal breakpoints. *Genomics* 12:738–744.

86. Szepetowski P, Courseaux A, Carle GF, Theillet C, Gaudray P (1992) Amplification of 11q13 DNA sequences in human breast cancer: D11S97 identifies a region tightly linked to BCL1 which can be amplified separately. *Oncogene* 7:751–755.

87. Lammie GA, Fantl V, Smith R, Schuuring E, Brookes S, Michalides R, Dickson C, Arnold A, Peters G (1991) D11S287, a putative oncogene on chromosome 11q13, is amplified and expressed in squamous cell and mammary carcinomas and linked to BCL-1. *Oncogene* 6:439–444.

166

88. Gillett C, Fantl V, Smith R, Fisher C, Bartek J, Dickson C, Barnes D, Peters G (1994) Amplification and overexpression of cyclin D1 in breast cancer detected by immunohistochemical staining. *Cancer Res* 54:1812–1817.

89. Bartkova J, Lukas J, Strauss M, Bartek J (1995) Cyclin D1 oncoprotein aberrantly accumulates in malignancies of diverse histogenesis. *Oncogene* 10:775–778.

90. Theillet C, Adnane J, Szepetowski P, Simon M-P, Jeanteur P, Birnbaum D, Gaudray P (1990). *BCL*-1 participates in the 11q13 amplification found in breast cancer. *Oncogene* 5:147–149.

91. Borg A, Sigurdsson H, Clark GM, Ferno M, Fuqua SA, Olson H, Kilander D, McGuire WL (1991) Association of INT2/HST coamplification in primary breast cancer with hormone-dependent phenotype and poor prognosis. *Br J Cancer* 63:136–142.

92. Tang RP, Kacinski B, Validire P, Beuvon F, Sastre X, Benoit P, dela Rochefordiere A, Mosseri V, Pouillart P, Scholl S (1990) Oncogene amplification correlates with dense lymphocyte infiltration in human breast cancers: A role for hematopoietic growth factor release by tumor cells? *J Cell Biochem* 44:189–198.

93. Tsuda H, Hirohashi S, Shimosato Y, Hirota T, Tsugane S, Yamamoto H, Miyajima N, Toyoshima K, Yamamoto T, Yokota J, Yoshida T, Sakamoto H, Terada M, Sugimura T (1989) Correlation between long-term survival in breast cancer patients and amplification of two putative oncogene-coamplification units: hst-1/int-2 and c-erbB-2/ear-1. *Cancer Res* 49:3104–3108.

94. Henry JA, Hennessy C, Levett DL, Lennard TW, Westley BR, May FE (1993) INT-2 amplification in breast cancer: Association with decreased survival and relationship to amplification of c-erbB-2 and c-myc. *Int J Cancer* 53:774–780.

95. Adnane J, Gaudray P, Simon MP, Simony-Lafontaine J, Jeanteur P, Theillet C (1989) Proto-oncogene amplification and human breast tumor phenotype. *Oncogene* 4:1389–1395.

96. Motokura T, Arnold A (1993) Cyclins and oncogenesis. *Biochim Biophys Acta* 1155:63–78.

97. Lovec H, Sewing A, Lucibello FC, Müller R, Möröy T (1994) Oncogenic activity of cyclin D1 revealed through cooperation with Ha-*ras*: Link between cell cycle control and malignant transformation. *Oncogene* 9:323–326.

98. Bodrug S, Warner BJ, Bath ML, Lindeman GJ, Harris AW, Adams JM (1994) Cyclin D1 transgene impedes lymphocyte maturation and collaborates in lymphomagenesis with the *myc* gene. *EMBO J* 13:2124–2130.

99. Hinds PW, Dowdy SF, Eaton EN, Arnold A, Weinberg RA (1994) Function of a human cyclin gene as an oncogene. *Proc Natl Acad Sci USA* 91:709–713.

100. Wang TC, Cardiff RD, Zukerberg L, Lees E, Arnold A, Schmidt EV (1994) Mammary hyperplasia and carcinoma in MMTV-cyclin D1 transgenic mice. *Nature* 369:669–671.

101. Lovec H, Grzeschiczek A, Kowalski M-B, Möröy T (1994) Cyclin D1/*bcl*-1 cooperates with *myc* genes in the generation of B-cell lymphoma in transgenic mice. *EMBO J* 13:3487–3495.

102. Kato J-Y, Sherr CJ (1993) Inhibition of granulocyte differentiation by G_1 cyclins D2 and D3 but not D1. *Proc Natl Acad Sci USA* 90:11513–11517.

103. Harper JW, Adami GR, Wei N, Keyomarsi K, Elledge SJ (1993) The p21 Cdk-interacting protein Cip1 is a potent inhibitor of G_1 cyclin-dependent kinases. *Cell* 75:805–816.

104. Xiong Y, Hannon GJ, Zhang H, Casso D, Kobayashi R, Beach D (1993) p21 is a universal inhibitor of cyclin kinases. *Nature* 366:701–704.

105. Li R, Waga S, Hannon GJ, Beach D, Stillman B (1994) Differential effects by the p21 CDK inhibitor on PCNA-dependent DNA replication and repair. *Nature* 371:534–537.

106. Sheikh MS, Li XS, Chen JC, Shao ZM, Ordonez JV, Fontana JA (1994) Mechanisms of regulation of WAF1/CIP1 gene expression in human breast carcinoma: Role of p53-dependent and independent signal transduction pathways. *Oncogene* 9:3407–3415.

107. Xiong Y, Zhang H, Beach D (1993) Subunit rearrangement of the cyclin-dependent kinases is associated with cellular transformation. *Genes Dev* 7:1572–1583.

108. Zhang H, Hannon GJ, Beach D (1994) p21-containing cyclin kinases exist in both active and inactive states. *Genes Dev* 8:1750–1758.

167

109. Michieli P, Chedid M, Lin D, Pierce JH, Mercer WE, Givol D (1994) Induction of WAF1/CIP1 by a p53-independent pathway. *Cancer Res* 54:3391–3395.
110. Parker SB, Eichele G, Zhang P, Rawls A, Sands AT, Bradley A, Olson EN, Harper WJ, Elledge SJ (1995) p53-independent expression of p21[CIP1] in muscle and other differentiating cells. *Science* 267:1024–1027.
111. Steinman RA, Hoffman B, Iro A, Guillouf C, Liebermann DA, el-Houseini, ME (1994) Induction of p21 (WAF-1/CIP1) during differentiation. *Oncogene* 9:3389–3396.
112. Jiang H, Lin J, Su ZZ, Collart FR, Huberman E, Fisher PB (1994) Induction of differentiation in human promyelocytic HL-60 leukemia cells activates p21, WAF1/CIP1, expression in the absence of p53. *Oncogene* 9:3397–3406.
113. Waga S, Hannon GJ, Beach D, Stillman B (1994) The p21 inhibitor of cyclin-dependent kinases controls DNA replication by interaction with PCNA. *Nature* 369:574–578.
114. Flores-Rozas H, Kelman Z, Dean FB, Pan ZQ, Harper JW, Elledge SJ, O'Donnell M, Hurwitz J (1994) Cdk-interacting protein 1 directly binds with proliferating cell nuclear antigen and inhibits DNA replication catalyzed by the DNA polymerase delta holoenzyme. *Proc Natl Acad Sci USA* 91:8655–8659.
115. Chen J, Jackson PK, Kirschner MW, Dutta A (1995) Separate domains of p21 involved in the inhibition of Cdk kinase and PCNA. *Nature* 374:386–388.
116. Chedid M, Michieli P, Lengel C, Huppi K, Givol D (1994) A single nucleotide substitution at codon 31 (Ser/Arg) defines a polymorphism in a highly conserved region of the p53-inducible gene WAF1/CIP1. *Oncogene* 9:3021–3024.
117. Li Y-J, Laurent-Puig P, Salmon RJ, Thomas G, Hamelin R (1995) Polymorphisms and probable lack of mutation in the WAF1-CIP1 gene in colorectal cancer. *Oncogene* 10:599–601.
118. Xiong Y, Zhang H, Beach D (1992) D type cyclins associate with multiple protein kinases and the DNA replication and repair factor PCNA. *Cell* 71:505–514.
119. Serrano M, Hannon GJ, Beach D (1993) A new regulatory motif in cell-cycle control causing specific inhibition of cyclin D/CDK4. *Nature* 366:704–707.
120. Parry D, Bates S, Mann DJ, Peters G (1995) Lack of cyclin D-Cdk complexes in Rb-negative cells correlates with high levels of p16 INK4/MTS1 tumour suppressor gene product. *EMBO J* 14:503–511.
121. Hannon GJ, Beach D (1994) p15[INK4B] is a potential effector of TGF-β-induced cell cycle arrest. *Nature* 371:257–261.
122. Nobori T, Miura K, Wu DJ, Lois A, Takabayashi K, Carson DA (1994) Deletions of the cyclin-dependent kinase-4 inhibitor gene in multiple human cancers. *Nature* 368:753–756.
123. Okamoto A, Demetrick DJ, Spillare EA, Hagiwara K, Hussian SP, Bennett WP, Forrester K, Gerwin B, Serrano M, Beach DH, Harris CC (1994) Mutations and altered expression of p16[INK4] in human cancer. *Proc Natl Acad Sci USA* 91:11045–11049.
124. Kamb A, Gruis NA, Weaver-Feldhaus J, Liu Q, Harshman K, Tavtigian SV, Stockert E, Day RS, Johnson BE, Skolnick MH (1994) A cell cycle regulator potentially involved in genesis of many tumor types. *Science* 264:436–440.
125. Cairns P, Mao L, Merlo A, Lee DJ, Schwab D, Eby Y, Tokino K, van der Riet P, Blaugrund JE, Sidransky D (1994) Rates of *p16* (*MTS1*) mutations in primary tumors with 9p loss. *Science* 265:415–416.
126. Spruck C, Gonzalez-Zulueta M, Shibata A, Simoneau AR, Lin MF, Gonzales Tsai YC, Jones PA (1994) p16 gene in uncultured tumours. *Nature* 370:183–184.
127. Caldas C, Hahn SA, da Costa LT, Redston MS, Schutte M, Seymour AB, Weinstein CL, Hruban RH, Yeo CJ, Kern SE (1994) Frequent somatic mutations and homozygous deletions of the p16 (MTS1) gene in pancreatic adenocarcinoma. *Nature Gene* 8:27–32.
128. Kamb A, Shattuck-Eidens D, Eeles R, Liu Q, Gruis NA, Ding W, Hussey C, Tran T, Miki Y, Weaver-Feldhaus J, McClure M, Aitken JF, Anderson DE, Bergman W, Frants R, Goldgar DE, Green A, MacLennan R, Martin NG, Meyer LJ, Youl P, Zone JJ, Skolnick MH, Cannon-Albright LA (1994) Analysis of the p16 gene (CDKN2) as a candidate for the chromosome 9p melanoma suseptibility locus. *Nature Gene* 8:23–26.

168

129. Hussussian CJ, Struewing JP, Goldstein AM, Higgins PA, Ally DS, Sheahan MD, Clark W Jr, Tucker MA, Dracopoli NC (1994) Germline p16 mutations in familial melanoma. *Nature Gene* 8:15–21.

130. Xu L, Sgroi D, Sterner CJ, Beauchamp RL, Pinney DM, Keel S, Ueki K, Rutter JL, Buckler AJ, Louis DN, Gusella JF, Ramesh V (1994) Mutational analysis of *CDKN2* (*MTS1*/p16[INK4]) in human breast carcinomas. *Cancer Res* 54:5262–5264.

131. Guan KL, Jenkins CW, Li Y, Nichols MA, Wu X, O'Keefe CL, Matera AG, Xiong Y (1994) Growth suppression by p18, a p16[INK4/MTS1]- and p14[INK4B/MTS2]-related CDK6 inhibitor, correlates with wild-type pRb function. *Genes Dev* 8:2939–2952.

132. Kato J-Y, Matsuoka M, Polyak K, Massague J, Sherr CJ (1994) Cyclic AMP-induced G_1 phase arrest mediated by an inhibitor (p27[KIP1]) of cyclin-dependent kinase 4 activation. *Cell* 79:487–496.

133. Ewen ME, Sluss HK, Whitehouse LL, Livingston DM (1993) TGF β inhibition of Cdk4 synthesis is linked to cell cycle arrest. *Cell* 74:1009–1020.

134. Firpo EJ, Koff A, Solomon MJ, Roberts JM (1994) Inactivation of a Cdk2 inhibitor during interleukin 2-induced proliferation of human T lymphocytes. *Mol Cell Biol* 14:4889–4901.

135. Polyak K, Lee M-H, Erdjument-Bromage H, Koff A, Roberts JM, Tempst P, Massagué J (1994) Cloning of p27[Kip1], a cyclin-dependent kinase inhibitor and a potential mediator of extracellular antimitogenic signals. *Cell* 78:59–66.

136. Polyak K, Kato JY, Solomon MJ, Sherr CJ, Massague J, Roberts JM, Koff A (1994) p27[KIP1], a cyclin-Cdk inhibitor, links transforming growth factor-beta and contact inhibition to cell cycle arrest. *Genes Dev* 8:9–22.

137. Slingerland JM, Hengst L, Pan C-H, Alexander D, Stampfer MR, Reed SI (1994) A novel inhibitor of cyclin-Cdk activity detected in transforming growth factor β-arrested epithelial cells. *Mol Cell Biol* 14:3683–3694.

138. Ewen ME, Sluss HK, Sherr CJ, Matsushime H, Kato J, Livingston DM (1993) Functional interactions of the retinoblastoma protein with mammalian D-type cyclins. *Cell* 73:487–497.

139. Knabbe C, Lippman ME, Wakefield LM, Flanders KC, Kasid A, Derynck R, Dickson RB (1987) Evidence that transforming growth factor-β is a hormonally regulated negative growth factor in human breast cancer cells. *Cell* 48:417–428.

140. Colletta AA, Wakefield LM, Howell FV, Danielpour D, Baum M, Sporn MB (1991) The growth inhibition of human breast cancer cells by a novel synthetic progestin involves the induction of transforming growth factor beta. *J Clin Invest* 87:277–283.

141. Sporn MB, Roberts AB (1991) Interactions of retinoids and transforming growth factor-beta in regulation of cell differentiation and proliferation. *Mol Endocrinol* 5:3–7.

142. Lee EY-HP, To H, Shew Y-Y, Bookstein R, Scully P, Lee W-H (1988) Inactivation of the retinoblastoma susceptibility gene in human breast cancers. *Science* 241:218–211.

143. Bartek J, Iggo R, Gannon J, Lane DP (1990) Genetic and immunohistochemical analysis of mutant p53 in human breast cancer cell lines. *Oncogene* 5:893–899.

144. T'Ang A, Varley JM, Chakraborty S, Murphree AL, Fung Y-KT (1988) Structural rearrangement of the retinoblastoma gene in human breast carcinoma. *Science* 242:263–266.

145. Wang J, Chenivesse X, Henglein B, Brechot C (1990) Hepatitis B virus integration in a cyclin A gene in a hepatocellular carcinoma. *Nature* 343:555–557.

146. Wang J, Zindy F, Chenivesse X, Lamas E, Henglein B, Brechot C (1992) Modification of cyclin A expression by hepatitis B virus DNA integration in a hepatocellular carcinoma. *Oncogene* 7:1653–1656.

147. Bagchi S, Raychaudhuri P, Nevins JR (1990) Adenovirus E1A proteins can dissociate heteromeric complexes involving the E2F transcription factor: A novel mechanism for E1A trans-activation. *Cell* 62:659–669.

148. Johnson DG, Schwarz JK, Cress WD, Nevins JR (1993) Expression of transcription factor E2F1 induces quiescent cells to enter S phase. *Nature* 365:349–352.

149. Mudryj M, Devoto SH, Hiebert SW, Hunter T, Pines J, Nevins JR (1991) Cell cycle regulation of the E2F transcription factor involves an interaction with cyclin A. *Cell* 65:1243–1253.

150. Singh P, Wong SH, Hong W (1994) Overexpression of E2F-1 in rat embryo fibroblasts leads to neoplastic transformation. *EMBO J* 13:3329–3338.
151. Arnold A, Kim HG (1989) Clonal loss of one chromosome 11 in a parathyroid adenoma. *J Clin Endorinol Metab* 69:496–499.
152. Friedman E, Bale AE, Marx SJ, Norton JA, Arnold A, Tu T, Aurbach GD, Spiegel AM (1990) Genetic abnormalities in sporadic parathyroid adenomas. *J Clin Endocrin Metab* 71:293–297.
153. Nisson PE, Watkins PC, Sacchi N (1992) Transcriptionally active chimeric gene derived from the fusion of the AML1 gene and a novel gene on chromosome 8 in t(8;21) leukemic cells. *Cancer Gen Cytogen* 63:81–88.
154. Hanna Z, Jankowski M, Tremblay P, Jiang X, Milatvich A, Francke U, Jolicoeur P (1993) The Vin-1 gene, identified by provirus insertional mutagenesis, is the cyclin D2. *Oncogene* 8:1661–1666.

170

9. Nuclear oncogenes in breast cancer

Don Dubik, Peter H. Watson, Marcello Venditti, and Robert P.C. Shiu

Introduction

The prevailing view of cancer is that it is a disease resulting from a number of sequential mutations in critical growth regulatory genes [1]. In the past 20 years it has been discovered that retroviral transforming genes, oncogenes, were actually modified growth regulatory genes derived from the viral host genome. In all cases the modifications in the viral oncogene yielded a growth regulatory gene that exhibited enhanced or unregulated activity when compared with its normal cellular counterpart. Growth regulatory genes may act to enhance or inhibit growth and encompass transactivators, including the steroid/retinoid/thyroid hormone receptors, cell cycle regulators, tumor suppressors, growth factors, and growth factor receptors.

This broad range of cellular regulators potentiates its effects through a number of different molecular pathways that may converge. Normal cell growth is a balance between progression through the cell cycle and programmed cell death (apoptosis), and cancer is a disease resulting from the disruption of this balance, allowing a cell to progress through the cell cycle unabated. It is evident that growth regulators control a small subgroup of genes that encode regulators of cell cycle progression or apoptosis. In this chapter we address one group of growth regulators, nuclear proto-oncogenes, as they relate to breast cancer. We review their functions and regulations, and attempt to define their role in the control of breast cell growth. We will limit our definition of proto-oncogenes to the cellular homologues of tumor-causing retroviral genes as opposed to any gene (e.g., cyclins) whose deregulated expression has the potential to cause tumorigenesis.

Nuclear oncogenes and tumor suppressor genes in the breast: c-*myc*, c-*fos*, c-*jun*, c-*myb*, Rb, and p53

To date more than 70 oncogenes have been characterized. Of these genes, more than a dozen encode proteins with a nuclear localization. For the most part, the products of these nuclear oncogenes encode *trans*-acting transcrip-

R. Dickson and M. Lippman (eds.) MAMMARY TUMOR CELL CYCLE, DIFFERENTIATION AND METASTASIS. 1996. Kluwer Academic Publishers. ISBN 0-7923-3905-3. All rights reserved.

tional factors. The nuclear oncogenes that have been studied with respect to their potential roles in the proliferation and development of normal and cancerous breast epithelium are c-*myc*, c-*fos*, c-*jun*, and c-*myb*. All of these proto-oncogenes are classified as *immediate early genes* since they are expressed transiently in the G_1 phase of the cell cycle and are involved in initiating the progression of the cells through the cell cycle. In breast epithelium, the expression of these genes has been found to be influenced by a variety of factors, including steroids, retinoids, peptide hormones, and growth factors. In addition to these proto-oncogenes, the nuclear tumor-suppressor genes (or antioncogenes) Rb and p53 have also been shown to be important in normal and cancerous breast physiology. In this review we limit the discussion to the above-mentioned genes.

c-myc

Although the c-*myc* proto-oncogene was one of the first to be identified, many aspects of its regulation, and the regulation, function, and mechanism of action of its protein product c-MYC, have only recently been discovered [2–4]. The c-*myc* proto-oncogene is one of three well-defined members (the others being N-*myc* and L-*myc*) of the MYC family. Each member codes for a nuclear phosphoprotein with structual similarity in the N- and C-terminal regions. The C-terminal region of each MYC protein contains a *helix-loop-helix*, *leucine zipper* motif through which it dimerizes with the nuclear protein MAX [4]. This MYC/MAX complex is a transactivator when bound to the E-box sequence [CA(C/T)GTG] of responsive genes [5,6]. To date more than a dozen genes have been reported to be regulated by MYC (Table 1). Among these MYC target genes are the G_1 cell cycle regulator cyclin D1, whose expression is enhanced upon short exposure to c-MYC and repressed upon chronic exposure [7], the transactivator E2F-2, one of a family of transactivators through which the tumor suppressor Rb acts [8], and the tumor suppressor p53 [9]. MYC also regulates its own activity through autorepression [10].

What is the evidence that c-MYC is involved in breast cancer? In vitro studies using human breast cancer cell lines indicate that c-MYC is important for cell growth and that it may play a role in the transition from hormone-dependent to hormone-independent growth [11]. In vivo studies in human breast tumors, focusing predominantly on c-*myc* amplification, have shown c-*myc* amplification is prevalent in 20–30% of breast carcinomas, although the degree of amplification is often low [12]. Furthermore, several of these studies, including some with large sample sizes [13,14], have shown c-*myc* amplification to be both a significant and independent prognostic indicator of early disease recurrence and poor outcome. Unlike hematopoietic malignancies, in breast carcinomas gross alteration of the c-*myc* gene through translocation is uncommon [15].

Aside from c-*myc* amplification and translocation, many aspects of c-*myc* expression in breast cancer, including changes in the regulation, changes in the

172

Table 1. List of proposed c-MYC regulated genes

Gene	Type of expression	Mechanism of expression	Ref.
c-*myc*	Repression	Autoregulation	10
Cyclin D1	Induction (short exposure)	3 E-box elements in promoter	104
	Repression (chronic exposure)	Inr element in promoter	51,105
Cyclin A	Induction	Unknown	51
Cyclin E	Induction	Unknown	51
E2F-2	Induction	3 E-box elements in promoter	8
p53	Induction	E-box element in exon 1	9
α-prothymosin	Induction	E-box element in intron 1	106,107
C/EBPα	Repression	Inr element	108
Dihydrofolate reductase	Induction	Tandem E-box elements	109
Ornithine decarboxylase	Induction	E-box element in promoter	110,111
ECA39	Induction	E-box element exon 1	112
c-*erbB*-2/*neu*	Repression	Transcriptional	113
N-CAM [by N-Myc]	Repression	Inr element	114
MHC class I	Repression	Inr element	115
LFA-1	Repression	Transcriptional/ post-transcriptional	116
CD44	Repression	Inr element	117,118
Pro-α1 (I) collagen Pro-α2 (I) collagen Pro-α3 (IV) collagen	Repression	Unknown	119
Albumin	Repression	Unknown	108
Gelatinase B	Induction	5 potential E-box elements, 2 in promoter region	120
PAI-1	Induction	Post-transcriptional	121,122
MIG 1	Induction	Unknown	123
MIG 11	Induction	Unknown	123

E-box = CACGTG; Inr = initiator sequence.

levels of expression, or the occurrence of alterations of c-*myc* within specific stages of tumor progression, have not been carefully examined. For example, altered regulation of c-*myc* expression at the level of mRNA stability can occur in breast cancer cell lines [11], and we have found that c-*myc* amplification can differ within components of breast carcinomas [12]. Furthermore, we have seen that amplification can occur at a comparatively early stage of tumor progression, and while this alteration exists in both the in situ and invasive components of tumors, it does not always persist in the corresponding nodal metastases [12]. Recent observations that MYC may regulate a number of genes involved in cell adhesion and proteolysis (see Table 1) have reaffirmed our suspicions that in breast cancer MYC may play a role in the transition from in situ to invasive carcinoma.

Perhaps the most compelling evidence of c-MYC's involvement in breast cancer is derived from studies of MMTV-*myc* or WAP-*myc* transgenic mice [16–18]. In the case of MMTV-*myc* transgenic mice, c-*myc* is expressed in breast cells and in lymphoid T cells and T-cell precursors. These mice develop breast tumors and occasional lymphomas, and tumors develop in 50% of female mice in less than a year [16,17]. Tumorigenesis can be greatly enhanced by coexpression of c-*myc* and c-*ras* [19]. In the case of c-*myc*/c-*ras* transgenic mice, within 46 days tumors formed in 50% of the females [19]. Furthermore, coexpression of c-*myc* with casein kinase II (CKII), which is a nuclear kinase that phosphorylates the MYC protein [20], results in the development of lethal lymphomas in neonatal and perinatal mice [21]. The early lethal effect of the cooperation between c-MYC and CKII on the hematopoietic cell lineage has precluded assessment of the effect on other tissues; however, it is possible that the same cooperative effects hold true in the breast. Therefore, deregulated MYC expression in the breast epithelium can lead to tumor formation, and the effect on tumorigenesis can be influenced by other cellular anomalies.

c-fos, c-jun

Both proto-oncogenes are members of larger gene families: c-*fos*, *fos*-B, *fra*-1, *fra*-2, and c-*jun*, *jun*-B, *jun*-D [22]. All encode nuclear phosphoproteins containing a *leucine zipper* dimerization domain. JUN proteins form homodimeric complexes and heterodimeric complexes with related family members, as well as heterodimeric complexes with FOS family members [23]. Dimeric complexes transactivate when bound to a phorbol ester response element (TRE, -TGACTCA-). Heterodimeric JUN/FOS (AP-1) complexes are efficient gene activators, while JUN homodimeric complexes transactivate poorly, and FOS homodimers fail to bind DNA [24,25]. The physiological function of different complexes varies, as does their tissue distribution, pathways, and sensitivity to different signal transductions [23]. There have been numerous reports of regulated expression of c-*fos* and c-*jun* after mitogen stimulation of breast cancer cells [22,23,26–28]. These studies have shown that c-*fos* and c-*jun* expression is influenced to varying degrees by growth factors including insulin, TGF-α, IGF-1, and EGF [22,28] and by steroid hormones [26,27]. Continuous expression of c-*fos* can transform fibroblasts and cause osteosarcomas in mice [29], suggesting a role in proliferation and differentiation. Surprisingly, targeted disruption of c-*fos* or c-*jun* in embryonic stem (ES) cells did not affect their growth and differentiation, suggesting that neither gene is essential for these processes [30,31]. This result suggests that other *fos* family members may be able to compensate for the absence of c-*fos* in ES cells. It should be noted, however, that mice with c-*jun* null mutations die at mid-gestation (12.5 days), suggesting that c-*jun* is critical to cells later in embryo development [32]. This result also suggest that various AP-1 factors act specifically and temporally with differing roles. The c-FOS/c-JUN complex is believed to regulate a variety of genes, including activation of *fra*-1, ornithine decarboxylase, cyclin D1, transin and collagenase and repression of *fra*-2, *jun*-D, and possibly c-*jun* [29].

174

Recently it has been proposed that the AP-1 complex might be an important regulator of vimentin expression in breast tumor cells [33], suggesting that expression of c-*fos* and c-*jun* could indirectly influence the development of the invasive phenotype that is associated with vimentin expression [34]. This observation suggests a possible association between c-*fos*/c-*jun* expression and tumor progression.

c-myb

The c-*myb* proto-oncogene also encodes a nuclear phosphoprotein. It was initially recognized to play a role in the proliferation and differentiation of hematopoietic precursor cells in which its expression was increased in late G_1 and S cells [35]. Subsequently, deregulated c-*myb* expression was recognized in a variety of cell types, including those in breast tumors [36]. In addition to c-*myb* there are at least two other family members, A-*myb* and B-*myb* [37,38]. The MYB protein is a transactivator that binds the consensus *cis*-acting element (C/Pu)(Py/A)Py AAC PyPu [39]. The c-*myc* gene has been proposed as a target of c-MYB and possibly B-MYB [39,40], and potential c-MYB binding sites have also been proposed in the DNA polymerase-α, cyclin D1, and cdc2 genes [41]. Alternatively, c-JUN and JUN-D may transactivate c-*myb* [42]. In breast cancer, c-*myb* mRNA expression was identified in at least one study in a high proportion of tumors (64%) and was associated with a positive estrogen receptor status [36].

Tumor suppressor genes in the breast

In addition to the nuclear oncogenes, two tumor suppressor genes, Rb and p53, have been shown to be important in breast physiology. Both are nuclear phosphoproteins and can suppress cell proliferation at the G_1 phase of the cell cycle.

p53

Mutation of p53 is believed to contribute to as much as 50% of human cancers. Runnebaum and colleagues examined 20 human breast cancer cell lines and 59 primary breast tumors, and concluded that p53 gene mutations are the most common single mutations found in human breast cancer [43]. Alteration of p53 occurs at several levels, including the gene itself, the mRNA transcript, or the p53 protein. Most p53 gene alterations result from a point mutation, but in breast cancer the p53 gene is also prone to small rearrangements, deletions, or insertions [43]. Transfection of an intact p53 into breast cancer cell lines harboring a p53 mutation was able to suppress the malignant phenotype [44]. Although the function of p53 is not as yet fully known, recent studies have suggested that its role in the cell is to attenuate cell progression through G_1 to allow DNA repair mechanisms the opportunity to function [45]. The mechanism of p53 action involves transactivation of its nuclear target p21 (also known as WAF1, CIP1, SDI1, CAP20, and PIC1), which in turn inactivates a number of cyclin-cdk complexes and PCNA (part of the DNA replication machinery) [7]. Mutation of p53 prevents it from entering the nucleus or from transactivating p21, the consequence of which is genomic instability and uncontrolled progression [7]. The mechanism of c-*myc* induced apoptosis is also believed to involve p53. As stated earlier, c-MYC transactivates p53, which will then, via p21, interrupt cell cycling. Depending on the growth stresses experienced by the cells, this p53-mediated cell cycle interruption can lead to G_1 arrest or to apoptosis [46].

Retinoblastoma susceptibility gene product, Rb

As with p53, mutations of the Rb gene are also prevalent in breast cancer, occurring in 20% of primary breast cancers and 25% of breast cancer cell lines [47]. Rb and related proteins, p107 and p130, are phosphoproteins that mediate their growth suppressor effects through an interaction with the E2F family of transcriptional activators and inhibit their function [48–50]. By blocking the activity of the E2F/DP transactivator, Rb is able to prevent the activation of cell cycle genes, such as cyclin A and cdc2 [50–52]. The mechanism or Rb action will be discussed in some detail later.

Regulation of nuclear oncogenes in the breast

Regulation by estrogens

Regulation of c-*myc* expression is complex because it is affected by a large number of factors, including steroid and peptide hormones and growth factors. This is due to the fact that c-*myc* is involved in many aspects of cell biology, including cell growth, differentiation, and apoptosis. Thus, changes in the expression of the c-MYC might conceivably affect many aspects of tumor progression.

The importance of estrogen in breast development is well established [53]. Estrogen together with other growth factors influence epithelial mitosis involved in ductal development [53]. Estrogen is also the principal hormone relevant to breast cancer, evidenced by the extremely low incidence of breast cancer in men and in women with dysfunctional ovaries [54,55]. The effects of estrogen and its mechanisms of action in both normal and cancerous tissue are vital to understanding breast cancer biology. In breast cancer cell lines, estrogen increases the activity of several genes involved in DNA replication, such as DNA polymerase, thymidine kinase, dihydrofolate reductase, thymidylate synthase, uridine kinase, carbamyl phosphate synthetase, aspartate transcarbamylase, and glucose-6-phosphate dehydrogenase [56]. Estrogen has also been shown to stimulate the expression of a variety of growth factors, including IGF-I, IGF-II, and TGF-α, all of which are breast cancer cell mitogens [56]. Estrogen also stimulates the expression of the progesterone receptor, and progesterone receptor levels are commonly used to assess estrogen receptor function in breast tumors [57]. Finally, our work and that of others has shown that estrogen can regulate the expression of the nuclear proto-oncogenes c-*myc* [58] and c-*myb* [59] in breast cancer cell lines and c-*fos* and c-*jun* in rat uterus [60].

In order to identify estrogen regulated genes involved in growth, we have focused on the MCF-7 breast cancer cell line, which is hormone responsive and contains functional estrogen receptors (ER). When MCF-7 cells are cultured in phenol red–free media containing charcoal-treated, steroid-depleted fetal bovine serum, they experience a distinct growth attenuation [58,61]. Treatment of these steroid-depleted cells with 17β-estradiol is sufficient to stimulate proliferation [58]. Associated with this proliferation is a rapid and transient induction in both c-*myc* mRNA and protein [58,62]. Pretreatment of the cells with cycloheximide, a translation inhibitor, does not inhibit the estrogen induction of c-*myc*, indicating that estrogen's effects on c-*myc* expression are independent of new protein synthesis. This result suggests the estrogen receptor complex transcriptionally regulates the c-*myc* gene, a conjecture that was confirmed by nuclear run-on transcriptional studies [11]. Our results have subsequently been reproduced by others [22,59].

We have also further examined the molecular mechanism of estrogen action on c-*myc* regulation. Using transient expression studies we were able to demonstrate that the P2 promoter of the human c-*myc* gene was essential to estrogen-regulated expression and that the estrogen response region of c-*myc* could be localized to a 116 bp fragment overlapping the P2 promoter [61]. Contained in the 116 bp region are two regulatory elements, ME1a1 and ME1a2: The former overlaps the binding site of the E2F and MAZ transcriptional factors [56]. The 116 bp region does not contain sequences resembling any known estrogen response elements. Furthermore, both gel retardation and DNaseI footprinting studies using the 116 bp region, and in vitro transcribed and translated ER failed to show a direct interaction of the ER complex with the 116 bp region. This failure of the ER complex to bind the 116 bp region may be an indication that the ER interaction is too weak to detect with standard DNA binding assays or that additional ER associated proteins may be necessary to permit DNA binding.

To date a number of ER associated proteins have been identified [63–65]. Not surprisingly, when MCF-7 nuclear extract was used in DNA binding studies, extensive retardation and footprinting of the 116 bp region was observed. We have yet to show that any of these complexes contain the ER. Alternatively, the lack of ER binding may point to an indirect ER function to activate existing transcriptional regulators of c-*myc*. Such transcriptional regulators may include the E2F family of transactivators that have been extensively studied in nonbreast cell types. Findings from these studies may be relevant to unraveling the events of c-*myc* regulation in the breast.

The E2F family consists of at least five members (E2F-1 through E2F-5), which, as heterodimeric complexes with factor DP (three members: DP-1 through DP-3), bind and transactivate from the E2F binding site [50]. E2F/DP heterodimeric transcription factors are believed to regulate a large number of genes, including c-*myc*, dihydrofolate reductase, cdc2, B-*myb*, cyclin A, and DNA polymerase α [66]. This regulation is carried out in conjunction with the tumor suppressor Rb and the related factors, p107 and p130 [50]. When complexed with Rb, p107, or p130, E2F is unable to transactivate [50]. In the E2F-Rb complex, phosphorylation of Rb, or Rb interaction with other factors such as E1A, lead to the generation of a 'free,' active E2F molecule [50,67]. Therefore, if ER was able to influence the dissociation of Rb from the E2F-Rb complex, it could render E2F active to transactivate c-*myc*. Experimental evidence to support ER activation of E2F, however, is lacking. There are no reports of ER triggering phosphorylation of Rb or the disruption of the E2F-Rb complex. Nonetheless, it should be noted that there is a two- to fourfold increase in the phosphorylation of the estrogen receptor in the presence of hormone [68,69] and that estradiol can, almost instantaneously and in a receptor-dependent manner, stimulate phosphorylation of other proteins in MCF-7 cells [70]. Also, there are at least two reports of enzymatic activity (kinase and protease) associated with immunopurified ER [71,72]. It is conceivable that these enzymatic activities are responsible for modifying the structure or function of other proteins.

Besides the lack of evidence that ER activates the E2F-Rb complex, there is also uncertainty regarding the importance of c-*myc* transactivation by E2F in vivo. It has been reported that E2F-1/DP-1 binds and transactivates the c-*myc* P2 promoter and that the inhibitory effects of Rb are associated with the E2F binding site [52]; however, there is also evidence to suggest that expression of E2F-1 occurs later in the G1 phase of the cell cycle, after c-*myc* activation [50]. It is still conceivable that other, more early expressed members of the E2F family (e.g., E2F-4 and E2F-5 [50]) could be responsible, at least in part, for the increased expression of c-*myc* following mitogen stimulation of cells. Even though the role of E2F transactivation of c-*myc* remains uncertain, recent work by Nevins and colleagues shows that MYC can transactivate E2F-2 but not E2F-1, defining another pathway through which c-*myc* expression leads to cellular proliferation [8].

To date not only the c-*myc* gene but also the c-*fos*, cathepsin D, progesterone receptor, ovalbumin, and creatine kinase genes have all been shown to exhibit unconventional mechanisms of ER transactivation [73–77]. Clearly the mechanism of estrogen receptor transactivation can vary widely for different genes in different cell types. Although estrogen activation of c-*myc* in hormone-responsive breast cancer cell lines is now well established, the precise mechanism of this activation is still unknown.

178

In addition to regulating c-*myc* expression, estrogen has also been reported to increase expression of c-*fos* and its partner c-*jun* in breast cancer cell lines [60]. This increased expression, however, appears to be dependent on the culture conditions. Under steroid-depleted culture conditions, we have observed a less than twofold induction of c-*fos* expression. Alternatively, addition of insulin results in a greater than fivefold induction in c-*fos* expression [56]. Similarly, Davidson et al. reported that estradiol had little effect on c-*fos*, c-*jun*, *jun*-B and *jun*-D expression in steroid-depleted MCF-7 cells synchronized by a double thymidine block [22]. They also showed that insulin, EGF, and TGF-α stimulate expression of c-*fos*, c-*jun*, and *jun*-B. Wilding et al. also confirmed that estrogen had a minimal effect on c-*fos* expression, whereas EGF and TGF-α stimulated expression up to sixfold [78]. These results together suggest that, unlike estrogen regulation of c-*myc* expression, the regulation of c-*fos* and c-*jun* in breast cancer cell lines is largely dependent on peptide hormones or growth factors. The inability of estrogen to activate the endogenous c-*fos* gene in breast cancer cells, even though it can stimulate CAT expression from the c-*fos* promoter in transient expression experiments [60], is probably an indication that the endogenous c-*fos* promoter is silent due to such processes as DNA methylation.

As mentioned earlier, c-*myb* has also been implicated as a direct estrogen target gene on the basis of in vitro studies and correlation of c-*myb* expression with estrogen receptor–positive tumors. It is also possible that c-*myb* lies upstream of c-*myc* in the pathway of estrogen action, because potential binding sites for c-*myb* have been found in the c-*myc*, cdc2, and cyclin D1 genes, and one report shows that c-*myb* and B-*myb* transactivate a c-*myc*–CAT construct [39]. A recent study by Gudas et al., however, does not confirm the above observations [59]. This latter study shows that in estrogen-depleted MCF-7 cells, addition of estradiol results in transient induction in c-*myb* expression, peaking at about 20-fold, 5 hours post–hormone addition and suggests a post-transcriptional level of c-*myb* regulation. Thus c-*myb* induction by estrogen occurs later than c-*myc* induction, suggesting that c-*myb* activation of c-*myc* expression, if it indeed occurs at all, is not an essential step in estrogen-regulated proliferation of breast cancer cells [59]. This conclusion is in agreement with our earlier studies of c-*myc* regulation by estrogen in the presence of a translational inhibitor cycloheximide, in which we showed that this regulation is a primary event not requiring de novo protein systhesis [11]. A recent study showed that the constitutive expression of B-*myb* can prevent p53-mediated growth arrest, suggesting that MYB may play a role in increasing the proliferative potential of stimulated cells by encouraging cells to cycle and protecting them from undergoing apoptosis [79].

Regulation by progrestins

In the normal breast, progesterone is a principal hormone involved in the stimulation of glandular epithelium, promoting ductal branching and lobuloalveolar development [53]. In breast cancer cells, the overall effect of progestins is to inhibit growth [26], and they have been used effectively in the therapeutic treatment of breast cancer patients [80]. The mechanism of this growth inhibition is for the most part unclear; however, several recent studies have identified the nuclear oncogenes c-*fos*, c-*jun*, and c-*myc* as targets of progestin action [26,81]. For the most part, these studies were done using the hormone-responsive human breast cancer cell line T-47D, although some of the experiments were repeated in the hormone-responsive MCF-7 breast cancer cell line with similar results. By culturing T-47D cells in serum-free medium supplemented with insulin, Musgrove et al. characterized a biphasic effect of progestin treatment [26]. This biphasic effect of progestin involved an initial stimulation of the progression of actively cycling cells through the cell cycle, followed by a blockage in G1 of the newly cycling cells.

Associated with the progestin-stimulated progression is a rapid transient induction in the expression of the proto-oncogenes c-*fos* and c-*myc*, which is maximal at 30 and 90 minutes, respectively. There is also an induction of EGF, TGF-α, and EGF receptors (EGF-R). Similar observations have been made by Murphy et al., who in addition showed a progestin specific induction of c-*jun* mRNA (maximal 3–6 hours post–hormone addition) and a progestin-specific reduction of TGF-β_1 mRNA levels [81]. Taken together, the increased expression of c-*fos*, c-*jun*, c-*myc*, EGF, EGF-R, and TGFα, with a corresponding decrease of TGF-β_1, are indicative of enhanced cellular proliferation and can explain the progestin-stimulated progression seen in T-47D and MCF-7 cells. What is not understood is the nature of the later growth-inhibitory effects of progestins. Some insight into this growth inhibition has been obtained through studies using antiprogestins, such as RU486 and ZK98299. Like progestins, antiprogestins inhibit cell proliferation of T-47D cells [81]. Adding to T-47D cells a 10- to 100-fold excess of RU486 simultaneously with progestin antagonizes progestin-stimulated gene expression [26,81]. However, when proliferating T-47D cells were treated with RU486, c-*myc* mRNA levels were lowered by approximately 80% [82]. Basal mRNA levels of c-*fos*, c-*jun*, EGF, EGF-R, TGF-α, and TGF-β_1 appeared to be unaffected by RU486 [81,82]. Although much work remains to be done to understand progestin action in breast cancer cells, it would seem that MYC is an important modulator of both the early cycle progression and later growth inhibitory effects of progestins, as well as the growth inhibitory effects of antiprogestins.

Regulation by retinoids

In general terms retinoids are classified as differentiating factors, and they are known to inhibit cell growth. In human breast cancer cell lines *all-trans* retinoic acid (RA) has been shown to block the growth of normal cycling cells as well as cell growth induced by estrogen and insulin-like growth factors [83]. In most cell types, differentiation triggered by RA is associated with a distinct

180

decrease in c-*myc* mRNA expression. In serum-deprived MCF-7 cells, however, RA has been shown not to decrease c-*myc* expression as expected, but rather to increase c-*myc* mRNA levels in a manner analogous to that seen with progestins [84]. Although further studies of the mechanism of growth inhibition by RA and progestins need to be done, it would appear that both compounds may share a common inhibitory mechanism, possibly involving MYC.

Regulation by growth factors

In breast cancer, insulin and a variety of growth factors, including IGF-I, IGF-II, TGF-α, EGF, and TGF-β, are believed to be important autocrine, paracrine, or endocrine factors. Each of these growth factors potentiates its effects by interacting with cell surface receptors to activate receptor-associated kinase activities, resulting in a phosphorylation cascade by several independent but interacting pathways [85–87].

Treatment of breast cancer cells with insulin or growth factors, such as EGF, TGF-α, IGF-I, and IGF-II, results in the increased expression of c-*fos*, c-*jun*, and c-*myc* [22,28,56,88]. Based on information obtained with many cell types, it is assumed that in breast cancer cells, this increased expression is a result of the actions of mitogen activated protein kinases (MAPK); thus, ERK1 and ERK2, via the activation of transcription factor Elk-1/TCP, are believed to activate c-*fos* expression [89–92]. Likewise, JNK1/p45 and JNK2/p55 are believed to activate c-JUN by phosphorylation [93–95]. c-JUN activation also triggers further c-*jun* expression through autoregulation [96]. With regard to c-MYC, the function of MAPKs is not clear. Phosphorylation events at Thr-58 (decreased phosphorylation) and Ser-62 (increased phosphorylation) are known to be important in c-MYC's transformation potential [97,98]. In vitro, MAPKs and glycogen synthase kinase-3 (GSK-3) phosphorylate Thr-58 and Ser-62 [99]. There is, however, some uncertainty as to whether MAPKs phosphorylate c-MYC in vivo and whether phosphorylation events at Thr-58 and Ser-62 are necessary for c-MYC transactivation via the E-box [98].

Casein kinase II (CKII) is also believed to phosphorylate MYC at several sites [20,100], as well as MYC's dimerization partner MAX at Ser-2 and Ser-11 [101]. This phosphorylation presumably enhances MYC activity, possibly by promoting the formation of MYC/MAX heterodimers instead of MAX/MAX homodimers [101]. That CKII is important in enhancing MYC activity is suggested by the MYC/CKII transgenic mice studies discussed earlier [21]. Nonetheless, it is at present not known whether CKII is a component of any peptide growth factor signal transduction pathway. Clearly, there is still a considerable amount of work to be done to elucidate the mechanism of the influence of growth factors on proto-oncogene expression in breast cancer cells.

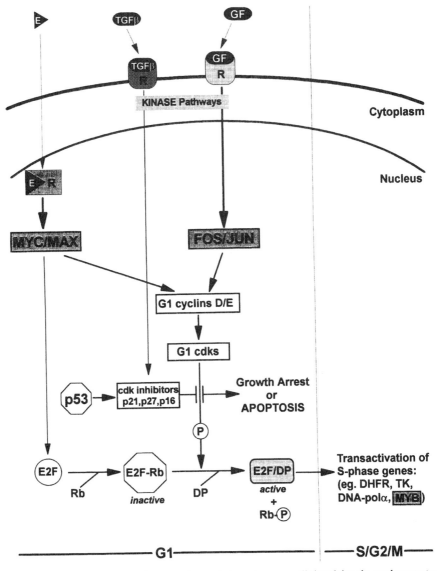

Figure 1. Potential growth regulatory pathways in breast cancer cells involving the nuclear proto-oncogenes. Activation of the estrogen receptor by binding estrogen leads to transactivation of c-*myc* (and to a lesser extent c-*fos* and c-*jun*), resulting in an active MYC/MAX or AP-1 (FOS/JUN) complex. These complexes are believed to influence expression of the G_1-phase cell cycle cyclins D1, D2, D3, and cyclin E. These cyclins, in turn, activate the respective cyclin dependent kinases (cdks), which can phosphorylate and activate other factors involved in cell cycle progression. One such factor may be Rb, which, upon phosphorylation, disassociates from E2F, thus triggering the formation of the active E2F/DP transactivator. Also, MYC is known to transcriptionally stimulate the expression of E2F-2, further augmenting total E2F activity. E2F/DP is known to transactivate a number of S-phase genes important for DNA synthesis, genes that include c-*myb*. In a similar manner, acting through membrane-bound receptors, growth factors (GF) trigger a phosphorylation cascade that also results in enhanced AP-1 and MYC/MAX activity. Growth inhibitors like p53 and TGF-β stimulate the expression of specific cdk inhibitors that block the action of G_1 cdks (cdk 2, 4, 5, 6). This blockage of G_1 cdks' activities leads to either growth arrest, or if the cell is stressed, to apoptosis. For more details see text. E = estradiol; R = receptor; cdk = cyclin-dependent kinase; DHFR = dihydrofolate reductase; TK = thymidine kinase; DNA polα = DNA polymerase α; P = phosphorylation.

Conclusions

In this short review, we have highlighted the current knowledge of nuclear proto-oncogene regulation and expression in human breast cancer. We have concentrated on c-*myc*, c-*fos*, c-*jun*, and c-*myb*, not because these are the only nuclear proto-oncogenes expressed in breast cancer, but because they are the best studied. In breast cancer cells, steroids, peptide hormones, or growth factors exert their influences by mechanisms that affect these nuclear oncogenes. In Figure 1 we have attempted to summarize potential growth and inhibition mechanisms that may exist in breast cancer cells. It would appear that there is considerable convergence between various regulatory pathways. For example, TGF-β potentiates its inhibitory effect on breast cancer cell growth through a pathway similar to that of p53, involving a cyclin-dependent kinase inhibitor [102]. Nonetheless, even if the effects of various steroids and growth factors are similar, the mechanisms resulting in these effects are, at least in part, distinctive and independent. For example, both IGF-I and estrogen stimulate cellular proliferation of breast cancer cells, and IGF-I receptor antibodies have been shown to inhibit the effects of IGF-I. However, these IGF-I receptor antibodies do not inhibit the effect of estrogen on cell growth, suggesting that the mechanisms of action of estrogen and IGF-I are distinct and independent [103]. The mechanisms by which mitogens and growth inhibitors influence nuclear oncogene activities in breast cancer remain to be defined. It is almost certain that many of the key intracellular regulators are now known, and the next few years will see a more complete definition of the pathways leading to the proliferation, differentiation, or apoptosis of breast cancer cells.

References

1. Fearon E, Vogelstein B (1990) A genetic model for colorectal tumorigenesis. *Cell* 61:759–767.
2. Luscher B, Eisenman RN (1990) New light on Myc and Myb. Part 1. Myc. *Genes Dev* 4:2025–2035.
3. Amati B, Brooks MW, Levy N, Littlewood TD, Evan GI, Land H (1993) Oncogenic activity of the c-Myc protein requires dimerization with Max. *Cell* 72:233–245.
4. Blackwood EM, Luscher B, Kretzner L, Eisenman RN (1991) The Myc: Max protein complex and cell growth regulation. *Cold Spring Harb Symp Quant Biol* 56:109–117.
5. Prendergast GC, Ziff EB (1991) Methylation-sensitive sequence-specific DNA binding by the c-myc basic region. *Science* 251:186–189.
6. Blackwood EM, Eisenman RN (1991) Max: A helix-loop-helix zipper protein that forms a sequence-specific DNA binding complex with Myc. *Science* 251:1211–1217.
7. Hunter T, Pines J (1994) Cyclins and cancer. II: Cyclin D and CDK inhibitors come of age [see comments]. *Cell* 79:573–582.
8. Nevins JR (1995) Cell cycle control and oncogenesis (abstr). *Proc Am Assoc Cancer Res* 36:685.
9. Reisman D, Elkind NB, Roy B, Beamon J, Rotter V (1993) c-Myc trans-activates the p53 promoter through a required downstream CACGTG motif. *Cell Growth Differ* 4:57–65.

10. Penn LJ, Brooks MW, Laufer EM, Land H (1990) Negative autoregulation of c-myc transcription. *EMBO J* 9:1113–1121.
11. Dubik D, Shiu RP (1988) Transcriptional regulation of c-myc oncogene expression by estrogen in hormone-responsive human breast cancer cells. *J Biol Chem* 263:12705–12708.
12. Watson PH, Safneck JR, Le K, Dubik D, Shiu RP (1993) Relationship of c-myc amplification to progression of breast cancer from in situ to invasive tumor and lymph node metastasis. *J Natl Cancer Inst* 85:902–907.
13. Borg A, Baldetorp B, Ferno M, Olsson H, Sigurdsson H (1992) c-myc amplification is an independent prognostic factor in postmenopausal breast cancer. *Int J Cancer* 51:687–691.
14. Berns EM, Klijn JG, van Putten WL, van Staveren IL, Portengen H, Foekens JA (1992) c-myc amplification is a better prognostic factor than HER2/neu amplification in primary breast cancer. *Cancer Res* 52:1107–1113.
15. Varley JM, Wainwright AM, Brammar WJ (1987) An unusual alteration in c-myc in tissue from a primary breast carcinoma. *Oncogene* 1:431–438.
16. Stewart TA, Pattenfale PK, Leder P (1984) Spontaneous mammary adenocarcinomas in transgenic mice that carry and express MMTV/myc fusion genes. *Cell* 38:627–637.
17. Leder A, Pattengale PK, Kuo O, Stewart TA, Leder P (1986) Consequences of widespread deregulation of the c-myc gene in transgenic mice: Multiple neoplasms and normal development. *Cell* 45:485–495.
18. Schoenenberger C, Andres A, Groner B, van der Valk M, LeMeur M, Gerlinger P (1988) Targeted c-myc gene expression in mammary glands of transgenic mice induces mammary tumours with constitutive milk protein gene transcription. *EMBO J* 7:169–175.
19. Sinn E, Muller W, Pattengale P, Tepler I, Wallace R, Leder P (1987) Coexpression of MMTV/v-Ha-ras and MMTV/c-myc genes in transgenic mice: Synergistic action of oncogenes in vivo. *Cell* 49:465–475.
20. Luscher B, Kuenzel EA, Krebs EG, Eisenman RN (1989) Myc oncoproteins are phosphorylated by casein kinase II. *EMBO J* 8:1111–1119.
21. Seldin DC, Leder P (1995) Casein kinase IIα transgene-induced murine lymphoma: Relation to theileriosis in cattle. *Science* 267:894–896.
22. Davidson NE, Prestigiacomo LJ, Hahm HA (1993) Induction of jun gene family members by transforming growth factor alpha but not 17 beta-estradiol in human breast cancer cells. *Cancer Res* 53:291–297.
23. Doucas V, Spyrou G, Yaniv M (1991) Unregulated expression of c-Jun or c-Fos proteins but not Jun D inhibits oestrogen receptor activity in human breast cancer derived cells. *EMBO J* 10:2237–2245.
24. O'Shea E, Rutkowski R, Stafford W, Kim P (1989) Preferential heterodimer formation by isolated leucine zippers from Fos and Jun. *Science* 245:646–648.
25. Chui R, Boyle W, Meek J, Smeal T, Hunter T, Karin M (1988) The c-Fos protein interacts with c-Jun/AP-1 to stimulate transcription of AP-1 responsive genes. *Cell* 54:541–552.
26. Musgrove EA, Lee CS, Sutherland RL (1991) Progestins both stimulate and inhibit breast cancer cell cycle progression while increasing expression of transforming growth factor alpha, epidermal growth factor receptor, c-fos, and c-myc genes. *Mol Cell Biol* 11:5032–5043.
27. Alkhalaf M, Murphy LC (1992) Regulation of c-jun and jun-B by progestins in T-47D human breast cancer cells. *Mol Endocrinol* 6:1625–1633.
28. Wosikowski K, Eppenberger U, Kung W, Nagamine Y, Mueller H (1992) c-fos, c-jun and c-myc expressions are not growth rate limiting for the human MCF-7 breast cancer cells. *Biochem Biophys Res Commun* 188:1067–1076.
29. Miao GG, Curran T (1995) Cell transformation by c-fos requires and extended period of expression and is independent of the cell cycle. *Mol Cell Biol* 14:4295–4310.
30. Hilberg F, Wagner EF (1992) Embryonic stem (ES) cells lacking functional c-jun: Consequences for growth and differentiation, AP-1 activity and tumorigenicity. *Oncogene* 7:2371–2380.
31. Randall SJ, Johnson RS, Mortensen RM, Papaioannou VE, Speigelman BM, Greenberg ME

(1992) Growth and differentiation of embryonic stem cells that lack an intact c-fos gene. *Proc Natl Acad Sci USA* 89:9306–9310.

32. Johnson RS, van Lingen B, Papaioannou VE, Speigelman BM (1993) A null mutation at the c-jun locus causes embryonic lethality and retarded cell growth in culture. *Genes Dev* 7:1309–1317.
33. Sommers CL, Skerker JM, Chrysogelos SA, Bosseler M, Gelmann EP (1994) Regulation of vimentin gene transcription in human breast cancer cell lines. *Cell Growth Differ* 5:839–846.
34. Thompson EW, Paik S, Brunner N, Sommers CL, Zugmaier G, Clarke R, Shima TB, Torri J, Donahue S, Lippman ME, et al. (1992) Association of increased basement membrane invasiveness with absence of estrogen receptor and expression of vimentin in human breast cancer cell lines. *J Cell Physiol* 150:534–544.
35. Luscher B, Eisenman RN (1990) New light on Myc and Myb. Part II. Myb. *Genes Dev* 4:2235–2241.
36. Guerin M, Sheng ZM, Andrieu N, Riou G (1990) Strong association between c-myb and oestrogen-receptor expression in human breast cancer. *Oncogene* 5:131–135.
37. Foos G, Grimm S, Klempnauer KH (1994) The chicken A-myb protein is a transcriptional activator. *Oncogene* 9:2481–2488.
38. Lam EW, Robinson C, Watson RJ (1992) Characterization and cell cycle-regulated expression of mouse B-myb. *Oncogene* 7:1885–1890.
39. Nakagoshi H, Kanei Ishii C, Sawazaki T, Mizuguchi G, Ishii S (1992) Transcriptional activation of the c-myc gene by the c-myb and B-myb gene products. *Oncogene* 7:1233–1240.
40. Watson RJ, Robinson C, Lam EW (1993) Transcription regulation by murine B-myb is distinct from that by c-myb. *Nucleic Acids Res* 21:267–272.
41. Calabretta B, Nicolaides NC (1992) c-myb and growth control. *Crit Rev Eukaryot Gene Expr* 2:225–235.
42. Nicolaides NC, Correa I, Casadevall C, Travali S, Soprano KJ, Calabretta B (1992) The Jun family members, c-Jun and JunD, transactivate the human c-myb promoter via an Ap1-like element. *J Biol Chem* 267:19665–19672.
43. Runnebaum IB, Nagarajan M, Bowman M, Soto D, Sukumar S (1991) Mutations in p53 as potential molecular markers for human breast cancer. *Proc Natl Acad Sci USA* 88:10657–10661.
44. Runnebaum IB, Yee JK, Kieback DG, Sukumar S, Friedmann T (1994) Wild-type p53 suppresses the malignant phenotype in breast cancer cells containing mutant p53 alleles. *Anticancer Res* 14:1137–1144.
45. Eyfjord JE, Thorlacius S, Steinarsdottir M, Valgardsdottir R, Ogmundsdottir HM, Amanthawat-Jonnson K (1995) p53 abnormalities and genomic instability in primary human breast carcinomas. *Cancer Res* 55:646–651.
46. Hoffman B, Leibermann DA (1994) Molecular controls of apoptosis: Differentiation/growth arrest primary response genes, protooncogenes, and tumor suppressor genes as positive & negative modulators. *Oncogene* 9:1807–1812.
47. Wang NP, To H, Lee WH, Lee EY (1993) Tumor suppressor activity of RB and p53 genes in human breast carcinoma cells. *Oncogene* 8:279–288.
48. Schwarz JK, Devoto SH, Smith EJ, Chellappan SP, Jakoi L, Nevins JR (1993) Interactions of the p107 and Rb proteins with E2F during the cell proliferation response. *EMBO J* 12:1013–1020.
49. Cobrink D, Whyte P, Peeper DS, Jacks T, Weinberg RA (1993) Cell cycle-specific association of E2F with the p130 E1A-binding protein. *Genes Dev* 7:2392–2404.
50. Sardet C, Vidal M, Cobrink D, Geng Y, Onufryk C, Chen A, Weinberg RA (1995) E2F-4 and E2F-5, two members of the E2F family, are expressed in the early phases of the cell cycle. *Proc Natl Acad Sci USA* 92:2403–2407.
51. Jansen Durr P, Meichle A, Steiner P, Pagano M, Finke K, Botz J, Wessbecher J, Draetta G, Eilers M (1993) Differential modulation of cyclin gene expression by MYC. *Proc Natl Acad Sci USA* 90:3685–3689.
52. Oswald F, Lovec H, Moroy T, Lipp M (1994) E2F-dependent regulation of human MYC:

185

Trans-activation by cyclins D1 and A overrides tumour suppressor protein functions. *Oncogene* 9:2029–2036.

53. Topper YJ, Freeman CS (1980) Multiple hormone interactons in the developmental biology of the mammary gland. *Physiol Rev* 60:1049–1106.

54. Wilhelm MC, Wanebo HJ (1991) Cancer of the male breast. In *The Breast: Comprehensive Management of Benign and Malignant Diseases*. KI Bland, EM Copeland (eds). Philadelphia: W.B. Saunders, pp 1030–1033.

55. Mant D, Vessey MP (1995) Epidemiology and primary prevention of breast cancer. In *The Breast: Comprehensive Management of Benign and Malignant Diseases*. KI Bland, EM Copeland (eds). Philadelphia: W.B. Saunders, pp 235–261.

56. Dubik D, Watson PH, Shiu RPC (1994) Estrogen, c-myc, and the breast. In *Protooncogenes and Growth Factors in Steroid Hormone Induced Growth and Differentiation*. SA Khan, GM Stancel (eds). Boca Raton, FL: CRC Press, pp 175–186.

57. McGuire WL (1980) Steroid hormone receptors in breast cancer treatment strategy. *Recent Prog Horm Res* 36:135–145.

58. Dubik D, Dembinski TC, Shiu RP (1987) Stimulation of c-myc oncogene expression associated with estrogen-induced proliferation of human breast cancer cells. *Cancer Res* 47:6517–6521.

59. Gudas JM, Klein RC, Oka M, Cowan KH (1995) Posttranscriptional regulation of the c-myb proto-oncogene in estrogen receptor-positive breast cancer cells. *Clin Cancer Res* 1:235–243.

60. Weisz A, Bresciani F (1993) Estrogen regulation of proto-oncogenes coding for nuclear proteins. *Crit Rev Oncog* 4:361–388.

61. Dubik D, Shiu RP (1992) Mechanism of estrogen activation of c-myc oncogene expression. *Oncogene* 7:1587–1594.

62. Watson PH, Pon RT, Shiu RPC (1991) Inhibition of c-myc expression by phosphorothioate antisense oligonucleotide identifies a critical role for c-myc in the growth of human breast cancer. *Cancer Res* 51:3996–4000.

63. Gaub MP, Bellard M, Scheuer I, Chambon P, Sassone Corsi P (1990) Activation of the ovalbumin gene by the estrogen receptor involves the fos-jun complex. *Cell* 63:1267–1276.

64. Halachmi S, Marden E, Martin G, MacKay H, Abbondanza C, Brown M (1994) Estrogen receptor-associated proteins: Possible mediators of hormone-induced transcription. *Science* 264:1455–1458.

65. Baniahmad C, Nawaz Z, Banianhman A, Gleeson MAG, Tsai M, O'Malley BW (1995) Enhancement of human estrogen receptor activity by SPT6: A potential coactivator. *Mol Endocrinol* 9:34–43.

66. Xu G, Livingston DM, Krek W (1995) Multiple members of the E2F transcription factor family are the products of oncogenes. *Proc Natl Acad Sci USA* 92:1357–1361.

67. Hiebert SW, Blake M, Azizkhan J, Nevins JR (1991) Role of E2F transcription factor in E1A-mediated trans activation of cellular genes. *J Virol* 65:3547–3552.

68. Kuiper GG, Brinkmann AO (1994) Steroid hormone receptor phosphorylation: Is there a physiological role? *Mol Cell Endocrinol* 100:103–107.

69. Denton RR, Koszewski NJ, Notides AC (1992) Estrogen receptor phosphorylation. *J Biol Chem* 267:7263–7268.

70. Migliaccio A, Pagano M, Auricchio F (1993) Immediate and transient stimulation of protein tyrosine phosphorylation by estradiol in MCF-7 cells. *Oncogene* 8:2183–2191.

71. Baldi A, Boyle DM, Wittliff JL (1986) Estrogen receptor is associated with protein and phospholipid kinase activity. *Biochem Biophys Res Commun* 135:597–606.

72. Puca GA, Abbondaza C, Nigro C, Armetta I, Medici N, Molinari AM (1986) Estrogen receptor has proteolytic activity that is responsible for its own transformation. *Proc Natl Acad Sci USA* 83:5367–5371.

73. Weisz A, Rosales R (1990) Identification of an estrogen response element upstream of the human c-fos gene that binds the estrogen receptor and the AP-1 transcription factor. *Nucleic Acids Res* 18:5097–5106.

74. Hyder SM, Stancel GM, Nawaz Z, McDonnell DP, Loose Mitchell DS (1992) Identification of an estrogen response element in the 3'-flanking region of the murine c-fos protooncogene. *J Biol Chem* 267:18047–18054.
75. Augereau P, Miralles F, Cavaillès V, Gaudelet C, Parker M, Rochefort H (1994) Characterization of the proximal estrogen-responsive element of human cathepsin D gene. *Mol Endocrinol* 8:693–703.
76. Kraus WL, Montano MM, Katzenellenbogen BS (1994) Identification of multiple, widely spaced estrogen-responsive regions in the rat progesterone receptor gene. *Mol Endocrinol* 8:952–969.
77. Wu Peng XS, Pugliese TE, Dickerman HW, Pentecost BT (1992) Delineation of sites mediating estrogen regulation of the rat creatine kinase B gene. *Mol Endocrinol* 6:231–240.
78. Wilding G, Lippman ME, Gelmann EP (1988) Effects of steroid hormones and peptide growth factors on protooncogene c-fos expression in human breast cancer cells. *Cancer Res* 48:802–808.
79. Lin D, Fiscella M, O'Connor PM, Jackman J, Chen M, Luo LL, Sala A, Travali S, Appella E, Mercer WE (1994) Constitutive expression of B-myb can bypass p53-induced Waf1/Cip1-mediated G1 arrest. *Proc Natl Acad Sci USA* 91:10079–10083.
80. Santen RJ, Manni A, Harvey H, Redmond C (1990) Endocrine treatment of breast cancer in women. *Endocr Rev* 11:221–265.
81. Murphy LC, Alkhalaf M, Dotzlaw H, Coutts A, Haddad Alkhalaf B (1994) Regulation of gene expression in T-47D human breast cancer cells by progestins and antiprogestins. *Hum Reprod* 9(Suppl 1):174–180.
82. Musgrove EA, Hamilton JA, Lee CS, Sweeney KJ, Watts CK, Sutherland RL (1993) Growth factor, steroid, and steroid antagonist regulation of cyclin gene expression associated with changes in T-47D human breast cancer cell cycle progression. *Mol Cell Biol* 13:3577–3587.
83. Li XS, Chen JC, Sheikh MS, Shao ZM, Fontana JA (1994) Retinoic acid inhibition of insulin-like growth factor I stimulation of c-fos mRNA levels in a breast carcinoma cell line. *Exp Cell Res* 211:68–73.
84. Sheikh MS, Shao ZM, Chen JC, Ordonez JV, Fontana JA (1993) Retinoid modulation of c-myc and max gene expression in human breast carcinoma. *Anticancer Res* 13:1387–1392.
85. Chrysogelos SA, Dickson RB (1994) EGF receptor expression, regulation, and function in breast cancer. *Breast Cancer Res Treat* 29:29–40.
86. Marshall CJ (1995) Specificity of receptor tyrosine kinase signaling: transient versus sustained extracellular signal-regulated kinase activation. *Cell* 80:179–185.
87. Leinhard GE (1994) Life without the IRS. *Nature* 372:128–129.
88. Sutherland RL, Lee CS, Feldman RS, Musgrove EA (1992) Regulation of breast cancer cell cycle progression by growth factors, steroids and steroid antagonists. *J Steroid Biochem Mol Biol* 41:315–321.
89. Westwick JK, Cox AD, Der CJ, Cobb MH, Hibi M, Karin M, Brenner DA (1994) Oncogenic Ras activates c-Jun via a separate pathway from the activation of extracellular signal-regulated kinases. *Proc Natl Acad Sci USA* 91:6030–6034.
90. Hipskind RA, Buscher D, Nordheim A, Baccarini M (1994) Ras/MAP kinase-dependent and -independent signaling pathways target distinct ternary complex factors. *Genes Dev* 8:1803–1816.
91. Janknecht R, Ernst WH, Pingoud V, Nordheim A (1993) Activation of ternary complex factor Elk-1 by MAP kinases. *EMBO J* 12:5097–5104.
92. Marais R, Wynne J, Treisman R (1993) The SRF accessory protein Elk-1 contains a growth factor-regulated transcriptional activation domain. *Cell* 73:381–393.
93. Minden A, Lin A, Smeal T, Derijard B, Cobb M, Davis R, Karin M (1994) c-Jun N-terminal phosphorylation correlates with activation of the JNK subgroup but not the ERK subgroup of mitogen-activated protein kinases. *Mol Cell Biol* 14:6683–6688.
94. Sluss HK, Barrett T, Derijard B, Davis RJ (1994) Signal transduction by tumor necrosis factor mediated by JNK protein kinases. *Mol Cell Biol* 14:8376–8384.
95. Abate C, Baker SJ, Lees Miller SP, Anderson CW, Marshak DR, Curran T (1993) Dimeriza-

tion and DNA binding alter phosphorylation of Fos and Jun. *Proc Natl Acad Sci USA* 90:6766–6770.

96. Deng T, Karin M (1994) c-Fos transcriptional activity stimulated by H-Ras-activated protein kinase distinct from JNK and ERK. *Nature* 371:171–175.

97. Gupta S, Seth A, Davis RJ (1993) Transactivation of gene expression by Myc is inhibited by mutation at the phosphorylation sites Thr-58 and Ser-62. *Proc Natl Acad Sci USA* 90:3216–3220.

98. Lutterbach B, Hann SR (1994) Hierarchical phosphorylation at N-terminal transformation-sensitive sites in c-Myc protein is regulated by mitogens and in mitosis. *Mol Cell Biol* 14:5510–5522.

99. Pulverer BJ, Fisher C, Vousden K, Littlewood T, Evan G, Woodgett JR (1994) Site-specific modulation of c-Myc cotransformation by residues phosphorylated in vivo. *Oncogene* 9:59–70.

100. Hagiwara T, Nakaya K, Nakamura Y, Nakajima H, Nishimura S, Taya Y (1992) Specific phosphorylation of the acidic central region of the N-myc protein by casein kinase II. *Eur J Biochem* 209:945–950.

101. Berberich SJ, Cole MD (1992) Casein kinase II inhibits the DNA-binding activity of Max homodimers but not Myc/Max heterodimers. *Genes Dev* 6:166–176.

102. Polyak K, Kato JY, Solomon MJ, Sherr CJ, Massague J, Roberts JM, Koff A (1994) p27Kip1, a cyclin-Cdk inhibitor, links transforming growth factor-beta and contact inhibition to cell cycle arrest. *Genes Dev* 8:9–22.

103. Osborne CK, Clemmons DR, Arteaga CL (1990) Regulation of breast cancer growth by insulin-like growth factors. *J Steroid Biochem Mol Biol* 37:805–809.

104. Daksis JI, Lu RY, Facchini LM, Marhin WW, Penn LJ (1994) Myc induces cyclin D1 expression in the absence of de novo protein synthesis and links mitogen-stimulated signal transduction to the cell cycle. *Oncogene* 9:3635–3645.

105. Philipp A, Schneider A, Vasrik I, Finke K, Xiong Y, Beach D, Alitalo K, Eilers M (1994) Repression of cyclin D1: A novel function of MYC. *Mol Cell Biol* 14:4032–4043.

106. Gaubatz S, Meichle A, Eilers M (1994) An E-box element localized in the first intron mediates regulation of the prothymosin alpha gene by c-myc. *Mol Cell Biol* 14:3853–3862.

107. Eilers M, Schirm S, Bishop JM (1991) The MYC protein activates transcription of the alpha-prothymosin gene. *EMBO J* 10:133–141.

108. Li LH, Nerlov C, Prendergast G, MacGregor D, Ziff EB (1994) c-Myc represses transcription in vivo by a novel mechanism dependent on the initiator element and Myc box II. *EMBO J* 13:4070–4079.

109. Mai S, Jalava A (1994) c-Myc binds to 5′ flanking sequence motifs of the dihydrofolate reductase gene in cellular extracts; Role in proliferation. *Nucleic Acids Res* 22:2264–2273.

110. Bello-Fernandez C, Packham G, Cleveland JL (1993) The ornithine decarboxylase gene is a transcriptional target of c-MYC. *Proc Natl Acad Sci USA* 90:7804–7808.

111. Pena A, Reddy CD, Wu S, Hickok NJ, Reddy EP, Yumet G, Soprano DR, Soprano KJ (1993) Regulation of human ornithine decarboxylase expression by the c-Myc. Max protein complex. *J Biol Chem* 268:27277–27285.

112. Benvenisty N, Leder A, Kuo A, Leder P (1992) An embryonically expressed gene is a target for c-Myc regulation via the c-Myc-binding sequences. *Genes Dev* 6:2513–2523.

113. Suen TC, Hung MC (1991) c-myc reverses neu-induced transformed morphology by transcriptional repression. *Mol Cell Biol* 11:354–362.

114. Akeson R, Bernards R (1990) N-myc down regulates neural cell adhesion molecule expression in rat neuroblastoma. *Mol Cell Biol* 10:2012–2016.

115. Versteeg R, Noordermeer IA, Kruse-Wolters M, Ruiter DJ, Schrier PI (1988) c-myc down-regulates class I HLA expression in human melanomas. *EMBO J* 7:1023–1039.

116. Inghirami G, Grignani F, Sternas L, Lombardi L, Knowles DM, Dalla Favera R (1990) Down-regulation of LFA-1 adhesion receptors by C-myc oncogene in human B lymphoblastoid cells. *Science* 250:682–686.

188

117. Shtivelman E, Bishop JM (1991) Expression of CD44 is repressed in neuroblastoma cells. *Mol Cell Biol* 11:5446–5453.
118. Gross N, Beretta C, Peruisseau G, Jackson D, Simmons D, Beck D (1994) CD44H expression by human neuroblastoma cells: Relation to MYCN amplification and lineage differentiation. *Cancer Res* 54:4238–4242.
119. Yang BS, Geddes TJ, Pogulis RJ, de Crombrugghe B, Freytag SO (1991) Transcriptional suppression of cellular gene expression by c-Myc. *Mol Cell Biol* 11:2291–2295.
120. Dickinson Laing TMA, Gibson AW, Johnston RN, Edwards DR (1995) Role of c-myc in regulation of gelationase B expression (abstr). *Proc Am Assoc Cancer Res* 36:97.
121. Prendergast GC, Cole MD (1989) Posttranscriptional regulation of cellular gene expression by the c-myc oncogene. *Mol Cell Biol* 9:124–134.
122. Prendergast GC, Diamond LE, Dahl D, Cole MD (1990) The c-myc-regulated gene mrl encodes plasminogen activator inhibitor 1. *Mol Cell Biol* 10:1265–1269.
123. Wasfy G, Marhin W, Lu R, Daksis J, Penn LJZ (1995) Cloning and identification of Myc-regulated genes (abstr). *Proc Am Assoc Cancer Res* 36:521.

10. Antiprogestin–progesterone interactions

H. Michna, K.-H. Fritzemeier, K. Parczyk, Y. Nishino, and M.R. Schneider

Introduction

It was more than a decade ago that in 1889 Schinzinger was the first to propose that ovariectomy may be an effective treatment for breast cancer [1,2]. Until today the available treatment strategies for hormone-dependent breast cancer have mainly been based on estrogen-ablative principles, and improvements in the therapy for breast cancer are still sorely needed. A totally different strategy utilizes progesterone antagonists: This class of compounds targets the progesterone receptor in mammary carcinomas and therefore does not represent another enzyme or receptor blockade of estrogen action.

History and perspectives on progesterone antagonists

Progesterone antagonists were not originally developed for breast cancer but rather for pregnancy-related indications. The original lead compound, RU (38)486 (Mifepristone), was discovered and pharmacologically characterized by Herrmann et al. [3] in 1981 in the laboratories of Roussel Uclaf. The most characteristic feature of the steroidal progesterone antagonists is the 11β-aromatic side chain, with the exception of one example, in which the aromatic substituent is attached to C18 [4]. The clinical potential of this new class of compounds was evaluated by Baulieu [5]. Mifepristone was originally intended to be an antiglucocorticoid [6], and thus it is obvious that in other indications in which long-term treatment is necessary, the compound may suffer from the major drawback of having this endocrine profile, as was in fact detected by Klijn et al. [7] in clinical studies in postmenopausal patients with metastatic breast cancer. Nevertheless, this does not exclude its well-known and hotly debated use for the induction of medical abortion in more than 100,000 women [5,8].

Numerous applications of RU (38)486 are currently being investigated (Table 1). It is apparent that there are pregnancy-related indications for this compound, and several tumor indications exist as well, and breast cancer is certainly the main focus. Therefore, we have been investigating compounds

R. Dickson and M. Lippman (eds.) MAMMARY TUMOR CELL CYCLE, DIFFERENTIATION AND METASTASIS. 1996. Kluwer Academic Publishers. ISBN 0-7923-3905-3. All rights reserved.

Table 1. Applications for progesterone antagonists

Endocrine indication	
Cushing syndrome	C
Tumor indications	
Breast cancer	CT
Meningioma	CT
Endometrial carcinoma	?
Endometriosis	CT
Prostate cancer	EXP
Gastro intestinal cancers	EXP
Pregnancy-related indications	
Medical abortion	C
Intrauterine fetal death	C
Cervical ripening	EXP
Induction of labor	CT
Ectopic pregnancy	?
Stimulation of lactation	EXP
Leiomyomata	CT
Premenstrual syndrome	?
Cervical dilatation	CT
Early postcoital contraception	CT
Menses induction, late postcoital contraception	CT
Male fertility control	EXP

C = in clinical use; CT = in clinical trials; EXP = under preclinical evaluation; ? = theoretically to be considered.

with a better distinction between their antiprogestational and antigluco-corticoid activities. The 13-methyl compound, Onapristone (ZK 98.299), represents a new group of progesterone antagonists characterized by inversion of the junction between the C and D rings (Figure 1).

Pharmacology of progesterone antagonists

In our preclinical models for evaluating antiglucocorticoid activity, Onapristone showed less activity than Mifepristone and, most significantly, induced no remarkable antiglucocorticoid changes at a dose of 100 mg orally in a phase I clinical study in female volunteers (unpublished data).

Receptor binding studies

After the chemical breakthrough of synthesing 11β-substituted 19-nor steroids [9], it was interesting to discover that this class of compounds presented an unexpectedly high binding affinity to both progesterone and androgen receptors. Table 3 provides an overview of the relative binding affinities of Onapristone and Mifepristone in standard binding assays. In contrast to the excellent binding of both compounds to the progesterone and androgen receptors (Table 2), both antiprogestins displayed only marginal affinity to the

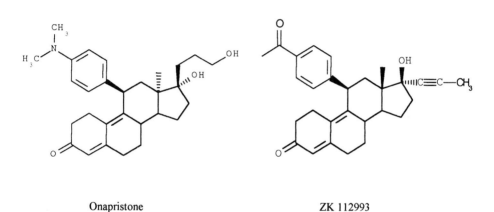

Progesterone

Mifepristone

Onapristone

ZK 112993

Figure 1. Chemical structure of progesterone antagonists.

Table 2. Relative binding affinities (RBA) of onapristone and mifepristone to the steroid hormone receptors

	PR (rabbit)	PR (rabbit)	GR (rat)	AR (rat)	MR (human)	ER (rat)	ER (human)
Incubation time (hours)	2 h	24 h	2 h	2 h	2 h	2 h	2 h
Mifepristone	143	667	334	5.9	n.c.	0.002	0.06
Onapristone	25	37	100	8.3	n.c.	0.012	0.06

[1] The reference compounds were progesterone for the progesterone receptor (PR), dexamethasone for the glucocorticoid receptor (GR), R1881 for the androgen receptor (AR), aldosterone for the mineralocorticoid receptor (MR) and estradiol for the estrogen receptor (ER). The RBA value of the respective reference compound was arbitrarily designed 100% (n.c. = no competition).

Hormone dependent MXT (+) mammary-carcinoma

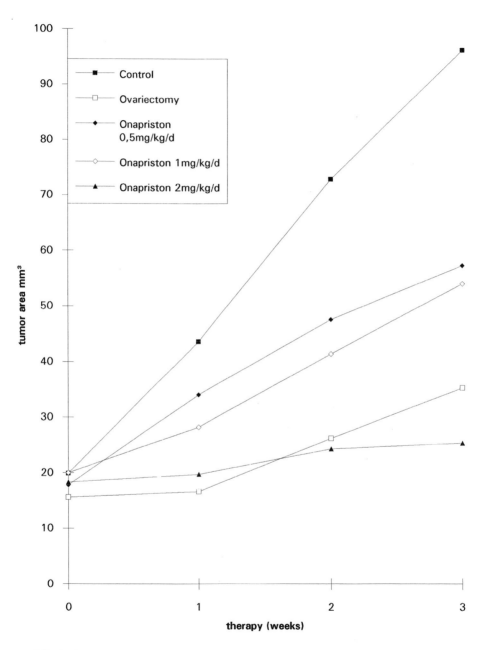

n = 10 mice/group; s.c.

Figure 2. Dose-dependent growth inhibition of the MXT mammary carcinoma of the mouse by Onapristone (daily subcutaneous treatment).

194

estrogen receptor [10]. In addition, in our hands (Table 2) in standard binding assays using the rat uterine estrogen receptor, the affinity of Onapristone was found to be 10,000-fold and that of mifepristone to be about 50,000-fold lower than that of estradiol. In binding studies with biotechnologically produced human estrogen receptor, both compounds exhibited about 4,000-fold lower affinity than the reference estradiol. Finally, the binding affinity of Onapristone to the glucocorticoid receptor is lower than that of Mifepristone (Table 2; Figure 2).

Progesterone antagonists and DNA interactions

Progesterone antagonists are divided into two classes of antihormones based on their molecular mechanism detected in some assays [11]. The antihormone receptor complex of the so-called type I progesterone antagonists, like Mifepristone, does bind to DNA but prevents transactivation of target genes, whereas type II compounds, such as Onapristone, block the progesterone receptor function by prohibiting its interaction with DNA [12]. On the other hand, in whole cell preparations, Delabre and colleagues [13] detected that both compounds act similarly on receptor binding, dimerization, and binding to hormone-responsive elements in dose-response studies. Based on these studies further experiments from the laboratories of Horwitz using progesterone receptors mutated in the DNA binding domain did not support the concept that all antiprogestins trigger binding of progesterone receptor to DNA [14].

Antiproliferative activity

Antiproliferative activity in vitro

Several independent investigators have reported that Mifepristone and Onapristone may inhibit cell cycle phase-specific growth of a panel of progesterone receptor–positive breast cancer cell lines [15–24]. However, it has also been reported that Mifepristone has a weak mitogenic effect on MCF-7 cells [25–28,29] and on the androgen-responsive Shionogi carcinoma [30]. A far higher increase in proliferation on T47D cells is described for Mifepristone than for Onapristone and Org 31806 and Org 31710 [29,31,32].

Antiproliferative activity in vivo

For the valid in vivo screening of progesterone antagonists, we established a proliferation assay in the normal mammary gland of ovariectomized rats [33]. The antiproliferative potency of progesterone antagonists in this bioassay depends on the inhibition of the effect of progesterone on the development of mammary gland buds [34–40], estimating the development of tubular-alveolar buds. Based on our experience we can conclude that this assay measures the potency of the compounds to competitively antagonize the effects of progesterone, and in fact, Mifepristone and Onapristone displayed strong antiproliferative potency in this assay. In our hands, there is a strong correlation of the antiproliferative potency of progesterone antagonists in this bioassay and in hormone-dependent experimental breast cancer models.

Mammary carcinoma inhibitory potential

The tumor inhibitory potential of progesterone antagonists was characterized in a panel of mammary carcinoma models that are described in detail elsewhere [41,42]. The tumor inhibitory potential of the progesterone antagonist Onapristone proved to be dose dependent; for example, in the MXT mammary carcinoma model (Figure 2), with an efficacy comparable or superior to the clinically established endocrine treatment strategies. As representative examples, homogenous growth inhibition of Onapristone compared with treatment with Mifepristone, tamoxifen, or megestrol acetate has been shown in the carcinogen-induced mammary carcinoma model (Figures 3 and 4). Also, in view of the mechanism of tumor inhibition, a key finding was that Onapristone was superior in efficacy than even supraphysiological doses of medroxyprogesterone acetate in the MXT tumor model [42,43]. These data agree with the experience of Klijn and colleagues [44,45] as well as that of Kloosterboer and colleagues [46] on the efficacy of antiprogestins.

In a second-line treatment regimen in the MXT (Figure 5), DMBA, and NMU (Figure 6) tumor model after a 2 or 3 week pretreatment with tamoxifen, the effectiveness of Onapristone (5 or 10 mg/kg/day s.c.) on tumor growth was compared with that of a further treatment with supraphysiological doses of medroxyprogesterone acetate (100 mg/kg/day s.c.). In this treatment regimen Onapristone proved to induce superior growth inhibition compared with treatment with tamoxifen and to be as effective as high-dose treatment with medroxyprogesterone acetate, which, in contrast to Onapristone, resulted in significant side effects (Figure 6; compare also Michna et al. [47]); in the second-line treatment regimen in the MXT tumor model, Onapristone was even more effective than medroxyprogesterone acetate (Figure 5).

Progesterone antagonists and estrogen-dependent functions

Progesterone antagonists, such as Mifepristone and Onapristone, may modulate reactions known to be mainly estrogen dependent. Our group [42,48–52] and others [53–55] have reported these effects, although no significant affinity of these progesterone antagonists for the estrogen receptor has been detected. Reactions in intact animals after treatment with antiprogestins considered to

196

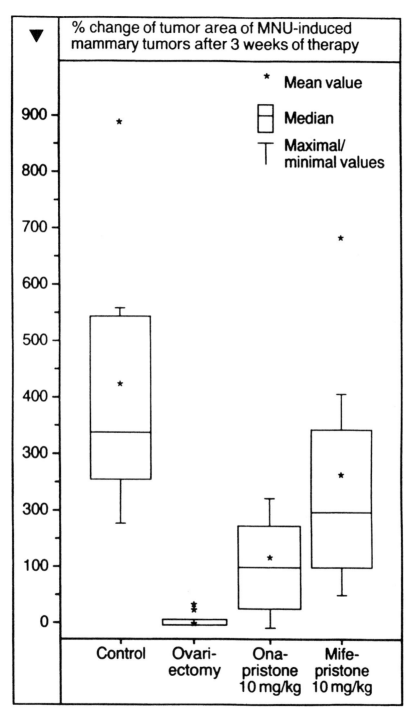

Figure 3. Growth inhibition of the progesterone antagonists Onapristone and Mifepristone in comparison with ovariectomy on MNU-induced mammary carcinomas (3 week therapy, compounds were administered 6 times a week subcutaneously; n >10/group; tumor area was set at 100% at the start of treatment).

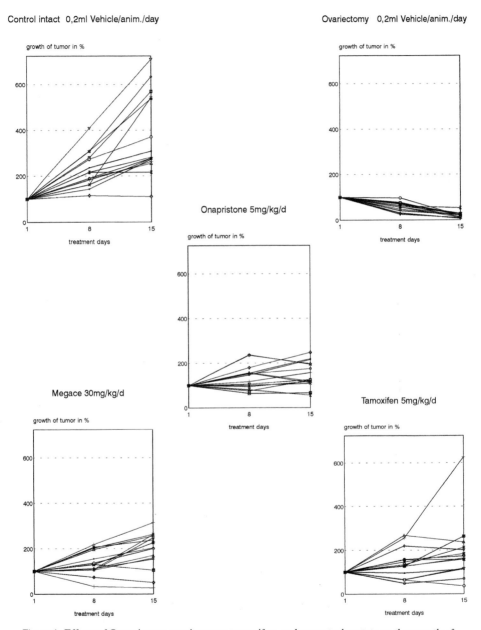

Figure 4. Effects of Onapristone, ovariectomy, tamoxifen, and megestrol acetate on the growth of the DMBA-induced mammary carcinoma of the rat. (See Thomas and Monet [21] and Bigaby and Cunha [61] for the experimental details. Note the very homogenous inhibition of tumor growth by Onapristone.

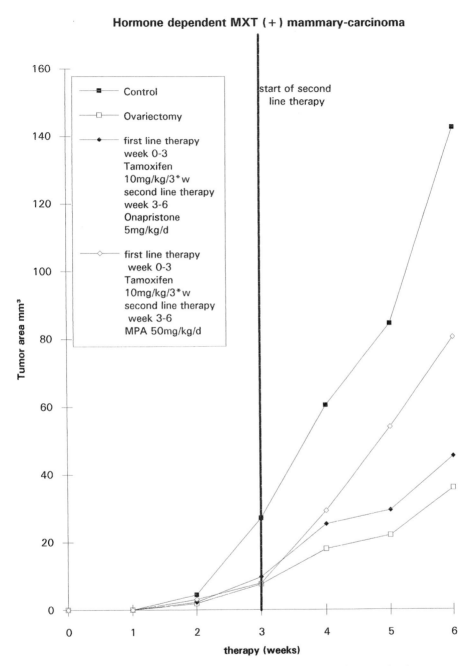

Hormone dependent MXT (+) mammary-carcinoma

Legend:
- ■ — Control
- □ — Ovariectomy
- ◆ — first line therapy week 0-3 Tamoxifen 10mg/kg/3*w second line therapy week 3-6 Onapristone 5mg/kg/d
- ◇ — first line therapy week 0-3 Tamoxifen 10mg/kg/3*w second line therapy week 3-6 MPA 50mg/kg/d

start of second line therapy

Tumor area mm³

therapy (weeks)

Figure 5. In a second-line treatment regimen in the MXT tumor model after 3 weeks of treatment with tamoxifen, the effectiveness of Onapristone on tumor growth was compared with that of a further high-dose treatment with medroxyprogesterone acetate. In this treatment regimen, Onapristone induced superior growth inhibition than treatment with medroxyprogesterone acetate.

Hormone dependent MNU mammary carcinoma

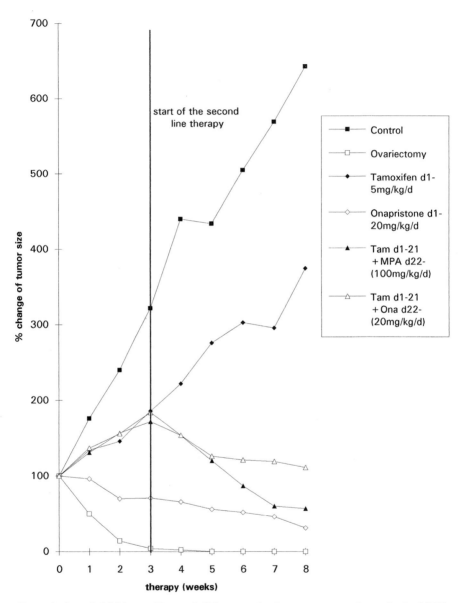

Figure 6. Growth inhibitory efficacy of different endocrine treatment regimens in the MNU-induced mammary carcinoma model. Long-term treatment over 8 weeks with Onapristone achieved the most significant blockade of tumor growth. In a second-line treatment regimen after 3 weeks of pretreatment with tamoxifen, the effectiveness of Onapristone on tumor growth was compared with that of further treatment with tamoxifen and high-dose treatment with medroxyprogesterone acetate. Both second-line regimens are equally effective statistically.

mimic 'estrogenicity' have been interpreted as *unopposed estrogenic effects* resulting from inhibition of the known estrogen antagonizing effect of progesterone [41,48,56–63], although responses opposing estrogen action were also reported [41,54,64–69].

In view of the reported estrogenic side effects of tamoxifen [70–76] and the use of progesterone antagonists in postmenopausal women, it was logical to analyze the 'pureness' of Onapristone in ovariectomized mammary carcinoma–bearing mice. In contrast to tamoxifen (Figure 7) [70–75,77–79], any tumor growth stimulatory effect of Onapristone on hormone-dependent carcinomas could be excluded in ovariectomized mice. Thus, Onapristone behaved in this model like the pure estrogen receptor antagonist ICI 164.384 (Figure 7) [compare also 76–80]. In this respect, it is also significant to consider that Onapristone may inhibit surgically induced endometriosis in rats [81,82] and that Mifepristone showed beneficial effects in woman suffering from endometriosis and uterine fibrosis [83,84].

To explain the tissue-specific noncompetitive estrogenic effects of progesterone antagonists, it should be considered that they may affect estrogen metabolism in a tissue-type specific manner or may interfere with the sensitivity of target tissue to estrogens. A molecular explanation is provided by studies of McDonnell [85], using a reconstituted estrogen-responsive transcription system, demonstrating that the A- form of the progesterone receptor plays a key role in modulating estrogen receptor function in cells in which both receptors are expressed. However, there is no convincing evidence that such estrogen-like effects are the consequence of direct activation of estrogen receptor–dependent transcriptional events, as we demonstrated in transactivation assays in which we transfected HeLa cells that are devoid of sex hormone receptors with an estrogen receptor expression vector (HEGO, 86), together with an estrogen-inducible reporter gene (Vit-TK-CAT, 87). In contrast to estradiol, Onapristone did not induce the Vit-TK-CAT reporter gene, even when it was applied at the extremely high dose of $10 \mu M$ (Figure 8). However, Mifepristone displayed estrogenic activity in the micromolar range (Figure 8), which agrees with the detection of an estrogenic action of Mifepristone at very high doses with a comparable assay by Meei-Huey et al. [28].

Mechanism of tumor inhibitory potential

We demonstrated that in ovariectomized mammary carcinoma–bearing animals, progesterone antagonists, like Onapristone and ZK112.993, completely antagonized the pronounced stimulation of estradiol [41]. In conclusion, these and further in vitro [17] and in vivo [41] data indicate that the mammary carcinoma–inhibiting mechanism of progesterone antagonists cannot be explained primarily by displacement of progesterone from its receptor, because after ovariectomy the level of circulating progesterone is below the detection limit [88, and unpublished data]. Because it is also well documented that the

MXT (+) Mammary Carcinoma of the mouse

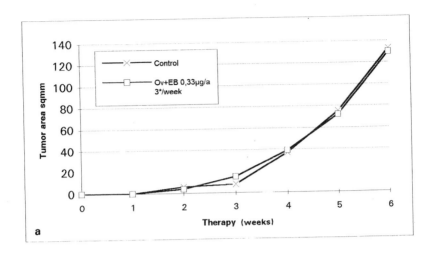

a

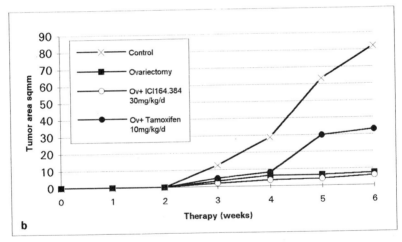

b

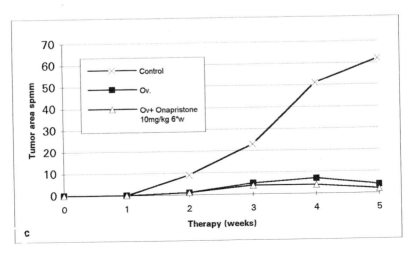

c

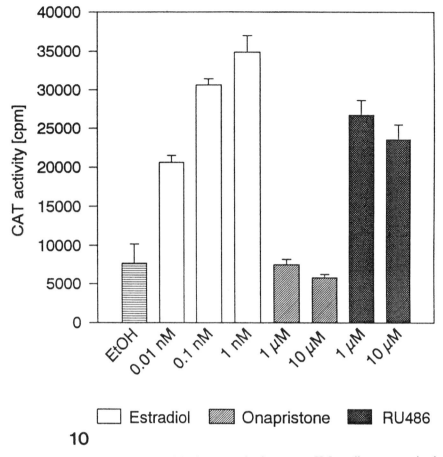

10

Figure 8. Analysis of estrogenic activity in transactivation assays. HeLa cells were transiently transfected with the human estrogen receptor (HEGO) and a Vit-TK-CAT reporter gene. Onapristone displayed no estrogenic action, whereas Mifepristone was estrogenic in the micromolar range. Estradiol represents the positve control.

progesterone receptor level is driven by estrogens [89], a progesterone receptor–dependent mechanism may be considered. In fact, it was demonstrated in vitro [17] and in vivo [41] that this potential depends on the availability of a sufficient number of progesterone receptors.

Detailed quantitative morphological studies revealed that treatment with

---

Figure 7. Analysis of the effects of tamoxifen (**a**), the pure estrogen receptor antagonist ICI 164.384 (**b**), and Onapristone (**c**) on the growth of the estrogen-dependent (a; EB = estradiol benzaote 0.33 μg/animal 3 times s.c./week) MXT mammary carcinoma in ovariectomized mice. No growth stimulation was induced by the pure ICI antiestrogen and Onapristone, whereas tamoxifen displayed estrogen-like stimulation of tumor growth.

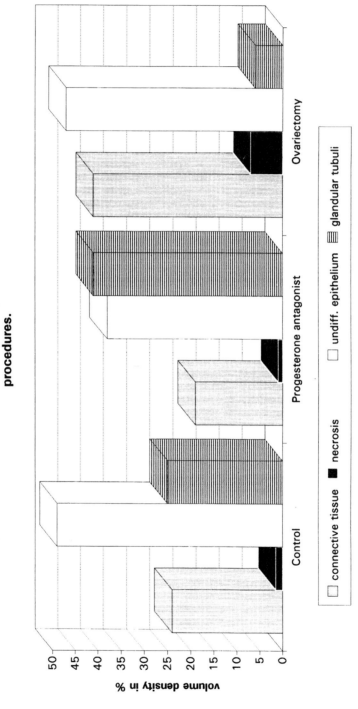

Figure 9. Morphometrical analysis of tissue distribution within DMBA-induced mammary carcinomas after treatment with Onapristone compared with ovariectomy. Note the reduced undifferentiated epithelial cell content and enhanced volume density of glandular structures induced by the progesterone antagonist.

204

Hormone dependent DMBA mammary-carcinoma

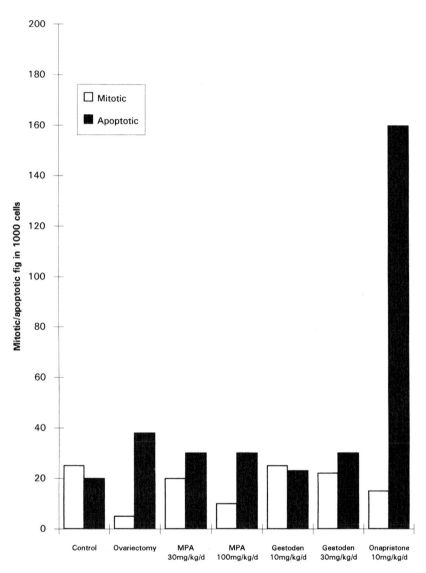

Figure 10. Morphometrical analysis of mitotic and apoptotic cell nuclei in semithin sections of DMBA-induced mammary carcinomas after treatment with different progestins (medroxyprogesterone acetate, gestoden) and Onapristone. Only Onapristone strongly enhanced the appearence of apoptotic cell nuclei.

Hormone dependent MNU mammary-ca
TGF ß1:immunhistochemical scoring

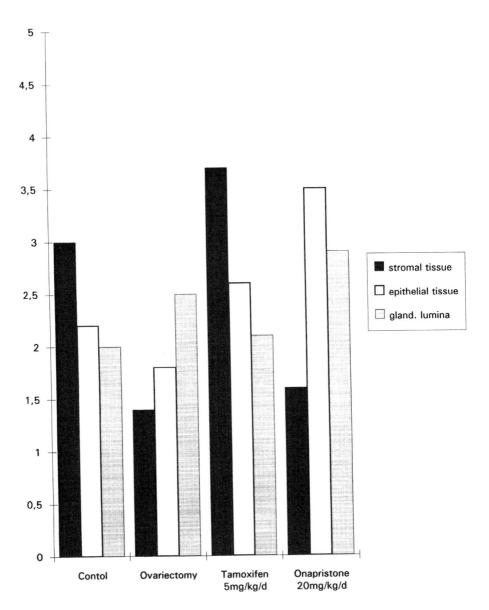

treatment 4 weeks

Figure 11. Immunohistochemical, semiquantitative scoring of the expression of TGF-β_1 in MNU-induced mammary carcinomas after treatment with tamoxifen and Onapristone. Whereas tamoxifen stimulated enhanced stromal localization of TGF-β_1, Onapristone enhanced epithelial localization.

206

the antiprogestins induces differentiation of mitotically active polygonal tumor cells toward dysplastic glandular structures (Figure 9) with massive sequestering of secretory products [48,90,91]. We also ensured this mechanism was taking place by using a new differentiation factor, estimating and relating the amount of undifferentiated tumor epithelial cells arranged into dysplastic, ductlike structures [91]. The same conclusion could be drawn using the classical grading systems, such as the WHO or Richardson grading system.

Simultaneously, morphometric data indicate the appearence of cells undergoing gene-directed death, or apoptotic cell death [92], but the mitotic pathway is not stimulated (Figure 10).

Because TGF-β_1 is colocalized in cells undergoing apoptosis, is a negative growth factor in human breast cancer cells [93], and has been found to induce apoptosis in cultured carcinoma cells [94], we studied the expression of TGF-$\beta_{1,2,3}$ within experimental mammary carcinomas at the mRNA and protein level. Only at the protein level could we detect higher expression of TGF-β_1 by semiquantitative immunohistochemical analysis (Figure 11). Whereas after treatment with tamoxifen a higher degree of TGF-β_1 immunostaining was localized in stromal cells in clinical specimens [95] and in experimental breast cancer models (Figure 11), after treatment with Onapristone greater staining was detected in tumor epithelial cells (Figure 11).

Finally, a differentiation-specific G_1 arrest in the cell cycle has already been proposed [96,97], and thus we decided to analyze changes in the distribution of tumor cells within the cell cycle. Treatment of hormone-dependent experimental breast cancers in vivo led to an accumulation of cells in G_0G_1 of the cell cycle, together with a significant and biologically relevant reduction in the number of the cells in the G_2M and S phases, whereas all other endocrine treatment strategies displayed no effects [43]. Since it is well accepted that the S-phase fraction is a highly significant predictor of disease-free survival among axillary node–negative patients with diploid mammary tumors [98,99], the ability of progesterone antagonists such as Onapristone to reduce the number of cells in the S- phase may offer a significant clinical advantage, which is now being evaluated in an ongoing phase III study in tamoxifen-relapsed, postmenopausal breast cancer patients.

Acknowledgment

Dr. L. Wakefield and Dr. M. Sporn kindly provided the antibodies against TGF$\beta_{1,2,3}$.

References

1. Schinzinger F (1889) Über Carcinoma Mammae. In *Verh Dtsch Ges Chirurgie*. Berlin: Hirschwald Verlag, Chap 18.

2. Beatson GT, Edin MD (1896) On the treatment of inoperable cases of carcinoma of the mamma: Suggestions for a new method of treatment, with illustrative cases. *Lancet* 18:107–108.

3. Herrmann W, Wyss R, Riondel A, Philibert D, Teutsch G, Sakiz E, Baulieu EE (1982) The effects of an antiprogesterone steroid in women: Interruption of the menstrual cycle and of early pregnancy. *C R Acad Sci Paris* 294:933–938.

4. Kloosterboer HJ, Deckers GHJ, Van der Heuvel MJ, Loozen HJJ (1988) Screening of antiprogestagens by receptor studies and bioassays. *J Steroid Biochem* 31:567–571.

5. Beaulieu EE (1993) RU486 — a decade on, today and tomorrow. In *Clinical Applications of Mifepristone RU486 and Other Antiprogestins.* MS Donaldson, L Dorflinger, SS Brown, LZ Benet (eds). Washington, DC: National Academy Press, pp 71–119.

6. Philibert D (1985) Pharmacological profile of RU 486 in animals. In *The Antiprogestin Steroid RU 486 in Human Fertility Control.* EE Baulieu, SJ Segall (eds). New York: Plenum Press, pp 49–68.

7. Klijn JGM, de Jong FH, Bakker GH, Lamberts SWJ, Rodenburg CJ, Aliexa-Figusch J (1989) Antiprogestins, a new form of endocrine therapy for human breast cancer. *Cancer Res* 49:2851–2856.

8. Ulmann A, Silvestre L, Chemama L, Rezvani Y, Renault M, Aguillaume J, Baulieu EE (1992) Medical termination of early pregnancy with RU486 (mifepristone) followed by a prostaglandin analogue: Study in 16,369 women. *Scand J Obstet Gynecol* 71:278–283.

9. Teutsch G, Belanger A (1979) Regional and stereospecific synthesis of 11β-substituted 19-nor-steroids. *Tetrahedron Lett* V17:2051–2054.

10. Bigsby RM, Young PCM (1992) Estrogen-like effects of the antiprogestin ZK 98.299. In *Proceedings of the 74th Annual Meeting of the Endocrine Society, San Antonio, Texas, June 24–27, 1992.* San Antonio, Endocrine Society, p 233.

11. Gronemeyer H, Benhamou B, Berry M, Bocquel MT, Gofflo D, Garcia T, Leronge T, Metzger D, Meyer ME, Tora L, Vergezac A, Chambon D (1992) Mechanism of antihormone action. *J Steroid Biochem Mol Biol* 41:217–221.

12. Takimoto GS, Tasset DM, Eppert AC, Horwitz KB (1992) Hormone-induced progesterone receptor phosphorylation consists of sequential DNA-independent and DNA-dependent stages: Analysis with zinc finger mutants and the progesterone antagonist ZK 98299. *Proc Natl Acad Sci USA* 98:3050–3054.

13. Delabre K, Guiochon-Mantel A, Milgrom E (1993) In vivo evidence against the existence of antiprogestins disrupting receptor binding to DNA. *Proc Natl Acad Sci USA* 90:4421–4425.

14. Horwitz KB, Takimoto GS, Tung L (1994) When steroid antagonists act like agonists: Issues of hormone resistance and tissue specificity. In *Program and abstracts, Dallas, IX International Congress on Hormonal Steroids,* September 1994, Dallas, Texas.

15. Bardon S, Vignon F, Chalbos D, Rochefort H (1985) RU 486, a progestin and glucocorticoid antagonist, inhibits the growth of breast cancer cells via progesterone receptor. *J Clin Endocrinol Metab* 60:692.

16. Horwitz KB (1985) The antiprogestin RU 38486: Receptor mediated progestin versus antiprogestin actions screened in estrogen-sensitive T 47 D10 human breast cancer cells. *Endocrinology* 116:2236–2245.

17. Bardon S, Vignon F, Montcourrier P, Rochefort H (1987) Steroid receptor-mediated cytotoxity of an antiestrogen and an antiprogestin in breast cancer cells. *Cancer Res* 47:1441–1448.

18. Gill P, Vignon F, Bardon S, Derocq S, Rochefort H (1987) Difference between R 5020 and the antiprogestin RU 486 on anti-proliferative effects on human breast cancer cells. *Breast Cancer Res Treat* 10:37–45.

19. Terakawa N, Shimizu I, Tanizawa O, Matsumoto K (1988) RU 486, a progestin antagonist, binds to progesterone receptors in a human endometrial cancer cell line and reverses the growth inhibition by progestins. *J Steroid Biochem* 31:161–166.

20. Van den Berg HW, Martin JHJ, Lynch M (1990) Progestin/anti-progestin action towards

208

human breast cancer cell lines differing in their progesterone receptor content. *Br J Pharmacol* 101(Suppl).

21. Thomas M, Monet JD (1992) Combined effects of RU 486 and Tamoxifen on the growth and cell cycle phases of the MCF-7 cell line. *J Clin Endocrinol Metab* 75:865–870.
22. Classen S, Possinger K, Pelka-Fleischer R, Wilmanns W (1993) Effect of Onapristone and medroxy-progesterone acetate on the proliferation and hormone receptor concentration of human breast cancer cells. *J Steroid Biochem Mol Biol* 45:315–319.
23. Van den Berg HW, Lynch M, Martin JHJ (1993) The relationship between affinity progestins and antiprogestins for the progesterone receptor in breast cancer cells (ZR-PR-LT) and ability to down-regulate the receptor: Modulation via the glucocorticoid receptor. *Eur J Cancer* 29A:1771–1775.
24. Maass N, Eidmann H, Arps H, Jonat W (1994) Progesterone antagonist ZK 98.299 (Onapristone) inhibits growth of the estrogen receptor (ER) and progesterone receptor (PR) positive breast cancer cell line MCF-7. *Tumordiagn Ther* 15:6–11.
25. Bowden TR, Hissom JR, Moore MR (1989) Growth stimulation of T47D human breast cancer cells by the antiprogestin RU 486. *Endocrinology* 124:2642–2646.
26. Jeng MH, Jordan VC (1992) Estrogenic actions of RU 486 in estrogen responsive human breast cancer MCF-7 cells. *Proc Am Assoc Cancer Res* 282, abstr 1684.
27. Jeng M-H, Langan-Fahey SM, Jordan VC (1993) Estrogenic actions of RU 486 in hormone-responsive MCF-7 human breast cancer cells. *Endocrinology* 132:2622–2630.
28. Meei-Huey J, Langan-Fahey SM, Jordan VC (1993) Estrogenic actions of RU 486 in hormone responsive MCF-7 human breast cancer cells. *Endocrinology* 132:2622–2630.
29. Herman M, Bhakta A, Underwood B, Kodali S, Moudgil VK (1993) Interaction of progesterone receptor from T47D human breast cancer cells with different progestins and antiprogestins. Abstract book, Endocrine Society, Las Vegas, abstract 957, p 290.
30. Lu J, Matsumoto K, Nishizawa Y, Tanaka A, Hirose T, Sato B (1991) Nonclassical androgen actions of RU 38.486 in androgen-responsive Shionogi carcinoma 115 cells in serum-free culture. *J Steroid Biochem Mol Biol* 39:329–335.
31. Kloosterboer HJ, Deckers GHV, Van der Heuvel MJ, Loozen HJJ (1988) Screening of antiprogestagens by receptor studies and bioassays. *J Steroid Biochem* 31:567–571.
32. Mizutani T, Bhakta A, Kloosterboer HJ, Moudgil VK (1992) Novel anti-progestins Org 31806 and Org 31710 interaction with mammalian progesterone receptor and DNA binding of antisteroid receptor complexes. *J Steroid Mol Biol* 42:695–704.
33. Michna H, Nishino Y, Schneider MR, Louton T, El Etreby MF (1991) A bioassay for the evaluation of antiproliferative potencies of progesterone antagonists. *J Steroid Biochem Mol Biol* 38:359–365.
34. Bargmann W, Fleischhauer K, Knopp A (1960) Über die Morphologie der Milchsekretion. II. *Z Zellforsch* 53:545–568.
35. Bargmann W, Welsch W (1969) On the ultrastructure of the mammary gland. In *Lactogenes*. M Reynolds, SJ Folley (eds). Philadelphia: University of Pennsylvania Press, pp 43–52.
36. Haslam SZ, Shyalama G (1981) Relative distribution of estrogen and progesterone receptors among the epithelial, adipose, and connective tissue components of the normal mammary gland. *Endocrinology* 108:825–830.
37. Russo H, Russo JH (1987) Development of the human mammary gland. In *The Mammary Gland*. MC Neville, CW Daniel (eds). New York: Plenum, pp 53–68.
38. Haslam SZ (1988) Progesterone effects on deoxyribonucleic acid synthesis in normal mouse mammary glands. *Endocrinology* 122:464–470.
39. Russo IH, Medado J, Russo J (1989) Endocrine influences on the mammary glands. In *Integument and Mammary Glands*. TC Jones, U Mohr, RD Hunt (eds). Berlin: Springer Verlag, pp 252–266.
40. Neumann U, Mendoza A, Kühnel W, Nishino Y, Michna H (1996) A new assay for progestins. *J Steroid Biochem Mol Biol*, in press.
41. Michna H, Schneider MR, Nishino Y, El Etreby MF (1989) The antitumor mechanism of

progesterone antagonists is a receptor mediated antiproliferative effect by induction of terminal cell death. *J Steroid Biochem* 34:447–453.

42. Schneider MR, Michna H, Nishino Y, El Etreby MF (1989) Antitumor activity of the progesterone antagonists ZK 98299 and RU486 in the hormone-dependent MXT mammary tumor model of the mouse and the DMBA- and MNU-induced mammary tumor model of the rat. *Eur J Cancer Clin Oncol* 25:691–701.

43. Michna H, Schneider MR, Nishino Y, El Etreby MF, McGuire WL (1990) Progesterone antagonists block the growth of experimental mammary tumors in G_0G_1. *Breast Cancer Res Treat* 17:155–156.

44. Bakker GH, Setyono-Han B, Portengen H, de Jong FH, Foekens JA, Klijn JGM (1990) Treatment of breast cancer with different antiprogestins: Preclinical and clinical studies. *J Steroid Biochem Mol Biol* 37:789–794.

45. Bakker GH, Setyono-Han B, de Jong FH, Klijn JGM (1987) Mifepristone in treatment of experimental breast cancer in rats. In *Hormonal Manipulation of Cancer: Peptides, Growth Factors and New (Anti-) Steroidal Agents*. JGM Klijn, R Paridaens, JA Foekens (eds). New York: Raven, pp 39–48.

46. Orlemans EOM, Deckers GH, Schoonen WGEJ, Kloosterboer HJ (1994) Pharmacology of the very selective antiprogestin Org 31710 and comparison with the antiprogestins RU38486 and ZK 98299. Program and abstracts, Dallas TX, International Congress on Hormonal Steroids, p 81.

47. Michna H, Schneider MR, Nishino Y, El Etreby MF (1989) Antitumor activity of the antiprogesterones ZK 98.299 and RU 38.486 in hormone dependent rat and mouse mammary tumors: Mechanistic studies. *Breast Cancer Res Treat* 14:275–288.

48. Michna H, Nishino Y, Schneider MR (1993) Effective sequential treatment of experimental mammary carcinomas with Tamoxifen and the progesterone antagonist Onapristone. *Proc Am Assoc Cancer Res* 34:25.

49. Rumpel E, Michna H, Kühnel W (1993) Morphology of the rat uterus after long-term treatment with progesterone antagonists. *Ann Anat* 175:141–149.

50. Michna H, Nishino Y, Hasan SH, Schneider MR (1993) Morphological and endocrine reactions of hormone dependent target organs to a progesterone receptor blockade by a progesterone antagonist. *Ann Anat* 175:303.

51. Nishino Y, Michna H, Hasan SH, Schneider MR (1991) The progesterone antagonist Onapristone modulates estrogen-dependent functions in different target organs in rats and mice. *Acta Endocrinol* 124(Suppl 1):160.

52. Nishino Y, Michna H, Hasan SH, Schneider MR (1992) Involvement of the adrenal gland in the prolactin rise induced in the femal rat to an antiprogestin, Onapristone. *J Steroid Biochem Mol Biol* 41:841–845.

53. Koering MJ, Healy DL, Hodgen GD (1986) Morphologic response of endometrium to a progesterone receptor antagonist, RU 486, in monkeys. *Fertil Steril* 45:280–287.

54. Wolf JP, Hsiu JG, Anderson TL, Ulman A, Baulieu EE, Hodgen GD (1989) Noncompetitive antiestrogenic effect of RU 486 in blocking the estrogen-stimulated luteinizing hormone surge and the proliferative action of estradiol on endometrium in castrated monkeys. *Fertil Steril* 52:1055–1060.

55. Bigsby RM, Young PCM (1994) Estrogenic effects of the antiprogestin Onapristone in the rodent uterus. *Am J Obstet Gynecol* 171:188–194.

56. Tachi C, Tachi S, Lindner HR (1972) Modification by progesterone of oestradiol-induced cell proliferation, RNA synthesis and oestradiol distribution in the rat uterus. *J Reprod Fertil* 31:59–76.

57. Clark BF (1973) The effect of estrogen and progesterone on uterine cell division and epithelial morphology in spayed-hypophysectomized rats. *J Endocrinol* 56:341–342.

58. Martin L, Finn CA, Tinder G (1973) Hypertrophy and hyperplasia in the mouse uterus after oestrogen treatment: An autoradiographic study. *J Endocrinol* 56:133–144.

59. Bigsby RM, Cunha GR (1985) Effects of progestins and glucocorticoids on deoxyribonucleic acid synthesis in the uterus of the neonatal mouse. *Endocrinology* 117:2520–2526.

60. Van der Schoot P, Bakker GH, Klijn JGM (1987) Effects of the progesterone antagonist RU 486 (mifepristone) on ovarian activity in the rat. *Endocrinology* 121:1375–1382.
61. Bigsby RM, Cunha GR (1988) Progesterone and dexamethasone inhibition of uterine epithelial proliferation in two models of estrogen-independent growth. *Am J Obstet Gynecol* 518:646–650.
62. Van der Schoot P, Uilenbroek JT, Slappendel EJ (1990) Effect of the progesterone antagonist mifepristone on the hypothalamo-hypophysial-ovarian axis in rats. *J Endocrinol* 124:425–432.
63. Jo T, Terada N, Saji F, Tanizawa O (1993) Inhibitory effects of estrogen, progesterone, androgen and glucocorticoid on death of neonatal mouse uterine epithelial cells induced to proliferate by estrogen. *J Steroid Biochem Mol Biol* 46:25–32.
64. Rauch M, Loosfeld H, Philibert D, Milgrom E (1985) Mechanism of action of an antiprogesterone, RU 468, in the rabbit endometrium. Effects of RU 468 on the progesterone receptor and on the expression of the uteroglobin gene. *Eur J Biochem* 148:213–18.
65. Van Uem JFHM, Hsiu JG, Chillik CF (1989) Contraceptive potential of RU 486 by ovulation inhibition. I. Pituitary versus ovarian action with blockade of estrogen-induced endometrial proliferation. *Contraception* 40:171–184.
66. Neulen J, Williams RF, Hodgen GD (1990) RU 486: Induction of dose dependent elevations of estradiol receptor in endometrium from ovariectomized monkeys. *J Clin Endocrinol Metab* 71:1074–1075.
67. Chwalisz K, Hegele-Hartung C, Fritzemeier KH, Beier HM, Elger W (1991) Inhibition of the estradiol-mediated endometrial gland formation by the antigestagen Onapristone in rabbits: Relationship to uterine estrogen receptors. *Endocrinology* 129:312–322.
68. Slayden OD, Brenner RM (1994) RU 486 action after estrogen priming in the endometrium and oviducts of rhesus monkeys (*Macaca mulatta*). *J Clin Endocrinol Metab* 78:440–448.
69. Slayden OD, Hirst JJ, Brenner RM (1993) Estrogen action in the reproductive tract of rhesus monkeys during antiprogestin treatment. *Endocrinology* 132:1845–1856.
70. Gottardis MM, Jordan VC (1988) Development of tamoxifen-stimulated growth of MCF-7 tumors in athymic mice after long-term antiestrogen administration. *Cancer Res* 48:5183–5187.
71. Reddel RR, Sutherland RL (1984) Tamoxifen stimulation of human breast cancer proliferation in vitro: A possible model for tamoxifen tumour flare. *Eur J Cancer Clin Oncol* 20:1419–1424.
72. Martin L (1981) Effects of antiestrogens on cell proferation in the rodent reproductive tract. In *Non-steroidal Antioestrogens. Molecular Pharmacology and Antitumor Activity*. RL Sutherland, VC Jordan (eds). New York: Academic Press, pp 47–55.
73. Howell A, Dodwell D, Laidlaw J, Anderson H, Anderson E (1990) Tamoxifen as an agonist for metastatic breast cancer. In *Endocrine Therapy of Breast Cancer IV*. A Goldhirsch (eds). Berlin: Springer Verlag, pp 49–58.
74. Osborne C (1993) Mechanisms for tamoxifen resistance in breast cancer: Possible role of tamoxifen metabolism. *J Steroid Biochem Mol Biol* 47:83–90.
75. Lahti E, Blanco G, Kauppila A, Apaja-Sarkkinen M, Taskinen P, Laatikainen T (1993) Endometrial changes in postmenopausal breast cancer patients receiving tamoxifen. *Obstet Gynecol* 81:660–664.
76. Wakeling AE, Bowler J (1987) Steroidal pure antiestrogens. *J Endocrinol* 112:R7–10.
77. Brunne N, Bronzert D, Vindelov L, Rygaard K, Spang-Thomsen M, Lippman ME (1989) Effect on growth and cell cycle kinetics of estradiol and tamoxifen on MCF-7 human breast cancer cells grown in vitro and in nude mice. *Cancer Res* 49:1515–1520.
78. Lamberts SWJ, Koper JW, de Jong FH (1991) The endocrine effects of long-term treatment with mifepristone (RU 486). *J Clin Endocrinol Metab* 73:187–191.
79. Jordan VC (1992) The role of tamoxifen in the treatment and prevention of breast cancer. *Curr Probl Cancer* 16:134–176.
80. Wakeling AE, Bowler J (1988) Biology and mode of action of pure antiestrogens. *J Steroid Biochem* 30:141–149.

211

81. Stöckemann K, Chwalisz K (1993) Effects of the new progesterone antagonist ZK 136799 on surgically-induced endometriosis. Program of the 40th Annual Meeting of Obstetrics, Toronto, abstract.

82. Stöckemann K, Chwalisz K (1993) Effects of the progesterone antagonist Onapristone and ZK 136799 on surgically-induced endometriosis in rats. Program of the 37th Symposium of the German Endocrine Society Berlin, abstract.

83. Kettel LM, Murphy AA, Mortola JF, Liu JH, Ulmann A, Yen SS (1991) Endocrine responses to long-term administration of the antiprogesterone RU 486 in patients with pelvic endometriosis. *Fertil Steril* 56:402–407.

84. Murphy AA, Kettel LM, Morales AJ, Roberts VJ, Yen SS (1993) Regression of uterine leiomyomata in response to the antiprogesterone RU486. *J Clin Endocrinol Metab* 76:513–517.

85. McDonnell DP, Goldman ME (1994) RU 486 exerts antiestrogenic activities through a novel progesterone receptor A-form mediated mechanism. *J Biol Chem* 269:1945–1949.

86. Tora A, Mullick A, Metzger D, Ponglikitmongkol M, Park I, Chambon P (1989) The cloned human oestrogen receptor contains a mutation which alters its hormone binding properties. *EMBO J* 49:1981–1986.

87. Klein-Hitpass L, Schorpp M, Wagner U, Ryffel GU (1986) An estrogen-responsive element derived from the 5' flanking region of the Xenopus vitellogenin A2 gene functions in trans-fected human cells. *Cell* 46:1053–1061.

88. Döhler KD, Wuttke W (1975) Changes with age in levels of serum gonadotropins, prolactin, and gonadal steroids in prepubertal male and female rats. *Acta Endocrinol* 97:898–916.

89. Horwitz KB, McGuire WL (1977) Progesterone and progesterone receptors in experimental breast cancer. *Cancer Res* 37:1733–1738.

90. Vollmer G, Michna H, Ebert K, Knuppen R (1992) Downregulation of tenascin expression by antiprogestins during terminal differentiation of rat mammary tumors. *Cancer Res* 52:4642–4648.

91. Gehring S, Michna H, Kühnel W, Nishino Y, Schneider MR (1991) Morphometrical and histochemical studies on the differentiation potential of progesterone antagonists in experi-mental mammary carcinomas. *Acta Endocrinol* 124:177.

92. Tenniswood M, Michna H (1995) *Apoptosis in Hormone-Dependent Cancers*. Berlin: Springer Verlag.

93. Knabbe C, Lippmann ME, Flanders KC, Kasid A, Derynck R, Dickson RB (1987) Evidence that transforming growth factor-beta is a hormonally regulated negative growth factor in human breast cancer cells. *Cell* 48:417–428.

94. Bursch W, Grasl-Kraupp B, Ellinger A, Török L, Kienzl H, Müllauer L, Schulte-Hermann R (1995) Active cell death and cancer. In M Tenniswood, H Michna (eds). *Apoptosis in Hor-mone Dependent Cancers*. Berlin: Springer Verlag, pp 83–103.

95. Colletta AA, Wakefield LM, Howell FV, van Roozendaal KE, Danielpour D, Ebbs SR, Sporn MB, Baum M (1992) Anti-estrogens induce the secretion of active transforming growth factor-beta from fetal fibroblasts. *Br J Cancer* 62:405–409.

96. Scott RE, Hoerl BJ, Wille JJ, Florine DL, Krawisz BR, Kankatsu Y (1982) Coupling of proadipocyte growth arrest and differentiation. II. A cell cycle model for the physiological control of cell proliferation. *J Cell Biol* 94:400–405.

97. Wille JJ, Maercklein PB, Scott RE (1982) Neoplastic transformation and defective control of cell proliferation and differentiation. *Cancer Res* 42:5139–5146.

98. Clark GM, Dressler LG, Owens MA, Pounds G, Oldaker T, McGuire WL (1989) Prediction of relapse or survival in patients with node-negative breast cancer by DNA flow cytometry. *N Engl J Med* 320:627–633.

99. McGuire WL, Dressler LG (1985) Emerging impact of flow cytometry in predicting recur-rence and survival in breast cancer patients. *J Natl Cancer Inst* 75:405–410.

11. Antiestrogen–estrogen receptor interactions

Malcolm G. Parker

Introduction

Estrogens function as mitogens primarily in the G_1 phase of the cell cycle by recruiting cells into the cycle and by shortening the length of their G_1 phase. Conversely, estrogen antagonists that inhibit cell proliferation reduce the proportion of cells in S phase [1]. The precise role of estrogen in cell growth and proliferation is poorly understood. Initially it was proposed that estrogens stimulate proliferation indirectly by increasing the production of growth factors such as transforming growth factor (TGF)-α [2] or reducing the secretion of growth inhibitory factors such as TGF-β [3,4]. Alternatively, since estrogens stimulate the expression of receptors for a number of growth factors, including those for insulin-like growth factor (IGF-I) and epidermal growth factor (EGF) [5,6], they might function by increasing the sensitivity of cells to growth factors produced either by tumor cells themselves or perhaps by surrounding stromal cells, thereby regulating cell proliferation by a paracrine mechanism [7].

More recently it has been suggested that genes, implicated in the G_1 phase of the cell cycle, might be primary targets for estrogen. For example, the products of a number of immediate early response genes, including members of the Fos and Myc families, which are associated with cell cycle progression, are increased in MCF-7 breast cancer cells following estrogen treatment [8,9]. The expression of these immediate early response genes is transient and, as transcription factors, they in turn probably regulate the expression of downstream target genes involved in cell proliferation. One such group are the cyclins and the cyclin-dependent kinases. The D-type cyclins may function at G_1 control points and, interestingly, the expression of cyclin D1 mRNA and protein is regulated by steroid hormones in breast cancer cells [10]. Given the number of target genes for estrogens that are implicated in cell proliferation, in has been very difficult to identify the most crucial ones. It is possible that the concept of a single rate-limiting step is inappropriate to explain the effects of various mitogens and that steroid hormones regulate several steps in the cell cycle or different stages in the development of a tumor. In any event, despite the uncertainty about the mechanism by which estrogen functions as a mito-

R. Dickson and M. Lippman (eds.) MAMMARY TUMOR CELL CYCLE, DIFFERENTIATION AND METASTASIS. 1996. Kluwer Academic Publishers. ISBN 0-7923-3905-3. All rights reserved.

gen, several types of estrogen antagonists have been discovered empirically. In this chapter, the molecular mechanisms of estrogen receptor action are described, followed by a review of the action of partial agonists/antagonists, such as tamoxifen, and pure antiestrogens, and a brief outline of potential mechanisms that have been suggested to account for tamoxifen insensitivity.

Molecular mechanisms of estrogen receptor action

Many, but not all, of the actions of estrogens in target cells are mediated by estrogen receptors functioning directly as transcription factors. Upon hormone binding, the receptor forms homodimers and binds to regulatory DNA sites in the vicinity of target genes [11]. In many cases, the sites are simple response elements consisting of inverted repeats that bind the receptor with relatively high affinity (Figure 1A). In other cases, at sites referred to as *composite response elements*, the receptor binds only in association with another transcription factor. One example is the presence of a site resembling that for activator protein 1 (AP-1), which binds either homodimers of the transcription factor Jun or Fos/Jun heterodimers [12] (Figure 1B). Simple response elements for estrogen receptors consist of inverted repeats of the sequence $^A/_G$GTCA, whose binding affinity for receptor varies depending on their precise sequence and number. The majority of estrogen response elements that have been characterized to date contain imperfect inverted repeats that function less well than the consensus sequence but, in some promoters, there are several such sites that increase the estrogen response [13].

In the absence of hormone, the estrogen receptor is detected predominantly in the cell nucleus as inactive oligomeric complexes containing a number of heat shock proteins, including hsp 90 (Figure 2). The role of hsp90 appears to be to maintain the receptor in an inactive state in the absence of ligand and it may also be important for folding of the receptor protein and/or transport across membranes [14]. In spite of its nuclear location under steady-state conditions, the receptor is not static but constantly shuttling between the nucleus and the cytoplasm. The receptor appears to diffuse passively into the cytoplasm but is rapidly transported back into the cell nucleus in an energy-dependent process [15]. Following hormone binding, the oligomeric complex dissociates and the receptor either binds to DNA response elements in the form of homodimers or interacts with other transcription factors. Since the hormone binding pocket is at or near the dimer interface, it appears that dimerization is stabilized in the presence of the hormone on the basis of hydrophobic shielding [16].

Transcriptional activation by steroid receptors is mediated by at least two distinct activation regions, at least on simple response elements. One of these, referred to as AF-1, is located in the N-terminal domain and another, AF-2, is in the hormone binding domain [17–19]. Their absolute and relative activities vary depending on the target promoter and the cell type. However, while the

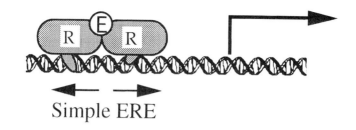

Simple ERE

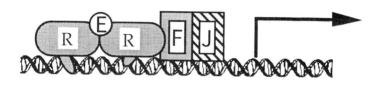

Composite Response Element

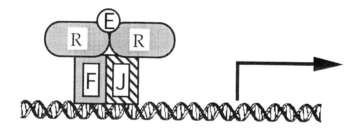

AP-1 site

Figure 1. Mechanisms of transcriptional activation by estrogen receptors. Classically estrogen receptors (R) occupied by estrogen (E) bind to simple response elements as homodimers, where they usually stimulate transcription. However, receptors can also function in combination with other transcription factors, such as AP-1, either on composite response elements, when both the receptor and AP-1 contact DNA, or on AP-1 sites, when the receptor forms protein–protein interactions with AP-1. AP-1 consists of either Fos/Jun heterodimers or Jun homodimers, and the precise composition of the complex seems to determine whether the receptor promotes or antagonizes the activity of AP-1.

two activation domains have the potential to act independently, they appear to interact with one another in some ill-defined way in the intact receptor. It is generally accepted that the rate at which RNA polymerase initiates gene transcription depends on the formation of a pre-initiation complex that includes a number of basic transcription factors and that one of the major roles

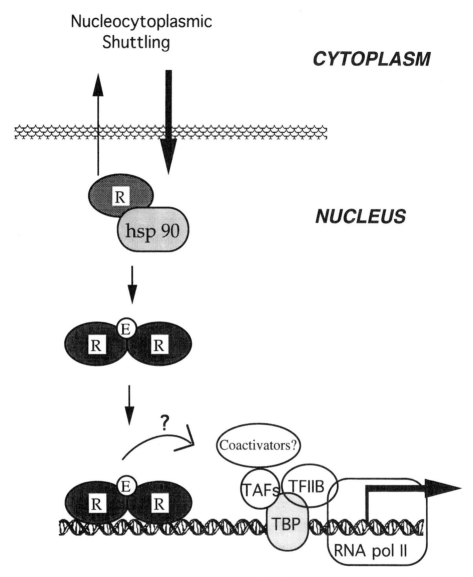

Figure 2. Scheme of estrogen receptor action upon binding to target genes. In the absence of hormone, estrogen receptors (R) passively diffuse into the cytoplasm but are actively transported back into the nucleus so that under steady-stage conditions they are predominantly nuclear proteins. Upon estrogen binding (E), the receptor is activated and, following the dissociation of heat shock proteins, forms homodimers and binds to target genes. Transcription by RNA polymerase II is then activated by an poorly defined mechanism that probably involves stabilization of the basic transcription machinery. This might be achieved by direct interactions between the receptor and basic transcription factors, such as TATA-box binding protein (TBP), TFIIB, or a TBP associated factor (TAF), or it might involve indirect interactions with coactivators.

216

of transcriptional activators is to stabilize this complex [20,21]. A number of activators, including steroid hormone receptors, have been shown to bind directly to basal transcription factors (see Figure 2), including TFIIB [22], the TATA-box binding protein, TBP [23], and TAF30 [24]. However, the significance of these interactions is unclear since they are unaffected by either hormone binding or mutations in the receptor that abolish its transcriptional activity. Thus we assume that there are additional targets for the estrogen receptor. Possible candidates include two receptor interacting proteins, RIP140 and RIP160, which have the properties expected of coactivator proteins and might mediate the transcriptional activity of the receptor [25].

As mentioned earlier in addition to binding to simple response elements, steroid hormone receptors also appear to bind to *composite response elements* only in association with another transcription factor. For example, the estrogen regulation of ovalbumin gene expression seems to involve the binding of AP-1 to an estrogen response element (Figure 1B) and may be a feature of many other hormone-sensitive genes. However, the receptor has also been reported to modulate AP-1 activity, either by stimulating the expression of Fos [8] or by modulating the activity of AP-1 without contacting DNA (Figure 1C). Moreover, it has been found that estrogens enhance and antiestrogens inhibit growth factor induced AP-1 activity in estrogen receptor–positive breast cancer cells [26]. One explanation for these effects, which were not accounted for by alterations in the levels of Fos or Jun, is that they involve protein–protein interactions between the estrogen receptor and AP-1 family members. Since AP-1 is implicated in many signaling pathways that regulate cell differentiation, proliferation, and transformation, its modulation by the estrogen receptor would be extremely important and will be discussed in more detail later.

Role of estrogen antagonists

While the relevant targets involved in mediating the mitogenic effects of estrogen have yet to be identified, antiestrogens have been developed empirically, some of which are in widespread clinical use. The best known of these is the nonsteroidal antiestrogen tamoxifen, which is the most commonly used first-line endocrine therapy in advanced breast cancer and has become established in adjuvant therapy after removal of the primary tumor [27]. Although tamoxifen is a potent antagonist, it retains partial agonist activity, which varies according to cell type and response. In some cases, the agonist activity of tamoxifen gives rise to beneficial side effects, including the maintenance of bone density and a reduction of mortality due to cardiovascular problems. While tamoxifen itself is a ligand for the estrogen receptor, it is metabolized in the liver and to some extent in target cells so that the majority of its actions are probably mediated by one of its metabolites, 4-hydroxytamoxifen, which has a higher affinity for the receptor than tamoxifen itself.

It view of the agonist activity of tamoxifen, which is probably associated with an increase in the incidence of endometrial cancer, attempts were made to synthesize antiestrogens devoid of any estrogenic activity. The steroidal antiestrogen ICI 164384 completely inhibited the stimulatory effects of estradiol on uterine weight and lacked agonist activity. Its effectiveness depends on an alkylamine side chain at the 7α-position of the B ring in the steroid, whose optimum length is 16–18 carbon atoms [28]. The hydrophobic nature of ICI 164384 limits its clinical use, but the introduction of fluorine atoms in the side chain to generate ICI 182780 appears largely to overcome the problem of solubility and also results in a slight increase in affinity for the receptor [29]. In view of the lack of agonist activity of ICI 164384 and ICI 182780, they are referred to as pure antiestrogens. It is doubtful whether ICI 182780 retains the beneficial side effects associated with tamoxifen treatment but may be useful for the treatment of patients who are insensitive to tamoxifen or acquire resistance to the treatment.

Tamoxifen–estrogen receptor interactions

Tamoxifen and its more potent metabolite, 4-hydroxytamoxifen, act as competitive inhibitors of estrogen action by binding to the estrogen binding site in the receptor. In studies of the mouse receptor, site-directed mutagenesis have indicated that a number critical amino acids are located between residues 518 and 525 in the C-terminal region of the hormone binding domain. Interestingly, although mutation of a glycine at position 525 (521 in the human receptor) and a methionine and/or serine at positions 521/522 essentially abolished estrogen binding activity, they had very little effect on the binding of 4-hydroxytamoxifen [30]. The mutant receptors retained the partial agonist activity exhibited by the wild-type receptor in the presence of 4-hydroxytamoxifen. Analysis of the human receptor has shown that mutation of lysines at positions 529 and 531 to glutamines reduced its affinity for estradiol 5- to 10-fold but had no effect on hydroxytamoxifen binding [31]. Thus a number of residues in the C-terminal region of the hormone binding domain are able to confer differential sensitivity to estrogen and 4-hydorxytamoxifen, indicating that while the binding sites overlap one another, they are not completely coincident.

Upon binding to the receptor, estrogen and 4-hydroxytamoxifen each induce different conformations and/or post-translational modifications, as shown by their protease digestion patterns and their electrophoretic mobilities when they are complexed with DNA [18,32–35]. These differences do not appear to affect either dimerization or high affinity DNA binding of the receptor but modify its transcriptional activity. Following the observation that there are two discrete transcriptional activation regions in the estrogen receptor, AF-1 and AF-2 [19,36], it was found that the activity of AF-2 is dependent on the binding of estrogen and is negligible in the presence of the tamoxifen. Since AF-1 has the potential to function constitutively, it has been proposed that it is likely to be active not only in the presence of agonists, but also antagonists that promote DNA binding [34,36]. Therefore in situations where AF-1 and AF-2 function independently of one another, 4-hydroxytamoxifen might act predominantly as an antagonist on gene promoters on which AF-2 contributed the most activity, but as an agonist when AF-1 was most active. If both AF-1 and AF-2 contributed activity, 4-hydroxytamoxifen is likely to act as a mixed agonist/antagonist.

However, it is doubtful whether antiestrogens function simply by antagonizing the effects of estradiol. Since they not only inhibit estrogen-induced cell growth but are also capable of blocking the mitogenic effects of growth factors such as EGF and IGF-1 [37], antiestrogens must elicit a growth inhibitory response in their own right. This might be achieved by an increase in the secretion of TGF-β, which is normally suppressed by estrogen [3,4]. Alternatively, it might involve the antagonism of another signaling pathway involved in cell proliferation. Candidates include those that modulate AP-1 activity [26], which, as mentioned earlier, can be regulated indirectly by protein–protein interactions between the estrogen receptor and AP-1 family members.

Mechanism of action of 'pure' estrogen antagonists

One of the most striking effects of the pure antiestrogens, ICI 164384 and ICI 182780, is to block nucleocytoplasmic shuttling of the estrogen receptor. Normally it appears that the receptor freely diffuses out of the cell nucleus but is actively taken up into the cell nucleus. This nuclear uptake does not occur in the presence of the pure antiestrogens and can be visualized by immunofluorescence. It is accompanied by a decrease in the cellular content of receptor protein brought about by a reduction in its half-life [38]. Since degradation was prevented by the presence of the lysosomal inhibitor chloroquine, it is likely to occur in lysosomes.

We have also suggested that the pure antiestrogens inhibit dimerization of the receptor and thereby reduce its DNA binding activity. We assume that ICI 164384 binds to a similar, if not identical, site to that of estradiol, which we have shown overlaps with a region involved in receptor dimerization [16]. As a consequence, we proposed that the antiestrogens, by means of their 7α side chains (Figure 2), sterically interfere with dimerization and as a consequence are able to reduce the affinity with which the receptor bound to DNA [39,40]. Moreover, we demonstrated that the ability of analogues of ICI 164384 with different side-chain lengths to inhibit DNA binding correlated with their ability to inhibit uterine growth in vivo [28,39]. We initially thought that this disruption in dimerization may be causally linked to the block in nuclear uptake, but subsequently it became evident that this is unlikely. We have found that dimerization-defective receptor mutants can still be detected in the cell nucleus and have a half-life resembling that of the wild-type receptor. Thus the alteration in subcellular localization of the receptor and its increased turnover is not simply a reflection of defective dimerization but is dependent on antiestrogen binding.

Although pure antiestrogens clearly inhibit the in vitro DNA binding activity of the receptor, their in vivo effects are controversial. Since ICI 164384 did not prevent DNA binding of the receptor in transiently transfected cells or when expressed in yeast, it has been argued that the antiestrogen must act at a step subsequent to DNA binding [19,41,42]. However, the significance of some of these experiments is unclear, given the recent finding that the uptake of pure antiestrogens by yeast is poor [43]. Another possibility is that the pure antiestrogens disrupt the interaction of the receptor with downstream target proteins that mediate transcriptional activity. To date the receptor has been shown to interact with the basal transcription factors TFIIB, TBP, and TAFII30 and a number of novel proteins, including RIP140 and RIP160. Although the precise role of the RIP proteins has yet to be elucidated, their interaction with the receptor was blocked in the presence of antiestrogens. Since their binding to mutant estrogen receptors to the RIP proteins is correlated with their transcriptional activity, it is possible that they act as coactivators and play a role in mediating hormone regulated transcription. Thus pure antiestrogens (and tamoxifen) might also inhibit estrogen-dependent transcription by interfering with the function of such proteins.

Tamoxifen insensitivity

Although overviews of randomized worldwide clinical trials indicate that the 5- and 10-year mortality rates of breast cancer patients can be reduced by 20–25% by using adjuvant tamoxifen therapy [44], as many half the patients whose tumors express estrogen receptors are insensitive to tamoxifen treatment, and many of those who initially respond eventually develop drug resistance. Since some of these tamoxifen-resistant patients still respond to alternative forms of endocrine therapy, such as the use of aromatase inhibitors to block estradiol production, it appears that estrogen receptors are still involved in the growth of this subset of tumors. Many mechanisms have been proposed to account for tamoxifen insensitivity based primarily on either alterations in tamoxifen metabolism or receptor function. Given the potential to generate tamoxifen insensitivity in vitro, it is likely that a number of alternative mechanisms may be involved. Those that involve the estrogen receptor are reviewed later.

A number of variant mRNAs generated by aberrant splicing have been described that have the potential to code for truncated and/or mutant receptors [45]. However, it has been difficult to determine whether or not such variant mRNAs are translated into stable protein products in vivo. Although the proteins have yet to be characterized with specific immunological reagents, one of the variants is of particular interest, namely, an exon 5 deletion that gives rise to a truncated receptor that lacks the hormone binding domain. This receptor retains some constitutive activity that is probably mediated by AF-1 in transfected cells, and so it might be capable of stimulating the transcription of estrogen target genes, even in the presence of tamoxifen [45]. However, upon exogenous expression of the exon 5 variant receptor in a number of MCF-7 human breast cancer cell line sublines, we have been unable to detect increased cell growth in the presence of tamoxifen. There is also no apparent increase in the expression of the variant mRNA in tamoxifen-resistant tumors compared with untreated tumors [46]. Thus, we conclude that the expression of this variant is unlikely to account for tamoxifen insensitivity in the absence of additional cellular alterations in the majority of breast cancer cases.

Another possibility is that mutations in the estrogen receptor gene might allow the receptor to function as a mitogen, even in the presence of antiestrogen. There is very little published information on the incidence of estrogen receptor mutations in breast cancer, perhaps indicating that they are uncommon. In one study of metastatic tumors from patients receiving adjuvant tamoxifen and from patients with stage III or IV metastatic disease, the receptor was normal in 18 of 20 cases, as determined by single-strand conformation analysis [47]. In the remaining two cases, the mutations in the gene would potentially give rise to receptors that were truncated in the hormone binding domain, but their functional activity has yet to be examined. From our own work we have established that amino acids between residues 518 and 535 are particularly important in ligand binding, as described earlier. Moreover, mutations exist that abolish estrogen binding activity [48], but mutant receptors incapable of binding tamoxifen have not been reported. However, mutations have been described that do not affect ligand binding but dramatically alter the pharmacology of estrogen antagonists [49]. These mutations are located between residues 538 and 552 in a region essential for estrogen-dependent transcriptional activity and are not part of the ligand binding site itself. Thus, both tamoxifen and the pure antiestrogens behave as agonists when these mutant receptors are expressed in mammalian cells, including breast cancer cells. In contrast to the wild-type receptor, the mutant receptors maintain nuclear localization and DNA binding activity in cells treated with ICI 164384. We are in the process of analyzing whether the mutant receptors alter growth properties on breast cancer cells.

It is quite possible that both the metabolism of tamoxifen and the expression of the receptor is unchanged and that the response of the receptor to tamoxifen altered by another signaling pathway that may or may not be normally cross-coupled. For example, activators of protein kinase A are capable of enhancing the agonist activity of partial agonist/antagonists, such as tamoxifen, at least in model system [50,51]. What is unclear is whether there is a change in protein kinase A activation in tumor cells that would account for the change in sensitivity to tamoxifen. Interestingly, dopamine, which increases intracellular cAMP levels, has been reported to stimulate the transcriptional activity of the estrogen receptor in the absence of estrogen binding [52]. Although breast cancer cells are not usually considered targets for dopamine, its effects in the presence of antiestrogens warrants further investigation. All the effects of tamoxifen described earlier relate to transcriptional activation by the estrogen receptor when it is bound to estrogen response elements. Since it is conceivable that the mitogenic effects of estrogens are mediated by AP-1, an alternative mechanism for generating tamoxifen insensitivity may involve signaling pathways that modulate AP-1 activity. Thus there are already several mechanisms that, at least in model systems, might account for insensitivity and resistance to tamoxifen, but there is little information about which, if any, occurs in breast tumors.

References

1. Brunner N, Bronzert D, Vindelov LL, Rygaard K, Spang-Thomsen M, Lippman ME (1989) Effect on growth and cell cycle kinetics of estradiol and tamoxifen on MCF-7 human breast cancer cells grown in vitro and in nude mice. *Cancer Res* 49:1515–1520.
2. Bates SE, Davidson NE, Valverius EM, Dickson RB, Freter CE, Tam JP, Kulow JE, Lippman ME, Salomon S (1988) Expression of transforming growth factor alpha and its messenger ribonucleic acid in human breast cancer, its regulation by estrogen and its possible functional significance. *Mol Endocrinol* 2:543–545.
3. Knabbe C, Lippman ME, Wakefield LM, Flanders KC, Kasid A, Derynck R, Dickson RB (1987) Evidence that transforming growth factor-β is a hormonally regulated negative growth factor in human breast cancer cells. *Cell* 48:417–428.
4. Roberts AB, Sporn MB (1992) Mechanistic interrelationships between two superfamilies: The steroid/retinod receptors and transforming growth factor-β. In *Cancer Surveys*, Vol 14. MG Parker (ed). Cold Spring Harbor, NY: Cold Spring Harbor Laboratory Press, pp 205–220.
5. Stewart AJ, Johnson MD, May FEB, Westley BR (1990) Role of insulin-like growth factors and the Type I insulin-like growth factor receptor in the estrogen-stimulated proliferation of human breast cancer cells. *J Biol Chem* 265:21172–21178.
6. Berthois Y, Dong XF, Martin PM (1989) Regulation of epidermal growth factor-receptor by estrogen and antiestrogen in the human breast cancer cell line MCF7. *Biochem Biophys Res Commun* 159:126–131.
7. Clarke R, Dickson RB, Lippman ME (1991) The role of steroid hormones and growth factors in the control of normal and malignant breast. In *Nuclear Hormone Receptors*. M Parker (ed). London: Academic Press, pp 297–319.
8. Wilding G, Lippman ME, Gelmann EP (1988) Effects of steroid hormones and peptide growth factors on proto-oncogene c-fos expression in human breast cancer cells. *Cancer Res* 48:802–805.
9. Dubik D, Dembinski TC, Shiu RPC (1987) Stimulation of c-myc oncogene expression associated with estrogen-induced proliferation of human breast cancer cells. *Cancer Res* 47:6517–6521.
10. Musgrove EA, Sutherland RL (1994) Cell cycle control by steroid hormones. In *Seminars in Cancer Biology*, Vol 5. M Parker (ed). London: Academic Press, pp 381–389.
11. Martinez E, Wahli W (1991) Characterization of hormone response elements. In *Nuclear Hormone Receptors. Molecular Mechanisms, Cellular Functions, Clinical Abnormalities*. MG Parker (ed). London: Academic Press, pp 125–154.
12. Diamond MI, Miner JN, Yoshinaga SK, Yamamoto KR (1990) Transcription factor interactions: Selectros of positive or negative regulation from a single DNA element. *Science* 249:1266–1272.
13. Martinez E, Wahli W (1989) Cooperative binding of estrogen receptor to imperfect estrogen-responsive DNA elements correlates with their synergistic hormone-dependent enhancer activity. *EMBO J* 8:3781–91.

14. Pratt WB (1993) Role of heat-shock proteins in steroid receptor function. In *Steroid Hormone Action*. MG Parker (ed). Oxford: IRL Press, pp 64–93.
15. Dauvois S, White R, Parker MG (1993) The antiestrogen ICI 182780 disrupts estrogen receptor nucleocytoplasmic shuttling. *J Cell Sci* 106:1377–1388.
16. Fawell SE, Lees JA, White R, Parker MG (1990) Characterization and colocalization of steroid binding and dimerization activities in the mouse estrogen receptor. *Cell* 60:953–962.
17. Tora L, White J, Brou C, Tasset D, Webster N, Scheer E, Chambon P (1989) The human estrogen receptor has two independent nonacidic trascriptional activation functions. *Cell* 59:477–487.
18. Lees JA, Fawell SE, Parker MG (1989) Identification of two transcativation domains in the mouse oestrogen receptor. *Nucleic Acids Res* 17:5477–5488.
19. Webster NJG, Green S, Jin JR, Chambon P (1988) The hormone-binding domains of the estrogen and glucocorticoid receptors contain an inducible transcription activation function. *Cell* 54:199–207.
20. Ptashne M (1988) How eukaryotic transcriptional activators work. *Nature* 335:683–689.
21. Mitchell PJ, Tjian R (1989) Transcriptional regulation in mammalian cells by sequence-specific DNA binding proteins. *Science* 245:371–378.
22. Ing NH, Beekman JM, Tsai SY, Tsai M-J, O'Malley BW (1992) Members of the steroid hormone receptor superfamily interact with TFIIB (S300-II). *J Biol Chem* 267:17617–17623.
23. Sadovsky Y, Webb P, Lopez G, Baxter JD, Cavailles V, Parker MG, Kushner PJ (1994) Transcriptional activators differ in their response to overexpression of TBP. *Mol Cell Biol*, in press.
24. Jacq X, Brou C, Lutz Y, Davidson I, Chambon P, Tora L (1994) Human TAF$_{11}$30 is present in a distrinct TFIID complex and is required for transcriptional activation by the estrogen receptor. *Cell* 79:107–117.
25. Cavaillès V, Dauvois S, Danielian PS, Parker MG (1994) Interaction of proteins with tran-scriptionally active estrogen receptors. *Proc Natl Acad Sci USA* 91:10009–10013.
26. Philips A, Chalbos D, Rochefort H (1993) Estradiol increases and anti-estrogens antagonize the growth factor-induced activator protein-1 activity in MCF7 breast cancer cells without affecting c-fos and c-jun synthesis. *J Biol Chem* 268:14103–14108.
27. Jordan VC (1984) Biochemical pharmacology of antiestrogen action. *Pharmacol Rev* 36:245–276.
28. Bowler J, Lilley TJ, Pittam JD, Wakelling AE (1989) Novel steroidal pure antiestrogens. *Steroids* 54:71–99.
29. Wakeling AE, Dukes M, Bowler J (1991) A potent specific pure antiestrogen with clinical potential. *Cancer Res* 51:3867–3873.
30. Danielian PS, White R, Lees JA, Parker MG (1992) Identification of a conserved region required for hormone dependent transcriptional activation by steroid hormone receptors. *EMBO J* 11:1025–1033.
31. Pakdel F, Katzenellenbogen BS (1992) Human estrogen receptor mutants with altered estro-gen and antiestrogen ligand discrimination. *J Biol Chem* 267:3429–3437.
32. Allan GF, Leng X, Tsai SY, Weigel NL, Edwards DP, Tsai M-J, O'Malley BW (1992) Hormone and anti-hormone induce distinct conformational changes which are central to steroid receptor activation. *J Biol Chem* 267:19513–19520.
33. Kumar V, Chambon P (1988) The estrogen receptor binds tightly to its responsive element as a ligand-induced homodimer. *Cell* 55:145–156.
34. Berry M, Metzger D, Chambon P (1990) Role of the two activating domains of the oestrogen receptor in the cell-type and promoter-context dependent agonistic activity of the anti-oestrogen 4-hydroxytamoxifen. *EMBO J* 9:2811–2818.
35. Brown M, Sharp PA (1990) Human estrogen receptor forms multiple protein-DNA com-plexes. *J Biol Chem* 265:11238–11243.
36. Meyer M-E, Pornon A, Ji J, Bocquel M-T, Chambon P, Gronemeyer H (1990). Agonistic and antagonistic activities of RU486 on the functions of the human progesterone receptor. *EMBO J* 9:3923–3932.

37. Chalbos D, Philips A, Rochefort H (1994) Genomic cross-talk between the estrogen receptor and growth factor regulatory pathways in estrogen target tissues. In *Seminars in Cancer Biology*, Vol 5. M Parker (ed). London: Academic Press, pp 361–368.

38. Dauvois S, Danielian PS, White R, Parker MG (1992) Antiestrogen ICI 164,384 reduces cellular estrogen receptor content by increasing its turnover. *Proc Natl Acad Sci USA* 89:4037–4041.

39. Arbuckle ND, Dauvois S, Parker MG (1992) Effects of antioestrogens on the DNA binding activity of oestrogen receptors in vitro. *Nucleic Acids Res* 20:3839–3844.

40. Fawell SE, White R, Hoare S, Sydenham M, Page M, Parker MG (1990) Inhibition of estrogen receptor-DNA binding by the 'pure' antiestrogen ICI 164,384 appears to be mediated by impaired receptor dimerization. *Proc Natl Acad Sci USA* 87:6883–6887.

41. Pham TA, Elliston JF, Nawaz Z, McDonnell DP, Tsai MJ, O'Malley BW (1991) Antiestrogen can establish nonproductive receptor complexes and alter chromatin structure at target enhancers. *Proc Natl Acad Sci USA* 88:3125–3129.

42. Reese JC, Katzenellenbogen BS (1992) Examination of the DNA-binding ability of estrogen receptor in whole cells: Implications for hormone-dependent transactivation and the actions of antiestrogens. *Mol Cell Biol* 12:4531–4538.

43. Zysk JR, Johnson B, Ozenberger BA, Bingham B, Gorski J (1995) Selective uptake of estrogenic compunds by *Saccharomyces cerevisiae*: A mechanism for antiestrogen resistance in yeast expressing the mammalian estrogen receptor. *Endocrinology* 136:1323–1326.

44. Bentley A, Fentiman IS, Rubens RD, Cuzick J, Crossley E, Durrand K, Harris A, Clarke M, Collins R, Godwin J, Gray R, Greaves E, Harwood C, Mead G, Peto R, Wheatley K (1992) Systemic treatment of early breast cancer by hormonal, cytotoxic, or immune therapy: 133 randomised trials involving 31000 recurrences and 24000 deaths among 75000 women. Part 2. *Lancet* 339:71–85.

45. Fuqua SA, Fitzgerald SD, Chamness GC, Tandon AK, McDonnell DP, Nawaz Z, O'Malley BW, McGuire WL (1991) Variant human breast tumor estrogen receptor with constitutive transcriptional activity. *Cancer Res* 51:105–109.

46. Daffada AAI, Johnston SRD, Smith IE, Detre S, King N, Dowsett M (1995) Exon 5 deletion variant estrogen receptor messenger RNA expression in relation to tamoxifen resistance and progesterone/receptor/pS2 status in human breast cancer. *Cancer Res* 55:288–293.

47. Karnik PS, Kulkarni S, Liu XP, Budd GT, Gukowski RM (1994) Estrogen-receptor mutations in tamoxifen-resistant breast-cancer. *Cancer Res* 54:349–353.

48. Danielian PS, White R, Hoare SA, Fawell SE, Parker MG (1993) Identification of residues in the estrogen receptor which confer differential sensitivity to estrogen and hydroxytamoxifen. *Mol Endocrinol* 7:232–240.

49. Mahfoudi A, Roulet E, Dauvois S, Parker MG, Wahli W (1995) Specific mutations in the estrogen receptor change the properties of antiestrogens to full agonists. *Proc Natl Acad Sci USA*, in press.

50. Chalbos D, Philips A, Galtier F, Rochefort H (1993) Synthetic antiestrogens modulate induction of pS2 and Cathepsin D messenger ribonucleic acid by growth factors and adenosine 3′,5′-monophosphate in MCF-7 cells. *Endocrinology* 133:571–576.

51. Fujimoto NaK BS (1994) Alteration in the agonist/antagonist balance of antiestrogens by activiation of protein kinase A signalling pathways in breast cancer cells: Antiestrogen-selectivity and promoter-dependence. *Mol Endocrinol* 8:296–304.

52. Smith CL, Conneely OM, O'Malley BW (1993) Modulation of ligand-independent activation of the human estrogen receptor by hormone and antihormone. *Proc Natl Acad Sci USA* 90:6120–6124.

C

Human breast cancer: Invasion, metastasis, angiogenesis, and immunology

12. Differentiation antigens in stromal and epithelial cells of the breast

Tahereh Kamalati, Birunthi Niranjan, Amanda Atherton,
Ramasawamy Anbazhaghan, and Barry Gusterson

Introduction

There is a large morphological spectrum of benign and malignant diseases that are specific to the human breast. The presence of stromal tumors (phyllodes) that are not found anywhere else in the body suggests that there may be functionally distinct fibroblasts associated with the intralobular stroma. The heterogeneity of benign and malignant breast diseases also indicates that the different types of lesions may reflect origins from cells that have different degrees of commitment to the main epithelial lineages. Some benign and malignant epithelial lesions have characteristic stromal changes associated with them that point to important stromal epithelial interactions in the pathogenesis of these conditions. At the present time, however, there is very little information on the normal development of the human breast, the normal lineage patterns, and the cellular origins of benign and malignant diseases. The functional interactions between the stroma and the epithelium in the normal human breast are observational, and how perturbations of such interactions may contribute to the pathogenesis of breast diseases is even more obscure.

In this chapter our current knowledge is described as it relates to the normal cell types in the human breast and what is known about their possible contributions to diseases of the breast. Throughout the course of the text, the critical gaps in our knowledge are stressed, together with the some suggested approaches to their further investigation. Cross references are made to the mouse where appropriate.

Breast development

The human mammary gland begins to develop in utero but is still immature at birth and undergoes further growth and differentiation throughout the first 2 years of life [1]. During the latter part of this postnatal period, the breast undergoes involutional changes similar to that seen in the postmenopausal woman [1]. The next significant stage of development is during puberty, when

R. Dickson and M. Lippman (eds.) MAMMARY TUMOR CELL CYCLE, DIFFERENTIATION AND METASTASIS. 1996. Kluwer Academic Publishers. ISBN 0-7923-3905-3. All rights reserved.

the ducts elongate and branch, leading to rapid development of the mammary tree [2,3]. The factors that control this morphogenesis are unclear.

In contrast, considerable progress has been made in understanding the development of the rodent gland, in which the mesenchyme determines the fate of the mammary epithelium in the embryo [4] and is important for the sequential events in organogenesis [5,6]. Classical studies by Kratochwil [7], and later by Sakakura et al. [8], clearly demonstrated the continuing essential role of the stroma in determining glandular morphogenesis in rodents. In the human relatively little is known, but morphological studies would indicate that similar interactions between the epithelium and the stroma are important [9,10].

Breast development in utero

At 16–18 weeks of intrauterine life, the breast bud becomes recognizable as a down growth of the overlying periderm. At this stage a distinct condensation of mesenchymal cells is present around the bud. These stromal cells express high concentrations of the BCL-2 protein [10], suggesting that this protein, through inhibition of apoptosis, contributes to the expansion of this specialized mesenchyme that may be the precursor of the intralobular stroma of the infant and adult breast. At the same time, there are associated changes in the cytoskeleton of the epithelial bud as the basal (myoepithelial) layer becomes recognizable at the ultrastructural and immunohistochemical level.

Cytoskeletal antigens have proven to be very useful markers of breast epithelial differentiation. Muscle proteins were first demonstrated in myoepithelial cells in 1968 using an antibody prepared for an actomyosin preparation of colonic smooth muscle. Later an antibody specific to the alpha isoform of smooth muscle actin was developed [11] that shows a high degree of specificity for myoepithelial cells. This actin isoform also occurs in the myofibroblasts of benign and malignant breast disease, but these cells are distinguishable from the myoepithelial cells because they do not contain cytokeratins. Electrophoretic studies of the cytoskeleton of human mammary epithelial cells show that they contain cytokeratins, 5, 7, 8, 14, 15, 17, 18, and 19. Detailed studies with antibodies that are monospecific for the individual cytokeratins reveal that luminal cells contain the cytokeratins of simple epithelium (cytokeratins 8 and 18), whilst the myoepithelial cells contain cytokeratins typical of the undifferentiated layers of stratified epithelium (cytokeratins 5 and 14) [12,13].

The myoepithelial layer is first recognizable at the ultrastructural level at 20 weeks of gestation, although at this time the basal layer of the breast primordium does not stain for smooth muscle actin [14]. The cytokeratin profile indicates that when the bud forms, as a downgrowth from the periderm, the myoepithelial cytokeratins (5 and 14) are absent, but by birth the adult pattern is established (Figure 1). It must be presumed that the cells in the basal layer of the breast primordium, which are negative for cytokeratins 5 and 14, and

228

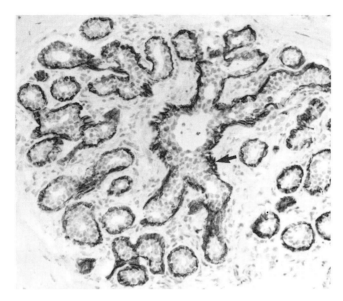

Figure 1. Human breast lobule in which the peptidase NEP is demonstrated on the myoepithelial cells (arrow). The enzyme is not present on either the myoepithelial cells nor the stromal cells. Magnification ×260.

strongly positive for BCL-2, are the precursors of the entire mammary tree, including any potential stem cells. It is also of interest that these cells are strongly positive for both transforming growth factor (TGF-α) and epidermal growth factor receptor (EGFR), suggesting an autocrine stimulation of proliferation in these cells [15].

It is essential that we know more about the structure and development of the human breast at this critical stage of development. Evidence is accumulating that factors affecting development in utero may play an important role in the predisposition of the breast to develop cancer in the adult [16,17]. In particular, it is important that we understand the role of hormones in the control of breast development, the cellular fate of the cells in the epithelial bud, and the role of the mesenchyme.

Development in the infant and at puberty

There is very little evidence for major differences in breast development in the sexes in humans up until 2 years after birth (the only period studied in any detail) [1]. While there are no data on the structural development of the breast during the third trimester of intrauterine life, studies of newborn infants of both sexes indicate that there are wide variations in the 'maturity' of the breast at birth [1], when the breast epithelium varies from well-defined lobular structures to simple tubes. However, milk proteins and secretory activity are present regardless of the degree of glandular differentiation. Studies of large numbers of cases from birth to two years have also provided some interesting data on the development of the stromal components of the breast and their relationship to the morphogenesis of the ductal and lobular framework. Development of the breast epithelium is seen in association with areas of embryonal adipose tissue [18]. Another interesting observation is that extramedullary hemopoiesis is concentrated on the developing intralobular stroma, supporting the view that it has specific functional attributes [19].

Developing stroma. There are two stromal components in the human adult breast: the intralobular stroma surrounding the terminal ductular units (TDLUs) and the interlobular stroma that lies between the epithelium of the ducts and the lobules. Within these two stromal areas, the fibroblasts can be clearly defined by the exclusive expression of a cell surface peptidase, dipeptidyl peptidase IV (DPPIV), on the interlobular fibroblasts [20]. It is also worth noting that another cell surface peptidase, neutral endopeptidase (NEP), is a specific marker of myoepithelial cells (Figure 1) [21,22]; aminopeptidase W is a marker of luminal cells; aminopeptidase A is a marker of blood vessels, with a differential high expression on intralobular fibroblasts compared with interlobular fibroblasts [Atherton and Gusterson, unpublished observation]; and aminopeptidase N (APN) is expressed on all fibroblasts [23]. The importance of these enzymes as functional markers will be discussed in more detail later.

After 1 month of age, DPPIV-positive stromal cells can be detected between the ducts, which are separated from the epithelium by a clearly defined population of DPPIV-negative cells. It is a reasonable working hypothesis that these cells may be the precursors of the future intralobular stroma. As the lobules develop, the presence of a DPPIV-negative stromal population is apparent [9]. Aminopeptidase N is present on all fibroblasts from the earliest samples studies with the typical adult pattern of expression, while NEP is expressed on all basal cells (myoepithelial cells) at all stages of development.

Role of cell surface peptidases. The presence of several cell surface peptidases within the developing breast raises interesting questions regarding the possible role of these enzymes in the local control of growth and differentiation [24]. These enzymes have specificities for certain amino acid residues, but little is known of their function either in vivo or in vitro. It is of interest that TGF-β_1 is a potential substrate for DPPIV, particularly as this peptide is synthesized by breast fibroblasts [25]. In relation to NEP, oxytocin is a good substrate for this enzyme, which may be relevant to the observation that oxytocin is trophic for myoepithelial cells [26]. Recent studies in the developing lung may have relevance to the role of NEP in the breast [27,28]. Bombesin and related peptides have a critical role in lung morphogenesis [28]. The effect of this peptide can be reversed by NEP, which hydrolyzes the peptide. There are, however, specific inhibitors available for these enzymes that will facilitate studies of the in vitro and in vivo function of these enzymes [29].

Epithelial differentiation. In parallel with the stromal changes, the epithelium organizes into the adult pattern of ducts and lobules, although after 2 months the breast begins to involute so that by 2 years of age, in both sexes, only rudimentary ducts remain. As the breast involutes, apocrine changes and cystic involution occur [1], similar to those observed in the postmenopausal breast.

In the first few months after birth in humans and in the first 10 weeks in mice, active growth and elongation can be observed. During this period, there are changes that give clues to the possible epithelial lineages. In rodents the major growth points are seen in structures called *terminal end buds*. Similar structures are not seen in humans, but we have identified solid areas at the ends of ducts and ductules that are probably, from a functional point of view, the human equivalents. These solid areas of epithelium have a high rate of proliferation, and the cytoskeletal profile suggests that they contain cells that are the precursors of both luminal and myoepithelial cells. In association with the migrating edge of these end buds, there is a loss of the characteristic adult pattern of integrin staining, together with reduced expression of tenascin [Anbazhagan and Gusterson, unpublished observation].

Very few studies have examined the human breast during the peripubertal period, but as in the period immediately after birth, end bud–like structures are present that contain cells with an undifferentiated phenotype [15]. The developing mammary tree has similar markers as the adult breast. There is an acute need to pool samples from many laboratories to study in detail the changes that take place in this stage of development that are likely to be critical in relation to the primary effect of carcinogens.

The infant breast goes through a series of changes that are initially modulated by maternal hormones. It is difficult to understand why the breast still undergoes active proliferation and growth after birth and the factors that are responsible for this. Also, the signals that are required for involution are obscure. It can be concluded that there is still much to learn about the early stages of human breast development.

Adult human breast

In the adult breast, the mammary tree is clearly defined into two major epithelial components: the ducts and the functional lobulo-alveolar units, which produce milk during lactation. The lobules have a clearly defined intralobular stroma with a specialized fibroblast population that is the precursor for the stromal component of both fibroadenomas and of phyllodes tumors [20]. In the newborn infant, although a morphological distinction can be drawn between the ducts and lobular structures, all luminal epithelial cells, including those of terminal end buds, have the capacity to produce milk proteins [Anbazhagan and Gusterson, unpublished observation]. Thus all cells can functionally respond to maternal hormones, in contrast to the adult tissue, in which the ducts have a limited response to both proliferative and secretory stimuli. It is also worth noting that in the adult breast, the individual lobules appear to behave as independent functional units, such that during pregnancy some lobules can be secretory whilst others are quiescent. This indicates that it may be necessary for the lobules to be primed for full secretory activity via the interactions of both local and systemic factors. This lobular heterogeneity is also seen in the proliferative activity of the normal gland in vivo [30] and the response of the gland to exogenous growth factors in vitro [31].

The luminal cells of the adult breast have been defined by a number of markers, but epithelial membrane antigen (EMA) [32] has proved to be one of the most useful. This antigen is a large glycoconjugate or mucin [38], which forms part of the apical membrane of all luminal cells and has thus found utility both as a marker to identify metastatic breast cancers [33,34] and as a tool to separate luminal cells for in vitro studies [35]. The other major markers of the resting virgin luminal cell population are keratins 8, 18, and 19 [36].

Because the majority of breast carcinomas appear to be of a luminal cell phenotype, the myoepithelial (basal) cell has been relatively neglected. This cell type was first identified over 150 years ago when work with Masson trichrome stains and phosphotungstic acid hematoxylin emphasized the similarity to muscle. Recently phalloidin, which specifically binds to F-actin, has been used as a marker, but the cytoskeletal antigens referred to earlier have proved preferable markers for in vivo and in vitro studies. As reviewed earlier [37,38], enzyme histochemistry clearly defined the myoepithelial cells as a functionally distinct population with high concentrations of sodium-potassium ATPase, adenyl cyclase, carbonic anhydrase, and alkaline phosphatase. As considered previously, neutral endopeptidase (endopeptidase 24.11) is a specific marker for all basal cells in the adult breast [39], and this may have significance for the growth control of the luminal and myoepithelial cell populations. The presence of this broad range of enzyme activities suggests that the myoepithelial cell may have a very specific role in the breast outside of the context of lactation.

A large number of external factors influence the development and secretory function of the breast. Static, in vivo observations of staining patterns, however, tell us little about the lineage pathways in the breast. Organ culture studies of dissected lobules indicate that in the normal breast the luminal cells and an electron microscopically defined population of basal clear cells [40] are the major proliferating cell types [41]. In vivo the myoepithelial cells have a relatively slow rate of turnover, which is of interest because they have the highest levels of EGFR [42]. All evidence, including the orientation of mitotic figures in vivo, would indicate that if there is a breast stem cell, then it is present in the luminal cell population. Electron microscopic studies predict that there is a population of the basal clear cells in the region of the human terminal ductal lobulo-alveolar unit that may be the precursor of the mature myoepithelial cell population [40]. Unfortunately there have been no ultra-structural studies of the cytokeratin profile of the basal clear cells. Analyses of benign and malignant tumors arising in the human breast indicate the potential complexity of the lineages. In vitro studies of clonal populations of isolated luminal and myoepithelial cells also throw some further light on this question.

In order to understand the potential role of cell surface peptidases in the breast, we have studied their distribution in the premenopausal and postmeno-pausal state. Aminopeptidase N was strongly expressed on the delimiting fibroblasts around lobules that are negative for DPPIV [Atherton and Gusterson, unpublished observation]. There was an apparent upregulation of NEP on myoepithelial cells in the postmenopausal breast. It is of interest that coincident with the upregulation of NEP, there is a striking reduction in immunoreactive laminin [Atherton and Gusterson, unpublished observation]. There is some evidence that these cell surface metalloproteases may be in-volved in interactions with the extracellular matrix [43].

As stated earlier, in the developing breast there are distinct populations of interlobular and intralobular fibroblasts that can be defined on the basis of DPPIV immunoreactivity [20]. In addition, fibroblasts in the interlobular stroma are strongly positive for fibronectin, whilst the intralobular fibroblasts are very low expressers of this extracellular matrix protein [Atherton and Gusterson, unpublished observation]. This is most clearly seen when direct comparisons are made with the staining pattern with antibodies to APN, where all fibroblasts are uniformly labeled [23]. The distribution of cell surface peptidases in the breast is summarized in Table 1.

Table 1. Cell surface peptidases present in the normal human breast

Enzyme	Location in the breast					
	Myo	Epi	Int F	Int E	Ina F	Ina E
APN	−	+/−	+	−	+	−
DPPIV	−	−	+	+/−	−	*
NEP	+	−	−	−	−	−
APW	+/−	+	−	−	−	−
PDPA	−	−	−	+	−	*
MDP	+	+	+	+	+	+
PABA	−	−	−	−	−	−

*indicates on occasional positive cell.
Myo = myoepithelial cells; Epi = epithelial cells; Int F = interlobular fibroblasts; Int E = endothelial cells of vessels in the interlobular stroma; Ina = intralobular; Ina F = intralobulr fibroblasts; Ina E = endothelial cells of vessels in the intralobular stroma; APN = aminopeptidase N; DPPIV = dipeptidyl peptidase IV; NEP = neutral endopeptidase; APW = aminopeptidase W; PDPA = peptidyl dipeptidase A; MDP = microsomal dipeptidase; PABA = para-amino benzoic acid hydrolase.

Benign and malignant tumors arising in the human breast

Although recent publications have attempted to justify the use of rodent models of breast cancer based on correlations between rat and human diseases of the breast, there are some striking differences in the two [43]. In rats, it is clear from morphological studies of the tumors that they have well-differentiated luminal and myoepithelial components, and some workers have interpreted in vitro studies of cell lines derived from these tumors as showing that there is a common stem cell for luminal cells and myoepithelial cells [44]. No such evidence exists for human malignant tumors, but in benign breast disease there is clear evidence that both myoepithelial and luminal cells form important components [45]. In fact, benign human lesions have much in common with the malignant rodent tumors, which rarely metastasize as primary induced tumors. The majority of human breast cancers have a luminal cell phenotype, although some rare tumors contain myosin (Figure 2) and smooth muscle actin–positive cells. A few tumors are positive for neutral endopeptidase [22], but in a recent study of 28 infiltrating breast carcinomas, only 2 were weakly positive in the epithelial component. It would thus appear that in human benign breast lesions either both luminal cells and basal cells proliferate to generate a mixed tumor or the lesions arise from an as yet undefined pluripotential cell. In the case of malignant epithelial lesions, it would appear that the carcinogenic damage occurs in a cell that is committed to the luminal cell phenotype.

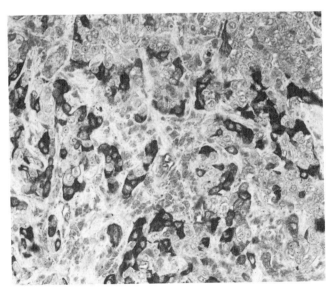

Figure 2. Immunohistochemical staining of an invasive breast carcinoma for myosin. Note the strong positive cells scattered throughout the tumor. Magnification ×400.

234

Another striking feature of breast carcinomas is the upregulation of NEP on a subpopulation of stromal cells in 50% of cases. DPPIV-positive cells are rare in the tumors, suggesting that the majority of the stroma may be derived for the intralobular fibroblasts [Atherton and Gusterson, unpublished observation]. It is very clear that fibroadenomas and phyllodes tumors are derived from this intralobular cell population. These two tumor types are also of interest because they are associated with a spectrum of chromosomal changes [46,47], that may in the future indicate the underlying molecular abnormalities responsible for them.

Cell culture of normal human breast cells

In order to understand the cell lineages within the human breast, it has been necessary to develop methods to isolate these cells and to culture them. This was originally carried out using cell sorting on the basis of the exclusive expression of EMA on luminal cells and NEP on myoepithelial (basal) cells [35], but recently immunomagnetic methods have proved more useful for large-scale purification [48]. In parallel, methods have been developed for the isolation of interlobular and intralobular fibroblasts [49] that will enable future investigation into the roles of these individual populations in epithelial/mesenchymal interactions. In vitro these subpopulations of fibroblasts maintain their phenotype for a limited number of passages and can synthesize a broad range of extracellular matrix molecules [50] and metalloproteases [51].

A striking observation is that cultured luminal and myoepithelial cells, when plated at clonal density, give rise to colonies that are all of one type [35] (Figure 3A and 3B). This is true for cells isolated from purified ducts and lobules [52] and from human milk [O'Hare, personal communication]. It is of interest that human milk contains cells with both basal and luminal characteristics, which is important when considering the phenotype of cells that have been immortalized from this source. In clonal studies of cells derived from ducts and lobules, it was shown that of 1932 studied with cytokeratin markers for basal (cytokeratin 14) and luminal cells (cytokeratins 18 and 19), only 3 contained cells that marked for both cell types and only two colonies had cells that simultaneously expressed cytokeratins 14 and 18.

The conclusions that can be drawn from these studies are that the incidence of potential stem cells is very low in the population that could be cultured under the conditions that were used. In addition, intermediate cells that have been recognized by others in studies of both rodent and human derived cell lines are not an easily recognizable population. The other striking feature of these in vitro studies is that the luminal cells appear to have a very limited in vitro capacity to proliferate, whilst the myoepithelial cells grow very rapidly [35,52]. This is particularly important when considering the studies currently underway throughout the world using primary breast cultures. Perhaps this observation may explain why it is so difficult to establish new cell lines from

235

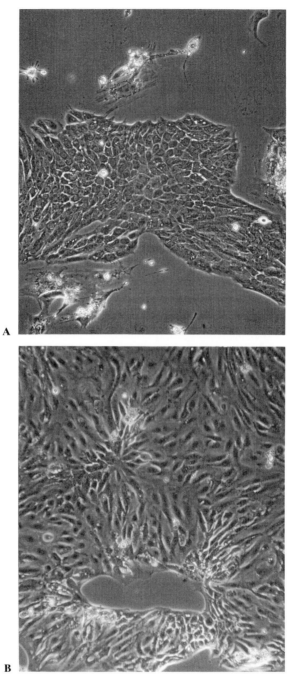

Figure 3. Phase contrast photographs of colonies of myoepithelial cells (**A**) and luminal cells (**B**). Note the cuboidal uniform nature of the myoepithelial cells. Magnification ×125.

236

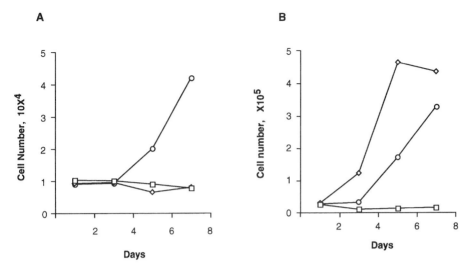

Figure 4. Growth of human mammary epithelial cells. **A**: Human mammary luminal cells grown in RPMI 1640 supplemented with 10% FCS, I (5 μg/ml), CT (100 ng/ml), and H (5 μg/ml), □; RPMI 1640 supplemented with 1% FCS, I, CT, and H, ◇; and Ham's F12 supplemented with 10% FCS, I, CT, H, and EGF, ○. **B**: Human mammary myoepithelial cells grown in RPMI 1640 supplemented with 10% FCS, I, CT, and H, □; RPMI 1640 supplemented with 1% FCS, I, CT, and H, ◇; and CDM5 media, ○.

primary breast cancers because they have the phenotype of these poorly growing luminal cells and perhaps the same in vitro growth requirements that have yet to be optimized. These results were carried out using a medium that contained 10% fetal calf serum (FCS) and the additives hydrocortisone (H), insulin (I), and cholera toxin (CT). More recently, using separated cells it has been possible to produce culture conditions that favour the growth of luminal cells or myoepithelial cells.

In studying the growth characteristics of human mammary epithelial cells, we have examined the growth response of human luminal cells and myoepithelial cells in a variety of media. We have found that luminal cells do not grow in media containing H, I, and CT in the presence of 1% or 10% FCS (Figure 4A). However, addition of EGF at 10 ng/ml to the above-mentioned media, in the presence of 10% FCS, improves the growth rate of luminal cells significantly (Figure 4A). We have recently demonstrated that hepatocyte growth factor/scatter factor (HG/SF) is a potent cytokine to human mammary luminal cells, improving the growth rate of these cells by nine fold when the cells are grown in media containing the above-mentioned cocktail of growth factors and 1% FCS [53]. In parallel with these observations, we have demonstrated the cell types that produce HGF/SF in the breast and that express *met*, its receptor (Table 2).

Human myoepithelial cells also demonstrate poor growth when grown in media supplemented with 10% FCS (Figure 4B). Interestingly, the growth of

Table 2. Expression of HGF/SF and its cellular receptor, c-met, in human mammary cell populations

	HGF/SF	c-met
Fibroblast	+	−
Luminal	−	+
Myoepithelial	−	+

(−) indicates absence of expression.

Table 3. Biological effects of HGF/SF on human mammary cell populations

	Mitogenic	Motogenic	Morphogenic
Fibroblast	−	−	−
Luminal	+	+	−
Myoepithelial	−	+	+

(−) indicates lack of response.

these cells is dramatically improved when the serum content of the medium is dropped to 1%. Myoepithelial cell growth is also improved when the cells are grown in CDM5, a serum-free media [54]. However, myoepithelial cells appear to grow more efficiently in the former media (Figure 4B). Our previous data have demonstrated that HGF/SF has no mitogenic effect on myoepithelial cells [53]. It has also been noted that HGF/SF induces tubular structures in a pure myoepithelial cell population when grown in collagen gels and increases myoepithelial cell motility (Table 3).

An interesting observation has been made that may have relevance to the interaction between the luminal cells and the myoepithelial cells. When mixed cultures of the two populations are put in suspension culture, they rapidly re-aggregate with homotyic preferential binding that is probably the result of cell type preferential cadherin expression. After 6 days the cells produce organized structures with the development of lumina. At this stage tritiated thymidine pulse labeling demonstrates high labeling of luminal cells and low labeling of myoepithelial cells. Thus, when these two cell types are combined in a three-dimensional structure, they proliferate as they would in vivo, suggesting that there are important interactions between these two cell populations that are dependent on their juxtaposition. The importance of the spatial arrangement is supported by the fact that conditioned medium from the pure populations of cells does not have a significant effect on the proliferation of the other cell type in monolayer culture.

These data, when taken together, raise the interesting possibility that the myoepithelial cells may form the 'ductal skeleton' down which the luminal cells migrate during development and that in the adult they act as a biological niche, being interdependent. This would suggest that studies of luminal/myoepithelial cell interactions may lead to a better understanding of the biology of the breast, and if they are interdependent it may lead to new findings in the evolution of early breast cancer.

Cell lines derived from cell-separated or primary mixed cultures of human breast cells, using retroviral infection with a temperature-sensitive SV40 T-antigen construct [55,56] or with a wild-type large T antigen gene [57], retain many of the features of the primary cells. The cell lines produced using the temperature-sensitive system were derived using cells that were sorted on the basis of their cell surface characteristics prior to immortalization. Thus only cells that expressed the luminal marker EMA were infected. The cell line referred to as 4a is positive for keratins 18 and 7, and predominantly negative for keratin 14, thus retaining the markers of a typical luminal cell. Another clone, designated 2a, expresses keratins 14, 18, and 7 [Kamalati, unpublished observation], similar in phenotype to the rare clones that were seen in the primary cultures referred to earlier. The 4a cells have similar growth characteristics as the normal luminal cells [Kamalati, unpublished observation].

Summary and future perspectives

It is obvious that our current knowledge about the normal lineage pathways in the human breast and their relationship to the phenotype of benign and malignant breast disease is largely unknown. It is also becoming increasingly apparent that there are specific functional subpopulations of stromal cells in the breast that contribute to morphogenesis, differentiation, and growth control of the epithelial cells. In addition, it would appear that the myoepithelial and luminal cells form a functional niche. It is essential that future studies are directed to understanding normal breast development and the dissection of the complex cellular interactions that take place during this process. Also, it is important that more effort be placed on understanding the contribution made by the myoepithelial cells to the normal homeostasis of the luminal cell population.

Acknowledgments

The work of the authors referred to in this chapter was supported by the Cancer Research Campaign. We thank Dr. O'Hare for the use of Figure 3.

References

1. Anbazhagan R, Bartek J, Monaghan P, Gusterson BA (1991) Growth and development of the human infant breast. *Am J Anat* 192:407–417.

2. Monghan P, Perusinghe NP, Cowen P, Gusterson BA (1990) Peripubertal human breast development. *Anat Record* 226:501–508.
3. Russo J, Gusterson B, Rogers AE, Russo IH, Wellings SR, van Zwieten J (1990) Biology of disease: Comparative study of human and rat mammary tumorigenesis. *Lab Invest* 62:244–278.
4. Propper AY (1968) Relations epidermo-meseodermiques dans la differentiation de l'ebauche mammaire d'embryon de lapin. *Ann Embryol Morphogen* 2:151–160.
5. Sakakura T (1987) Mammary embryogenesis. In *The Mammary Gland*. MC Neville, CW Daniels (eds). New York: Plenum Press, pp 37–65.
6. Sakakura T (1991) New aspects of stroma-parenchyma relations in mammary gland differentiation. *Int Rev Cytol* 125:165–202.
7. Kratchowil K (1969) Organ specificity in mesenchymal induction demonstrated in the embryonic development of the mammary gland of the mouse. *Dev Biol* 20:46–71.
8. Sakakura T, Nishizuka Y, Dawe CJ (1976) Mesenchyme-dependent morphogenesis and epithelium-specific cytodifferentiation in mouse mammary gland. *Science* 194:1439–1441.
9. Atherton AJ, Anbazhagan R, Monaghan P, Bartek J, Gusterson BA (1994) Immunolocalisation of cell surface peptidases in the developing human breast. *Differentiation* 56:101–106.
10. Nathan B, Anbazhagan R, Clarkson P, Bartkova J, Gusterson BA (1994) Expression of bcl-2 in the developing human foetal and infant breast. *Histopathology* 24:73–76.
11. Skalli O, Ropraz P, Trzeciak A, Benzonana G, Gillessen D, Gabbiani G (1986) A new monoclonal antibody against alpha-smooth muscle actin: A new probe for smooth muscle differentiation. *J Cell Biol* 103:2787–2796.
12. Nagle RB, Bocker W, Davis JR, Heid HW, Kanfman M, Lucas DO, Jarasch ED (1986) Characterization of breast carcinomas by two monoclonal antibodies distinguishing myoepithelial from luminal epithelial cells. *J Histochem Cytochem* 34:869–881.
13. Dairkee SH, Blayney C, Smith HS, Hackett AJ (1985) Monoclonal antibody that defines human myoepithelium. *Proc Natl Acad Sci USA* 82:7409–7413.
14. Anbazhagan R, Bartkova J, Nathan B, Lane EB, Gusterson BA (1995) The development of epithelial phenotypes in the human fetal and infant breast. *Lab Invest*, submitted.
15. Anbazhagan R, Colletta A, Bartek J, Nathan B, Clarkson P, Sakakura T, Gusterson BA (1995) Immunolocalisation of growth factors and extracellular matrix proteins in the developing human breast. *Lab Invest*, submitted.
16. Anbazhagan R, Nathan B, Gusterson BA (1992) Prenatal influences and breast cancer [letter], *Lancet* 340:1477–1478.
17. Anbazhagan R, Gusterson BA (1993) Prenatal factors may influence predispostion to breast cancer. *Eur J Cancer* 30A:1–3.
18. Anbazhagan R, Gusterson BA (1995) Ultrastructure and immunohistochemistry of the embryonic type of fat identified in the human infant breast. *Anat Rec* 241:129–135.
19. Anbazhagan R, Bartkova J, Nathan B, Gusterson BA (1992) Extramedullary haematopoiesis in the human infant breast. *Breast* 1:182–186.
20. Atherton AJ, Monaghan P, Warburton MJ, Robertson D, Kenny AJ, Gusterson BA (1992) Dipeptidyl peptidase IV expression identified a function subpopulation of breast fibroblasts. *Int J Cancer* 50:15–19.
21. Gusterson B, Laurence D, Anbazhagan R, Atherton A, O'Hare M (1994) The breast myoepithelial cell and its significance in physiology and pathology. *Curr Diagn Pathol* 1:203–211.
22. Gusterson BA, Monaghan P, Mahendran R, Ellis J, O'Hare MJ (1986) Identification of myoepithelial cells in human and rat breasts by anti-common acute lymphoblastic leukaemia antigen antibody A12. *J Natl Cancer Inst* 77:343–349.
23. Atherton AJ, Monaghan P, Warburton MJ, Gusterson BA (1992) Immunocytochemical localization of the ectoenzyme aminopeptidase N in the human breast. *J Histochem Cytochem* 40:705–710.

24. Kenny AJ, O'Hare MJ, Gusterson BA (1989) Cell surface peptidases as modulators of growth and differentiation. *Lancet* 2(8666):785–787.
25. Butta A, MacLennan K, Flanders KC, Sacks NPM, Smith I, McKinna A, Dowsett M, Wakefield LM, Sporn MB, Baum M, Colletta AA (1992) Induction of transforming growth factor β₁ in human breast cancer in vivo following tamoxifen treatment. *Cancer Res* 52:4261–4264.
26. Sapino A, Macri L, Tonda L, Bussolati G (1993) Oxytocin enhances myoepithelial cell differentiation and proliferation in the mouse mammary gland. *Endocrinology* 133:838–842.
27. Sunday ME, Hua J, Torday J, Reyes B, Shipp MA (1992) CD10/neural endopeptidase 24.11 in developing human fetal lung: Patterns of expression and modulation of peptide-mediated proliferation. *J Clin Invest* 90:2517–2525.
28. King KA, Drazen JM, Hua J, Graham S, Torday JS, Shipp MA (1993) CD10/neural endopeptidase 24.11 regulates murine fetal lung growth and maturation. *J Clin Invest* 91:1969–1973.
29. Kenny AJ, Stephenson SL, Turner AJ (1987) Cell surface peptidases. In *Mammalian Ectoenzymes*. AJ Kenny, AJ Turner (eds). Amsterdam: Elsevier, pp 169–210.
30. Anderson TJ, Battersby S (1989) The involvement of oestrogen in the development and function of the normal breast: Histological evidence. *Proc R Soc Edinburgh* 95B:23–32.
31. Perusinghe N, Monaghan P, O'Hare MJ, Ashley S, Gusterson BA (1992) Effects of growth factors on proliferation of basal and luminal cells in human breast epithelial explants in serum free culture. *In Vitro Cell Dev Biol* 28A:90–96.
32. Imrie SF, Sloane JP, Ormerod MG, Styles J, Dean CJ (1990) Detailed investigation of the diagnostic value in tumour histopathology of ICR-2, a new monoclonal antibody to epithelial membrane antigen. *Histopathology* 16:573–581.
33. Mansi JL, Berger U, McDonnell T, et al. (1989) The fate of bone marrow micrometastases in patients with primary breast cancer. *J Clin Oncol* 7:445–449.
34. Mansi JL, Easton D, Berger U, et al. (1991) Bone marrow metastases in primary breast cancer: Prognostic significance after 6 years follow up. *Eur J Cancer* 27:1552–1555.
35. O'Hare MJ, Ormerod MG, Monaghan P, Lane EB, Gusterson BA (1991) Characterization in vitro of luminal and myoepithelial cells isolated from the human mammary gland by cell sorting. *Differentiation* 46:209–221.
36. Taylor-Papadimitriou J, Lane EB (1987) In *The Mammary Gland: Development Regulation and Function*. MC Neville, CS Daniel (eds). New York: Plenum Press, pp 181–195.
37. Gusterson B, Laurence D, Anbazhagan R, Atherton A, O'Hare M (1994) The breast myoepithelial cell and its significance in physiology and pathology. *Curr Diagno Patholo* 1:203–211.
38. Laurence DJ, Monaghan P, Gusterson BA (1991) The development of the normal human breast. In *Oxford Reviews of Reproductive Biology*, Vol 13. SR Milligan (ed). Oxford University Press, pp 149–174.
39. Metzgar RS, Borowitz MJ, Jones NH, Dowell BL (1981) Distribution of common acute lymphoblastic leukemia antigen in nonhematopoietic tissues. *J Exp Med* 54:1249–1254.
40. Smith CA, Monaghan P, Neville AM. Basal clear cells of the normal human breast. *Virchows Arch A Pathol Anat* 402:319–329.
41. Joshi K, Smith JA, Perusinghe N, Monaghan P. Cell proliferation in the human mammary epithelium. Differential contribution by epithelial and myoepithelial cells. *Am J Pathol* 124:199–206.
42. O'Hare MJ, Ormerod MG, Monaghan P, Cooper CS, Gusterson BA (1989) Differentiation and growth in the human breast parenchyma. *Biochem Soc Trans* 17:589–591.
43. Piazza FA, Callanan HM, Mowery J, Hixson DC (1989) Evidence for a role of dipeptidyl peptidase IV in fibronectin-mediated interaction of hepatocytes with extracellular matrix. *Biochem J* 262:327–334.
44. Rudland PS, Gusterson BA, Hughes CM, Ormerod EJ, Warburton MJ (1982) Two forms of tumors in nude mice generated by a neoplastic rat mammary stem cell line. *Cancer Res* 42:5196–5208.

45. Gusterson BA, Warburton MJ, Mitchell D, Ellison M, Neville AM, Rudland PS (1982) Distribution of myoepithelial cells and basement membrane proteins in the normal breast and in benign and malignant breast disease. *Cancer Res* 42:4763–4770.

46. Birdsall SH, MacLennan K, Gusterson BA (1992) t(6;12)(q23;q13) and t(10;16)(q22;p11) in phyllodes tumour of the breast. *Cancer Genet Cytogenet* 60:74–77.

47. Birdsall S, Summersgill BM, Egan M, Fentiman IS, Gusterson BA, Shipley JM (1995) Additional copies of 1q in sequential samples from phyllodes tumor of the breast. *Cancer Genet Cytogenet*, in press.

48. Clarke C, Titley J, Davies S, O'Hare MJ (1994) An immunomagnetic separation method using superparamagnetic (MACS) beads for large-scale purification of human mammary luminal and myoepithelial cells. *Epith Cell Biol* 3:38–46.

49. Atherton AJ, O'Hare MJ, Buluwela L, Titley J, Monaghan P, Paterson HF, Warburton MJ, Gusterson BA (1994) Ectoenzyme regulation by phenotypically distinct fibroblast sub-populations isolated from the human mammary gland. *J Cell Sci* 107:2931–2939.

50. Atherton AJ, Warburton MJ, O'Hare MJ, Monaghan P, Schuppan D, Gusterson BA (1995) Human breast intralobular and interlobular fibroblasts synthesise stromal and basement membrane extracellular matrix proteins in vitro. *Cell Biol*, submitted.

51. Atherton AJ (1992) *Cell Surface Peptidases and Human Breast*, PhD thesis. University of London.

52. O'Hare MJ, Davies SC (1995) Clonal analysis in vivo of human mammary ducts and lobules: Evidence for the extreme rarity of 'intermediate' or multipotental 'stem' cell types in the non-lactating adult human breast. *J Cell Sci*, submitted.

53. Niranjan B, Yant J, Perusinghe N, Atherton A, Phippard D, Dale T, Gusterson B, Buluwela L, Kamalati T (1995) HGF/SF: A potent cytokine for mammary growth, morphogenesis and development. *Development* 121:2897–2908.

54. Pandis N, Heim S, Bardi G, Limon J, Mandahl N, Mitelman F (1992) Improved technique for short-term and cytogenetic analysis of human breast cancer. *Genes Chromosom Cancer* 5:14–20.

55. Jat PS, Sharp PA (1989) Cell lines established by a temperature sensitive Simian virus 40 large T antigen are growth restricted at the nonpermissive temperature. *Mol Cell Biol* 9:1672–1681.

56. Stamps AC, Davies SC, Burman J, O'Hare MJ (1994) Analysis of proviral integration in human mammary epithelial cell lines immortalised using retroviral infection with a temperature-sensitive SV40 T-antigen construct. *Int J Cancer* 57:865–874

57. Bartek J, Bartkova J, Kyprianou N, Lalani E-N, Staskova Z, Shearer M, Chang S, Taylor-Papadimitriou J (1991). Efficient immortalization of luminal epithelial cells from human mammary gland by introduction of simian virus 40 large tumor antigen with a recombinant retrovirus. *Proc Natl Acad Sci USA* 88:3520–3524.

242

13. Models of progression spanning preneoplasia and metastasis: The human MCF10AneoT.TGn series and a panel of mouse mammary tumor subpopulations

Fred R. Miller

Introduction

Progression in human breast cancer is often depicted as the loss of estogen receptor expression as cancers shift from hormone-responsive/dependent to hormone-independent phenotypes. The narrowness of this definition stems from the obvious importance of this stage in progression in terms of prognosis and hormonal therapeutic approaches. Other investigators tend to view progression as initiation and promotion events, loss of contact inhibition and/or anchorage dependence in vitro, changes in growth factor requirements in vitro, acquirement of invasive capabilities, acquirement of metastatic phenotype, or transition from hyperplastic preneoplastic to neoplastic lesions. Of course, progression is a continuum of all these events from the first alteration of a normal epithelial cell, to the preneoplastic cell, to the ultimately lethal metastatic cell. We have developed two models that span the full spectrum of progression, one a human preneoplastic model and one a panel of closely related sister subpopulations derived from a single mouse mammary tumor that metastasize by different routes or fail to metastasize at different sequential steps of metastasis.

MCF10AneoT.TGn: Human preneoplastic model

Preneoplasia and progression in mammary biology have been defined almost solely by studies of mouse hyperplastic alveolar nodules (HANs). These lesions are stromal dependent and must be transplanted into mammary fat pads [1]. Medina has described a number of HAN lines that progress to carcinoma at different rates and at a different final incidence [2]. Morphologically, the HAN lesions in normal mice are similar to normal mammary tissue in pregnant mice but are hormone independent. Thus, carcinomas arise sporadically from a homogeneous field of morphologically normal, albeit preneoplastic, alveolar-ductule tissue. Although these mouse mammary models have been the basis for much information regarding the basic biology of mammary cancer, a number of differences in the histology and biology of mouse and

R. Dickson and M. Lippman (eds.) MAMMARY TUMOR CELL CYCLE, DIFFERENTIATION AND METASTASIS. 1996. Kluwer Academic Publishers. ISBN 0-7923-3905-3. All rights reserved.

human mammary lesions exist. Indeed, whether or not a preneoplastic lesion exists in the development of human breast cancer is still a point of contention.

In the human breast, a spectrum of microscopic changes has been termed *proliferative breast disease* (PBD). Although hyperplastic lesions are observed in human breast, their role in disease progression is not understood. The progression of histopathological features of PBD has been correlated with increased risk for the development of invasive carcinoma. One in eight women will be diagnosed with breast cancer within their lifetimes. The risk is increased by a factor of four for those women in which atypical hyperplastic lesions are recovered from breast biopsy specimens [3] and 10-fold for those women in which carcinoma in situ is recovered [4]. At present, we are unable to determine which lesions with increased relative risk are the most likely to progress to carcinoma. Indeed, it is not clear whether these lesions are precursor lesions or simply markers for breasts with high risk. At the time of diagnosis, not all breast carcinomas are associated with lesions typical of proliferative breast disease, suggesting that such stages are not prerequisite. Such lesions, of course, may have been present earlier in the development of the disease. Follow-up studies of women with proliferative breast disease, such as atypical hyperplasia and lobular carcinoma in situ, have found that carcinoma is as likely to occur in the contralateral breast as it is to occur in the breast from which the high risk lesion was recovered [3]. On the other hand, ductal carcinoma in situ seems more likely to be a direct precursor because invasive cancers frequently occur at the site of biopsy [5].

Recently we have established a new and unique model of early human breast cancer progression. This model, which is called *MCF10AneoT*, is a line of preneoplastic human breast epithelial cells that are able to grow in immunedeficient mice, where they undergo a sequence of progressive histological changes, culminating in cases of frank neoplasia in about 25% of the animals [6]. Thus, MCF10AneoT is a transplantable, xenograft model of human PBD with proven neoplastic potential. Immortalized human breast epithelial MCF-10A cells [7] are unable to survive long term in immune-deficient nude/beige mice. Transfection of these cells with the mutated human T24 HRAS gene, however, resulted in cells with a transformed phenotype [8]. These cells, MCF10AneoT cells, have lost anchorage dependence in vitro [8] and form palpable lesions in nude/beige mice that persist indefinitely [6]. This model should not be confused with the related MCF10F series of carcinogen-treated and ras-transfected lines described by Russo et al. [9–12], which do not produce xenograft lesions with characteristics of human breast and are tumorigenic rather than preneoplastic.

Lesions

Unlike the murine HAN models in which homogeneous lobuloalveolar lesions consistently give rise to rapidly growing adenocarcinomas within a few

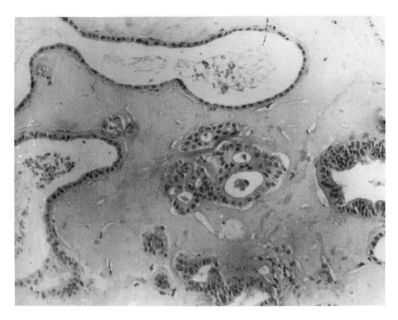

Figure 1. Benign day 223 MCF10AneoT lesion with heterogeneous display of simple dilated ducts, multilayering, and early bridging.

months, breasts of women with high risk PBD are heterogeneous and early breast cancer grows slowly. MCF10AneoT cells implanted into immune-deficient mice generate interlesional and intralesional heterogeneity, and give rise to a variety of slowly growing ductal carcinomas.

The initial histology of MCF10AneoT xenografts is benign. Simple ducts and cysts with simple epithelium coexist with ducts displaying tufting or papillary infolding (Figure 1). These structures may persist in the mice for over a year, with no indication of progression. However, on five occasions thus far (three in one experiment and two in a repeat experiment), carcinomas have arisen from persistent lesions in nude/beige mice. Unlike the preneoplastic mouse HAN models, which progress to histologically similar adeno-carcinomas, the five human carcinomas were of different histologic types (Figure 2). The first MCF10AneoT tumor was removed after 50 days in the animal and was an undifferentiated carcinoma with a few normal ducts included in the mass of the tumor; the second MCF10AneoT tumor, removed at day 100, was a squamous cell carcinoma; and the other three were invasive adenocarcinomas removed after 142, 367, and 393 days.

Cells derived from the carcinoma removed from a mouse 100 days after injecting MCF10AneoT cells, named *MCF10AneoT.TG1*, represent a more advanced preneoplastic state than MCF10AneoT. Although the final inci-dence of carcinomas formed from TG1 lesions is no higher than for MCF10AneoT lesions, TG1 cells initially form simple ducts, which then

245

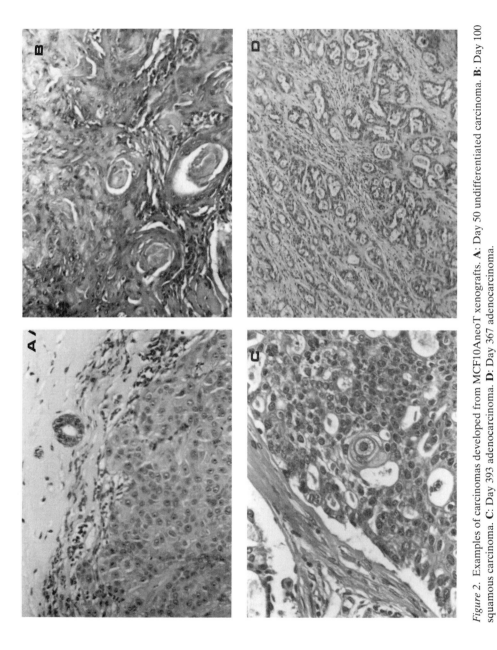

Figure 2. Examples of carcinomas developed from MCF10AneoT xenografts. **A**: Day 50 undifferentiated carcinoma. **B**: Day 100 squamous carcinoma. **C**: Day 393 adenocarcinoma. **D**: Day 367 adenocarcinoma.

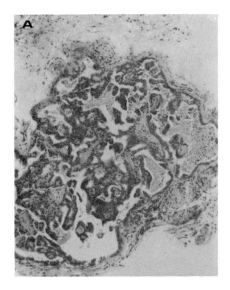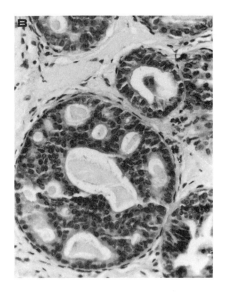

Figure 3. Examples of atypical hyperplastic lesions in xenografts. **A**: papillary pattern in day 128 MCF10AneoT.TG4JJ lesion. **B**: Cribriform pattern in day 190 MCF10AneoT.TG3B lesion.

progress to form atypical hyperplastic lesions within 5 months after implanting cells in Matrigel into nude/beige mice (Figure 3).

MCF10AneoT.TG2B cells derived from a TG1 lesion form atypical hyperplastic lesions in 3 months from which carcinomas develop at an incidence of 25–30%. MCF10AneoT.TG3B cells derived from a TG2B lesion give rise to focal cribriform ducts within a month, which progress to ductal carcinoma in situ at high frequency and ultimately to invasive carcinomas. The hyperplastic lesions formed are themselves quite heterogeneous. Both papillary and cribriform atypical hyperplastic lesions develop in xenografts of TG3B cells (Figure 4).

Other variant lines have been derived from advanced lesions, but upon xenografting simple ducts first form, followed by hyperplastic patterns and carcinomas at sporadic intervals. Thus, whether cells are derived from hyperplastic lesions or carcinomas, the progressive sequence is recapitulated upon transplanting into immunedeficient mice (Figure 5). This suggests that the preneoplastic stem cell has a growth advantage in vitro over malignant cells, and we turned to media that had been reported to selectively grow human breast cancer cells [13,14] and media we normally use for MCF10A minus all growth factors but insulin. All recovered variants were preneoplastic regardless of the media used for primary culture. We are now attempting to clone directly from the advanced lesions so that cancer cells may be immediately separated from the apparently dominant preneoplastic stem cell.

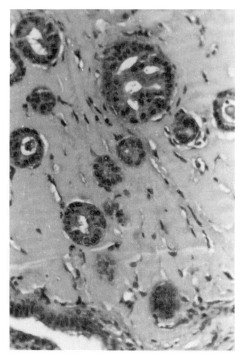

Figure 4. Day 29 MCF10AneoT.TG3B lesion depicting early microfocus of cribriforming.

Estrogen receptor

MCF10AneoT cells, but not normal parental MCF10A cells, express estrogen receptor (Figure 6) [15], which is functional, as determined by response to estradiol in transient CAT transfection assays [Shekhar, unpublished]. Unlike the estrogen receptor–positive MCF7 carcinoma cell line, MCF10AneoT cells are not hormone dependent in situ. It is not clear at this time if the model is hormone responsive. Perhaps estrogen supplementation of the mice to approximate human estrogen levels will alter progression to high risk hyperplastic lesions and/or from atypical hyperplasia to invasive carcinoma, but preliminary data comparing a low estrogen environment (female mice) with no estrogen (male mice) suggest that progression to hyperplasia may be independent of estrogen but progression from hyperplasia to carcinoma may be hormonally influenced.

MCF10AneoT lesions persist in xenografts in male mice as well as in female mice, and progress to carcinoma in approximately the same fraction (Figure 7). The transplant derived lines (MCF10AneoT.TGn) form long-term hyperplastic lesions that are not apparent in MCF10AneoT lesions. Figure 8 depicts grades of xenograft MCF10AneoT.TG1 lesions in nude/beige mice. Progression to hyperplasia was not different in males and females, but

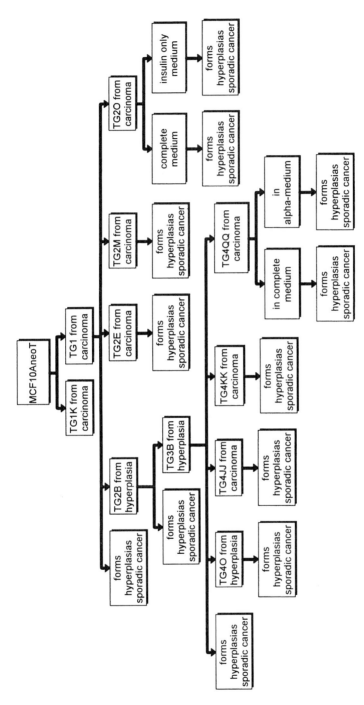

Figure 5. Evolutionary tree of lesions and variants from alternating in vivo and in vitro transplant generations.

249

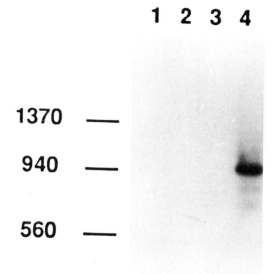

1 2 3 4

1370 —

940 —

560 —

Figure 6. Expression of estrogen receptor (ER) by MCF10AneoT but not by MCF10A. Two micrograms of total RNA extracted from MCF10A-derived lines were reverse transcribed, and the oligonucleotides flanking the human ER cDNA sequence from base 276 to 1241 corresponding to exons 1 through 6 were used for amplification by PCR. The primers were sense 5'-GCCCGCGGCCACGGACCATGACCAT-3', and antisense 5'-TGACCATCTGGTCGGCCGTC-3'. The identity of the 966 bp ER cDNA fragment amplified from MCF10AneoT was confirmed by Southern blot hybridization analysis with a full-length human ER cDNA probe. Lane 1, MCF10A; lane 2, MCF10Aneo (control transfectant); lane 3, MCF10AneoN (transfected with normal Hras and neo); lane 4, MCF10AneoT.

progression to carcinoma occurred in four females, with no carcinomas detected in the males. Numbers are insufficient to draw any conclusions from these experiments, and, as previously mentioned, the low level of estrogen found in mice relative to humans may be insufficient to produce an effect. However, the presence of a functional estrogen receptor clearly offers the opportunity to assess the efficacy of antiestrogens in preventing the progression of high risk breast lesions as well as the effect of estrogenic environmental xenobiotics.

Stem cell characteristics

The cells of MCF10AneoT and TG*n* appear to be atypical breast epithelial stem cells, capable of indefinite proliferation with a wide range of differentiation potential from normal to atypical. Ductule structures that develop in xenografts consist of myoepithelial cells, as defined by shape, location, and staining with smooth muscle actin [Miller and Tait, unpublished data], as well as luminal epithelium. With prolonged xenograft growth, the ductule epithelia

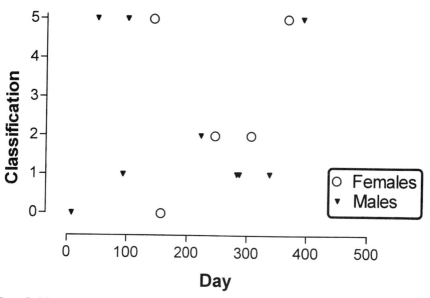

Figure 7. Distribution frequency of different grades of progression for MCF10AneoT in male and female mice.

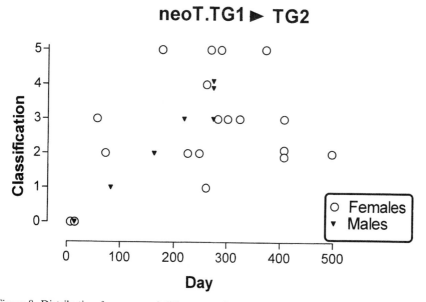

Figure 8. Distribution frequency of different grades of progression for MCF10AneoT.TG1 in male and female mice.

sporadically evolve to a fully malignant histological appearance, strengthening the perception of progression from hyperplasia, to atypical hyperplasia, to invasive breast carcinoma. In the period immediately after transplant, the generative cells give rise to 'normal' proliferating ductal epithelium, which, possibly because of genetic instability, is permissive of evolution to atypical and malignant epithelium. We expect that the MCF10AneoT and TG*n* model will facilitate construction of a genetic model comparable with the colorectal paradigm of Fearon and Vogelstein [16].

Genetic progression

The p53 gene is not mutated in the MCF10AneoT.TGn system [17]. An unusual feature of the MCF10AneoT model is the presence of a mutated H-*ras* gene. Although overexpression of *ras* is common in human breast cancer, *ras* mutations are not [18]. However, the importance of the mutated *ras* in the model is unclear. We have found that mutated *ras* is not sufficient to produce the persistent, premalignant phenotype in MCF10A cells; a number of clones of MCF10AneoT derived by random chimney cloning techniques do not form persistent lesions in immune-deficient mice [Miller, unpublished]. It is interesting that transfection of a mutated *ras* gene into rat fibroblasts did not transform the cells but the frequency of spontaneous transformation was increased [19]. Perhaps comparison of TG*n* cells with the nonpersistent neoT clones will elucidate genetic defects directly responsible for the preneoplastic phenotype.

We have found that the karyotype of MCF10AneoT variants is not changing with progressive transplant generations but remains 47xx, t(3;9), t(9;9;5), 6p+, t(3;17), 9+, as described for MCF10AneoT and MCF10AneoT.TG1 [6,8]. In addition to monitoring karyotypes, genes that are differentially expressed in the progressive variants of MCF10AneoT.TG are being identified. We now have cDNA libraries for MCF10AneoT, neoT.TG1, and neoT.TG3B, from which differentially expressed genes are to be cloned. Genes are first identified by RT-PCR and differential display methods. Because of the common genetic background of the progressive variants, only a few differences in gene expression are evident (Figure 9) [K. Reddy, unpublished]. Cloned genes will be sequenced and then inserted into MCF10 variants with retrovirus methodology to determine if the gene has a role in progression. A gene that becomes expressed with progression will be transduced into an earlier stage cell (e.g., MCF10A or MCF10AneoT), and the stage of progression is determined by xenografting. A gene that is lost with progression will be transduced into the more advanced variant and xenografted to determine if the transduced cell is less advanced. A second approach that we have initiated is to introduce known genes implicated in breast cancer progression, such as *erb*B2 and *bcl*2, into MCF10AneoT cells, or to knockout suppressor genes such as p53, to determine if a more malignant variant is produced.

252

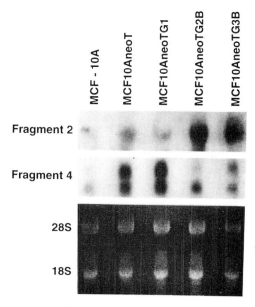

Figure 9. Differential gene expression by parental MCF10A, and preneoplastic MCF10AneoT, MCF10AneoT.TG2B, and MCF10AneoT.TG3B. Fifteen micrograms of total RNA was isolated frome each cell line, subjected to electrophoresis on a 1% formaldehyde-agarose gel, and transferred to a nylon membrane. Reamplified differentially expressed cDNA fragments were used as probes, individually, for Northern hybridization. Fragment 2, a 4.0 kb transcript, increases with progression and fragment 4, a 2.4 kb transcript, decreases with progression, as evidenced by the kinetics of formation of high risk lesions in immune-deficient mice. DNA sequencing followed by computer search against Genbank and EMBL DNA databases indicate that these two clones are novel.

Invasion

The use of a silver stain to detect loss of basement membrane demonstrates the heterogeneous disruption of that important structure during progression to carcinoma (Figure 10). This method provides a means of classifying areas within heterogeneous progressive lesions for colocalization studies utilizing FISH and immunohistochemical methods for microdissection for RT-PCR analyses [20]. We have not yet unequivocally observed metastasis in the MCF10AneoT.TGn model. One MCF10AneoT.TG3B xenografted mouse did have a draining lymph node in which the breast epithelial cells were growing, but the cytologic features of those cells within the lymph node did not appear to be malignant (Figure 11). Future xenograft generations may provide metastatic variants, but we continue to rely upon a mouse model for analysis of the sequential steps of metastasis.

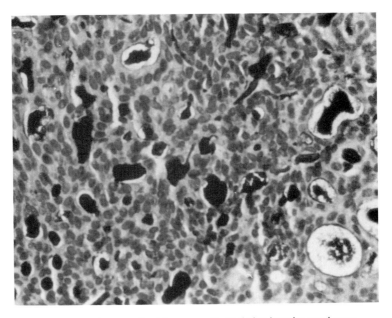

Figure 10. Basement membrane stained in xenografts depicting invasive carcinoma.

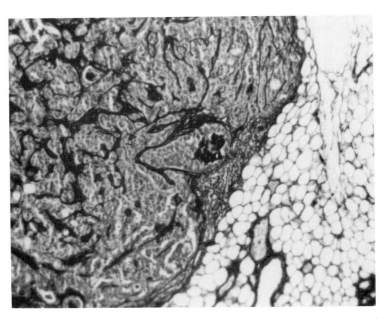

Figure 11. Lymph node in normal mammary gland of nude/beige mouse bearing the MCF10AneoT.TG3B subcutaneous xenograft.

Mouse model for metastatic analysis

Metastasis is a multistep event that is thought to require the acquisition of a number of functions by a cancer cell for completion of the process. Cells must be able to invade and intravasate, survive transport trauma, arrest in distant organs, extravasate, and grow at the distant site. It is generally thought that a number of genetic changes must occur for a cell to become fully metastatic.

Genes involved in metastasis have generally been evaluated on the basis of their effects on the *end point* of the metastatic process by determining the number of metastases and/or the sizes of metastatic nodules at death. Investigators often suggest the step in metastasis at which they believe a 'metastasis gene' acts based on in vitro assays. Increased levels of proteases suggest increased invasiveness; motility factors might increase the ability of cells to intravasate/extravasate; lectins might increase cell aggregation, leading to enhanced arrest or survival during transport; matrix component receptors might enhance arrest; expression of various growth factor receptors might change the ability of cells to grow in different organ environments; and antigenic changes might enable tumor cells to escape from host-resistance mechanisms at various stages of the metastatic cascade.

At this time the data regarding the roles of various genes in specific steps in the metastatic cascade are conflicting and confusing. This confusion is likely due to unappreciated genetic background differences among the different cell models studied. If a cell is unable to intravasate, introduction of a gene that increases survival during transport will have little effect on metastasis of that cell from a primary tumor, although it may increase lung colonization potential following intravenous injection. That same gene placed into a cell unable to survive in the lung parenchyma would likely have no effect on either spontaneous or experimental metastatic potential. Likewise, a gene that enables a cell to grow in the lung would not be expected to alter the metastatic potential of cells unable to reach the lung and extravasate into the parenchyma; an additional complication could be the requirement of a second genetic event, that is, growth in the lung might be promoted only in cells coexpressing complementary genes. Thus, transfection into two different cancer cells, each able to accomplish all initial steps of the cascade but only one coexpressing the essential complementary gene, could lead to different conclusions regarding the role of that gene in metastasis. Furthermore, interactions among tumor cells may result in the metastasis of a subpopulation unable, by itself, to complete all steps of the cascade. Nonmetastatic cells have occasionally been shown to metastasize in the presence of metastatic cells [21,22]. It is conceivable that two nonmetastatic cell subpopulations could be complimentary such that both metastasize from mixtures. Thus, cells isolated from metastases may not be independently metastatic and genetic analysis could be misleading.

A panel of closely related mammary tumor subpopulations with different metastatic potential and defined deficiencies would provide the means to

255

discern which steps in the metastatic cascade are actually altered by transfection of (1) 'metastasis genes' into tumor cell subpopulations that are deficient at different steps in the cascade or (2) 'antimetastasis genes' into tumor cell subpopulations that are metastatic.

The model

Subpopulations of a single spontaneously arising BALB/cfC3H mouse mammary tumor differ in a number of phenotypes, including metastatic potential [23,24]. We selected for drug-resistant variants of both metastatic and nonmetastatic subpopulations and developed a sensitive method to study metastasis by determining the number of clonogenic tumor cells present in various tissues of mice injected with mammary tumor cells [25–29].

The sequential spread of metastatic tumor cells has been difficult to measure quantitatively. By prelabeling cells with ^{125}IUdR [30,31] or fluorescein isothiocyanate [32], it has been possible to determine the initial arrest and short-term redistribution of tumor cells in organs following intravenous injection of the tumor cells. Cytochemical methods have been described for the detection of melanoma cells [33] and tumor cells transfected with the bacterial β-galactosidase gene [34] in spontaneous metastasis. These methods detect the presence of tumor cells but do not provide information regarding the growth potential of those cells detected. Our method defines the kinetics of metastasis by the recovery of clonogenic tumor cells from host tissues at multiple time points following implantation of tumor cells into the mammary gland, tail vein, or spleen.

The recovery of colony forming tumor cells after plating enzymatically dispersed tissues in selective media provides a highly sensitive method to detect occult metastases in a quantitative manner. Growth rates, that is, doubling time of the clonogenic tumor population, in these organs can be determined. The method has successfully delineated the time course of the sequential spread of tumors growing in the mammary gland to the regional lymph node or blood, then to the lung, and finally to the liver. In addition, cell kill can be closely monitored after intravenous injection by comparing the radiolabeled tumor cell present with their clonogenic capacity. Because human cancers are poorly immunogenic, we have selected poorly immunogenic variants for these studies. Of the five subpopulations constituting the model, *only* line 4TO7 is sufficiently immunogenic to cause a delay in growth of a challenge inoculum following surgical removal of an initial primary growth. Utilizing the relative antigenic strength (RAS) criteria proposed by Reif [35], in which highly immunogenic tumors that grow only in immune-deficient animals are assigned a value of 9.9, line 4TO7 has a RAS score of less than 1; 67, 168 and 66cl4 score less than 0.1; and 4T1 scores less than 0.01. Thus, with the exception of 4TO7, these lines are all weakly antigenic to totally non-antigenic.

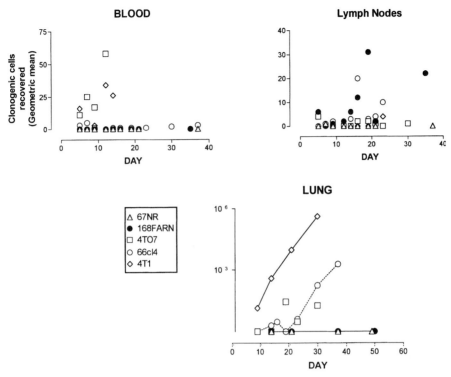

Figure 12. Recovery of clonogenic tumor cells from mice bearing primary tumors in mammary fat pads. At the indicated intervals, groups of mice were bled and then sacrificed, and lymph nodes and lungs were removed. Single cell suspensions were prepared and plated in selective media, and were cultured for 10–14 days before fixing, staining, and counting colonies developed from clonogenic drug-resistant tumor cells.

Spontaneous metastasis

The model includes variants that do not spontaneously metastasize for different reasons (i.e., fail at different steps in the cascade) and metastatic variants that spread by different routes (lymphatic vs. hematogenous) and to different organs (Figure 12). The 67NR cells form large tumors but do not invade and intravasate; clonogenic cells cannot be recovered from blood or draining regional lymph nodes of 67NR-bearing syngeneic BALB/c mice. Like 67NR, 168FARN does not form visible metastases and clonogenic cells are never recovered from lungs or blood. However, in contrast to 67NR, clonogenic 168FARN cells are frequently recovered from the regional draining lymph node.

A third subpopulation that does not metastasize spontaneously to the lung, line 4TO7, does reach the lung, principally by a hematogenous route, but does not form visible nodules. If primary 4TO7 tumors are removed, clonogenic

257

cells quickly disappear from the lung, indicating that cells detected are recent arrivals from the primary. When seeding is terminated by removal of the primary cancer, clonogenic cells already present are eliminated within a day. Thus, these three nonmetastatic subpopulations fail at different steps in metastasis. Two metastatic variants, 66cl4 and 4T1 cells, form visible nodules in the lung. Figure 12 depicts that the preferential route of metastasis by 66cl4 is via the lymph node, while 4T1 typically metastasizes via the blood. Clonogenic cells can eventually (after first appearing in lung digests) be recovered from livers of mice bearing 4T1 and 66cl4 [29], demonstrating the metastatic cascade sequence from the lung generalizing site to the secondary liver site [36].

Experimental metastasis

To analyze differences among subpopulations at steps of metastasis following transport, the arrest event is synchronized by injecting cells intravenously. All of these subpopulations will colonize the lung and liver if sufficient numbers of cells are injected into a tail vein or spleen, respectively. Once arrested, the fate of the malignant cell remains bleak, as indicated by the rapid loss, or clearance, of [125]IUdR-labeled cells within a few hours after arrest. The typical clearance of [125]IUdR-labeled neoplastic cells follows a biphasic curve, with an initial rapid exponential decline for a few hours, followed by a second more gradual exponential declining phase. Liotta and DeLisi [37] proposed a mathematical model to interpret the biphasic clearance kinetics of tumor cells. This model assumes that the number of cells ([125]IUdR label) remaining in the lung after initial arrest is a function of three first-order rate constants: (1) death or dislodgement of intravascular cells, (2) extravasation, and (3) death of cells after extravasation. Because not all arrested neoplastic cells extravasate simultaneously, there is no time that divides postarrest phenomena exclusively into intravascular and extravascular states, but the time of transition between the two logarithmic clearance curves is thought to reflect the time during which extravasation is largely accomplished.

We have validated the Liotta and DeLisi model to define the time of extravasation with our mouse mammary tumor line 4TO7 [28]. Clearance of [125]IUdR-labeled 4TO7 cells suggested that a major portion of the tumor cells extravasate between 8 and 12 hours postarrest. Histological examination of serial sections of lungs removed 6, 24, and 168 hours after injection of tumor cells intravenously generally supported the Liotta and DeLisi model. For each timed sacrifice group, a number of sections of lungs were scanned so that at least 50 tumor cell loci could be observed. The percent of loci in which the cell(s) were located extravascularly increased from 9% at 6 hours to 62% at 24 hours and 86% at 168 hours. The number of loci in which the cell(s) appeared to be extravasating decreased from 36% at 6 hours to 13% at 24 hours and to 7% at 168 hours. Further supporting evidence for the Liotta and DeLisi model includes the finding that benign mouse cells continue to be cleared at a rapid

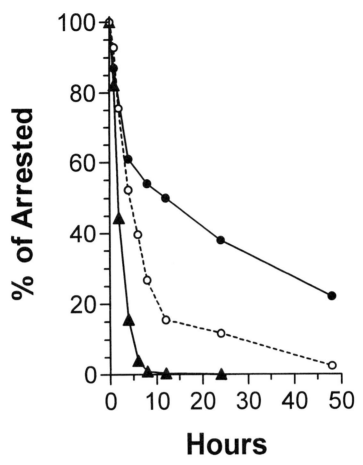

Figure 13. Clearance of [125]IUdR-labeled tumor cells in the lungs after intravenous injection. Mice injected intravenously at time 0 with prelabeled cells were killed at the indicated times, and the total label in lungs was determined. Each point represents the median of three to four mice. ●, 4TO7; ○, 66cl4; ▲, 168FARN.

rate with no deflection, presumably because the benign cells are unable to extravasate [38].

Our criteria for determining the postarrest survival of intravascular cells is the change in clonogenic potential of cells recovered during the first decay component of the radiolabel clearance curve. We have constructed these curves for six of our sublines (Figure 13 depicts the clearance kinetics of three of them) and, although the slopes of both decay curves vary between lines, all begin to deflect from the initial logarithmic curve at 8–12 hours and enter the second decay curve by 24 hours postarrest. The rapid clearance of the nonmetastatic 168FARN cells indicates a profound deficiency in this line at this step in metastasis. However, 4TO7 cells are more resistant than the metastatic 66cl4 cells.

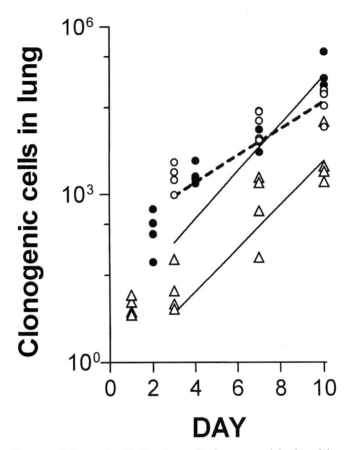

Figure 14. Recovery of clonogenic cells from lungs after intravenous injection of three mammary tumor subpopulations at time 0. Mice were killed at the indicated days postinjection, lungs were removed and dissociated, and cell suspensions were plated in the appropriate selective media to determine the total number of clonogenic cells that could be recovered. Regression analysis was used to determine the clonogenic population doubling time. ●, 4TO7 (doubling time = 20 hours); ○, 66cl4 (DT = 36 hours); △, 4T1 (DT = 24 hours).

Figure 14 depicts the growth of three subpopulations in the lung after extravasation. The nonmetastatic subpopulation 4TO7 grows as rapidly as the highly metastatic line 4T1 and more rapidly than the metastatic 66cl4. Line 4TO7 is, in fact, as efficient as 4T1 and grows rapidly in the lung following intravenous injection [27]. Taken together, our analysis of spontaneous and experimental metastasis of 4TO7 indicates that there is no deficiency at the tumor cell level because cells reach the lung in the spontaneous model and extravasate and grow rapidly in the experimental metastasis model. The failure of 4TO7 to metastasize from fat pads is likely due to the development of host immunity during the initial local growth. Thus, by the time cells reach the lung, sufficient immunity has developed to prevent metastatic growth. We

260

have used this model to demonstrate that specific concomitant immunity is able to slow the growth of extravasated 4TO7 cells without altering arrest or initial killing of arrested cells [28]. On the other hand, tumor cells arrested in the lung are initially quite susceptible to NK cells [28].

Initial genetic analysis of this panel indicates that, with increasing malignancy, *ras* expression increases (*ras* is normal, not mutated) and p53 expression decreases, but nm 23 expression is not lost [39–42]. This battery of subpopulations with defined deficiencies should allow the validation of many characteristics implicated in metastasis and the determination of the steps at which positive and negative 'metastasis genes' act.

Summary

The two models described offer an opportunity to determine relevant genetic alterations during progression from preneoplasia to metastatic disease while avoiding genetic noise among individuals (patients and mice) and independent cancers. The human preneoplastic MCF10AneoT.TGn model allows the identification of altered genes as progression occurs sporadically and affords a method of directly testing the gene affect by introduction into non-expressing variants. The model also will allow testing suspected oncogenes and suppressor genes identified in other cancers. However, its value in the latter studies may be limited because genes may not alter MCF10AneoT phenotypes due to other unidentifiable differences between the MCF10 model and the cancer in which the gene was identified.

The mouse model allows similar cause and effect studies to determine at which specific steps metastasis genes might be important. The model also provides an opportunity to determine which host response elements are important deterrents at each step in metastasis and in different organ sites. Together, these models have the potential to elucidate a genetic sequence of progression in breast comparable with that being constructed for colon carcinoma [16].

Acknowledgments

This work supported by CA28366, CA61230, core grant CA22453, and the Elsa U. Pardee Foundation. I thank my collaborators, Dr. P.V.M. Shekhar for Figure 6, depicting expression of estrogen receptor by MCF10AneoT cells, and Dr. K. Reddy for Figure 9, depicting differential gene expression among MCF10A and neoT variants.

References

1. DeOme KB, Faulkin LJ Jr, Bern HA, Blair PB (1959) Development of mammary tumors from hyperplastic alveolar nodules transplanted into gland-free mammary fatpads of female C3H mice. *Cancer Res* 19:515–520.

2. Medina D (1973) Preneoplastic lesions in mouse mammary tumorigenesis. *Methods Cancer Res* 7:3–53.
3. Dupont WD, Page DL (1985) Risk factors for breast cancer in women with proliferative breast disease. *N Eng J Med* 312:146–151.
4. Page DL, Kidd TE Jr, Dupont WD, Simpson JF, Rogers LW (1991) Lobular neoplasia of the breast: Higher risk for subsequent invasive cancer predicted by more extensive disease. *Hum Pathol* 22:1232–1239.
5. Page DL, Dupont WD, Rogers LW (1982) Intraductal carcinoma of the breast: Follow-up after biopsy only. *Cancer* 49:751–758.
6. Miller FR, Soule HD, Tait L, Pauley RJ, Wolman SR, Dawson PJ, Heppner GH (1993) Xenograft model of progressive human proliferative breast disease. *J Natl Cancer Inst* 85:1725–1732.
7. Soule HD, Maloney TM, Wolman SR, Peterson WD Jr, Brenz R, McGrath CM, Russo J, Pauley RJ, Jones RF, Brooks SC (1990) Isolation and characterization of a spontaneously immortalized human breast epithelial cell line, MCF-10. *Cancer Res* 50:6075–6086.
8. Basolo F, Elliott J, Tait L, Chen XQ, Maloney T, Russo IH, Pauley R, Momiki S, Caamano J, Klein-Szanto AJP, Koszalka M, Russo J (1991) Transformation of human breast epithelial cells by c-Ha-ras oncogene. *Mol Carcinogene* 4:25–35.
9. Calaf G, Russo J (1993) Transformation of human breast epithelial cells by chemical carcinogens. *Carcinogenesis* 14:483–492.
10. Pauley R, Henry N, Reddy K, Calaf G, Russo J, Soule H, Wei W (1995) Differential gene expression during breast cancer development. *Proc Am Assoc Cancer Res* 36:622.
11. Barnabas NJ, Alvarado ME, Adesina K, Moraes RCB, Estrada S, Calaf G, Russo J (1995) Role of p53 and mdm2 in the transformation of human breast epithelial cell line MCF 10F treated with chemical carcinogens. *Proc Am Assoc Cancer Res* 36:624.
12. Barnabas NJ, Calaf G, Brilliant M, Russo J (1995) Detection of genomic DNA changes using endogenous human LTR-like elements in human breast epithelial cells transformed by chemical carcinogens. *Proc Am Assoc Cancer Res* 36:624.
13. Taylor-Papadimitriou J, Stampfer M, Bartek J, Lewis A, Boshell M, Lane EB, Leigh IM (1989) Keratin expression in human mammary epithelial cells cultured from normal and malignant tissue: Relation to in vivo phenotypes and influence of medium. *J Cell Sci* 94:403–413.
14. Band V, Sager R (1989) Distinctive traits of normal and tumor-derived human mammary epithelial cells expressed in a medium that supports long-term growth of both cell types. *Proc Natl Acad Sci USA* 86:1249–1253.
15. Shekhar PVM, Chen M-L, Werdell J, Heppner GH, Miller FR, Christman JK (1995) Activation of the endogenous estrogen receptor (ER) gene in MCF10AneoT cells, a potential factor in neoplastic progression of MCF10AneoT xenografts. *Proc Am Assoc Cancer Res* 36:1523.
16. Fearon ER, Vogelstein B (1990) A genetic marker for colorectal tumorigenesis. *Cell* 61:759–767.
17. Shekhar PVM, Welte RA, Sarkar F, Jones R, Pauley RJ, Christman JK (1995) Role of p53 in neoplastic progression of MCF10AneoT in a xenograft model for human breast cancer. *Proc Am Assoc Cancer Res* 36:573.
18. Bos JL (1988) The ras gene family and human carcinogenesis. *Mutat Res* 195:255–268.
19. Finney RE, Bishop JM (1993) Predisposition to neoplastic transformation caused by gene replacement of H-ras1. *Science* 260:1524–1527.
20. Tait L, Dawson PJ, Heppner GH, Miller FR (1995) Identification of microinvasiveness during progression in preneoplastic human breast xenograft model. *Proc Am Assoc Cancer Res* 36:77.
21. Miller FR (1983) Tumor subpopulation interactions in metastasis. *Invasion Metastasis* 3:234–242.
22. Waghorne C, Thomas M, Lagarde A, Kerbel RS, Breitman ML (1988) Genetic evidence for progressive selection and overgrowth of primary tumors by metastatic cell subpopulations. *Cancer Res* 48:6109–6114.

23. Dexter DL, Kowalski HM, Blazar BA, Fligiel Z, Vogel R, Heppner GH (1978) Heterogeneiety of tumor cells from a single mouse mammary tumor. *Cancer Res* 38:3174–3178.
24. Miller FR, Miller BE, Heppner GH (1983) Characterization of metastatic heterogeneity among tumor subpopulations of a single mouse mammary tumor: heterogeneity in phenotypic stability. *Invasion Metastasis* 3:22–31.
25. Miller FR, McInerney DJ, Rogers C, Aitken DR, Wei WZ (1986) Use of drug resistance markers to recover clonogenic tumor cells from occult metastases in host tissue. *Invasion Metastasis* 6:197–208.
26. Miller BE, Aslakson CJ, Miller FR (1990) Efficient recovery of clonogenic stem cells from solid tumors and occult metastatic deposits. *Invasion Metastasis* 10:101–112.
27. Aslakson CJ, Rak JW, Miller BE, Miller FR (1991) Differential influence of organ site on three subpopulations of a single mouse mammary tumot at two distinct steps of metastasis. *Int J Cancer* 47:466–472.
28. Aslakson CJ, McEachern D, Conaway DH, Miller FR (1991) Inhibition of lung colonization at two different steps steps in the metastatic sequence. *Clin Exp Metastasis* 9:139–150.
29. Aslakson CJ, Miller FR (1992) Selective events in the metastatic process defined by analysis of the sequential dissemination of subpopulations of a mouse mammary tumor. *Cancer Res* 52:1399–1405.
30. Fidler IJ (1970) Quantitative analysis of distribution and fate of tumor emboli labeled with [125]IUdR. *J Natl Cancer Inst* 45:773–782.
31. Proctor JW, Auclair BG, Rudenstam CM (1976) The distribution and fate of blood-borne [125]IUdR-labelled tumor cells in immune syngeneic rats. *Int J Cancer* 18:255–262.
32. Potter KM, Juacaba DF, Price JE, Tarin D (1983) Observations on organ distribution of fluorescein-labelled tumour cells released intravascularly. *Invasion Metastasis* 3:221–233.
33. Hisano G, Hanna N (1982) A cytochemical procedure for the in vivo identification of melanoma micrometastases. *Invasion Metastasis* 2:299–312.
34. Lin W, Pretlow TP, Pretlow TG II, Culp LA (1990) Development of micrometastases: Earliest events detected with bacterial lacZ gene-tagged tumor cells. *J Nat Cancer Inst* 82:1497–1503.
35. Reif AE (1985) Some key problems for success of classical immunotherapy. In *Immunity to Cancer*. AE Reif, MS Mitchell (eds). New York: Academic Press, pp 3–16.
36. Viadana E, Bross IDJ, Pickren W (1978) Cascade spread of blood-borne metastases in solid and non-solid cancers of humans. In *Pulmonary Metastasis*. L Weiss, HA Gilbert (eds). Boston: GK Hall, pp 143–167.
37. Liotta LA, DeLisi C (1977) Method for quantitating tumor cell removal and tumor cell-invasive capacity in experimental metastases. *Cancer Res* 37:4003–4008.
38. Liotta LA, Vembu D, Saini RK, Boone C (1978) In vivo monitoring of the death rate of artificial murine pulmonary micrometastases. *Cancer Res* 38:1231–1236.
39. Shekhar PVM, Aslakson CJ, Miller FR (1993) Molecular events in metastatic progression. *Semin Cancer Biol* 4:193–204.
40. Shekhar PVM, Miller FR. (1995) Correlation of differences in modulation of ras expression with metastatic competence of mouse mammary tumor subpopulations. *Invasion Metastasis* 14:27–37.
41. Shekhar PVM, Werdell J, Christman JK, Miller FR. (1995) Heterogeneity in p53 mutations in mouse mammary tumor subpopulations with different metastatic potential from the orthotopic site. *Anticancer Res* 15:815–820.
42. Shekhar PVM, Lane MA, Werdell J, Christman JK, Miller FR. Correlation of alterations in structure and expression of c-Ha-ras, p-53, and nm23 with metastatic potential of mouse mammary tumor subpopulations from the orthotopic site. *Cancer Molecular Biology*, in press.

14. Angiogenesis in breast cancer

Noel Weidner

Introduction

This chapter reviews the basic concepts of tumor angiogenesis as well as the role of measuring intratumoral microvessel density as an independent prognostic indicator for predicting tumor growth and metastasis, not only in breast carcinoma, but also in other solid tumors. For a tumor to grow, the tumor cells must proliferate and the benign host tissues must form around the tumor cells. Moreover, to metastasize a variety of critically important interactions must occur between tumor cells and the non-neoplastic vasculature, immune system, and connective tissues. Tumor angiogenesis refers to the growth of new vessels toward and within the tumor. This tumor neovascularization is caused by factors released by the tumor cells and/or associated inflammatory cells. Initially, many investigators thought that tumor hyperemia resulted from expansion of pre-existing vessels [1,2], but during the last two to three decades it has become clear that tumor growth is dependent upon the growth of new vessels [3].

Angiogenesis is necessary for tumor growth

Folkman in 1971 proposed that tumor growth is angiogenesis dependent (i.e., once tumor take has occurred, every further increase in tumor cell population must be preceded by an increase in new capillaries, which converge upon the tumor) [4] (Figure 1). In addition, he suggested that tumor cells and blood vessels composed an integrated ecosystem, that endothelial cells could be 'switched' from a resting state to rapidly growing state by a diffusible signal from tumor cells or associated inflammatory cells, and that 'anti-angiogenesis' could become an effective anticancer therapy.

Both indirect (Table 1) and direct (Table 2) evidence exists showing that tumor growth is angiogenesis dependent. The indirect evidence is that tumors grown in vitro or in avascular rabbit cornea attain a limited size at which passive diffusion no longer provides adequate nutrients or allows waste products to exit into the adjacent medium [5–7]. At equilibrium the diameter of the

R. Dickson and M. Lippman (eds.) MAMMARY TUMOR CELL CYCLE, DIFFERENTIATION AND METASTASIS. 1996. Kluwer Academic Publishers. ISBN 0-7923-3905-3. All rights reserved.

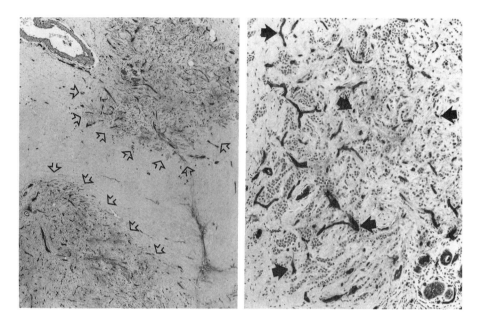

Figure 1. Invasive breast carcinoma with microvessels highlighted after immunostaining for factor VIII–related antigen. **Left**: Two foci of invasive carcinoma are shown (i.e., outlined by open arrows). The section is immunohistochemically stained with antibody to factor VIII–related antigen. Microvessels are represented by dark clusters, which stand -out from invasive carcinoma cells and connective tissue. Note the greater microvessel density within the invasive carcinoma foci relative to the adjacent benign fibrous stroma. [Diaminobenzidine (DAB)-immunoperoxidase stain with anti–factor VIII–related antigen plus hematoxylin counterstain, original magnification [OM] ×5]. **Right**: Invasive carcinoma shown at left with relatively high angiogenesis (i.e., metastasizing tumor). Solids arrows indicate five representative microvessels (DAB-immunoperoxidase stain with anti–factor VIII–related antigen plus hematoxylin counterstain, OM ×50). (Reprinted with permission from W.B. Saunders Co, Philadelphia, PA; from Weidner N, *Semin Diag Pathol* 1993;302–313.

avascular spheroids is up to 4 mm in vitro [8] and up to 2 mm in vivo [9,10]. Continued growth and metastases do not occur unless the spheroids become vascularized [3,9–18]. Moreover, human retinoblastoma metastatic to the anterior chamber vitreous are avascular and growth restricted, although they remain viable; and metastatic ovarian carcinoma to the peritoneal surface grow as tiny avascular seeds, unless neovascularization occurs [3]. Additional indirect evidence is that in breast carcinoma intratumoral endothelial cells proliferate 45 times faster than endothelial cells in adjacent benign stroma [19], and the rate of tumor progression is associated with increased intratumoral microvessel density, a morphologic measure of tumor angiogenesis [20,21].

The direct evidence supporting that tumor growth is angiogenesis dependent is that various methods of inhibiting angiogenesis, which are not cytostatic to tumor cells in vitro, inhibit tumor growth in vivo [22-31]. First, a

Table 1. Indirect evidence that tumor growth is angiogenesis dependent

Tumors grown in vitro or in avascular cornea attain a limited size (1–4 mm diameter) (Folkman [3]).

Retinoblastoma metastatic to the avascular vitreous of the anterior chamber are growth restricted (Folkman [3]).

Metastatic ovarian carcinoma to the peritoneal surface grow as tiny, granular nodules until neovascularization occurs (Folkman [3]).

Rate of tumor growth, spread, and/or patient survival are associated with increasing intratumoral microvessel density (Weidner [20]; Weidner [21]).

In breast carcinoma intratumoral endothelial cells proliferate 45 times faster than endothelial cells in adjacent benign stroma (Vartanian [19]).

Table 2. Direct evidence that tumor growth is angiogenesis dependent

Angiogenesis inhibitors (AGM-1470 or TNP-470), which are not cytostatic to tumor cells in vitro, inhibit tumor growth in vivo (Ingber [25]; Toi [100]; Yamaoka [109]).

Implanted colon carcinoma in mice respond to bFGF by increase in tumor size and density of tumor blood vessels, but neutralizing antisera against the bFGF retards tumor growth. Tumor cells lack receptor for bFGF (Gross [26]).

A specific antibody to bFGF, which is not cytostatic to tumor cells in vitro, causes ~70% inhibition of growth of a mouse tumor, which relies on bFGF as its main mediator of angiogenesis (Hori [28]).

A specific antibody to VEGF, which is not cytostatic to tumor cells in vitro, causes 'significant or dramatic' inhibition of 3 different implanted human tumors (in nude mice), which rely on VEGF as their main mediator of angiogenesis (Kim [27]).

Tumor angiogenesis and growth are inhibited when a retrovirus vector encoding a dominant nonfunctional mutant of the VEGF receptor (flk-1) is used to infect tumor endothelial cells in vivo (Millauer [29]).

Induction of angiogenesis promotes vascular cell entry into the cell cycle and expression of alpha$_v$beta$_3$ integrin. Antagonists of this integrin cause regression of transplanted human tumors (Brooks [30]).

synthetic analogue of fumagillin, a naturally secreted antibiotic of *Aspergillus fumigatus fresenius*, inhibits endothelial proliferation in vitro and tumor-induced angiogenesis in vivo [25], and this 'angioinhibin' (as AGM-1470 or TNP-470) will suppress tumor growth with few side effects. Indeed, this drug and other angiogenesis inhibitors [i.e., bryostatin, thalidomide, platelet factor 4, alpha interferon, carboxyaminotriazole, metalloproteinase inhibitor (BB94), and D-gluco-D-galactan sulfate (DS4152)], are now in various phases of clinical trials as chemotherapeutic agents for a variety of malignant solid tumors, leukemias, and infantile hemangiomas [23,24].

Second, a human colon carcinoma cell line implanted in mice was shown to respond to infusions of basic fibroblast growth factor (bFGF) by a twofold increase in tumor size and a concomitant increase in the density and branching of tumor blood vessels [26]. Cells of this line lacked receptors for bFGF, a strong angiogenic factor, and were unresponsive to bFGF in vitro. Yet, bFGF receptors were shown to be present on endothelial cells, and when the tumor-bearing mice also received neutralizing antisera against the bFGF, tumor growth was significantly retarded. Clearly, this experiment showed that changes in vessel growth rate can directly determine tumor growth rate. Likewise, Hori et al. [28] have shown that a specific antibody to bFGF, which is not cytostatic to tumor cells in vitro, causes ~70% inhibition of growth of a mouse tumor, which relies on bFGF as its main mediator of angiogenesis.

Third, Kim et al. [27] have shown that inhibition of vascular endothelial growth factor (VEGF)–induced angiogenesis suppresses tumor growth in vivo. These investigators injected human rhabdomyosarcoma, glioblastoma multiforme, or leiomyosarcoma cell lines into nude mice, and they found that treatment of these mice with a monoclonal antibody specific for VEGF inhibited the growth of the tumors but had no effect on the growth rate of the tumor cells in vitro. The density of tumor vessels was decreased in the antibody-treated mice, and the researchers concluded that inhibition of the action of an angiogenic factor (VEGF) spontaneously produced by tumor cells may suppress tumor growth in vivo. Likewise, Millauer et al. [29] have shown that tumor growth is markedly suppressed by introduction of defective VEGF receptors into tumor endothelial cells. The latter investigators showed that tumor angiogenesis and tumor growth are inhibited when a retrovirus vector encoding a dominant-negative, nonfunctional mutant of the VEGF receptor (flk-1) is used to infect tumor endothelial cells in vivo.

Recently, Brooks et al. [30] have reported that a single intravascular injection of antagonists of alpha^{v}beta^3 integrin (i.e., either a cyclic peptide antagonist or monoclonal antibody) disrupts ongoing angiogenesis on the chick chorioallantoic membrane. This leads to the rapid regression of histologically distinct human tumors transplanted onto the chorioallantoic membrane. Also, induction of angiogenesis by a tumor or cytokine promotes vascular cell entry into the cell cycle and expression of alpha^{v}beta^3 integrin. After angiogenesis is initiated, antagonists of this integrin induce apoptosis (programmed cell death) of the proliferative angiogenic vascular cells, leaving pre-existing quiescent blood vessels unaffected. These findings are consistent with a role for integrin in a signaling event critical to the survival, and ultimately differentiation, of vascular cells undergoing angiogenesis in vivo.

Obviously, tumor neovascularization allows growth because the new vessels allow exchange of nutrients, oxygen, and waste products by a crowded cell population for which simple diffusion of these substances across its outer surfaces is no longer adequate. It is also becoming apparent that, in addition to this 'perfusion effect,' endothelial cells may release important 'paracrine' growth factors for tumor cells (e.g., bFGF, insulin growth factor-2, platelet derived growth factor, and colony stimulating factors) [31–34]. Also, the invasive chemotactic behavior of endothelial cells at the tips of growing capillaries is facilitated by their secretion of collagenases, urokinases, and plasminogen activator [35,36]. These degradative enzymes likely facilitate the spread of tumor cells into and through the adjacent fibrin-gel matrix and connective tissue stroma. Indeed, elevated levels of urokinase-type plasminogen activator (uPA) and plasminogen activator inhibitor-1 (PA-1) in breast carcinomas have been shown to be independent predictors of poor prognosis. It is important that Fox et al. [35] have shown a significant association of uPA and PA-1 with intratumoral microvessel density. As a consequence, these investigators concluded that the poor prognosis in breast carcinomas associated with elevated uPA and PA-1 might be due to an interaction between endothelial and tumor cells using the uPA enzyme system.

Thus, the additive impact of the 'perfusion and paracrine' tumor effects, plus the endothelial-cell derived invasion-associated enzymes, all likely contribute to a phase of rapid tumor growth and signal a 'switch' to a potentially lethal angiogenesis phenotype. As will be shown, these same effects likely contribute to a much higher metastatic potential by facilitating entry of tumor cells into the lymphatic-vascular system.

Tumor angiogenesis: Probable mechanisms

The sequence of events of angiogenesis include (1) growth of endothelial cells from small venules lacking a muscle wall, (2) secretion of collagenases and degradation of basement membranes and connective-tissue stroma, (3) movement of endothelial cells toward the source of the angiogenic stimulus, (4) proliferation of endothelial cells, (5) elongation of the endothelial sprout, (6) joining of one sprout with another to form a capillary loop, (7) formation of a cytoplasmic vacuole with subsequent complete lumen formation and blood flow, and (8) deposition of a new (initially fragmented and leaky) basement membrane. Our study in human breast carcinomas showed that the intratumoral endothelial-cell proliferation index (mean 2.7%) was 45-fold greater than that observed in surrounding benign breast [19]; however, there was no correlation of intratumoral endothelial-cell proliferation with intratumoral microvessel density and tumor-cell proliferation, an observation suggesting that they may be regulated by different mechanisms. Furthermore, the value of 2.7% is unexpectedly low, especially given the much higher intratumor microvessel density compared with adjacent benign stroma. This suggests that a significant component of the angiogenic process is due to endothelial-cell migration, capillary budding, establishment of capillary loops, and/or neovascular remodeling [37–40].

Certainly, some tumor angiogenesis can occur without active endothelial proliferation. For instance, Auerbach et al. [41] observed that the onset and initial pattern of angiogenesis were similar in both irradiated and non-irradiated tumors grafted intracorneally into adult rabbits. The radiation doses were sufficient to prevent the normally observed growth and cell division of grafted tumors, but active capillary circulation at the periphery of the tumors was, nonetheless, observed within 24–28 hours. In a study of inflammation-induced neovascularization of rat cornea, Sholley et al. [42] observed that vascular sprouting at 2 days was similar in non-irradiated and irradiated cornea, even though the irradiated cornea showed no endothelial-cell proliferation. However, in contrast to non-irradiated controls, this neovascular growth decreased between 2 and 4 days, and ceased thereafter, implying that endothelial-cell proliferation soon becomes essential to continued growth [42]. Because tumor angiogenesis requires both DNA synthesis and vascular remodeling, the most effective antiangiogenesis therapies should target both components of the neovascularization process.

The process of tumor neovascularization shares many features with normal wound healing [43] and is likely to be mediated by similar and specific angiogenic molecules (e.g., VEGF), which are released by the tumor cells and/ or host immune cells into the tumor stroma or possibly are mobilized from a bound inactive state within the tumor stroma (e.g., acidic and basic FGF) [8,23,44,45]. Of relevance, my colleagues and I [46] recently reported that some breast ducts containing duct carcinoma in situ (DCIS) may also have a cuff or ring of microvessels around the duct (Figure 2). The close proximity of this cuff of neovascularization to the DCIS cells suggested that it formed in response to angiogenic factor(s) released by the DCIS cells. This microvessel rim was limited to ducts containing DCIS and did not correlate with periductal inflammation, suggesting that the angiogenic stimulus may be a diffusible

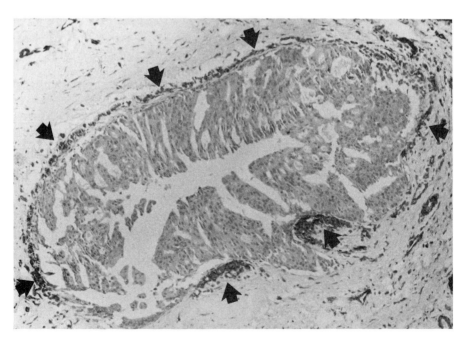

Figure 2. Ductal carcinoma in situ (intermediate-grade) with a cuff of periductal angiogenesis. Shown is a breast duct filled with ductal carcinoma in situ, which has been immunostained to highlight microvessels with anti–factor VIII–related antigen. A dark staining cuff of microvessels (closed arrows) is found in the stroma immediately adjacent to the basement membrane.

substance coming directly from the DCIS cells and not from associated inflammatory cells.

Guidi et al. [47] studied 55 cases of DCIS of the breast and found two patterns of peri-DCIS neovascularization, a diffuse microvessel pattern and an immediately adjacent, microvessel cuffing pattern. The diffuse pattern correlated with comedo-type DCIS, periductal desmoplastic stromal reaction, high DCIS proliferation index, and HER2/neu expression by DCIS cells. The microvessel cuffing pattern was found in 38% of cases and was not significantly associated with histologic type of DCIS, HER2/neu expression, or proliferation rate. Clearly, tumor angiogenic activity can occur independently of stromal invasion. Likewise, Smith-McCune et al. [48] found that microvessels were markedly and significantly increased in the cervix immediately beneath cervical intraepithelial neoplasia (CIN), when compared with adjacent normal epithelium. Yet, the neovascularization (CIN angiogenesis) was not related to the number of macrophages within the CIN lesions, indicating that the production of the angiogenic factor(s) is likely a property of the dysplastic epithelial cells themselves [48].

Nonetheless, in addition to tumor cells, inflammatory cells may be important in tumor angiogenesis. Stimulated macrophages can secrete angiogenic factors, such as transforming growth factor-alpha (TGF-α), angiotropin, tumor necrosis factor-alpha (TNF-α), and bFGF [8,44,45,49–54]. Clearly, many tumors have associated macrophages, which may amplify tumor angiogenesis, especially when activated by high intratumoral lactate levels caused by tumor hypoxia [54]. Also, some human tumors are heavily infiltrated by mast cells, often in significant numbers before tumor angiogenesis occurs [56,57] or during maximal growth in developing hemangiomas [58]. Mast cells are rich in heparin, a substance known to mobilize the angiogenic substance bFGF from the extracellular matrix, to protect it from degradation, and to potentiate its angiogenic effects [59]. Moreover, when tumors were implanted in mast cell–deficient mice (W/W^v), angiogenesis and tumor growth were inhibited to less than 60% of that observed in mice having normal mast cell numbers [60]. It is important that tumor angiogenesis and tumor growth increased when these mast cell–deficient mice were injected with exogenous mast cells along with the original bolus of tumor cells. Finally, stimulated tumor-infiltrating lymphocytes may also play a role in tumor angiogenesis by secreting cytokines that activate other inflammatory cell types, and/or chemoattractants for other immune cells. Thus far, lymphocytes themselves have not been found to directly secrete an angiogenic factor.

Although the factor(s) and/or cell(s) causing tumor angiogenesis remain incompletely understood, the current leading candidates for this role include basic FGF [61,62] and vascular endothelial growth factor (VEGF) [27]. Other possible angiogenic factors include: acidic FGF, TGF-α, TGF-β, platelet-derived endothelial cell growth factor (PD-ECGF), vascular permeability factor (VPF), folliculostellate-derived growth factor (FSDGF), granulocyte colony stimulating factor, placental growth factor, interleukin-8, hepatocyte growth factor, angiotropin, angiogenin, and TNF-α [23,8,44,45]. The amino acid sequences of VEGF, VPF, and FSDGF are nearly identical and likely represent that same substance. In fact, VEGF is often designated VPF/VEGF. With the exception of angiogenin, most of the angiogenic molecules were first purified on the basis of some unrelated activity and then were only later shown to be angiogenic [8,44,50].

VEGF (a well-studied permeability and selective endothelial-cell growth factor) is likely to be an important tumor angiogenic factor. Brown et al. [63,64] have shown in a variety of solid tumor types that tumor cells express high levels of VEGF protein and mRNA, the expression of which was accentuated in tumor cells close to areas of necrosis. In contrast, tumor endothelial cells express VEGF protein but not VEGF mRNA. Yet the same endothelial cells expressed high levels of mRNA for the VEGF receptors flk-1 and kdr, indicating that the endothelial-cell staining likely reflects binding of VEGF protein secreted by adjacent tumor cells. It is important that endothelial cells away from the tumor did not express these proteins or mRNAs.

Moreover, VEGF has been shown to induce in endothelial cells expression of plasminogen activator, plasminogen activator inhibitor, interstitial collagenase, and procoagulant activity [63]. VEGF promotes extravasation of plasma fibrinogen, leading to fibrin deposition within the tumor matrix, a process that promotes the ingrowth of macrophages, fibroblasts, and endothelial cells [65]. As mentioned earlier, the work of Kim et al. [27] and Millauer et al. [29] also support the importance of VEGF, a key tumor angiogenic factor, and work by Goto et al. [66] suggests that VEGF and bFGF act in a synergistic manner to cause tumor angiogenesis.

Also, various low molecular weight, nonpeptide angiogenic factors have been reported. These include 1-butyryl-glycerol, prostaglandins (PGE1 and PGE2), nicotinamide, adenosine, nitric oxide, hyaluronic acid degradation products, and an arachidonic acid metabolite named 12(R)-hydroxyeicosatrienoic acid (12[R]-HETrE) [8,44,67,68]. Of interest, when endothelial cells had been stimulated by 12(R)-HETrE, the proto-oncogenes c-*myc*, c-*jun*, and c-*fos* were activated [68]. Like the polypeptides, the actual role of the nonpeptide angiogenic factors under natural conditions remains incompletely studied, but nitric oxide and 12(R)-HETrE may prove to be very important molecules in the angiogenic process [8,44].

Thus far, the angiogenic factors described earlier have been stimulatory, but inactivation of a suppressor gene resulting in loss of an angiogeneic suppressor substance may allow tumor angiogenesis to proceed. Indeed, the switch to active angiogenesis and the rate of the angiogenic process are likely the net effect of both stimulatory and inhibitory factors. For example, it has been shown that inactivation of a suppressor gene during carcinogenesis results in increased angiogenesis that parallels increased tumorigenicity [69,70]. During this process there is a 10-fold decrease in the secretion of a 140-kD glycoprotein, called thrombospondin, an inhibitor of angiogenesis [71]. Next,

Zajchowski et al. [72] have shown that somatic hybrid cells, produced by fusion of MCF-7 human breast-carcinoma cells with normal immortalized human mammary epithelial cells, are suppressed in their ability to form tumors in nude mice. The hybrids had, among other traits of their normal parent cells, the ability to increase the expression of the angiogenesis inhibitor thrombospondin, supporting the concept that angiogenic capability contributes to tumorigenicity in human breast carcinoma.

Also, Dameron et al. [73] showed that the 'switch' to the angiogenic phenotype by fibroblasts cultured from Li-Fraumeni patients coincided with loss of the wild-type allele of the p53 tumor suppressor gene and to be the result of reduced expression of thrombospondin-1. Finally, O'Reilly et al. [74] have reported that a novel angiogenesis inhibitor, *angiostatin*, is released by the primary tumor mass of a Lewis lung carcinoma. When the primary tumor is present, metastatic tumor growth is suppressed by this angiostatin; but, after primary tumor removal, the metastases neovascularize and grow. The angiostatin activity copurifies with a 38 kD plasminogen fragment. This mechanism may explain one form of *dormancy*, but some metastatic deposits appear to remain dormant in spite of the fact that the primary tumor had been previously removed. Possibly, the latter deposits do not grow until they *switch* to a more angiogenic phenotype [75]. Other reported endogenous negative regulators of endothelial proliferation include: platelet factor 4, tissue inhibitors of metalloproteinases, a 16 kD fragment of prolactin, bFGF soluble receptor, and TGF-β [23].

Angiogenesis is necessary for metastasis of solid tumors

To metastasize, a tumor cell must successfully negotiate a series of obstacles, as well as present and respond to several growth factors or cytokines. In most primary tumors, less than one cell in 1000 or 10,000 has all of these abilities [76–78]. Tumor cells must gain access to the vasculature from the primary tumor, survive the circulation, escape immune surveillance, localize in the microvasculature of the target organ, escape from (or grow from within) the vasculature into the target organ, and induce tumor angiogenesis [76–87]. Tumor growth and spread are further amplified geometrically, when the newly established metastasis sheds additional tumor cells to form even more metastases by following the same cascade of events [77]. If the metastasis is already highly angiogenic, then its daughter metastases (clones) are likely to be highly angiogenic as well.

Angiogenesis is necessary at the beginning of this journey because without it tumor cells are only rarely shed into the circulation [79,84,85]. New proliferating capillaries have fragmented basement membranes and are leaky, making them more accessible to tumor cells than mature vessels [80]. Furthermore, the invasive chemotactic behavior of endothelial cells at the tips of growing capillaries is facilitated by their secretion of collagenases, urokinases, and plasminogen activator [81]. These degradative enzymes may also facilitate the escape of tumor cells into the tumor neovasculature. Indeed, the 'invading' capillaries may actively participate in the metastatic process by engulfing, and thus facilitating, the entry of tumor cells into vascular spaces, allowing systemic spread. Indeed, Sugino et al. [88] observed, in a naturally occurring mouse mammary carcinoma model (C3H/He mice), that intravasating tumor cells and tumor emboli within blood vessel lumina retained their nested architecture within a continuous basement membrane and were also invested by an endothelial-cell layer. These investigators believed the findings indicated a 'passive' mechanism of tumor cell intravasation, distinct from invasive properties of tumor cells, in which endothelial cells in sinusoidal vessels can envelop tumor cell nests, which then become detached into the blood. Arrest of such encapsulated emboli in pulmonary arterioles downstream could form new metastatic tumor foci.

Also, supporting this concept is the observation that India ink injected into the rabbit cornea will stay at the injection site indefinitely as a tattoo, unless neovascularization is induced in the cornea [56,82]. As new capillaries approach the ink spot, the ink fragments and reappears in the ipsilateral lymph nodes. Invasion into lymphatics can occur by invasion of tumors cells into adjacent lymphatics forming concomitantly with blood capillaries or, possibly, by passage of tumor cells from the blood stream into the lymphatics via lymphaticovenous junctions [8,83]. Also, tumor angiogenesis may facilitate this process by increasing tumor volume, thus, enhancing tumor cell–lymphatic contact at the growing edge of the tumor, and/or by increasing the numbers of lymphaticovenous junctions, allowing more intravascular micrometastases to enter the lymphatic spaces.

It has been shown that greater numbers of tumor vessels increase the opportunity for tumor cells to enter the circulation. Liotta et al. [84,85] showed, in a transplantable mouse fibrosarcoma model, that tumor cells shed into the blood stream increased from 1.4×10^3 cells per 24 hours on day 5 after tumor implantation to 1.5×10^5 cells per 24 hours on day 15, and this increase correlated very closely with increasing intratumoral microvessel density, especially with those intratumoral microvessels that were over 30 microns in diameter. Also, it became clear from these studies that the establishment of successful lung metastases depends upon increasing numbers of cells shed into the circulation [8,84,85]. These experimental data strongly suggest that intratumoral microvessel density might correlate with aggressive tumor behavior.

Angiogenesis is also necessary at the end of the metastatic cascade of events. Because of the clonal origin of metastases [86], a primary tumor containing a high proportion of angiogenic tumor cells will seed the blood stream with tumor cells that are already angiogenic when they arrive in their target organ. Indeed, tumors have been shown to be heterogeneous in the ability of their individual tumor cells to be angiogenic [87]. As with the pri-

IMPACT OF ANGIOGENESIS IN BREAST CARCINOMA

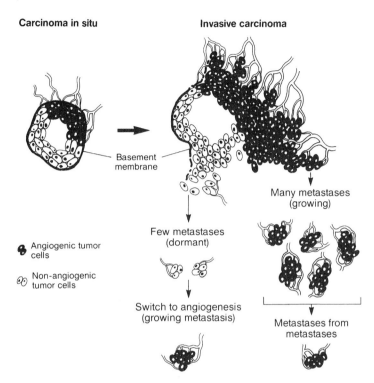

Figure 3. Angiogenic process and its contribution to tumor growth and metastasis. This artist's depiction shows the vascular response to angiogenic clones (blackened tumor cells) of breast carcinoma when the angiogenic clones are located in duct carcinoma in situ, when invasive into periductal stroma, and after metastatic clones are established at distant body sites. The angiogenic clones stimulate abundant microvessel growth, metastasize more frequently, and grow rapidly relative to the non-angiogenic cells (nonblackened tumor cells). Also shown are 'dormant' non-angiogenic metastatic clones, which can 'switch' to an angiogenic phenotype and produce growing metastatic deposits. This switch may occur after the primary is removed and an angiogenic inhibitor previously secreted by the primary is removed from the circulation.

mary tumor, angiogenesis will be necessary to establish a growing metastatic deposit, which will then give rise to additional metastatic deposits, thus amplifying the process of growth and dissemination (Figure 3).

It is important to emphasize that tumor angiogenesis is not sufficient for metastasis to occur, because tumor cells must also proliferate, penetrate host tissues, survive within vessels, escape the host's immune system, and begin growth at a new body site. The behavior of typical bronchial carcinoids illustrates this point, since they are highly vascular tumors, yet rarely do they metastasize to distant sites.

Tumor prognosis is related to tumor angiogenesis

Brem et al. [89] were among the first to suggest that the intensity of intratumoral tumor angiogenesis may correlate with tumor grade and aggressiveness. For this purpose, they defined a microscopic angiogenesis grading system (MAGS) based on an index incorporating vascular density, endothelial-cell hyperplasia, and endothelial cytology. Yet, the first clear-cut evidence that tumor angiogenesis could predict the probability of metastasis from a solid human tumor was reported for cutaneous melanoma. Srivastava et al. [90] studied the vascularity of 20 intermediate thickness skin melanomas (0.76–4.0 mm levels of invasion). Vessels were highlighted with *Ulex europaeus* 1 agglutinin conjugated with peroxidase, and the stained histologic sections were analyzed with a semi-automatic image analysis system. The 10 cases that developed metastases showed a vascular area at the tumor base that was more than twice that seen in the 10 cases without metastases (p = 0.025). Age, sex, Breslow's tumor thickness, and Clark's level of invasion were similar in the two groups.

Intratumoral microvessel density as a prognostic factor in breast carcinoma

Does the extent of angiogenesis (i.e., measured by intratumoral microvessel density) in human breast carcinoma correlate with metastasis, and can the quantitation of intratumoral microvessel density on a biopsy specimen be carried out rapidly and reproducibly so as to be useful in predicting the prognosis or the potential for metastasis at the time of diagnosis? If true, such information might prove valuable in selecting subsets of breast carcinoma patients for aggressive adjuvant therapies. For this to be true, it is important that a spectrum of intratumoral microvessel densities exists within the spectrum of invasive breast carcinomas. Indeed, when the microvessel counts in a number of invasive breast carcinomas are sorted in ascending order of vessel count on a log scale, the spectrum of low to high microvessel densities becomes apparent (Figure 4). The densities are an evenly distributed continuum, extending from about 10 to 200 microvessels per $0.74 \, mm^2$ ($200\times$) field.

To further address these questions, my colleagues and I examined primary tumor specimens from 49 unselected patients with invasive breast carcinoma (26 node-positive and 23 node-negative); four of the node-negative patients subsequently developed distant metastases and died from cancer [91]. All microvessels were highlighted by immunostaining endothelial cells for factor VIII–related antigen/von Willebrand's factor (F8RA/vWF), using a standard immunoperoxidase technique in which tissue sections are treated with trypsin or trypsin plus microwave-based antigen unmasking (in citrate buffer) prior to application of the anti-F8RA/vWF (Figure 2). This markedly increases the sensitivity of anti-F8RA/vWF in highlighting endothelial cells, while often decreasing background [92,93]. Hematoxylin and eosin (H&E) stained sec-

Breast Cancer Neovascularization

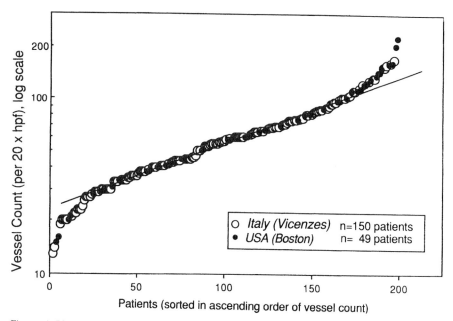

Figure 4. Plot showing the spectrum of microvessel densities of invasive breast carcinomas. Shown is a log -plot of the microvessel densities in 199 unselected invasive breast carcinomas sorted in ascending order of microvessel density. Note that there is a continuum extending from about 10 to 200 microvessels per 0.74 mm² (200× field of an Olympus microscope model BH-2). The spectrum of neovascularization in invasive breast carcinoma increases exponentially, suggestsing that tumor vascularization follows the arterial architectural network, characterized by dichotomous branching or budding, as opposed to venous segmental branching. (Reprinted with permission of Mosby Year Book; St. Louis, MO; from Weidner N, *Adv Pathol Lab Med* 1992;5:101–121.

tions of breast tumor were used to choose one paraffin-embedded tissue block representative of the invasive carcinoma, and only one 5 μm thick section was stained for F8RA/vWF.

Intratumoral microvessel density was assessed by light microscopic analysis for areas of the tumor that contained the most capillaries and small venules (microvessels; so-called neovascular hot spots). Finding the neovascular hot spot is critical to accurate assessment of a particular tumor's angiogenic potential. This is expected, because there is considerable evidence that, like tumor proliferation rate, tumor angiogenesis is heterogeneous within tumors (Table 3) [34,61,90,91,94]. The technique for identifying these hot spots is very similar to that for finding the hot spots for assessing mitotic figure content within breast tumors; thus, it is likely subject to the same kinds of interobserver and intraobserver variability. Sclerotic, hypocellular areas within tumors and im-

Table 3. Evidence that angiogenesis is heterogeneous within tumors (neovascular hot spots and cold spots)

Islet-cell tumors in transgenic mice develop angiogenic activity at 6–7 weeks in 10% of preneoplastic clones, which then grow (Folkman [75]).

Multifocal fibrosarcomas in transgenic mice develop angiogenic activity in only a subset of tumors, which then grow (Kandel [61]).

Individual tumor cells isolated from a single tumor (sarcoma) and then grown in vitro may or may not be mitogenic for endothelial cells (Folkman [34]).

Angiogenic activity usually occurs focally in early cutaneous melanoma (Srivastava [90]).

Solid tumors (e.g., breast, prostate cancer, etc.) show variable angiogenic activity (Weidner [20]; Weidner [111]).

Table 4. Technique for counting microvessels

Step	Procedure for counting intratumoral microvessels
1	Examine all histologic slides from the tumor and select a slide showing a generous cross section of representative tumor.
2	Have the block from which the selected slide was made used to make a 5 μm thick section for immunostaining.
3	Immunostain the section with an endothelial marker to highlight the microvessel density (e.g., anti-F8RA, anti-CD31, anti-CD34, etc.).
4	Scan the immunostained section at low magnification (~40–100×) and select areas of clear-cut, invasive carcinoma with the greatest numbers of distinctly highlighted microvessels (i.e., neovascular hot spot).
5	Count all vessels within a 0.74 mm² area of this neovascular hot spot.

mediately adjacent to benign breast tissue were not considered in intratumoral microvessel density determinations. Yet, microvessels in these latter areas served as internal controls for the quality of the F8RA/vWF staining. Only tumors that produced a high quality and distinct microvessel immunoperoxidase staining pattern (with low background staining) were included in this or subsequent studies. This is very important because the quality of immunoperoxidase staining can vary considerably between laboratories, and before measuring intratumoral microvessel density, high quality immunoperoxidase staining must be consistently achieved.

Just as their mitotic figure contents vary, so too are breast tumors frequently heterogeneous in their intratumoral microvessel density. Areas of highest neovascularization were found by scanning the tumor sections at low power (40× and 100× total magnification), and selecting those areas of invasive carcinoma with the greatest numbers of distinct F8RA/vWF-staining (brown) microvessels per 0.74 mm² area (Table 4). These high neovascular areas could occur anywhere within the tumor, but most frequently appeared at the margins of the carcinoma. After the area of highest neovascularization was identified, individual microvessel counts were made on a 200× field (20× objective and 10× ocular, Olympus BH-2 microscope, 0.74 mm² per field, with

278

the field size measured with an ocular micrometer). Any brown-staining endothelial cell or endothelial-cell cluster, clearly separate from adjacent microvessels, tumor cells, and other connective-tissue elements, was considered a single, countable microvessel. Even those distinct clusters of brown-staining endothelial cells, which might be from the same microvessel 'snaking' its way in and out of the section, were considered distinct and countable as separate microvessels. Vessel lumens, although usually present, were not necessary for a structure to be defined as a microvessel, and red cells were not used to define a vessel lumen. Results were expressed as the highest number of microvessels in any single 200× field. Averaging of multiple fields was not performed.

Invasive breast carcinomas from patients with metastases had a mean microvessel count of 101 per 200× field (SD = 49.3, range 16–220). For those carcinomas from patients without metastases, the corresponding value was 45 per 200× field (SD = 21.1, range 15–100). Univariate analysis revealed these differences to be statistically significant (p = 0.003). Also, we plotted the percent of patients with metastatic disease in whom a vessel count was carried out within progressive 33 vessel increments (Figure 5). The plot showed that the incidence of metastatic disease increased with the number of microvessels, reaching 100% for patients having invasive carcinomas with >100 microvessels per 200× field. The careful application of these counting techniques yielded data that, by multivariate analysis, indicated that intratumoral microvessel density was a better predictor for metastasis than tumor grade and tumor size.

To further define the relationship of intratumoral microvessel density to overall and relapse-free survival and to other reported prognostic indicators in breast carcinoma, a blinded study of 165 consecutive carcinoma patients was performed using identical techniques to measure intratumoral microvessel density [95]. The other prognostic indicators evaluated were metastasis to axillary lymph nodes, patient age, menopausal status, tumor size, histologic grade (i.e., Scarff-Bloom-Richardson criteria), peritumoral lymphatic-vascular invasion (PLVI), flow DNA ploidy analysis, flow S-phase fraction, growth fraction by Ki-67 binding, c-erbB2 oncoprotein expression, pro-cathepsin-D content, estrogen-receptor content, progesterone-receptor content, and EGFR expression. We found a highly significant association of intratumoral microvessel density with overall survival and relapse-free survival in all patients, including node-negative and node-positive subsets (Figures 6 and 7). All patients with breast carcinomas having >100 microvessels per 200× field experienced tumor recurrence within 33 months of diagnosis, compared with <5% of patients who had <33 microvessels per 200× field. Moreover, intratumoral microvessel density was the only significant predictor of overall and relapse-free survival among node-negative women. Weidner et al. [95] concluded that intratumoral microvessel density in the area of most intense neovascularization in invasive breast carcinoma is an independent, highly significant, and accurate prognostic indicator in predicting metastasis, as

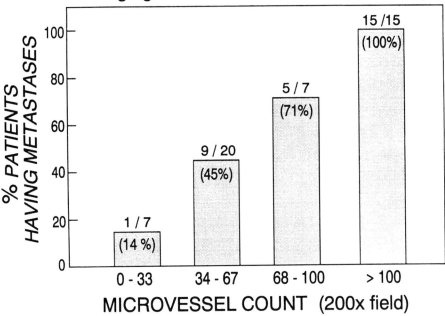

INVASIVE BREAST CARCINOMA
Angiogenesis and Metastasis (49 Patients)

Figure 5. Plot showing percent of breast carcinoma patients with metastasis by microvessel count. Shown is the plot of the percent of patients with metastatic disease in whom a vessel count was carried out within progressive 33 vessel increments. This plot reveals that the incidence of metastatic disease increases as microvessel density increases, becoming 100% for patients having invasive carcinomas containing microvessel counts of >100 per 200× field. (Reprinted with permission from W.B. Saunders Co, Philadelphia, PA; from Weidner N, *Semin Diagn Pathol* 1993;302–313.)

well as overall and relapse-free survival in patients with stage I to II breast carcinoma. Such an indicator would be useful in the selection of high-risk, node-negative patients with breast carcinoma for systemic adjuvant therapy.

Bosari et al. [96] were the first to confirm that quantitation of microvessels within invasive breast carcinomas was associated with prognosis. These investigators studied 151 node-negative and 32 node-positive breast carcinoma patients, who had a minimum follow-up of 9 years. Microvessels were highlighted after immunostaining with anti-F8RA/vWF in 5-μm thick sections from all tumor-containing blocks, and microvessels were counted in three 200× fields, which were considered to have the highest vascularization. The highest and average counts of the three 200× fields were recorded for correlation with outcome. The differences from the highest count to the average count varied from 12.8% to 14%. The value of using anti-ABH (blood group antigens) to highlight microvessels was also studied, but this approach was

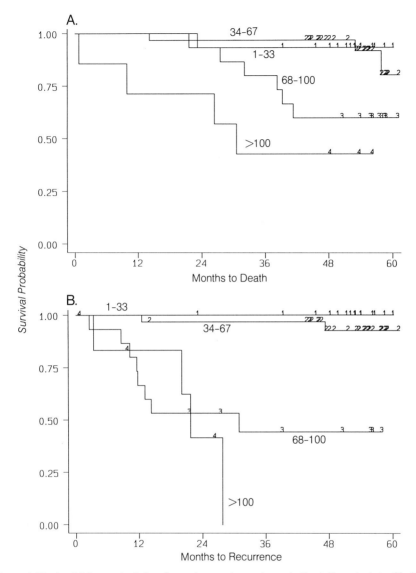

Figure 6. Kaplan-Meier survival plots for node-negative patients. **A**: Overall survival stratified by microvessel count. Note the decreasing overall survival associated with increasing microvessel counts in areas of invasive breast carcinoma ($p \leq 0.001$). **B**: Relapse-free survival stratified by microvessel count. Note the decreasing relapse-free survial associated with increasing microvessel counts in areas of invasive breast carcinoma ($p \leq 0.001$).

rejected because ABH antigens were frequently expressed by tumor cells, hampering microvessel counting. Likewise, carcinoma cells frequently show *Ulex europaeus*-1 lectin binding [97]. Node-positive carcinomas demonstrated significantly higher intratumoral microvessel density than did node-negative

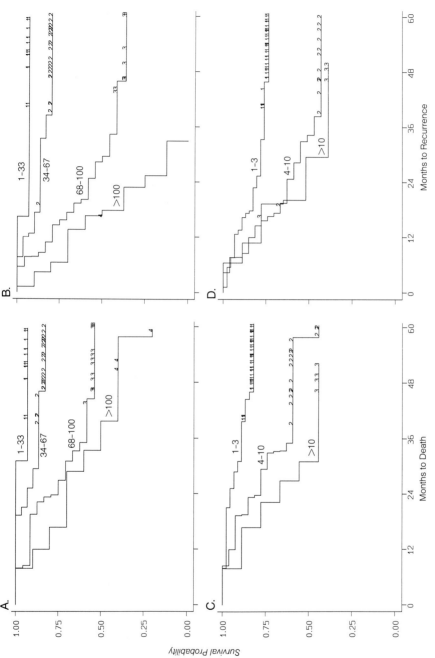

Figure 7. Kaplan-Meier survival plots for node-positive patients. **A**: Overall survival stratified by microvessel count. Note the decreasing overall survival associated with increasing microvessel counts in areas of invasive breast carcinoma (p ≤ 0.001). **B**: Relapse-free survival stratified by microvessel count. Note the decreasing relapse-free survival associated with increasing microvessel counts in areas of invasive breast carcinoma (p ≤ 0.001). **C**: Overall survival stratified by number of positive axillary nodes. Note the decreasing overall survival associated with increasing numbers of positive axillary lymph nodes (p ≤ 0.005). **D**: Relapse-free survival stratified by number of positive

282

carcinomas ($p < 0.001$), and patients with node-negative tumors who experienced distant relapse had higher intratumoral microvessel density than did those node-negative patients who remained disease free ($p = 0.01$). With the exception of peritumoral lymphatic-vascular invasion, intratumoral microvessel density was independent of traditional histologic parameters, ploidy status, and flow S-phase fraction. Moreover, multivariate analysis showed that intratumoral microvessel density and peritumoral lymphatic-vascular invasion were the two best independent predictors of outcome.

Horak et al. [98], using immunostaining to highlight microvessels with anti-CD31 (anti–platelet-endothelial cell adhesion molecules or PECAM), counted microvessels in tumors from 103 patients with breast carcinoma (64 node-negative and 39 node-positive). Anti-CD31 (JC70 antibody) was chosen after an evaluation of seven antibodies, including those to F8RA/vWF, CD34, and CD36. They found that the JC70 antibody to CD31 consistently stained more vessels than the others, although some plasma cell were also highlighted by JC70. They counted intratumoral microvessel density in areas of highest neovascularity and used the highest count of three distinct fields, each measuring $0.384 \, mm^2$ and extrapolated to microvessels per mm^2. Next, they compared their findings for intratumoral microvessel density to lymph node status, tumor grade, tumor size, tumor type, estrogen-receptor status, c-erbB2 protein expression, epidermal growth factor receptor expression (EGFR), and detection of mutant p53. Only 2 of 50 tumors with <99 microvessels/mm^2 were node positive, whereas 31 of 39 tumors with >140 per mm^2 were node positive ($p < 0.0001$). Tumor size ($p < 0.004$) and grade ($p < 0.028$) also correlated with node metastasis, and intratumoral microvessel density significantly increased with tumor size and grade. But multivariate analysis showed that intratumoral microvessel density alone ($p = 0.0001$) explains the association of size and grade with node metastasis. Of the other markers studied, EGFR status ($p < 0.01$), node status ($p < 0.02$), and ER status ($p < 0.05$) correlated with survival (30 months follow-up), but determination of intratumoral microvessel density was the most significant in predicting poor survival ($p < 0.006$). These results suggested that angiogenesis is closely linked to metastasis and that counting newly formed microvessels within the invasive carcinomas may be an effective means of early detection of metastatic potential and for selecting patients for whom anti-angiogenesis drugs might be beneficial.

Likewise, Gasparini et al. [99] used anti-CD31 to determine intratumoral microvessel density in node-negative breast cancer patients and found that anti-CD31 was more sensitive than anti-F8RA/vWF in highlighting intratumoral microvessels. Again, results correlated highly with overall and relapse-free survival by both univariate and multivariate analysis, but the stratification appeared no better than when anti-F8RA/vWF was used to highlight microvessels for intratumoral microvessel density determination [95]. Moreover, Gasparini et al. [99] showed that nuclear immunostaining of p53 protein and tumor size provided additional independent information to that already provided by intratumoral microvessel density (Figures 8 and 9).

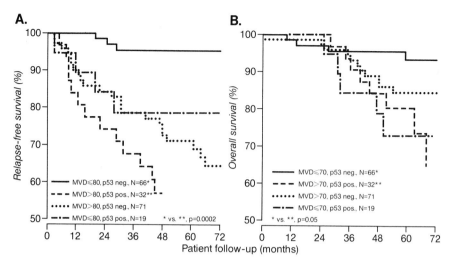

Figure 8. Kaplan-Meier survival plots for node-negative patients stratified according to microvessel density and nuclear p53 immunostaining. **A**: Relapse-free survival. Note the marked difference in survial between patients with low microvessel densities (≤80) and negative p53 immunostaining and those with high microvessel densities (>80) and positive p53 immunostaining (p = 0.0002). **B**: Overall survival. Again, note the marked difference in survival between patients with low microvessel densities (≤70) plus negative p53 immunostaining and those with high microvessel densities (>70) plus positive p53 immunostaining (p = 0.05). (Reprinted with permission from W.B. Saunders Co., Philadelphia, PA; Gasparini G, *J Clin Oncol* 1994;12:454–466.)

Toi et al. [100] have found an association between intratumoral microvessel density and outcome in breast carcinoma. They studied 125 breast cancer patients and found that intratumoral microvessel density (using either anti-F8RA/vWF or anti-CD31) was a significant predictor of relapse-free survival in both node-negative and node-positive patients, even more so than nodal status. Intratumoral microvessels in the areas considered to be most active for neovascularization, and immunostained cells, were counted in three fields (200×) and the average was calculated. These investigators found that the statistical value of intratumoral microvessel density by anti-F8RA/vWF immunostaining was more portent than evaluation by anti-CD31. Yet, there appeared to be a close correlation between CD31 immunostaining and F8RA/vWF immunostaining, each providing about the same intratumoral microvessel densities, suggesting that both were reliable methods for quantifying angiogenesis in tumor tissues.

Visscher et al. [101] combined image morphometry and vessel highlighting with anti-type IV collagen (basal lamina) and correlated survival and intratumoral microvessel density in 58 patients with stage-heterogenous breast carcinomas. They found that the short-term, disease-free survival was significantly related to intratumoral microvessel density for all patients (p = 0.001),

284

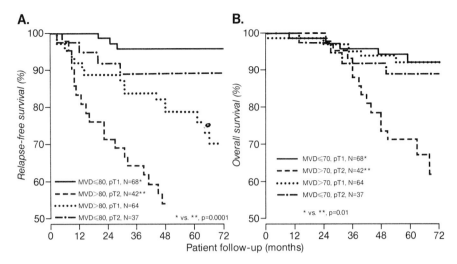

Figure 9. Kaplan-Meier survival plots for node-negative patients stratified according to microvessel density and tumor size. **A**: Relapse-free survival. Note the marked difference in survival between patients with low microvessel densities (≤ 80) and pT1 tumors, and those with high microvessel densities (>80) and pT2 tumors (p = 0.0001). **B**: Overall survival. Again, note the marked difference in survival between patients with low microvessel densities (≤ 70) plus pT1 tumors, and those with high microvessel densities (>70) plus pT2 tumors (p = 0.01). (Reprinted with permission from W.B. Saunders Co., Philadelphia, PA; Gasparini G, *J Clin Oncol* 1994;12:454–466.)

as well as in node-negative (p = 0.005) and node-positive (p = 0.02) subgroups. Furthermore, tumors recurred in 87% of patients with intratumoral microvessel density >30 vessels/mm² versus only 15% with counts <10 vessels/mm². The authors concluded that image morphometric quantitation of vascular basal lamina was an objective means of assessing angiogenic capacity in breast tumors that correlated strongly with disease aggressiveness in short-term follow-up (mean follow-up 52 months). Caution, however, should be observed when using anti–type IV collagen to highlight vessels, because this protein is also found in most basal lamina, especially around tumor cell nests [102].

Also, Sneige et al. [103], Sahin et al. [104], Obermair et al. [105], and Bundred et al. [106] have all reported associations of intratumoral microvessel density with survival in breast carcinoma patients (Table 5). Among the most recent to publish in this area, Obermair et al. [105] studied 64 patients with breast carcinoma and followed for 5 year recurrence-free survival (RFS). Using an ocular raster, they found that patients with a vessel density of more than 10 vessels per raster had an RFS of 42.7% versus those with fewer than 10 vessels per raster, who had an RFS of 97.8% (p = 0.0011). This effect was independent of nodal status.

Table 5. Journal reports of positive association of tumor angiogenesis and tumor aggressiveness: Breast carcinoma

1	Weidner et al.	*N Engl J Med*	1991;324:1–8
2	Bosari et al.	*Hum Pathol*	1992;23:755–71
3	Horak et al.	*Lancet*	1992;340:1120–1124
4	Weidner et al.	*J Natl Cancer Inst*	1992;84:1875–1887
5	Visscher et al.	*Anal Quant Cytol Histol*	1993;15:88–92
6	Toi et al.	*Int J Cancer*	1993;55:341–374
7	Obermair et al.	*Onkologie*	1994;17:44–49
8	Fox et al.	*Breast Cancer Res Treat*	1994;29:109–116
9	Gasparini et al.	*J Clin Oncol*	1994;12:454–466
10	Gasparini et al.	*Int J Oncol*	1994;4:155–162

Those authors whose names are underlined indicate studies based on different patient databases that have been analyzed by different groups of investigators located at geographically separate medical centers.

Role of microvessel density in other solid tumors

Further support for the value of determining intratumoral microvessel density in breast carcinoma is the finding of the same correlations of intratumoral microvessel density with metastases and/or clinical outcome in other solid-tumor systems (Table 6). Macchiarini et al. [107], using identical techniques as Weidner et al. [91,95] and Bosari et al. [96], studied early stage, non–small-cell lung carcinomas (87 patients all pT1N0M0) and found that the likelihood of metastasis increased as the intratumoral microvessel density increased (p < 0.0001). Also, the authors evaluated the prognostic associations of tumor size and tumor proliferative activity by immunostaining for proliferating cell nuclear antigen (PCNA, monoclonal PC10) and by mitosis counting. On multivariate analysis, the intratumoral microvessel density count was the only independent predictor of metastasis. Macchiarini et al. [108] have now extended their observations to non–small-cell lung cancer patients with tumor invading the thoracic inlet. Results of univariate and multivariate analysis of survival and the disease-free interval identified the degree of angiogenesis as the only independent and significant predictor of the disease-free interval. Aslo evaluated were tumor proliferative activity, p53 expression, tumor grade, tumor size, and vascular-space invasion. Yamazaki et al. [109] studied intratumoral microvessel density in lung adenocarcinomas from 42 patients and concluded that microvessel density correlated with relapse after surgical resection and hematogenous metastasis in all stages of lung adenocarcinoma, but they found no correlation with lymph node metastases.

Focusing on prostate carcinoma, Wakui et al. [110] highlighted endothelial cells with anti-vimentin and quantitated intratumoral angiogenesis with a computerized image analysis system. They determined the blood capillary density ratio (BCDR) in the entire tumor area of the section. The BCDR was

Table 6. Journal reports of positive, association of tumor angiogenesis and tumor aggressiveness

Lung carcinoma

1. Macchiarini et al.	*Lancet*	1992;340:145–146
2. Macchiarini et al.	*Ann Thorac Surg*	1994;57:1534–1539
3. Yamazaki et al.	*Cancer*	1994;74:2245–2251
4. Yuan et al.	*Am J Resp Crit Care Med*	1995;152:2157–2162

Prostate carcinoma

1. Wakui et al.	*J Pathol*	1992;168:257–262
2. Weidner et al.	*Am J Pathol*	1993;143:401–409
3. Fregene et al.	*Anticancer Res*	1993;13:2377–2381
4. Brawer et al.	*Cancer*	1994;73:678–687
5. Vesalainen et al.	*Anticancer Res*	1994;14:709–714

Squamous (head-and-neck) carcinoma

1. Mikami et al.	*Nip Jib Gak Kai*	1991;96:645–650
2. Gasparini et al.	*Int J Cancer*	1993;55:1–6
3. Albo et al.	*Ann Plast Surg*	1994;32:588–594
4. Williams et al.	*Am J Surg*	1994;168:373–380

Rectal carcinoma

1. Saclarides et al.	*Dis Colon Rectum*	1994;37:921–926

Central nervous system tumors

1. Li et al.	*Lancet*	1994;334:82–86

Testicular germ-cell tumors

1. Olivarez et al.	*Cancer Res*	1994;54:2800–2802

Bladder carcinoma

1. Jaeger et al.	*J Urol*	1995;154:59–71

Ovarian carcinoma

1. Hollingsworth et al.	*Am J Pathol*	1995;147:33–41

Multiple myeloma

1. Vacca et al.	*Br J Haematol*	1994;7:87:503–508

Cervical carcinoma

1. Bremer et al.	*Am J Obstet Gynecol*	1996, in press

Malignant melanoma

1. Srivastava et al.	*Eur J Can Clin Oncol*	1986;22:1205–1209
2. Srivastava et al.	*Am J Pathol*	1988;133:419–423
3. Fallowfield et al.	*J Pathol*	1991;164:241–244
4. Barnhill et al.	*Lab Invest*	1992;67:331–337
5. Barnhill et al.	*Am J Pathol*	1993;143:99–104
6. Graham et al.	*Am J Pathol*	1994;145:510–514
7. Cockerell et al.	*Am J Dermatopathol*	1994;16:9–13

Those authors whose names are underlined indicate studies based on different patient databases that have been analyzed by different groups of investigators located at geographically separate medical centers.

the ratio of the blood capillary area (x) to the tumor area (y) minus the luminal area of the tumor glands (z) [BCDR = $x/(y - z)$]. They found that in Gleason's low and intermediate grade tumors, the BCDR was significantly higher in prostate carcinomas that developed bone marrow metastasis than those that did not ($p < 0.001$).

Likewise, to determine how intratumoral microvessel density correlated with metastasis in prostate carcinoma, my colleagues and I used our own previously developed technique [91,95] and counted microvessels within the

287

initial invasive carcinomas of 74 patients (29 with metastasis, 45 without) [111]. The mean number of microvessels in tumors from patients with metastases was 76.8 microvessels per $200\times$ field (median, 66; SD, 44.6). The counts within carcinomas from patients without metastases were significantly lower, 39.2 (median, 36; SD, 18.6) ($p < 0.0001$). Intratumoral microvessel density increased with increasing Gleason's score ($p < 0.0001$), but this increase was present predominantly in the poorly differentiated tumors. Although Gleason's score also correlated with metastasis ($p = 0.01$), multivariate analysis showed that Gleason's score added no additional information to that provided by intratumoral microvessel density alone. Thus, assay of intratumoral microvessel density within invasive tumors may prove valuable in selecting patients for aggressive adjuvant therapies in early prostate carcinoma. Fregene et al. [112] then quantitated microvessels in 23 nonmalignant and 34 malignant prostatectomy speicmens. The findings were correlated with Whitmore-Jewitt stage and, based on the number of microvessels, the authors were able to distinguish stage D from all other pathologic stages ($p = 0.004$). They concluded that tumor angiogenesis in prostate cancer may have both clinical and pathological significance. Most recently, Brawer et al. [113] confirmed these observations in 32 patients with prostate cancer using a computer-aided image analysis system to measure intratumoral microvessel density after immunostaining with anti-F8RA/vWF. Their field size measured $1.71\,mm^2$, and the validity of the image analysis method was verified by comparing manual counts obtained by two of the authors with the computer counts ($p < 0.001$, $r = 0.98$, $n = 20$ fields compared).

In addition to these published reports, many other studies have shown an association between increasing intratumoral microvessel density and various other measures of tumor aggressiveness. In fact, the increasing number of publications is becoming difficult to follow. Gasparini et al. [114], Mikami et al. [115], Albo et al. [116], and Williams et al. [117] have found associations of intratumoral microvessel density with clinical outcome in squamous carcinomas of the head and neck. These observations are consistent with the reported observations by Petruzzeli et al. [118] that head-and-neck squamous carcinomas can induce an angiogenic response in vivo. Vasalainen et al. [119] have also confirmed, by univariate analysis, the association of increasing intratumoral microvessel density with higher Gleason's grade and poorer outcome in prostate carcinoma, and Saclarides et al. [120] have shown an association with decreased survival and relatively high intratumoral microvessel density for rectal carcinomas. Olivarez et al. [121] have shown a correlation of aggressive tumor behavior and intratumoral microvessel density in testicular carcinomas, and Hollingworth et al. [122] have noted an association of intratumoral microvessel density with disease-free survival for ovarian carcinomas. Moreover, Jaeger et al. [123] have shown an association of intratumoral microvessel density in invasive urothelial carcinomas with the presence or absence of metastases.

Both Barnhill et al. [124,125] and Nasser et al. [126] have reported a gradual rise in vascularity with tumor progression in the melanocytic system and onset of angiogenesis during the radial growth phase of cutaneous malignant melanoma. Fallowfield et al. [127] reported a significant relationship between the percentage vascular volume and maximum tumor thickness in 64 melanomas, suggesting that low tumor vascularity could correlate with a relatively favorable outcome in cutaneous melanoma, and Cockerell et al. [128] noted that intratumoral microvessel density was much greater in various malignant melanomas compared with all forms of Spitz nevi. These authors concluded that intratumoral microvessel density may be useful, together with clinical and histologic findings, in distinguishing melanoma from Spitz nevus in selected cases. Graham et al. [129] found that in thin melanomas (<0.75 mm invasion depth) high intratumoral microvessel density was associated with a greater chance of metastases and death from tumor. Examining soft tissue tumors, Ewaskow et al. [130] reported significantly increased vessel density in malignant fibrous histiocytoma and malignant nerve sheath tumors compared with their benign counterparts (p = 0.036). Li et al. [131] have documented that greater intratumoral microvessel density predicts poorer outcome in CNS tumors, and Vacca et al. [132] have found an association of increasing microvessel area with more rapidly progressing cases of multiple myeloma and also with those having the highest proliferating (DNA S-phase) fractions.

Other results with microvessel density measurements

Not all reports have found this association between intratumoral microvessel density and prognosis in solid tumors (Table 7). Van Hoef et al. [133] recently published a study of intratumoral microvessel density (using anti-F8RA/vWF to highlight microvessels) in the carcinomas of 93 node-negative breast carcinoma patients. These investigators found no correlation between relapse-free

Table 7. Journal reports of no association of tumor angiogenesis and tumor aggressiveness

Breast carcinoma		
1. Van Hoef et al.	*Eur J Cancer*	1993;29A:1141–1145
2. Hall et al.	*Surg Oncol*	1992;1:223–229
Malignant melanoma		
1. Carnochan et al.	*Br J Cancer*	1991;64:102–107
Tongue carcinoma		
1. Leedy et al.	*Otolaryrgol Head Neck Surg*	1994;111:417–422

Those authors whose names are underlined indicate studies based on different patient databases that have been analyzed by different groups of investigators located at geographically separate medical centers.

or overall survival and intratumoral microvessel density. However, the number of microvessels reported in their study appeared much higher than those obtained by Weidner et al. [91,93], even though the latter employed larger counting areas and the same immunostaining techniques. The mean and median (range) microvessel counts from the Weidner et al. [95] study were 60 and 56 (range 8–167), respectively, using a $0.74 \, mm^2$ counting area. In contrast, Van Hoef et al. [133] observed microvessels counts of 80 and 72 (range 32–156), respectively, using a $0.476 \, mm^2$ counting area, or 64% of the field used by Weidner [95]. Furthermore, they reported an intratumoral microvessel density count of 30 and a median of 28 (range 11–66) using a $0.1225 \, mm^2$ counting area, or 16.6% of that used by Weidner [95]. In fact, the microvessel densities obtained by Van Hoef et al. [133] are in a range greater than would be expected when using anti-CD31 to highlight microvessels, and Horak et al. [98] found anti-CD31 to be the most sensitive endothelial marker for highlighting intratumoral microvessels. These discrepancies suggest possible methodological problems.

Hall et al. [134] were unable to find an association with intratumoral microvessel density and metastasis in breast carcinoma. These authors reported microvessel counts using a $0.1256 \, mm^2$ microscopic field, which is much smaller than the optimal $0.74 \, mm^2$ field used in our studies. Significance of the intratumoral microvessel density drops when the field size is smaller than $0.19 \, mm^2$ [91]. They also excluded as vessels single cells that stained for anti-F8RA/VWF, believing that a lumen was necessary for it to be classified as a vessel, and that single cells were frequently not of vascular origin. This is a significant deviation from the Weidner et al. [91,93] procedure for determining intratumoral microvessel density; we have found that anti-F8RA/vWF immunostaining is very specific for endothelial cells (see later). Furthermore, Hall et al. [134] studied 87 breast carcinoma patients, 50 of whom had only 1.5 years median follow-up and, of the 50 node-negative patients, only three (6%) developed axillary or distant recurrence. A 6% incidence of disease relapse is far less than the expected 20–30% rate expected in node-negative breast carcinoma patients. It is important that published protocols [91,93] be followed carefully. Furthermore, considerable experience (i.e., at the senior staff pathologist level) is needed not only to oversee the immunostaining of endothelial cells, such that all microvessels can be clearly identified, but also for selecting the neovascular hot spot. Moreover, accurate staging and adequate follow-up are needed to determine those patients who will develop tumor relapses.

Carnochan et al. [135] and Leedy et al. [136] failed to show a relation of tumor-related microvessel density with outcome in patients with malignant melanoma and lymph nodal metastases in patients with squamous carcinoma of the tongue, respectively. Also, Leedy et al. [136] failed to show a relationship of p53 protein accumulation and lymph node status. Why these reports are contradictory to other reports is not clear.

Additional considerations in measuring intratumoral microvessel density

Because counting microvessels is based on a standard immunohistochemical assay wherein endothelial cells (and thus microvessels) are highlighted with an antibody to F8RA/vWF, the test can be performed using technology and reagents available in many pathology laboratories. Indeed, counting microvessels has been proven to be reproducible [91,98,112], especially following a period of training [137]. Brawer et al. [1132] compared manual intratumoral microvessel determinations with those determined by automated counting (i.e., Optimas Image Analysis) and found a very tight correlation ($r^2 = 0.98$, $p < 0.001$).

F8RA/vWF and Weibel-Palade bodies have been found in lymphatic endothelial cells, and possibly some of the intratumoral microvessels are lymphatics. But the overwhelming majority of the microvessels counted have proven to be capillaries and postcapillary venules based on their morphology and F8RA/vWF staining intensity. In many studies it has been shown that F8RA/vWF stains the endothelial cells of blood vessels more reliably than those of lymphatics [138–146]. In these studies, the investigators used the same basic techniques that were used in our studies [91,95]. These published observations and our own experience indicate that F8RA/vWF is not a reliable means of staining lymphatic microvessels. For example, Ordonez et al. [144] state that when F8RA/vWF is 'applied as a marker for lymphatics, staining of endothelial cells is weak or absent, even if the staining is done on enzymatically treated tissue sections.' Moreover, Lee et al. [139] stated that 'most reports indicate that small lymphatic vessels are negative [for F8RA/vWF] and that F8RA/vWF may be utilized to distinguish between blood vessel capillaries and lymphatic capillaries.' They also noted that they 'have found that lymphatic endothelium is occasionally positive after trypsin treatment, but the results have been inconsistent and unreliable' [139]. It is important that we have measured intratumoral microvessel density within invasive breast carcinoma, and there is good evidence to suggest that there are no (at least not functional) lymphatics within tumors [147–150]. Tanigawa et al. [148] concluded that there were no lymphatic vessels in cancerous regions by their lymphangiographic procedure, even in the early stages of cancer. Other studies, in which dyes were injected into the lymphatic vessels or interstitial space [149,150], yielded similar results.

Morphologically, with the current technology it can be difficult to determine if a single endothelial cell belongs to a lymphatic or blood microvessel [147,151]. Barsky et al. [152] reported that the distinction can be made by the presence of basal lamina around blood microvessels, but not around lymphatics. Unfortunately, some newly formed microvessels within tumors have poorly formed, discontinous, or even absent basal lamina. Accordingly, it would be inaccurate to claim that lymphatic microvessels were reliably included in our counts [91,95]. On the contrary, by using F8RA/vWF immunostaining, we may be missing some of the blood microvessels, rather

291

than including significant numbers of lymphatic microvessels, which are the least likely microvessels to immunostain reliably with F8RA/vWF.

Clealry, no endothelial marker developed to date has been 'perfect.' Yet we have found that F8RA/vWF has been the most specific endothelial marker, providing very good contrast between microvessels and other tissue components. Unfortunately, anti-F8RA/vWF may not highlight all intratumoral microvessels, and it may be diminished or even absent from some tumor capillaries [153]. Although apparently more sensitive, CD31, in our experience, crossreacts to a mild degree with fibroblasts and even with some tumor cells (as does CD34) [154–157], and it strongly crossreacts with plasma cells. Indeed, the crossreactivity of CD31 with plasma cells can significantly obscure the microvessels in those tumors with a prominent inflammatory background containing plasma cells, thus complicating accurate microvessel counts. CD34 is an acceptable alternative, but CD34 will highlight perivascular stromal cells and has been noted to stain a wide variety of stromal neoplasms. Like antibodies to F8RA/vWF, antibodies to CD31, CD34, and PAL-E also do not immunostain all intratumoral microvessels [158].

Wang et al. [158,159] have developed a monoclonal antibody (Mab E9), which was raised against proliferating or 'activated' endothelial cells of human umbilical-vein origin and grown in tissue culture. Mab E9 strongly reacted with endothelial cells of all tumors, fetal organs, and in regenerating and/or inflamed tissues, but it only rarely and weakly immunostained endothelial cells or normal tissues. Unfortunately, Mab E9 immunoreacted only in frozen tissue sections, although microwave antigen-retrieval techniques applied to formalin-fixed, paraffin-embedded tissues were not mentioned. Nonetheless, antibodies such as Mab E9 may provide the most sensitive staining of intratumoral microvessels by preferentially immunostaining 'activated or proliferating' endothelial cells. Thus the overall staining intensity may correlate best with active tumor angiogenesis and, hence, tumor aggressiveness. Automated ('machine') immunostaining and application of computer-aided image analysis may help to standardize microvessel counts and help eliminate interobserver and even intraobserver variables, such as inexperience and hot spot selection biases [160]. The latter approach may make determination of intratumoral microvessel density a simple, reliable, and reproducible prognostic factor in a variety of solid tumors, not just in breast carcinoma.

Actually, measuring intratumoral microvessel density may prove to be a relatively crude method for estimating a tumor's angiogenic capacity. Other methods may prove more reliable and reproducible, such as measuring serum or urine levels of angiogenic molecules or directly measuring angiogenic molecules or inhibitors from tumor extracts (i.e., in a manner similar to hormone receptor assays). Indeed, using an immunoassay, Watanabe et al. [161] and Nguyen et al. [162] reported elevated levels of bFGF in the serum and urine of patients with a wide variety of solid tumors, including breast carcinoma. Higher levels were found in patients with metastatic disease versus those with localized disease. Moreover, Li et al. [131] have measured bFGF in the cere-brospinal fluids of children with a variety of brain tumors and have correlated increasing fluid bFGF levels with greater intratumoral microvessel density and increased likelihood of recurrence.

Final comments

Tumor angiogenesis is necessary for tumor growth and metastasis. Thus far, the overwhelming majority of published reports show a significant correlation between the density of intratumoral microvessels of invasive breast carcinoma and the incidence of metastases and/or patient survival. Similar associations are now reported for patients with melanoma, prostate carcinoma, testicular carcinoma, ovarian carcinoma, rectal carcinoma, bladder carcinoma, central nervous system tumors, multiple myeloma, non–small-cell lung carcinomas, and squamous carcinoma of the head and neck (see Table 5).

The association between intratumoral microvessel density and various mea-sures of tumor aggressiveness could be explained in a number of ways. First, a highly angiogenic primary tumor with a high intratumoral microvessel density is more likely to seed distant sites with highly angiogenic clones [155]. Second, solid tumors are composed of two discrete yet interdependent components (i.e., the malignant cells and the stroma they induce), and measuring intratumoral microvessel density could be a valid measure of the success that a particular tumor has in forming this very important stromal compartment. Also, the endothelial cells of this stromal component may be stimulating the growth of the tumor cells in a 'reverse' paracrine fashion. Third, the density of the microvessel bed within a tumor is likely to be a direct measure of the size of the vascular 'window' through which tumor cells pass to spread to distant body sites. The larger that window, the greater the number of circulating tumor cells from which a metastasis could develop. Finally, if it is true that endothelial cells play a very active role in the metastatic process (i.e., engulfing tumor cells) and that tumor cells are actually more passive than previously thought, then intratumoral microvessel density could be a direct measure of those endothelial-derived forces promoting metastases. I believe all of these factors are acting together to encourage tumor growth and metastasis. Indeed, it is no surprise that intratumoral microvessel density correlates with various measures of tumor aggressiveness.

Nonetheless, it remains to be seen whether the findings and techniques reviewed here will be universally reproducible and continue to hold up as a predictor of metastasis when utilized in a prospective manner by pathologists in many different centers. Moreover, as tumor therapies become more effec-tive in preventing tumor recurrence, the ability of a prognostic test to stratify patients into various prognostic categories becomes more diminished. With a 100% cure rate, all prognostic tests for predicting tumor recurrence become meaningless. In any event, the findings reviewed here have increased our understanding about the critical role of angiogenesis in human tumor growth and metastasis.

References

1. Coman DR, Sheldon WF (1946) The significance of hyperemia around tumor implants. *Am J Pathol* 22:821–826.
2. Day ED (1964) Vascular relationships of tumor and host. *Prog Exp Tumor Res* 4:57–97.
3. Folkman J (1990) What is the evidence that tumors are angiogenesis-dependent? *J Natl Cancer Ins* 82:4–6.
4. Folkman J (1971) Tumor angiogenesis: Therapeutic implications. *N Engl J Med* 285:1182–1186.
5. Folkman J, Hochberg M, Knighton D (1974) Self-regulation of growth in three dimensions: The role of surface area limitations. In *Control of Animal Cell Proliferation*. B Clarkson, R Baserga (eds). Cold Spring Harbor, NY: Cold Spring Harbor Laboratory Press, pp 833–842.
6. Sutherland RM (1988) Cell and environment interactions in tumor microregions: The multicell spheroid model. *Science* 240:177–184.
7. Sutherland RM, McCredie JA, Inch WR (1971) Growth of multicell spheroids in tissue culture as a model of nodular carcinomas. *J Natl Cancer Inst* 46:113–120.
8. Blood CH, Zetter BR (1990) Tumor interactions with the vasculature: Angiogenesis and tumor metastasis. *Biochim Biophysi Acta* 1032:89–118.
9. Gimbrone MA, Leapman S, Cotran RS, Folkman J (1972) Tumor dormancy in vivo by prevention of neovascularization. *J Exp Med* 136:261–276.
10. Gimbrone MA, Cotran Leapman J (1974) Tumor growth neovascularization: An experimental model using rabbit cornea. *J Natl Cancer Inst* 52:413–427.
11. Antonelli-Orlidge A, Saunders KB, Smith SR, D'Amore PA (1989) An activated form of transforming growth factor-beta is produced by co-cultures of endothelial cells and pericytes. *Proc Natl Acad Sci USA* 86:4544–4588.
12. Ausprunk DH, Folkman J (1977) Migration and proliferation of endothelial cells in preformed and newly formed blood vessels during tumor angiogenesis. *Microvasc Res* 14:53–65.
13. Adam JA, Maggelakis AA (1990) Diffusion regulated growth characteristics of a spherical prevascular carcinoma. *Bull Math Biol* 52:549–582.
14. Roberts AB, Sporn MB, Assoian RK, Smith JM, Roche NS, Wakefield LM, Heine UI, Liotta LA, Falanga V, Kehrl JH, Fauci AS (1986) Transforming growth factor type-beta: Rapid induction of fibrosis and angiogenesis in vivo and stimulation of collagen formation in vitro. *Proc Natl Aca Sci USA* 83:4167–4171.
15. Knighton D, Ausprunk D, Tapper D, Folkman J (1977) Avascular and vascular phases of tumor growth in the chick embryo. *Br J Cancer* 35:347–356.
16. Lien W, Ackerman N (1970) The blood supply of experimental liver metastases. II. A microcirculatory study of normal and tumor vessels of the liver with the use of perfused silicone rubber. *Surgery* 68:334–340.
17. Thompson WD, Shiach KJ, Fraser RA, McIntosh LC, Simpson JG (1987) Tumors acquire their vasculature by vessel incorporation, not vessel ingrowth. *J Pathol* 151:323–332.
18. Skinner SA, Tutton PJM, O'Brien PE (1990) Microvascular architecture of experimental colon tumors in the rat. *Cancer Res* 50:2411–2417.
19. Vartanian R, Weidner N (1994) Correlation of intratumoral endothelial-cell proliferation with microvessel density (tumor angiogenesis) and tumor-cell proliferation in breast carcinoma. *Am J Pathol* 144:1188–1194.
20. Weidner N, Semple JP, Welch WR, Folkman J (1991) Tumor angiogenesis and metastasis — correlation in invasive breast carcinoma. *N Engl J Med* 324:1–8.

21. Weidner N, Folkman J, Pozza F, Bevilacqua P, Allred EN, Moore DH, Meli S, Gasparini G (1992) Tumor angiogenesis: A new significant and independent prognostic indicator in early-stage breast carcinoma. *J Natl Cancer Inst* 84:1875–1887.
22. Folkman J (1985) Angiogenesis and its inhibitors. In *Important Advances in Oncology*. VT DeVita, S Hellman, SA Rosenberg (eds). Philadelphia: JB Lippincott, pp 42–62.
23. Folkman J (1995) Clinical applications of angiogenesis research. *N Engl J Med*, in press.
24. Harris AL, Fox S, Bicknell R, Leek R, Relf M, LeJeune S, Kaklamanis L (1994) Gene therapy through signal transduction pathways and angiogenic growth factors as therapeutic targets in breast cancer. *Cancer* 74(Suppl):1021–1025.
25. Ingber D, Fujita T, Kishimoto S, Katsuichi S, Kanamaru T, Brem H, Folkman J (1990) Synthetic analogues of fumagillin that inhibit angiogenesis and suppress tumor growth. *Nature* 348:555–557.
26. Gross JL, Herblin WF, Dusak BA, Czerniak P, Diamond M, Dexter DL (1990) Modulation of solid tumor growth in vivo by bFGF. *Proc Am Assoc Cancer Res* 31:79.
27. Kim KJ, Li B, Winer J, Armanini M, Gillett N, Phillips HS, Ferrara N (1993) Inhibition of vascular endothelial growth factor-induced angiogenesis suppresses tumor growth in vivo. *Nature* 362:841–844.
28. Hori A, Sasada R, Matsutani E, et al. (1991) Suppression of solid tumor growth by immunoneutralizing monoclonal antibody against human basic fibroblast growth factor. *Cancer Res* 51:6180–6184.
29. Millauer B, Shawver LK, Plate KH, Risau W, Ullrich A (1994) Glioblastoma growth inhibited in vivo by a dominant-negative Flk-1 mutant. *Nature* 367:576–579.
30. Brooks PC, Montgomery AMP, Rosenfeld M, Reisfeld RA, Hu T, Ilier G, Cheresh DA (1994) Integrin αvβ3 antagonists promote tumor regression by inducing apoptosis of angiogenic blood vessels. *Cell* 79:1157–1164.
31. Nicosia RF, Tchao R, Leighton J (1986) Interactions between newly formed endothelial channels and carcinoma cells in plasma clot culture. *Clin Exp Metastasis* 4:91–104.
32. Rak JW, Hegmann EJ, Lu C, Kerbel RS (1994) Progressive loss of sensitivity to endothelium-derived growth inhibitors expressed by human melanoma cells during disease progression. *J Cell Physiol* 159:245–255.
33. Hamada J, Cavanaugh PG, Lotan O (1992) Separable growth and migration factors for large-cell lymphoma cells secreted by microvascular endothelial cells derived from target organs for metastasis. *Br J Cancer* 66:349–354.
34. Folkman J (1994) Angiogenesis and breast cancer. *J Clin Oncol* 12:441–443.
35. Fox SB, Stuart N, Smith K, Brunner N, Harris AL (1993) High levels of uPA and PA-1 are associated with highly angiogenic breast carcinomas. *J Pathol* 170(Suppl):388a.
36. Moscatelli D, Gross J, Rifkin D (1981) Angiogenic factors stimulate plasminogen activator and collagenase production by capillary endothelial cells. *J Cell Biol* 91:201a.
37. Folkman J, Klagsbrun M (1987) Angiogenic factors. *Science* 235:442–447.
38. Furcht LT (1986) Critical factors controlling angiogenesis: Cell products, cell matrix, and growth factors. *Lab Invest* 55:505–509.
39. Denekamp J (1993) Review article: Angiogenesis, neovascular proliferation and vascular pathophysiology as targets for cancer therapy. *Br J Radiol* 66:181–196.
40. Mahadevan V, Hart IR (1990) Metastasis and angiogenesis. *Rev Oncol* 3:97–103.
41. Auerbach R, Arensman R, Kubai L, Folkman J (1975) Tumor-induced angiogenesis: Lack of inhibition by irradiation. *Int J Cancer* 15:241–245.
42. Sholley MN, Ferguson GP, Seibel HR, Montour JL, Wilson JD (1984) Mechanisms of neovascularization. Vascular sprouting can occur without proliferation of endothelial cells. *Lab Invest* 51:624–634.
43. Dvorak HF (1986) Tumors: Wounds that do not heal. Similarities between tumor stroma generation and wound healing. *N Engl J Med* 315:1650–1659.
44. Folkman J, Klagsbrun M (1987) Angiogenic factors. *Science* 235:442–447.
45. Polverini PJ, Leibovich SJ (1984) Induction of neovascularization in vivo and endothelial proliferation in vitro by tumor associated macrophages. *Lab Invest* 51:635–642.

46. Weidner N, Semple JP, Welch WR, Folkman J (1991) Tumor angiogenesis and metastasis — correlation in invasive breast carcinoma. *N Engl J Med* 324:1–8.
47. Guidi AJ, Fisher L, Harris JR, Schnitt SJ (1994) Microvessel density and distribution in ductal carcinoma in situ of the breast. *J Natl Cancer Inst* 86:614–619.
48. Smith-McCune KK, Weidner N, Bishop JM (1993) Cervical intraepi-thelial neoplasia (CIN) is angiogenic. *Proc Am Assoc Cancer Res* 34:74.
49. Baird A, Mormede P, Bohlen P (1985) Immunoreactive fibroblast growth factor in cells of peritoneal exudate suggests its identity with macrophage-derived growth factor. *Biochiem Biophys Res Commun* 126:358–364.
50. Frater-Schroder M, Risau W, Hallmann R, Gautschi P, Bohlen P (1987) Tumor necrosis factor type a, a potent inhibitor of endothelial cell growth in vitro, is angiogenic in vivo. *Proc Natl Acad Sci USA* 84:5277–5281.
51. Liebovich SJ, Plverini PJ, Shepard HM, Wiseman DM, Nusseir SVN (1987) Macrophage-induced angiogenesis is mediated by tumor necrosis factor-a. *Nature* 329:630–632.
52. Schreiber AB, Winkler ME, Derynck R (1986) Transforming growth factor-alpha: A more potent angiogenic mediator than epidermal growth factor. *Science* 232:1250–1253.
53. Hockel M, Jung W, Vaupel P, Rabes H, Khaledpour C, Wissler JH (1988) Purified mono-cyte-derived angiogenic substance (angiotropin) induces controlled angiogenesis associated with regulated tissue proliferation in rabbit skin. *J Clin Invest* 82:1075–1090.
54. Folkman J, Klagsbrun M, Sasse J, Wadzinski M, Ingber D, Vlodavsk I (1988) Heparin-binding angiogenic protein — basic fibroblast growth factor — is stored within basement membrane. *Am J Pathol* 130:393–400.
55. Knighton D, Hunt T, Scheuenstuhl H, Halliday BJ, Werb Z, Banda MJ (1983) Oxygen tension regulates the expression of angiogenesis factor by macrophages. *Science* 221:1283–1285.
56. Smolin G, et al. (1971) Lymphatic drainage from vasculrized rabbit cornea. *Am J Opthalmol* 72:147–151.
57. Kessler D, Langer R, Pless N, Folkman J (1976) Mast cells and tumor angiogenesis. *Int J Can* 18:703–709.
58. Glowacki J, Mulliken J (1982) Mast cells in hemangiomas and vascular malformations. *Pediatrics* 70:48–51.
59. Thornton S, Mueller S, Levine E (1983) Human endothelial cells: Use of heparin in cloning and long-term serial cultivation. *Science* 222:623–625.
60. Dethlefsen SM, Matsuura N, Zetter BR (1990) Tumor growth and angiogenesis in wild type mast cell deficient mice. *FASEB* 4:A623.
61. Kandel J, Bossy-Wetzel E, Radvani F, Klagsburn M, Folkman J, Hanahan D (1991) Neovascularization is associated with a switch to the export of bFGF in the multi-step development of fibrosarcoma. *Cell* 66:1095–1104.
62. Nguyen M, Watanabe H, Budson AE, Richie JP, Folkman J (1993) Elevated levels of the angiogenic peptide basic fibroblast growth factor in urine of bladder cancer patients. *J Natl Cancer Ins* 85:241–242.
63. Brown LF, Berse B, Jackman RW, Tognazzi K, Manseau EJ, Dvorak HF, Senger DR (1993) Increased expression of vascular permeability factor (vascular endothelial growth factor) and its receptors in kidney and bladder carcinomas. *Am J Pathol* 143:1255–1262.
64. Brown LF, Berse B, Jackman RW, Tognazzi K, Manseau EJ, Senger DR, Dvorak HF (1993) Expression of vascular permeability factor (vascular endothelial growth factor) and its receptors in adenocarcinomas of the gastrointestinal tract. *Cancer Res* 53:4727–4735.
65. Senger DR, Van De Water L, Brown LF, Nagy JA, Yeo K-T, Yeo T-K, Berse B, Jackman RW, Dvorak AM, Dvorak HF (1993) Vascular permeability factor (VPF, VEGF) in tumor biology. *Cancer Metab Rev* 12:303–324.
66. Goto F, Goto K, Weindel K, Folkman J (1993) Synergistic effects of vascular endothelial growth factor and basic fibroblast growth factor on the proliferation and cord formation of bovine capillary endothelial cells within collagen gels. *Lab Invest* 69:508–517.
67. Leibovich SJ, Polverini PJ, Fong TW, Harlow LA, Koch AE (1994) Production of angiogenic

acitivity by human monocytes requires an L-arginine/nitric oxide-synthase-dependent effector mechanism. *Proc Natl Acad Sci USA* 91:4190–4194.

68. Laniado-Schwartzman M, Lavrovsky Y, Stotlz RA, Conners MS, Falck JR, Chauhan K, Abraham NG (1994) Activation of nuclear factor kappa B and oncogene expression by 12(R)-hydroxyeicosatrienoic acid, an angiogenic factor in microvessel endothelial cells. *J Biol Chem* 269:2432–2437.

69. Bond MD, Vallee BL (1990) Replacement of residues of 8–22 of angiogenin with 7–21 of RNASE-A selectively affects protein-synthesis inhibition and angiogenesis. *Biochemistry* 29:3341–3349.

70. Bouck N, Stoler A, Polverini PJ (1986) Coordinate control of anchorage independence, actin cytoskeleton and angiogenesis by human chromosome 1 in hamster-human hybrids. *Cancer Res* 46:5101–5105.

71. Rastinegjad F, Polverini PF, Bouck NP (1989) Regulation of the activity of a new inhibitor of angiogenesis by a cancer suppressor gene. *Cell* 56:345–355.

72. Zajchowski DA, Band V, Trask DK, Kling D, Connoly JL, Sager R (1990) Suppression of tumor-forming ability and related traits in MCF -7 human breast cancer cells by fusion with immortal mam-mary epithelial cells. *Proc Natl Acad Sci USA* 87:2314–2318.

73. Dameron KM, Volpert OV, Tainsky MS, Bouck N (1994) Control of angiogenesis in fibroblasts by p53 regulation of thrombospondin-1. *Science* 265:1582–1584.

74. O'Reilly MS, Holmgren L, Shing Y, Chen C, Rosenthal RA, Moses M, Lane WS, Cao Y, Sage EH, Folkman J (1994) Angiostatin: A novel angiogenesis inhibitor that mediates the suppression of metastases by a Lewis lung carcinoma. *Cell* 79:315–328.

75. Folkman J (1995) Angiogenesis in cancer, vascular, rheumatoid, and other disease. *Nature Med* 1:27–31.

76. Fidler IJ, Gersten DM, Hart IR (1978) The biology of cancer invasion and metastasis. *Adv Cancer Res* 28:149–250.

77. Nicolson G (1979) Cancer metastasis. *Sci Am* 240:66–76.

78. Weiss L (1976) Biophysical aspects of the metastatic cascade. In *Fundamental Aspects of Metastasis*. L Weiss (ed). Amsterdam: North Holland, pp 51–70.

79. Bernstein LR, Liotta LA (1994) Molecular mediators of interactions with extracellular matrix components in metastasis and angiogenesis. *Curr Opin Oncol* 6:106–113.

80. Nagy JA, Brown LF, Senger DR, Lanir N, Van de Water L, Dvorak AM, Dvorak HF (1989) Pathogenesis of tumor stroma generation: A critical role for leaky blood vessels and fibrin deposition. *Biochim Biophys Acta* 948:305–26.

81. Moscatelli D, Gross J, Rifkin D (1981) Angiogenic factors stimulate plasminogen activator and collagenase production by capillary endothelial cells. *J Cell Biol* 91:201a.

82. Folkman J (1987) Angiogenesis. In *Thrombosis and Haemostasis*. M Verstraete, J Vermylen, R Lijnan, J Arnout (eds). Leuven: Leuven University Press, 24:583–596.

83. Liotta LA, Stracke ML (1988) In *Breast Cancer: Cellular and Molecular Biology*. ME Lippman, RB Dickson (eds). Boston: Kluwer Academic Publishers, pp 223–238.

84. Liotta L, Kleinerman J, Saidel G (1974) Quantitative relationships of intravascular tumor cells, tumor vessels, and pulmonary metastases following tumor implantation. *Cancer Res* 34:997–1004.

85. Liotta L, Saidel G, Kleinerman J (1976) The significance of hematogenous tumor cell clumps in the metastatic process. *Cancer Res* 36:889–894.

86. Kerbel RS, Waghorne C, Korczak B, Lagarde A, Breitman ML (1988) Clonal dominance of primary tumours by metastatic cells: Genetic analysis and biological implications. *Cancer Surv* 7:597–629.

87. Folkman J (1992) Tumor angiogenesis. In *Cancer Medicine*, 3rd ed. JF Holland, E Frei, RC Bast, DW Kufe, DL Morton, RR Weichselbaum (eds). Melbourne, PA: Lea & Febiger, Chap. 11.

88. Sugino T, Kawaguchi T, Suzuki T (1995) Stromal invasion is not essential to blood-borne metastasis in mouse mammary carcinoma. Scientific Program Booklet of the Pathological Society of Great Britain and Ireland, 170th Meeting, January 1995, abstract #161.

89. Brem S, Cotran R, Folkman J (1972) Tumor angiogenesis: A quantitative method for histologic grading. *J Natl Cancer Inst* 48:347–356.
90. Srivastava A, Laidler P, Davies R, Horgan K, Hughes LE (1988) The prognostic significance of tumor vascularity in intermediate-thickness (0.76–4.0 mm thick) skin melanoma. *Am J Pathol* 133:419–23.
91. Weidner N, Semple JP, Welch WR, Folkman J (1991) Tumor angiogenesis and metastasis — correlation in invasive breast carcinoma. N Engl J Med 324:1–8.
92. McComb RD, Jones TR, Pizzo SV, Bigner D (1982) Specificity and sensitivity of immunohistochemical dectection of factor VIII/von Villebrand factor antigen in formalin-fixed paraffin-embedded tissue. *J Histochem Cytochem* 30:371–377.
93. Gown AM, de Wever N, Battifora H (1993) Microwave-based antigenic unmasking. A revolutionary new technique for routine immunohistochemistry. *Appl Immunohistochem* 1:256–266.
94. Folkman J, Watson K, Ingber D, Hanahan D (1989) Induction of angiogenesis during the transition from hyperplasia to neoplasia. *Nature* 399:58–61.
95. Weidner N, Folkman J, Pozza F, Bevilacqua P, Allred EN, Moore DH, Meli S, Gasparini G (1992) Tumor angiogenesis: A new significant and independent prognostic indicator in early-stage breast carcinoma. *J Natl Cancer Inst* 84:1875–1887.
96. Bosari S, Lee AKC, DeLellis RA, et al. (1992) Microvessel quantitation and prognosis in invasive breast carcinoma. *Hum Pathol* 23:755–761.
97. Longacre TA, Rouse RV (1994) CD31: A new marker for vascular neoplasia. *Adv Anat Pathol* 1:16–20.
98. Horak E, Leek R, Klenk N, LeJeune S, Smith K, Stuart N, Greenall M, Stepniewska K, Harris AL (1992) Angiogenesis, assessed by platelet/endothelial cell adhesion molecule antibodies, as indicator of node metastases and survival in breast cancer. *Lancet* 340:1120–1124.
99. Gasparini G, Weidner N, Bevilacqua P, Maluta S, Dalla Palma P, Caffo O, Barbareschi M, Boracchi P, Marubini E, Pozza F (1994) Tumor microvessel density, p53 expression, tumor size, and peritumoral lymphatic vessel invasion are relevant prognostic markers in node-negative breast carcinoma. *J Clin Oncol* 12:454–466.
100. Toi M, Kashitani J, Tominaga T (1993) Tumor angiogenesis is an independent prognostic indicator of primary breast carcinoma. *Int J Cancer* 55:371–374.
101. Visscher DW, Smilanetz S, Drozdowicz S, Wykes SM (1993) Prognostic significance of image morphometric microvessel enumeration in breast carcinoma. *Anal Quant Cytolol Histol* 15:88–92.
102. Arihiro K, Inai K, Kurihara K, Takeda S, Kaneko M (1993) Distribution of laminin, type IV collagen, and fibronectin in the invasive component of breast carcinoma. *Acta Pathol Jpn* 43:758–764.
103. Sneige N, Singletary E, Sahin A, et al. (1992) Multiparameter analysis of potential prognostic factors in node negative breast cancer patients. *Mod Pathol* 5:18a.
104. Sahin AA, Sneige N, Ordonez GN, et al. (1993) Tumor angiogenesis detected by *Ulex europaeus* agglutinin 1 lectin (UEA1) and factor VIII immunostaining in node-negative breast carcinoma (NNBC) treated by mastectomy: Prediction of tumor recurrence. *Mod Pathol* 6:19a.
105. Obermair A, Czerwenka K, Kurz C, Buxbaum P, Schemper M, Sevela P (1994) Influence of tumoral microvessel density on the recurrence-free survival in human breast cancer: Preliminary results. *Onkologie* 17:44–49.
106. Bundred NJ, Bowcott M, Walls J, Faragher DD, Knox F (1994) Angiogenesis in breast cancer predicts node metastases and survival. *Br J Surg* 81:768.
107. Macchiarini P, Fontanini G, Hardin MJ, Hardin MJ, Squartini F, Angeletti CA (1992) Relation of neovasculature to metastasis of non-small-cell lung cancer. *Lancet* 340:145–146.
108. Macchiarini P, Fontanini G, Dulmet E, de Montpreville V, Chapelier AR, Cerrin J, Le Roy Ladurie F, Dartevelle PG (1994) Angiogenesis: An indicator of metastasis in non-small-cell lung cancer invading the thoracic inlet. *Ann Thorac Surg* 57:1534–1539.

109. Yamazaki K, Abe S, Takekawa H, Sukoh N, Watanabe N, Ogura S, Nakajima I, Isobe H, Inoue K, Kawakami Y (1994) Tumor angiogenesis in human lung adenocarcinoma. *Cancer* 74:2245–2250.
110. Wakui S, Furusato M, Itoh T, Sasaki H, Akiyama A, Kinoshita I, Asano K, Tokuda T, Aizawa S, Ushigome S (1992) Tumor angiogenesis in prostatic carcinoma with and without bone marrow metastasis: A morphometric study. *J Pathol* 168:257–262.
111. Weidner N, Carroll PR, Flax J, Blumenfeld W, Folkman J (1993) Tumor angiogenesis correlates with metastasis in invasive prostate carcinoma. *Am J Pathol* 143:401–409.
112. Fregene TA, Khanuja PS, Noto AC, Gehani SK, Van Egmont EM, Luz DA, Pienta KJ (1993) Tumor-associated angiogenesis in prostate cancer. *Anticancer Res* 13:2377–2381.
113. Brawer MK, Deering RE, Brown M, Preston SD, Bigler SA (1994) Predictors of pathologic stage in prostate carcinoma. *Cancer* 73:678–687.
114. Gasparini G, Weidner N, Bevilacqua P, Maluta S, Boracchi P, Testolin A, Pozza F, Folkman J (1993) Intratumoral microvessel density and p53 protein: Correlation with metastasis in head-and-neck squamous-cell carcinoma. *Int J Cancer* 55:739–744.
115. Mikami Y, Tsukuda M, Mochimatsu I, Kokatsu T, Yago T, Sawaki S (1991) Angiogenesis in head and neck tumors. *Nip Jib Gak Kai* 96:645–50.
116. Albo D, Granick MS, Jhala N, Atkinson B, Solomon MP (1994) The relationship of angiogenesis to biological activity in human squamous cell carcinomas of the head and neck. *Ann Plast Surg* 32:588–594, 1994.
117. Williams JK, Carlson GW, Cohen C, Derose PB, Hunter S, Jurkiewicz MJ (1994) Tumor angiogenesis as a prognostic factor in oral cavity tumors. *Am J Surg* 168:373–380.
118. Petruzzelli GJ, Snyderman CH, Johnson JT, Myers EN (1993) Angiogenesis induced by head and neck squamous cell carcinoma xenografts in the chick embryo chorioallantoic membrane model. *Ann Otol Rhinol Laryngol* 102:215–221.
119. Vesalainen S, Lipponen P, Talja M, Alhava E, Syrjanen K (1994) Tumor vascularity and basement membrane structure as prognostic factors in T1-2M0 prostatic adenocarcinoma. *Anticancer Res* 14:709–714.
120. Saclarides TJ, Speziale NJ, Drab E, Szeluga DJ, Rubin DB (1994) Tumor angiogenesis and rectal carcinoma. *Dis Colon Rectum* 37:921–926.
121. Olivarez D, Ulbright T, DeRiese W, Foster R, Reister T, Einhorn L, Sledge G (1994) Neovascularization in clinical stage A testicular germ cell tumor: Prediction of metastatic disease. *Cancer Res* 54:2800–2802.
122. Hollingworth HC, Steinberg SM, Kohn E, Bryant B, Merino MJ (1994) Tumor angiogenesis advanced stage ovarian cancer. *Mod Pathol* 7:89a.
123. Jaeger TM, Weidner N, Chew K, Moore DH, Kerschmann RL, Waldman FM, Carroll PR (1994) Tumor angiogenesis and lymph node metastases in invasive bladder carcinoma. *J Urol* 151:348A.
124. Barnhill RL, Fandrey K, Levy MA, Mihm MC, Hyman B (1992) Angiogenesis and tumor progression of melanoma. Quantitation of vascularity in melanocytic nevi and cutaneous melanoma. *Lab Invest* 67:331–337.
125. Barnhill RL, Levy MA (1993) Regressing thin cutaneous malignant melanomas (≤1.0 mm) are associated with angiogenesis. *Am J Pathol* 143:99–104.
126. Nasser I, Tahan S (1993) Angiogenesis in malanocytic lesions and its relationship to tumor progression. *Mod Pathol* 6:35A.
127. Fallowfield ME, Cook MG (1991) The vascularity of primary cutaneous melanoma. *J Pathol* 164:241–244.
128. Cockerell CJ, Sonnier G, Kelly L, Patel S (1994) Comparative analysis of neovascularization in primary cutaneous melanoma and Spitz nevus. *Am J Dermatopathol* 16:9–13.
129. Graham CH, Rivers J, Kerbel RS, Stankiewicz KS, White WL (1994) Extent of vascularization as a prgnostic indicator in thin (<0.76 mm) malignant melanomas. *Am J Pathol* 145:510–514.
130. Ewaskow SP, Collins CA, Conrad EU, Gown AM, Schmidt RA (1993) Quantitative assessment of blood vessel density and size in soft-tissue tumors. *Mod Pathol* 6:6A.

131. Li VW, Folkerth RD, Watanabe H, Yu C, Rupnick M, Barnes P, Scott RM, Black PM, Sallan SE, Folkman J (1994) Microvessel count and cerebrospinal fluid basic fibroblast growth factor in children with brain tumors. *Lancet* 334:82–86.

132. Vacca A, Ribatti D, Roncali L, Ranieri g, Serio G, Silvestris F, Dammacco F (1994) Bone marrow angiogenesis and progression in multiple myeloma. *Br J Haematol* 87:503–508.

133. Van Hoef MEHM, Knox WF, Dhesi SS, Howell A, Schor AM (1993) Assessment of tumor vascularity as a prognostic factor in lymph node negative invasive breast cancer. *Eur J Cancer* 29A:1141–1145.

134. Hall NR, Fish DE, Hunt N, Goldin RD, Guillou PJ, Monson JRT (1992) Is the relationship between angiogenesis and metastasis in breast cancer real? *Surg Oncol* 1:223–229.

135. Carnochan P, Briggs JC, Westbury G, Davies AJ (1991) The vascularity of cutaneous melanoma: A quantitative histologic study of lesions 0.85–1.25 mm in thickness. *Br J Cancer* 64:102–107.

136. Leedy DA, Trune DR, Kronz JD, Weidner N, Cohen JI (1994) Tumor angiogenesis, the p53 antigen, and cervical metastasis in squamous carcinoma. *Otolaryngol Head Neck Surg* 111:417–422.

137. Weidner N (1992) The relationship of tumor angiogenesis and metastasis with emphasis on invasive breast carcinoma. In *Advances in Pathology and Laboratory Medicine*, Vol 5. RS Weinstein (ed). Chicago: Mosby Year Book, pp 101–121.

138. Ordonez NG, Batsakis JG (1984) Comparison of *Ulex europaeus* I lectin and factor VIII-related antigen in vascular lesions. *Arch Pathol Lab Med* 108:129–132.

139. Lee AKC, DeLillis RA, Wolfe HJ (1986) Intramammary lymphatic invasion in breast carcinomas. Evaluation using ABH isoantigens as endothelial markers. Am J Surg Pathol 10:589–594.

140. Bettelheim R, Michell D, Gusterson BA (1984) Immunocytochemistry in the identification of vascular invasion in breast cancer. J Clin Pathol 37:364–366.

141. Kiyoshi M, Rosai J, Burgdorf WHC (1980) Localization of factor VIII-related antigens in vascular endothelial cells using an immunoperoxidase method. Am J Surg Pathol 4:273–276.

142. Mukai K, Rosai J (1984) Factor VIII-related antigen: An endothelial marker. In *Advances in Immunohistochemistry*. RA DeLellis (ed). New York: Masson Publishing USA, pp 253–261.

143. Nagle RB, Witte MH, Martinez AP, Witte CL, Hendrix MJC, Way D, Reed K (1987) Factor VIII-associated antigen in human lymphatic endothelium. *Lymphology* 20:20–24.

144. Lee AKC, DeLellis RA, Silverman ML, Wolfe HJ (1986) Perspectives in pathology. Lymphatic and blood vessel invasion in breast carcinoma: A useful prognostic indicator. *Hum Pathol* 17:984–987.

145. Svanholm H, Nielsen K, Hauge P (1984) Factor VIII-related antigen and lymphatic collecting vessels. *Virchows Arch A Pathol Anat* 404:223–228.

146. Ordonez NG, Brooks T, Thompson S, Batsakis JG (1987) Use of *Ulex europaeus* agglutinin I in the identification of lymphatic and blood vessel invasion in previously stained microscopic slides. *Am J Surg Pathol* 11:543–550.

147. Jain RK (1989) Delivery of novel therapeutic agents in tumors: Physiologic barriers and strategies. *J Natl Cancer Inst* 81:570–576.

148. Tanigawa N, Kanazawa T, Satomura K, et al. (1981) Experimental study on lymphatic vascular changes in the development of cancer. *Lymphology* 14:149–154.

149. Zeidman I, Copeland B, Warren S (1955) Experimental studies on the spread of cancer in the lymphatic system. II. Absence of lymphatic supply in carcinoma. *Cancer* 8:123–127.

150. Gilchrist RK (1950) Surgical management of advanced cancer of the breast. *Arch Surg* 61:913–929.

151. Papadimitriou JM, Woods AE (1975) Structural and functional characteristics of the microcirculation in neoplasms. *J Pathol* 116:65–72.

152. Barsky SH, Baker A, Siegal GP, Togo S, Liotta LA (1983) Use of anti-basement membrane antibodies to distinguish blood vessel capillaries from lymphatic capillaries. *Am J Surg Pathol* 7:667–677.

153. Schlingemann RO, Rietveld FJR, Kwaspen F, van de Kerkhof PCM, de Waal RMW, Ruiter DJ (1991) Differential expression of markers for endothelial cells, pericytes, and basal lamina in the microvasculature of tumors and granulation tissue. *Am J Pathol* 138:1335–1347.

154. Traweek ST, Kandalaft PL, Mehta P, Battifora H (1991) The human hematopoietic progenitor cell antigen (CD34) in vascular neoplasia. *Am J Clin Pathol* 96:25–31.

155. Herlyn M, Clark WH, Rodeck U, Mancianti ML, Jambrosic J, Koprowski H (1987) Biology of tumor progression in human melanocytes. *Lab Invest* 56:461–474.

156. DeYoung BR, Wick MR, Fitzgibbon JF, Sirgi KE, Swanson PE (1993) CD31: An immunospecific marker for endothelial differentiation in human neoplasms. *Appl Immunohistochem* 1:97–100.

157. van de Rijn M, Rouse RV (1994) CD34: A review. *Appl Immunohistochem* 2:71–80.

158. Wang JM, Kumar S, Pye D, Haboubi N, Al-Nakib L (1994) Breast carcinoma: Comparative study of tumor vasculature using two endothelial-cell markers. *J Natl Cancer Inst* 86:386–388.

159. Wang JM, Kumar S, Pye D, van Agthoven AJ, Krupinski J, Hunter RD (1993) A monoclonal antibody detects heterogeneity in vascular endothelium of tumors and normal tissues. *Int J Cancer* 54:363–370.

160. Barbareschi M, Gasparini G, Weidner N, Morelli L, Forti S, Eccher C, Fina P, Leonardi E, Mauri F, Bevilacqua P, Dalla Palma P (199••) Microvessel density quantification in breast carcinomas: Assessment by manual vs. a computer-assisted image analysis system. *Appl Immunohistochem*, in press.

161. Watanabe II, Nguyen M, Schizer M (1992) Basic fibroblast growth factor in human serum — a prognostic test for breast cancer. *Mol Biol Cell* 3:324a.

162. Nguyen M, Watanabe II, Budson AE (1994) Elevated levels of an angiogenic peptide, basic fibroblast growth factor, in the urine of patients with a wide spectrum of cancers. *J Natl Cancer Inst* 86:356.

15. Cell motility in breast cancer

Jason D. Kantor and Bruce R. Zetter

Introduction

Tumor growth and metastasis involve a complex interaction between tumor and nontumor cells, characterized by alterations in the regulation of cell behavior. The earliest stage of tumor formation is proliferation. Through genetic mutations, a cell or group of cells becomes refractory to normal growth regulation. The resultant mass of cells exerts pressure on surrounding tissue but does not cross tissue boundaries. Noninvasive tumors have been termed *benign* and can often be easily removed. The progression from a benign to a malignant tumor entails a series of steps involving both tumor cells and the surrounding tissue.

The first step toward malignant transformation is local invasion. Metastatic tumor cells possess the capacity to detach from neighboring cells, to degrade basement membrane and connective tissue, and to migrate and invade into neighboring tissue. As a result, tumor cells invade the stroma, lymph, and vasculature. Tumors that have invaded local tissues are more difficult to remove and can often compromise normal organ functions by disrupting tissue architecture.

Second, as a tumor grows it becomes nutrient limited. To meet the growing nutritional needs of the tumor, it must recruit new blood vessels. To do this, tumors secrete soluble factors that cause both directed migration and proliferation of capillary endothelial cells. Angiogenesis, the growth of new blood vessels, is necessary for tumor growth beyond the critical size of approximately 2 mm in diameter, the limit of nutrient diffusion [1]. The process by which endothelial cells vascularize tumors is analogous to the process by which tumor cells invade neighboring tissue. Endothelial cells respond to angiogenic factors by degrading subendothelial basement membrane and adjoining connective tissue, migrating toward the tumor, and proliferating. The consequence is the formation of new blood vessels supplying the tumor.

Third, tumor cells enter the vasculature and disperse throughout the body. Entry of tumor cells into the vasculature is largely dependent on angiogenesis. The abundance of newly formed capillaries in and around the tumor, and the increased permeability of these new vessels, provides ample opportunity for

R. Dickson and M. Lippman (eds.) MAMMARY TUMOR CELL CYCLE, DIFFERENTIATION AND METASTASIS. 1996. Kluwer Academic Publishers. ISBN 0-7923-3905-3. All rights reserved.

motile cells to escape the primary site. Intravasation, the process of entering the vasculature, is highly efficient, such that a 1 cm diameter murine mammary carcinoma can shed two million cells into the blood stream in 24 hours [2]. Once in the vasculature, cells must both evade the immune system and survive long enough to exit the vasculature. Extravasation, the process by which tumor cells exit the vasculature across the endothelial cell layer, is a normal function of leukocytes, involving adhesion to endothelial cells, degradation of extracellular matrix, and cell motility [3]. For tumor cells, extravasation is less efficient than intravasation because the intact vessels in normal tissue present a greater barrier to the passage of tumor cells than do the permeable, angiogenic blood vessels at the primary tumor site. Finally, cells that have successfully escaped the primary site and exited the vasculature migrate into the tissue of the secondary site and must again establish a source of nutrients through the recruitment of new blood vessels.

Central to the process of tumor metastasis is the phenomenon of cell motility. Local invasion, angiogenesis, intravasation, and extravasation all require active motility of tumor and endothelial cells. The source of stimulation and the nature of the motile response define three types of cell motility: chemotaxis, chemokinesis, and haptotaxis (Figure 1). *Chemotaxis* refers to the directional migration of a cell in response to a gradient of a soluble factor, such as peptide growth factors and fragments of extracellular matrix molecules. Tumor cell chemotaxis has been proposed to play a role in local invasion and site-specific metastasis [4–6]. In an analogous system, angiogenic factors such as VEGF are chemotactic for endothelial cells, causing local invasion of new blood vessels [7]. To recruit new vessels, tumor cells secrete angiogenic factors, creating a point source and establishing a chemotactic gradient that can be sensed by nearby endothelial cells expressing the proper receptor; these cells then migrate in the direction of the tumor. The relationship between motility and the concentration of chemoattractant exemplifies the underlying mechanism of chemotaxis. Migration of cells in the direction of a chemotactic gradient increases as the dose of chemoattractant increases, but at very high chemoattractant doses motility is inhibited. The resultant bell-shaped dose-response curve is a hallmark of chemotaxis. Cells may 'sense' the gradient of chemoattractant by the differential stimulation of membrane receptors across the cell surface. Chemotaxis occurs when a cell migrates in the direction of greater stimulation. As a cell moves up a concentration gradient or the chemoattractant concentration is artificially increased, cell surface receptors saturate and the resulting homogeneous stimulation does not elicit a motile response. Chemotaxis will not occur in cells exposed to a homogeneous concentration of chemoattractant.

Chemokinesis refers to the stimulation of randomly directed motility due to either an increased rate of cellular translocation or an increased distance traveled between direction changes. Chemokinesis is also stimulated by the activation of membrane-bound receptors by their ligands, but unlike chemoattractants, chemokinetic factors will maximally stimulate cell motility

Chemotaxis   Soluble concentration gradient

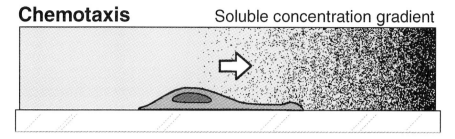

Chemokinesis   Uniform concentration

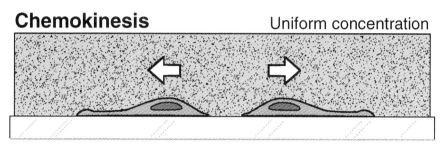

Haptotaxis

Immobilized
gradient

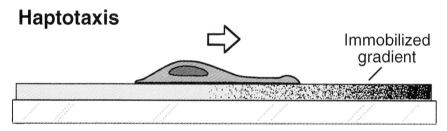

Figure 1. Three types of cell motility are defined by their source of stimulation. Chemotaxis is induced by a soluble concentration gradient. Chemokinesis is stimulated by soluble factors in the absence of a concentration gradient. Haptotaxis occurs when cells encounter an insoluble gradient of attractant.

in the absence of a soluble gradient. Chemokinetic factors, such as HGF/SF [8,9] and AMF [10], stimulate cell motility in tumor cells expressing the appropriate receptors and contribute to the process of local tissue invasion by promoting the radial spread of tumor cells away from the tumor. Cells exhibiting enhanced random motility will wander further from their initial position than cells that are less motile, and cells at the tumor margins are inhibited from moving back into the tumor by the high density of cells.

Haptotaxis refers to the directed migration of cells in response to a gradient of immobilized extracellular matrix. This term is frequently applied to the motility of cells placed on a substratum containing a gradient of a known adhesion molecule but can also be applied to movement in response to other immobilized attractants. Since many cells can respond to both soluble and insoluble extracellular matrix molecules, determining the contribution of

305

chemotaxis and haptotaxis can be difficult. Brandley and Schnaar have shown that it is possible to generate a solid phase gradient of attractant molecules in vitro [11]. Cells plated at uniform density will redistribute preferentially in the direction of increased attractant concentration after several hours [12,13]. This migration can be quantified and represents haptotaxis. Cells in vivo are more likely to be presented with a combination of soluble and insoluble attractants. For example, adhesive extracellular matrix molecules may be immobilized in a network or solubilized in fragments, and soluble growth factors may be free in solution or tightly bound to insoluble extracellular matrix molecules. Hence, the direction a cell moves may depend on the balance between chemotaxis and haptotaxis.

In this review, the relationship between cell motility and breast cancer is discussed with an emphasis on the molecules known to positively and negatively affect the regulation of cell motility in breast cancer. In addition, the methods for measuring cell motility and the distinction between random and directed migration are discussed.

Methods of measuring motility

Many methods are available to study cell motility, and each assay has its advantages and limitations. An understanding of these methods is essential in interpreting the literature. In this section, we describe a variety of methods commonly employed in the study of cell motility [14]. Direct observation by time lapse microscopy has been used to study chemokinesis and random unstimulated motility. When viewed at 360 times normal speed, aspects of cell motility can be observed and subjectively scored. The ability to separately quantify translocation, pseudopod extension, membrane ruffling, and cell shape is a unique advantage of this technique and has proven useful in predicting, for example, the metastatic potential of Dunning rat prostate carcinoma cell lines [15,16]. Although this method has been shown to produce consistent results independent of the observer [17], the subjective basis of scoring motility is a distinct disadvantage. Computer Fourier analysis of cell shape can substitute for subjective human grading and provide quantitative measurements of cell motility [18]. The wealth of morphological data produced by this technique can be useful, but the expense of the system is a disadvantage.

In vitro 'wound healing' assays are also used to study chemokinesis and random unstimulated motility. In this assay, a confluent monolayer of cells is 'wounded' by scraping away a thin line of cells, and the rate at which cells enter the denuded zone is used as a measurement of cell motility. Depending on the size of the wound, this assay can take days and has the added complication that proliferation can contribute to wound healing. In addition, cells in a monolayer may be in G_0 and/or inhibited in their motility by close contact with neighboring cells. As a result, differences in wound healing between cell types may reflect differences unrelated to motility. However, the simplicity of this assay is an advantage.

The phagokinetic track assay measure chemokinesis and random unstimulated motility based on the ability of migrating cells to phagocytose small gold or plastic particles as they move across a dish [19]. Cells are plated sparsely on a coated surface, and after many hours cell motility is quantified by measuring the average area that a single cell clears. The shape of the area cleared by a cell can provide additional information. For example, a cell moving rapidly but changing directions frequently may clear a circular region of gold particles. In contrast, a cell making infrequent direction changes will clear jagged tracks of particles.

To separately measure the effect of chemotaxis and random motility, a modified Boyden chamber is often used. In this assay, two chambers (upper and lower well) are separated by a porous filter. Cells are placed in the top well and the chemotattractant or chemokinetic factor is placed in either the top well, the bottom well, or both. The membrane serves as a limited barrier to the cells and establishes a soluble concentration gradient by slowing diffusion between the two chambers. After an incubation of 4–5 hours, the filter is removed and the 'cell side' of the filter is scraped. Cells that migrate to the other side of the filter are fixed, stained, and counted. In this assay, a chemoattractant will stimulate cells to cross the membrane only if it is at a higher concentration in the lower chamber, whereas a chemokinetic factor will stimulate cells to cross the filter when the factor is in either the top or the bottom well. The measurement of the effect of different concentrations of attractant in both the bottom and top well is often called a *checkerboard* analysis [20]. The Boyden chamber assay has the advantage of providing a quantitative distinction between chemotaxis and chemokinesis.

The Transwell assay utilizes the same two-chamber principle as Boyden chambers, but in this assay the top well and filter are a unit placed in a tissue culture dish. Like the Boyden chamber, the Transwell assay allows quantifiable measurements of chemotaxis and chemokinesis. In addition, cells can be grown in the bottom chamber, and the production of motility factors can be measured by the motility of cells placed in the top chamber. The size and structure of the chamber permit motility analysis of a greater number of cells, facilitating biochemical analysis of cells in the top chamber. However, the increased volume can be a disadvantage when studying motility factors that are expensive or difficult to purify.

The under-agarose assay utilizes the diffusion retardation properties of agarose to establish a two-dimensional concentration gradient of a chemotactic factor across the surface of a tissue culture dish. A tissue culture plate is covered with a thin layer of agarose in which three small wells are cut. Cells are plated in the central well, medium containing a motility factor is placed in a neighboring well, and the third well contains control medium. Without motility stimulators present, cells will spread radially due to unstimulated random migration. If, however, the neighboring well contains a chemoattractant, cells will migrate preferentially toward the chemoattractant. The difference between the migration distance in the direction of the chemoattractant well and the distance in the direction of the control well provides a measurement of chemotaxis. Like the wound healing assay, the under-agarose assay can take several days and can be complicated by the effects of concomitant proliferation.

Haptotaxis is not often measured precisely. Brandley and Schnaar described an assay to measure haptotaxis of melanoma cells on an adhesive gradient of immobilized RGD peptides [12]. The integrin binding peptide Arg-Gly-Asp (RGD) is immobilized in a polyacrylamide gel. Cells are plated uniformly on the gel, and after several hours the distribution of cells on the gel is analyzed by computer. The results indicate that melanoma cells redistribute in the direction of increasing insoluble RGD peptide. In other cases, the Boyden chamber assay has been used under conditions in which adhesion molecules are coated onto only one side of the filter, creating a step gradient [21]. One caveat with this approach is that some portion of the adsorbed attractant may become solubilized during the course of the assay and may act as a conventional chemotactic stimulus.

Tumor cell motility

The relationship between motility and metastasis has been well described for the Dunning R3327 rat prostatic adenocarcinoma model. Mohler and Coffey analyzed cells using time-lapse video microscopy [15–17]. By viewing these cells in culture at 360 times normal speed, an observer could grade (from 0 to 5) the amount of membrane ruffling, pseudopod extensions, and cell translocation. When this analysis was applied to Dunning cell lines of different metastatic potential that were otherwise indistinguishable, each of the three motility grades could predict high or low metastatic potential. The best accuracy (96%) was obtained when both cell translocation and pseudopod extension were considered. Subsequent analysis of these cells using Fourier analysis to quantify cell motility also accurately predicted metastatic potential [18]. These results strongly suggest a link between tumor cell motility and metastatic potential.

In normal adult breast tissue, cell motility is tightly regulated and is largely limited to macrophages and lymphocytes. Abnormal regulation of tumor cell and endothelial cell motility can result from (1) a local increase in production and secretion of motility factors by tumor cells, (2) production of motility factors by nontumor cells locally at the site of the tumor, (3) increased systemic production of motility factors, (4) alterations in the expression of intracellular proteins that regulate cell motility, and (5) alterations in the expression and activation of enzymes that modify and degrade the basement membrane. In each of these cases, motility can be regulated both positively and negatively, and the balance between stimulation and inhibition deter-

308

mines the direction and extent of cell motility. The consequences of increased cell motility include increased tumor vascularization and tumor invasion.

Local motility-stimulating cytokines

Production of cell motility–stimulating cytokines by tumor cells and tumor-associated stromal cells provides a local environment that promotes invasion and/or angiogenesis. Autocrine motility factors and scatter factor both act locally in breast tumors to support motility and may play a role in malignant progression. Autocrine stimulation of tumor cell motility occurs in cells that both produce and respond to the same factor. Both human breast and melanoma cells produce autocrine motility factors [22,23,24], and it is believed that the production of these factors promotes tumor invasion by increasing the random motility of tumor cells. Liotta and colleagues originally purified a 55 kD tumor cell autocrine motility factor (AMF) from melanoma cell conditioned media [23]. Checkerboard analysis indicated that AMF stimulates chemokinesis in the cells that produce it. Microscopic analysis revealed that stimulation of breast tumor cells with AMF leads to the formation of pseudopod extensions enriched in receptors for the extracellular matrix molecules laminin and fibronectin [25]. Although AMF is defined by its ability to stimulate motility in cells that produce it, the production of AMF by a cell or a subpopulation of cells in a tumor may also promote the motility of nearby nonproducing tumor cells. In addition to the 55 kD AMF, a number of different molecules have been identified that have autocrine motility activity. Most recently, Liotta and colleagues purified autotaxin from human melanoma conditioned media [22]. Autotaxin is functionally similar to previously characterized autocrine motility factors, but its size and partial amino acid sequence identify it as a novel factor.

Stimulation of tumor cell motility by members of the AMF family of molecules may contribute to tumor metastasis. Production of AMF by highly metastatic rat mammary adenocarcinoma cell lines was greater than in low metastatic lines [24]. In addition, high levels of AMF in the urine of patients with bladder cancer correlate with increased tumor progression [26]. Although a direct link between AMF production and human breast cancer metastasis has not been established, the current data support a role for AMF in increased motility and invasiveness of breast tumor cells.

Tumor cell motility can also be stimulated by parcrine factors produced by nontumor cells. For example, fibroblasts can produce a cytokine, known as hepatocyte growth factor or scatter factor (HGF/SF), that dissociates epithelial cells by stimulating cell motility and promoting detachment of cell–cell contacts [27]. Recent work describing the production and action of HGF/SF in breast cancer provides a working model for the role of HGF/SF in breast cancer metastasis. Production and secretion of HGF/SF by tumor-associated fibroblasts are stimulated by the production of an unknown low-molecular-weight factor by breast tumor cells [28,29]. HGF/SF stimulates chemokinesis in murine breast tumor cells [29], and this effect may be greater in poorly differentiated breast tumors that have been shown to express the c-met receptor [30]. Activation of cells by HGF/SF is dependent on the cell surface expression of the c-met tyrosine kinase receptor [31]. HGF/SF may also promote metastasis by recruiting new blood vessels to the tumor. Angiogenesis is stimulated by HGF/SF, a response that is due in part to the stimulation of endothelial cell chemotaxis and random motility by HGF/SF [32–35]. Additionally, high levels of HGF/SF in the lungs of BalbC mice [29] may promote extravasation of mouse mammary tumors into the lung, a preferred site of metastasis for many mouse mammary tumors.

The importance of HGF/SF in breast tumor metastasis is further supported by clinical and experimental animal observations. High levels of HGF/SF in samples of human breast tumors correlate with shorter relapse-free and overall survival time [36]. In addition, injection of mammary tumor cells that have been pretreated with HGF/SF into the tail vein of BalbC mice produces a small but significant increase in lung tumors compared with control, untreated cells [29].

Systemic cytokines

In addition to locally acting motility factors, cytokines produced by a variety of cell types may influence tumor formation and progression systemically by affecting the motility of tumor cells and/or nontumor cells. Migration-stimulating factor (MSF) and interleukin-6 provide two such examples. Migration-stimulating factor is produced by fetal fibroblasts and induces the motility of either adult or fetal fibroblasts into three-dimensional collagen gels. As a result, fetal fibroblasts can invade collagen gels through autocrine stimulation by MSF, while adult fibroblasts do not significantly invade collagen gels without the addition of exogenous MSF. Tumor-derived fibroblasts from approximately 50% of sporadic human breast tumors and 90% of familial tumors have migratory phenotypes similar to fetal fibroblasts [37]. Moreover, Haggie et al. reported that skin-derived fibroblasts from over 90% of patients with familial breast cancer and 50% of their unaffected first-degree relatives displayed the fetal-fibroblast phenotype [38]. Migration-stimulating factor could also be detected in the serum of breast cancer patients both before and after tumor resection, and no MSF could be detected in control serum. Because MSF persists after tumor resection and fetal-like fibroblasts are present in the skin of both tumor patients and people predisposed to breast tumors, it has been hypothesized that a systemic effect of MSF persists in the absence of primary tumor mass and may precede and contribute to tumor formation [39].

Although it is too early to say conclusively whether fetal-like fibroblasts and MSF production predispose one to breast cancer, Sakakura reported in 1983 that implantation of fetal fibroblasts into rat mammary tissue could induce hyperplasia [40]. This phenomenon was not observed when adult fibroblasts were similarly injected. Recently, however, the distinction between the adult and fetal fibroblast phenotypes has become obscure [41], making it difficult to assign a role for MSF in tumor progression and cell motility. In fact, Schor et al. reported that the effect of MSF on cell motility may be indirect and may require the synthesis of hyaluronic acid [42]. The relationship between MSF and motility requires further clarification. All studies of MSF employed the collagen invasion assay, which does not directly measure motility. Boyden chamber analysis of MSF may help to determine whether the effect on fibroblasts is due to random motility, chemotaxis, or haptotaxis.

Interleukin-6 (IL-6), another systemic cytokine, may have a more direct effect on breast tumor cells. In response to inflammation-associated cytokines, IL-6 is produced by a wide variety of cells, including fibroblasts, keratinocytes, endothelial cells, smooth muscle cells, and monocyte/macrophages [43]. IL-6 acts systemically and can be detected in the circulation of patients with infection, injury, or tumors. Among its numerous and pleitropic effects, IL-6 acts directly on breast tumor cells, affecting both growth and motility. IL-6 is a potent inhibitor of breast tumor cell proliferation. Treatment of breast tumor cells with IL-6 will cause dissociation of epithelial-like cell clusters, due to the loss of cell–cell adhesions and an increase in random motility 44]. IL-6–treated breast tumor cells viewed in culture using time-lapse photography exhibit increased filopodial extensions and increased cellular translocation. All this said, however, it remains unclear what effect IL-6 has on the progression and metastasis of breast tumors in vivo.

Tumor cell motility genes

The presence of motility factors in and around tumors is not sufficient to produce metastasis. As tumor cells progress from a benign lesion to a malignant tumor, gene expression changes as a result of genetic mutations and clonal selection. By identifying genes that are differentially expressed between high and low metastatic tumors of the same origin, it has been possible to determine some of the cellular processes that are important in providing selective advantage to metastatic cells. Two examples that implicate cell motility in metastasis are presented here.

Mts-1 was identified as a result of its overexpression in highly metastatic mouse mammary carcinoma cells compared with the low metastatic parental line [45]. Mts-1 is a member of the S100 family of Ca^{2+} binding proteins. Its expression is highest in the spleen, thymus, bone marrow, and lymphocytes [46,47]. Mts-1 is homologous to a rat protein, p9Ka, whose expression is also upregulated in metastatic mammary carcinoma cells [48]. Overexpression of p9Ka in a rat mammary epithelial cell line results in an increase in metastasis to the lung [48–50]. Conversely, overexpression of an mts-1 antisense construct in mouse metastatic mammary carcinoma cells leads to a reduction in metastatic potential [46]. These results strongly support the hypothesis that mts-1 and p9Ka function as positive regulators of mammary tumor metastasis.

Overexpression of mts-1 has been correlated with an increase in cell motility [51,52]. In that study, random motility measured by phagokinesis was increased in cell lines that expressed high levels of mts-1 as a result of transformation or transfection. Similarly, high levels of mts-1 expression are normally found in nontumor cells that exhibit high rates of cell motility, including neutrophils, T lymphocytes, and activated macrophages [46,51]. The mechanism by which mts-1 affects cell motility is not known, but recent studies indicate that mts-1 is associated with the actin cytoskeleton [48,53]. Specific binding interactions between mts-1 and both nonmuscle myosin [54,55] and nonmuscle tropomyosin [56] may provide the biochemical basis for the observed actin colocalization.

Another gene, nm23, was identified based on its differential expression between high and low metastatic murine melanoma cell lines [57]. In contrast to mts-1, nm23 was more highly expressed in the low metastatic lines. Of the two human homologues, nm23-H1 and nm23-H2, only nm23-H1 is differentially expressed between high and low metastatic tumors. In human breast carcinomas, decreased levels of nm23-H1 have been correlated with greater invasiveness [58] and lymph node metastasis [59–63], and two studies found nm23-H1 expression associated with a good prognosis [64,65]. Although some reports suggest that a decrease in nm23 expression is not correlated with breast tumor invasion [66], most evidence supports the observation that nm23-H1 expression is inversely correlated with breast cancer metastasis. Lastly, stable clones of metastatic human breast carcinoma [67] and mouse melanoma [68] cell lines overexpressing nm23-H1 (or mouse nm23) exhibited a significant reduction in tumor metastasis, supporting the hypothesis that nm23-H1 functions as a suppressor of the metastatic phenotype.

The mechanism by which nm23-H1 suppresses metastasis in breast carcinoma cells remains unknown. However, expression of nm23 in both human breast carcinoma and murine melanoma cell lines inhibits serum and growth factor–stimulated chemotaxis and chemokinesis without affecting basal random motility [69]. In addition, cells transfected with nm23-H1 remain responsive to the motility stimulating effects of lysophosphatidic acid (unpublished data). The loss of motility in response to several but not all motility factors indicates that nm23-H1 affects motility subsequent to receptor binding and does not cripple the motility machinery. The mechanism by which nm23-H1 inhibits stimulated cell motility remains unknown and is the focus of ongoing research. To date, the only molecule found to associate with nm23-H1 is nm23-H2, which has also been shown to bind to the c-*myc* promoter and to stimulate transcription [70,71]. Although the interraction of nm23-H2 with the promotor region of c-*myc* may be rather nonspecific [M Veron, personal communication], the association of nm23-H1 with nm23-H2 may have an effect on either the localization or the nuclear function of nm23-H2. Identifying the nuclear function of nm23-H2 may help one understand how nm23-H1 inhibits cell motility and tumor metastasis.

Although there is no clear explanation of how nm23 inhibits both metastasis and tumor cell motility, a great deal is known about this protein. Nm23-H1 and nm23-H2 (identical to human erythrocyte NDPK A and B) have molecular weights of 18,500 and 17,000, respectively, and exist as stable hexamers. These hexamers function as nucleoside diphosphate kinases (NDPK), transferring high-energy phosphates from NTP to NDP with a histidine-phosphorylated enzyme intermediate. In addition to its function as an NDPK, nm23 and its homologue in *Myxococcus xanthus* have both been reported to autophosphorylate on serine residues [72,73], and nm23-H1 autophosphorylation was observed to be a better predictor of metastatic potential than NDPK activity [72]. Recent work on nm23-H1, NDPK from *Dictyostelium discoideum*, and NDPK from *Myxococcus xanthus* questions the relevance of this serine autophosphorylation, arguing that the low stoichiometry of phosphate incorporation excludes a role of autophosphorylation in regulating overall enzyme activity [74].

It has been proposed that the opposing effects of mts-1 and nm23-H1 are due to changes in microtubule polymerization [75]. Although NDPK from pigs has been shown to shorten the lag time of in vitro tubulin polymerization [76], no direct interaction between nm23-H1 and either tubulin or microtubules has been observed [77]. Mts-1 appears to be closely associated with the actin/myosin cytoskeleton and not microtubules. An effect of nm23-H1 and mts-1 on microtubule polymerization cannot be ruled out, but strong evidence to support this hypothesis is lacking. The identification of both positive and negative regulators of metastasis, along with their connection to tumor cell motility, argues that tumor cell motility strongly influences the metastatic potential of breast tumors.

Angiogenesis

The formation of new tumor associated blood vessels facilitates solid tumor growth and metastasis to distant sites [78,79]. As a tumor mass grows, the availability of nutrients becomes diffusion limited, and the tumor seldom grows beyond 1–2 mm in diameter [1,80]. Further progression occurs when a subpopulation of cells within the tumor becomes angiogenic, and newly formed microvessels sprout from nearby capillaries and perfuse the tumor [81]. The availability of nutrients supports further tumor cell proliferation, and the permeability of newly forming microvessels increases the opportunity for tumor cells to metastasize. The importance of angiogenesis in the progression of breast cancer has been demonstrated by staining sections of primary human breast tumors with antibodies to endothelial cell–specific markers, such as factor VIII–related antigen or CD31. The number of endothelial cells counted in an area of high endothelial cell density within a tumor section provides a useful prognostic indicator of survival in both node-positive and node-negative breast cancer patients [82–89].

The angiogenic phenotype is characterized by the release of angiogenic factors from tumor cells, tumor-associated cells, extracellular matrix molecules, and endothelial cells. Most angiogenic stimulators are polypeptides, many of which bind to heparin in the extracellular matrix. Notable exceptions include prostaglandins E_1 and E_2, derived from lipids, and the small cofactor molecule nicotinamide. Endothelial cells expressing the appropriate receptors will proliferate and/or migrate in response to angiogenic stimulation [90]. Tumor neovascularization may depend on the release of multiple angiogenic factors.

The process of tumor neovascularization is similar to tumor cell invasion of local tissue Endothelial cells responding to angiogenic stimulation degrade subendothelial basement membrane molecules, migrate into neighboring tissue, proliferate, form tubes and loops, and secrete new basement membrane. Inhibition in any one step is sufficient to reduce neovascularization. Endothelial cell motility is an early and ongoing process in the development of new blood vessels. Blocking endothelial proliferation will inhibit neovascularization but will not affect the formation of vascular sprouts, which form early in the angiogenic process and are believed to be dependent on cell motility [91]. The role of endothelial cell motility in the formation of capillary networks has been analyzed by computer modeling [92]. Stokes and Lauffenburger [92] concluded that endothelial cell migration is rate limiting in the formation of vascular networks; thus, the growth of a single vessel follows the path and progresses at the rate of the motile endothelial cell at the vessel tip. The extent to which the new blood vessels invade the neighboring tumor and form a network structure depends on the relative contribution of chemotaxis and chemokinesis to endothelial cell migration. For example, chemokinetic stimulation of endothelial cells by an angiogenic factor results in a disorganized distribution of vessels randomly oriented with respect to the tumor. On the other hand, stimulation of chemotaxis by a tumor-derived angiogenic factor causes vessels to grow in the direction of the tumor. A combination of chemotactic and chemokinetic motility may be required for proper vascularization to occur.

To understand the process of angiogenesis in human breast tumors, the angiogenic factors involved must be identified and characterized with respect to their effect on endothelial cell motility and proliferation. Three peptides have been identified as the most likely contributors to neovascularization of human breast tumors. Vascular endothelial growth factor (VEGF) is expressed by a majority of tested human breast tumor lines [93], and its expression is correlated with both increased microvessel density and early relapse in human breast tumors [83,94]. In addition, increased expression of VEGF receptors has been observed in small blood vessels adjacent to invasive breast tumors [95]. Basic fibroblast growth factor (bFGF) is a potent angiogenic factor detectable in elevated quantities in the serum of 6% of breast cancer patients and correlates with increased mortality [96]. Platelet-derived endo-thelial cell growth factor (PD-ECGF) is also expressed in most human breast tumor cell lines [93], but its involvement in human breast tumor progression is not well understood. All three factors stimulate endothelial cell motility [97–99,115]. VEGF is a potent stimulator of endothelial cell chemotaxis at doses as low as 1 ng/ml, and VEGF also stimulates endothelial cell chemokinesis. bFGF preferentially stimulates chemokinesis of endothelial cells at a dose of 1 ng/ml. The migration stimulation of endothelial cells by VEGF and bFGF is additive. PD-ECGF also stimulates endothelial cell chemotaxis, with no chemokinetic component at a dose of 10 ng/ml, higher than for either VEGF or bFGF. Although it is difficult to accurately measure the in vivo extracellular concen-tration of these angiogenic factors, the relative abundance of these factors influences the degree of tumor vascularization in human breast tumors by inducing endothelial cells to migrate both directionally and randomly.

Extracellular matrix

The relationship between the extracellular matrix (ECM) and migrating cells is complex. Extracellular matrix can serve as a source of 'traction' for cell locomotion, a barrier to further movement, a chemical or physical gradient for chemotactic and haptotactic motility, and an inhibitor of stimulated cell motil-ity. The basement membrane is a specialized form of extracellular matrix that underlies epithelial cells and surrounds blood vessels. Its major constituents include collagen, laminin, and fibronectin. Interactions between tumor cells and basement membrane include adhesion via integral membrane proteins such as integrins, active degradation by specific cell associated proteinases, inhibition of proteinases by cell-secreted proteinase inhibitors, and active deposition of new matrix molecules. Invasive tumors are characterized by a disruption of basement membrane integrity, and breast tumor cell lines have been shown to possess basement membrane degradation activity, which is increased in highly metastatic cells relative to low metastatic cells [100–102].

Degradation of basement membrane proteins is dependent on the activity of four classes of proteinases: serine proteinases, aspartyl proteinases, cysteinyl proteinases, and metalloproteinases. Metalloproteinases, including interstitial collagenases, type IV collagenases, and stromelysins, are respon-sible for the degradation of the major basement membrane proteoglycans. In particular, type IV collagenases, which are unique in their ability to degrade the helical portion of type IV collagen, have been linked to breast tumor progression. Human breast tumors express increased amounts of type IV collagenase relative to nontumor cells, and type IV collagenase is further increased in invasive and metastatic breast tumors [103–105]. Type IV collage-nases are produced as latent proenzymes, lacking enzymatic activity, which form a complex with endogenous tissue inhibitors of metalloproteinases (TIMPs). Upregulation of type IV collagenase activity in metastatic breast cell lines can result from either an increase in proenzyme activation [106] or a decrease in expression of TIMP [107].

Local degradation of basement membrane proteins indirectly facilitates breast tumor cell motility. First, the basement membrane constitutes a cell impermeable barrier that must be breached to allow passage of migrating cells into neighboring tissue. Moreover, soluble fragments of collagen and soluble type I collagen are chemotactic for breast tumor cells [108]. Local collagen degradation may establish a concentration gradient of soluble collagen fragments, which can enhance tumor cell chemotaxis and promote invasion. Similarly, local degradation of extracellular matrix produces an adhesive gradient that may promote tumor cell haptotaxis. Inhibition of type IV collagenases by TIMPs may indirectly inhibit tumor cell motility by preventing the degradation of basement membrane. In addition, tissue inhibitors of metalloproteinases have been shown to play a direct role in regulating cell motility. Three TIMPs have been identified in humans: TIMP-1, TIMP-2, and TIMP-3. All three have been tested for their ability to inhibit endothelial cell migration. TIMP-1 inhibits adipocyte conditioned media stimulated endothelial cell motility with half-maximal inhibition at ~50 ng/ml [109]. TIMP-2 partially inhibits bFGF-stimulated motility of endothelial cells at a dose of 10 μg/ml [110]. This effect is limited to acute exposure to TIMP-2. Longer exposures (16 hours) produce no inhibition of motility. TIMP-3, however, is a potent inhibitor of both bFGF-induced chemokinesis and VEGF-stimulated chemotaxis of endothelial cells. Doses of TIMP-3 as low as 1.0 ng/ml inhibit motility as much as 50% with no pretreatment [B Anand-Apte, personal communication]. The production of TIMPs at the site of tumor formation can inhibit metastasis by disrupting endothelial cell motility.

Collagen deposition may also affect breast tumor motility. Alterations in the collagen composition of breast tissue have been described for ductal infiltrating carcinoma (DIC) [111,112]. DIC is associated with an increase in type I trimer collagen and type V collagen [113]. Interestingly, breast tumor cells grown in vitro on type I trimer collagen showed enhanced random motility compared with cells plated on type I collagen [114]. Further experiments are required to determine the role of matrix stimulated motility in breast cancer.

Conclusions

Tumor growth and metastasis involve a complex interaction between tumor and nontumor cells, characterized by alterations in the regulation of cell behavior. Stimulated cell motility is a complex process involving the production of motility factors, the recognition of motility factors by membrane receptors, and the subsequent coordinated cellular responses of pseudopod extension and cellular translocation. Cells respond both directionally (chemotaxis) and randomly (chemokinesis) to stimulation by soluble factors. The relative amount of chemotaxis and chemokinesis can have a dramatic effect on the direction and extent of the motile response.

Growth and metastasis of breast tumors are facilitated by increased cell motility. Endothelial cells migrate during the process of neovascularization, and tumor cells migrate during local invasion, intravasation, and extravasation. Factors acting locally in breast tumors to increase cell motility include AMF, HGF/SF, bFGF, VEGF, and PD-ECGF. Increased expression of these factors contributes to tumor cell motility (AMF and HGF/SF) and endothelial cell motility (HGF/SF, bFGF, VEGF, PD-ECGF), which together promote the growth and spread of breast tumors. Factors acting systemically to induce cell motility in breast cancer include MSF and IL-6. Elevated levels of these cytokines have been associated with breast tumors.

The increased ability of breast cancer cells to migrate in response to stimulation is associated with increased invasiveness. Proteins expressed intracellularly may act as positive or negative regulators of the motile response. In breast cancer, decreased expression of nm23-H1 and increased expression of mts-1 are associated with invasiveness and increased cell motility. The relative expression of positive and negative regulators of tumor cell motility may influence the progression of breast tumors.

Interactions between cells and the extracellular matrix can regulate cell motility. Collagen, fibronectin, and laminin can stimulated cell motility both as soluble fragments (chemotaxis) and as an insoluble gradient (haptotaxis). Expression and activation of matrix matalloproteinases and the expression of natural proteinase inhibitors, TIMPs, provides positive and negative regulation of the degradation of basement membrane proteins. In addition, metalloproteinases and their inhibitors can directly stimulate and inhibit motility of endothelial cells. The overall effect of proteinase activity on cell motility in vivo is difficult to determine, but increased activity of matrix metalloproteinases is associated with increased invasiveness in breast cancer.

The molecular basis of the regulation of tumor associated cell motility remains poorly understood. Ongoing efforts to identify new proteins relevant to both tumor metastasis and cell motility will provide new insights into tumor progression. The identification of proteins such as nm23-H1 and mts-1 stresses the necessity to understand intracellular mechanisms that regulate cell motility. The past decade has produced an invaluable wealth of information explaining how mitogenic signals can be transduced across the membrane and stimulate gene expression and mitogenesis. Many of the same stimuli that induce proliferation also induce cell motility, but often at significantly different doses. The molecular basis of signal transduction from membrane receptors to the intracellular motility machinery remains unclear and represents the future of motility research. By identifying the cellular components that regulate cell motility, it may be possible to design better therapies for the treatment of breast tumors.

References

1. Gimbrone M Jr, Leapman SB, Cotran RS, Folkman J (1972) Tumor dormancy in vivo by prevention of neovascularization. *J Exp Med* 136:261–276.
2. Butler TP, Gullino PM (1975) Quantitation of cell shedding into efferent blood of mammary adenocarcinoma. *Cancer Res* 35:512–516.
3. Downey GP (1994). Mechanisms of leukocyte motility and chemotaxis. *Curr Opin Immunol* 6:113–124.
4. Cerra RF, Nathanson SD (1989) Organ-specific chemotactic factors present in lung extracellular matrix. *J Surg Res* 46:422–426.
5. Ozaki T, Yoshida K, Ushijima K, Hayashi H (1971) Studies on the mechanisms of invasion in cancer. II. In Vivo effects of a factor chemotactic for cancer cells. *Int J Cancer* 7:93–100.
6. Hujanen ES, Terranova VP (1985) Migration of tumor cells to organ-derived chemoattractants. *Cancer Res* 45:3517–3521.
7. Koch AE, Harlow LA, Haines GK, Amento EP, Unemori EN, Wong WL, Pope RM, Ferrara N (1994) Vascular endothelial growth factor. A cytokine modulating endothelial function in rheumatoid arthritis. *J Immunol* 152:4149–4156.
8. Weidner KM, Hartmann G, Sachs M, Birchmeier W (1993) Properties and functions of scatter factor/hepatocyte growth factor and its receptor c-Met [review]. *Am J Respir Cell Mol Biol* 8:229–237.
9. Weidner KM, Hartmann G, Naldini L, Comoglio PM, Sachs M, Fonatsch C, Rieder H, Birchmeier W (1993) Molecular characteristics of HGF-SF and its role in cell motility and invasion [review]. *EXS* 65:311–328.
10. Nabi IR, Watanabe H, Raz A (1992) Autocrine motility factor and its receptor: Role in cell locomotion and metastasis [review]. *Cancer Metastasis Rev* 11:5–20.
11. Brandley BK, Schnaar RL (1988) Covalent attachment of an Arg-Gly-Asp sequence peptide to derivatizable polyacrylamide surfaces: Support of fibroblast adhesion and long-term growth. *Anal Biochem* 172:270–278.
12. Brandley BK, Schnaar RL (1989) Tumor cell haptotaxis on covalently immobilized linear and exponential gradients of a cell adhesion peptide. *Dev Biol* 135:74–86.
13. Brandley BK, Shaper JH, Schnaar RL (1990) Tumor cell haptotaxis on immobilized N-acetylglucosamine gradients. *Dev Biol* 140:161–171.
14. Manske M, Bade EG (1994) Growth factor-induced cell migration: Biology and methods of analysis. *Int Revi Cyto* 155:49–96.
15. Mohler JL, Partin AW, Coffey DS (1987) Prediction of metastatic potential by a new grading system of cell motility: Validation in the Dunning R-3327 prostatic adenocarcinoma model. *J Urol* 138:168–170.
16. Doyle GM, Sharief Y, Mohler JL (1992) Prediction of metastatic potential by cancer cell motility in the Dunning R-3327 prostatic adenocarcinoma in vivo model. *J Urol* 147:514–518.
17. Mohler JL, Partin AW, Isaacs WB, Coffey DS (1987) Time lapse videomicroscopic identification of Dunning R-3327 adenocarcinoma and normal rat prostate cells. *J Urol* 137:544–547.
18. Partin AW, Mohler JL, Coffey DS (1992) Cell motility as an index of metastatic ability in prostate cancers: Results with an animal model and with human cancer cells. *Cancer Treat Res* 59:121–130.
19. Albrecht-Buehler, G (1977) The phagokinetic tracks of 3T3 cells. *Cell* 11:395–404.
20. Zigmond, SH, Hirsch JG (1973) Leukocyte locomotion and chemotaxis: New methods for evaluation, and demonstration of a cell-derived factor. *J Exp Med* 137:387–410.
21. McCarthy JB, Palm SL, Furcht LT (1983) Migration by haptotaxis of a Schwann cell tumor line to the basement membrane glycoprotein laminin. *J Cell Biol* 97:772–777.
22. Stracke ML, Krutzsch, HC, Unsworth EJ, Arestad A, Cioce V, Schiffmann E, Liotta LA (1992) Identification, purification, and partial sequence analysis of autotaxin, a novel motility-stimulating protein. *J Biol Chemi* 267:2524–2529.
23. Liotta LA, Mandler R, Murano G, Katz DA, Gordon RK, Chiang PK, Schiffmann E (1986) Tumor cell autocrine motility factor. *Proc Natl Acad Sci USA* 83:3302–3306.

24. Atnip KD, Carter LM, Nicolson GL, Dabbous MK (1987) Chemotactic response of rat mammary adenocarcinoma cell clones to tumor-derived cytokines. *Biochem Biophys Res Commun* 146:996–1002.
25. Guirguis R, Margulies I, Taraboletti G, Schiffmann E, Liotta L (1987) Cytokine-induced pseudopodial protrusion is coupled to tumour cell migration. *Nature* 329:261–263.
26. Guirguis R, Schiffmann E, Liu B, Birkbeck D, Engel J, Liotta L (1988) Detection of autocrine motility factor in urine as a marker of bladder cancer. *J Natl Cancer Inst* 80:1203–1211.
27. Bhargava MM, Li Y, Joseph A, Jin L, Rosen EM, Goldberg ID (1993) HGF-SF: Effects on motility and morphology of normal and tumor cells [review]. *EXS* 65:341–349.
28. Seslar SP, Nakamura T, Byers SW (1993) Regulation of fibroblast hepatocyte growth factor/scatter factor expression by human breast carcinoma cell lines and peptide growth factors. *Cancer Res* 53:1233–1238.
29. Rosen EM, Knesel J, Goldberg ID, Jin L, Bhargava M, Joseph A, Zitnik R, Wines J, Kelley M, Rockwell S (1994) Scatter factor modulates the metastatic phenotype of the EMT6 mouse mammary tumor. *Int J Cancer* 57:706–714.
30. Byers S, Park M, Sommers C, Seslar S (1994) Breast carcinoma: A collective disorder. *Breast Cancer Res Treat* 31:203–215.
31. Weidner KM, Sachs M, Birchmeier W (1993) The Met receptor tyrosine kinase transduces motility, proliferation, and morphogenic signals of scatter factor/hepatocyte growth factor in epithelial cells. *J Cell Biol* 121:145–154.
32. Rosen EM, Grant D, Kleinman H, Jaken S, Donovan MA, Setter E, Luckett PM, Carley W, Bhargava M, Goldberg ID (1991) Scatter factor stimulates migration of vascular endothelium and capillary-like tube formation [review]. *EXS* 59:76–88.
33. Rosen EM, Grant DS, Kleinman HK, Goldberg ID, Bhargava MM, Nickoloff BJ, Kinsella JL, Polverini P (1993) Scatter factor (hepatocyte growth factor) is a potent angiogenesis factor in vivo. *Symp Soc Exp Biol* 47:227–234.
34. Bussolino F, Di Renzo MF, Ziche M, Bocchietto E, Olivero M, Naldini L, Gaudino G, Tamagnone L, Coffer A, Comoglio PM (1992) Hepatocyte growth factor is a potent angiogenic factor which stimulates endothelial cell motility and growth. *J Cell Biol* 119:629–641.
35. Grant DS, Kleinman HK, Goldberg ID, Bhargava MM, Nickoloff BJ, Kinsella JL, Polverini P, Rosen EM (1993) Scatter factor induces blood vessel formation in vivo. *Proc Natl Acad Sci USA* 90:1937–1941.
36. Yamashita J, Ogawa M, Yamashita S, Nomura K, Kuramoto M, Saishoji T, Shin S (1994) Immunoreactive hepatocyte growth factor is a strong and independent predictor of recurrence and survival in human breast cancer. *Cancer Res* 54:1630–1633.
37. Schor SL, Haggie JA, Durning P, Howell A, Smith L, Sellwood RA, Crowther D (1986) Occurrence of a fetal fibroblast phenotype in familiar breast cancer. *Int J Cancer* 37:831–836.
38. Haggie JA, Sellwood RA, Howell A, Birch JM, Schor SL (1987) Fibroblasts from relatives of patients with hereditary breast cancer show fetal-like behaviour in vitro. *Lancet* 1:1455–1457.
39. Schor SL, Schor AM (1990) Characterization of migration-stimulating factor (MSF): Evidence for its role in cancer pathogenesis [review]. *Cancer Invest* 8:665–667.
40. Sakakura T (1983) Epithelial-mesenchymal interactions in mammary gland development and its perturbation in relation to tumorigenesis. In *Understanding Breast Cancer*. MA Rich, JC Hager, P Furmanski (eds). New York: Marcel Dekker, pp 261–284.
41. Schor SL, Grey AM, Ellis I, Schor AM, Coles B, Murphy R (1993) Migration stimulating factor (MSF): Its structure, mode of action and possible function in health and disease [review]. *Symp Soc Exp Biol* 47:235–251.
42. Schor SL, Grey AM, Ellis I, Schor AM, Howell A, Sloan P, Murphy R (1994) Fetal-like fibroblasts: Their production of migration-stimulating factor and role in tumor progression. *Cancer Treatm Res* 71:277–298.

43. Krueger J, Ray A, Tamm I, Sehgal PB (1991) Expression and function of interleukin-6 in epithelial cells [review]. *J Cell Biochem* 45:327–334.

44. Tamm I, Cardinale I, Krueger J, Murphy JS, May LT, Sehgal PB (1989) Interleukin-6 decreases cell-cell association and increases motility of ductal breast carcinoma cells. *J Exp Med* 170:1649–1669.

45. Ebralidze A, Tulchinsky E, Grigorian M, Afanasyeva A, Senin V, Revazova E, Lukanidin E (1989) Isolation and characterization of a gene specifically expressed in different metastatic cells and whose deduced gene product has a high degree of homology to a Ca^{2+}-binding protein family. *Genes Dev* 3:1086–1093.

46. Grigorian MS, Tulchinsky EM, Zain S, Ebralidze AK, Kramerov DA, Kriajevska MV, Georgiev GP, Lukanidin EM (1993) The mtsl gene and control of tumor metastasis [review]. *Gene* 135:229–238.

47. Takenaga K, Nakamura Y, Sakiyama S (1994) Cellular localization of pEL98 protein, an S100-related calcium binding protein, in fibroblasts and its tissue distribution analyzed by monoclonal antibodies. *Cell Struct Funct* 19:133–141.

48. Barraclough R, Rudland PS (1994) The S-100-related calcium-binding protein, p9Ka, and metastasis in rodent and human mammary cells. *Euro J Cancer* 30A:1570–1576.

49. Davies BR, Davies MP, Gibbs FE, Barraclough R, Rudland PS (1993) Induction of the metastatic phenotype by transfection of a benign rat mammary epithelial cell line with the gene for p9Ka, a rat calcium-binding protein, but not with the oncogene EJ-ras-1. *Oncogene* 8:999–1008.

50. Davies BR, Barraclough R, Davies MP, Rudland PS (1993) Production of the metastatic phenotype by DNA transfection in a rat mammary model. *Cell Biol Int* 17:871–879.

51. Takenaga K, Nakamura Y, Endo H, Sakiyama S (1994) Involvement of S100-related calcium-binding protein pEL98 (or mts1) in cell motility and tumor cell invasion. *Jpn J Cancer Res* 85:831–839.

52. Takenaga K, Nakamura Y, Sakiyama S (1994) Expression of a calcium binding protein pEL98 (mts1) during differentiation of human promyelocytic leukemia HL-60 cells. *Biochem Biophys Res Commun* 202:94–101.

53. Gibbs FE, Wilkinson MC, Rudland PS, Barraclough R (1994) Interactions in vitro of p9Ka, the rat S-100-related, metastasis-inducing, calcium-binding protein. *J Biol Chem* 269:18992–18999.

54. Kriajevska MV, Cardenas MN, Grigorian MS, Ambartsumian NS, Georgiev GP, Lukanidin EM (1994) Non-muscle myosin heavy chain as a possible target for protein encoded by metastasis-related mts-1 gene. *J Biol Chem* 269:19679–19682.

55. Ford HL, Chakravarty R, Salim M, Silver D, Aluiddin V, Sellers J, Zain S (1995) The mts1 gene in metastasis and motility. *J Cell Biochem* 19b(Suppl):7.

56. Takenaga K, Nakamura Y, Sakiyama S, Hasegawa Y, Sato K, Endo H (1994) Binding of pEL98 protein, an S100-related calcium-binding protein, to nonmuscle tropomyosin. *J Cell Biol* 124:757–768.

57. Steeg PS, Bevilacqua G, Kopper L, Thorgeirsson UP, Talmadge JE, Liotta LA, Sobel ME (1988) Evidence for a novel gene associated with low tumor metastatic potential. *J Natl Cancer Inst* 80:200–204.

58. Kobayashi S, Iwase H, Itoh Y, Fukuoka H, Yamashita H, Kuzushima T, Iwata H, Masaoka A, Kimura N (1992) Estrogen receptor, c-erbB-2 and nm23/NDP kinase expression in the intraductal and invasive components of human breast cancers. *Jpn J Cancer Res* 83:859–865.

59. Tokunaga Y, Urano T, Furukawa K, Kondo H, Kanematsu T, Shiku H (1993) Reduced expression of nm23-H1, but not of nm23-H2, is concordant with the frequency of lymph-node metastasis of human breast cancer. *Int J Cancer* 55:66–71.

60. Noguchi M, Earashi M, Ohnishi I, Kinoshita K, Thomas M, Fusida S, Miyazaki I, Mizukami Y (1994) nm23 and c-erbB-2 expression in invasive breast cancer. *Oncol Rep* 1:523–528.

61. Noguchi M, Earashi M, Ohnishi I, Kinoshita K, Thomas M, Fusida S, Miyazaki I, Mizukami Y (1994) nm23 expression versus helix pomatia lectin binding in human breast cancer metastases. *Int J Oncol* 4:1353–1358.

320

62. Bevilacqua G, Sobel ME, Liotta LA, Steeg PS (1989) Association of low nm23 RNA levels in human primary infiltrating ductal breast carcinomas with lymph node involvement and other histopathological indicators of high metastatic potential. *Cancer Res* 49:5185–5190.

63. Noguchi M, Earashi M, Ohnishi I, Kitagawa H, Fusida S, Miyazaki I, Mizukami Y (1994) Relationship between nm23 expression and axillary and internal mammary liymph node metastases in invasive breast cancer. *Oncol Rep* 1:795–799.

64. Hennessy C, Henry JA, May FE, Westley BR, Angus B, Lennard TW (1991) Expression of the antimetastatic gene nm23 in human breast cancer: An association with good prognosis. *J Natl Cancer Inst* 83:281–285.

65. Hennessy C, Henry JA, May FE, Westley BR, Angus B, Lennard TW (1991) Expression of anti-metastatic gene nm23 [letter; comment]. *Br J Cancer* 63:1024.

66. Sastre-Garau X, Lacombe ML, Jouve M, Veron M, Magdelenat H (1992) Nucleoside diphosphate kinase/NM23 expression in breast cancer: Lack of correlation with lymph-node metastasis. *Int J Cancer* 50:533–538.

67. Leone A, Flatow U, VanHoutte K, Steeg PS (1993) Transfection of human nm23-H1 into the human MDA-MB-435 breast carcinoma cell line: Effects on tumor metastatic potential, colonization and enzymatic activity. *Oncogene* 8:2325–2333.

68. Leone A, Flatow U, King CR, Sandeen MA, Margulies IM, Liotta LA, Steeg PS (1991) Reduced tumor incidence, metastatic potential, and cytokine responsiveness of nm23-transfected melanoma cells. *Cell* 65:25–35.

69. Kantor JD, McCormick B, Steeg PS, Zetter BR (1993) Inhibition of cell motility after nm23 transfection of human and murine tumor cells. *Cancer Res* 53:1971–1973.

70. Postel EH, Berberich SJ, Flint SJ, Ferrone CA (1993) Human c-myc transcription factor PuF identified an nm23-H2 nucleoside diphosphate kinase, a candidate suppressor of tumor metastasis [see comments]. *Science* 261:478–480.

71. Postel EH, Ferrone CA (1994) Nucleoside diphosphate kinase enzyme activity of NM23-H2/PuF is not required for its DNA binding and in vitro transcriptional functions. *J Biol Chem* 269:8627–8630.

72. MacDonald NJ, De la Rosa A, Benedict MA, Freije JM, Krutsch H, Steeg PS (1993) A serine phosphorylation of nm23, and not its nucleoside diphosphate kinase activity, correlates with suppression of tumor metastatic potential. *J Biol Chem* 268:25780–25789.

73. Munoz-Dorado J, Almaula N, Inouye S, Inouye M (1993) Autophosphorylation of nucleoside diphosphate kinase from *Myxococcus xanthus*. *J Bacteriol* 175:1176–1181.

74. Bominaar AA, Tepper AD, Veron M (1994) Autophosphorylation of nucleoside diphosphate kinase on non-histidine residues. *FEBS Lett* 353:5–8.

75. Lakshmi MS, Parker C, Sherbet GV (1993) Metastasis associated MTS1 and NM23 genes affect tubulin polymerisation in B16 melanomas: A possible mechanism of their regulation of metastatic behaviour of tumors. *Anticancer Res* 13:299–303.

76. Huitorel P, Simon C, Pantaloni D (1984) Nucleoside diphophate kinase from brain — Purification and effect on microtubule assembly in vitro. *Eur J Biochem* 144:233–241.

77. Melki R, Lascu I, Carlier MF, Veron M (1992) Nucleoside diphosphate kinase does not directly interact with tubulin nor microtubules. *Biochem Biophys Res Commun* 187:65–72.

78. Weinstat-Saslow D, Steeg PS (1994) Angiogenesis and colonization in the tumor metastatic process: Basic and applied advances [review]. *FASEB J* 8:401–407.

79. Folkman J (1995) Tumor Angiogenesis. In *The Molecular Basis of Cancer*. J Mendelsohn, PM Howley, MA Israel, LA Liotta (eds). Phiadelphia: WB Saunders, pp 206–232.

80. Folkman J, Hochberg M (1973) Self-regulation of growth in three dimentions. *J Exp Med* 138:745–753.

81. Folkman J (1994) Angiogenesis and breast cancer [editorial; comment]. *J Clin Oncol* 12:441–443.

82. Toi M, Kashitani J, Tominaga T (1993) Tumor angiogenesis is an independent prognostic indicator in primary breast carcinoma. *Int J Cancer* 55:371–374.

321

83. Toi M, Hoshina S, Takayanagi T, Tominaga T (1994) Association of vascular endothelial growth factor expression with tumor angiogenesis and with early relapse in primary breast cancer. *Jpn J Cancer Res* 85:1045–1049.

84. Visscher DW, Smilanetz S, Drozdowicz S, Wykes SM (1993) Prognostic significance of image morphometric microvessel enumeration in breast carcinoma. *Anal Quant Cytol Histol* 15:88–92.

85. Horak ER, Leek R, Klenk N, LeJeune S, Smith K, Stuart N, Greenall M, Stepniewska K, Harris AL (1992) Angiogenesis, assessed by platelet/endothelial cell adhesion molecule antibodies, as an indicator of node metastases and survival in breast cancer. *Lancet* 340:1120–1124.

86. Weidner N, Folkman J, Pozza F, Bevilacqua P, Allred EN, Moore DH, Meli S, Gasparini G (1992) Tumor angiogenesis: A new significant and independent prognostic indicator in early-stage breast carcinoma [see comments]. *J Natl Cancer Inst* 84:1875–1887.

87. Gasparini G, Weidner N, Bevilacqua P, Maluta S, Dalla Palma P, Caffo O, Barbareschi M, Boracchi P, Marubini E, Pozza F (1994) Tumor microvessel density, p53 expression, tumor size, and peritumoral lymphatic vessel invasion are relevant prognostic markers in node-negative breast carcinoma [see comments]. *J Clin Oncol* 12:454–466.

88. Weidner N, Semple JP, Welch WR, Folkman J (1991) Tumor angiogenesis and metastasis — correlation in invasive breast carcinoma. *N Engl J Med* 324:1–8.

89. Harris AL, Fox S, Bicknell R, Leek R, Relf M, LeJeune S, Kaklamanis L (1994) Gene therapy through signal transduction pathways and angiogenic growth factors as therapeutic targets in breast cancer [review]. *Cancer* 74(Suppl):1021–1025.

90. Blood CH, Zetter BR (1990) Tumor interactions with the vasculature: Angiogenesis and tumor metastasis [review]. *Biochim Biophys Acta* 1032:89–118.

91. Sholley MM, Ferguson GP, Seibel HR, Montour JL, Wilson JD (1984) Mechanisms of neovascularization. Vascular sprouting can occur without proliferation of endothelial cells. *Lab Invest* 51:624–634.

92. Stokes CL, Lauffenburger DA (1991) Analysis of the roles of microvessel endothelial cell random motility and chemotaxis in angiogenesis. *J Theor Biol* 152:377–403.

93. Harris AL, Fox S, Bicknell R, Leek R, Relf M, LeJeune S, Kaklamanis L (1994) Gene therapy through signal transduction pathways and angiogenic growth factors as therapeutic targets in breast cancer [review]. *Cancer* 74(Suppl):1021–1025.

94. Zhang H-T, Craft P, Scott PAE, Ziche M, Weich HA, Harris AL, Bicknell R (1995) Enhancement of tumor growth and vascular density by transfection of vascular endothelial cell growth factor into MCF-7 human breast carcinoma cells. *J Natl Cancer Inst* 87:213–218.

95. Brown LF, Berse B, Jackman RW, Tognazzi K, Guidi AJ, Dvorak HF, Senger DR, Connolly JL, Schnitt SJ (1995) Expression of vascular permeability factor (vascular endothelial growth factor) and its receptors in breast cancer. *Hum Pathol* 26:86–91.

96. Watanabe H, Nguyen M, Schizer M, Li V, Hayes DF, Sallan S, Folkman J (1992) Basic fibroblast growth factor in human serum — A prognostic test for breast cancer. *Mol Biol Cell* 3(Suppl):234a.

97. Simorre-Pinatel V, Guerrin M, Chollet P, Penary M, Clamens S, Malecaze F, Plouet J (1994) Vasculotropin-VEGF stimulates retinal capillary endoethelial cells through an autocrine pathway. *Invest Ophthalmol Vis Sci* 35:3393–3400.

98. Terranova VP, DiFlorio R, Lyall RM, Hic S, Friesel R, Maciag T (1985) Human endothelial cells are chemotactic to endothelial cell growth factor and heparin. *J Cell Biol* 101:2330–2334.

99. Sato Y, Rifkin DB (1988) Autocrine activities of basic fibroblast growth factor: Regulation of endothelial cell movement, plasminogen activator synthesis, and DNA synthesis. *J Cell Biol* 107:1199–1205.

100. Yee C, Shiu PR (1986) Degradation of endothelial basement membrane by human breast cancer cell lines. *Cancer Res* 46:1835–1839.

101. Liotta LA, Tryggvason K, Garbisa S, Hart I, Foltz CM, Shafie S (1980) Metastatic potential correlates with enzymatic degradation of basement membrane collagen. *Nature* 284:67–68.

102. Nakajima M, Welch DR, Belloni PN, Nicolson GL (1987) Degradation of basement mem-

brane type IV collagen and lung subendothelial matrix by rat mammary adenocarcinoma cell clones of differing metastatic potentials. *Cancer Res* 47:4869–4876.

103. Monteagudo C, Merino MJ, San-Juan J, Liotta LA, Stetler-Stevenson WG (1990) Immuno-histochemical distribution of type IV collagenase in normal, benign, and malignant breast tissue. *Am J Pathol* 136:585–592.

104. Barsky SH, Togo S, Garbisa S, Liotta LA (1983) Type IV collagenase immunoreactivity in invasive breast carcinoma. *Lancet* 1:296–297.

105. D'Errico A, Garbisa S, Liotta LA, Castronovo V, Stetler-Stevenson WG, Grigiooni WF (1991) Augmentation of type IV collagenase, laminin receptor, and Ki67 proliferation anti-gen associated with human colon, gastric, and breast carcinoma progression. *Mod Pathol* 4:239–246.

106. Azzam HS, Arand G, Lippman ME, Thompson EW (1993) Association of MMP-2 activation potential with metastatic progression in human breast cancer cell lines independent of MMP-2 production. *J Natl Cancer Inst* 85:1758–1764.

107. Ponton A, Coulombe B, Skup D (1991) Decreased expression of tissue inhibitor of metalloproteinases in metastatic tumor cells leading to increased levels of collagenase activity. *Cancer Res* 51:2138–2143.

108. Mundy GR, DeMartino S, Rowe DW (1981) Collagen and collagen-derived fragments are chemotactic for tumor cells. *J Clin Invest* 68:1102–1105.

109. Johnson MD, Kim HR, Chesler L, Tsao-Wu G, Bouck N, Polverini PJ (1994) Inhibition of angiogenesis by tissue inhibitor of metalloproteinase. *J Cell Physiol* 160:194–202.

110. Murphy AN, Unsworth EJ, Stetler-Stevenson WG (1993) Tissue inhibitor of metal-loproteinases-2 inhibits bFGF-induced human microvascular endothelial cell proliferation. *J Cell Physiol* 157:351–358.

111. Pucci-Minafra I, Minafra S, Faccini AM, Alessandro R (1989) An ultrastructural evaluation of cell heterogeneity in invasive ductal carcinomas of the human breast. I. An in vivo study. *J Submicrosc Cytol Pathol* 21:475–488.

112. Pucci-Minafra I, Minafra S, Alessandro R, Faccini AM (1989) An ultrastructural evaluation of cell heterogeneity in invasive ductal carcinomas of the human breast. II. An in vitro study. *J Submicrosc Cytol Pathol* 21:489–499.

113. Pucci-Minafra I, Minafra S, Tomasino RM, Sciarrino S, Tinervia R (1986) Collagen changes in the ductal infiltrating (scirrhous) carcinoma of the human breast. A possible role played by type I trimer collagen on the invasive growth. *J Submicrosc Cytol* 18:795–805.

114. Luparello C, Sheterline P, Pucci-Minafra I, Minafra S (1991) A comparison of spreading and motility behaviour of 8701-BC breast carcinoma cells on type I, I-trimer and type V collagen substrata. Evidence for a permissive effect of type I-trimer collagen on cell locomotion. *J Cell Sci* 100:179–185.

115. Atsushi Y, Anand-Apte B, Zetter B (1996) Differential endothelial migration and prolifera-tion to basicfibroblast growth factor and vascular endothelial growth factor. *Growth Factors* 13:1–8.

16. Cathepsins D and B in breast cancer

Wei-Ping Ren and Bonnie F. Sloane

Introduction

The name *cathepsin* is derived from a Greek word meaning to digest and was used originally for acidic proteases, with the letters designating individual enzymes [1,2]. Examples of cathepsins are found in three classes of proteases, for example, cathepsin D is an aspartic protease, cathepsin B a cysteine protease, and cathepsin G is a serine protease. Although several cathepsins have collagenolytic activity, there are no cathepsins among the metalloproteases. Most cathepsins are lysosomal proteases with acidic pH optima ranging from the extremely acidic pH optimum of cathepsin D (i.e., pH 2.8) to the slightly acidic pH optimum of cathepsin B (i.e., pH 6.5). On the other hand, cathepsin E has an acidic pH optimum (i.e., pH 3.0) yet is not lysosomal [3], and cathepsin S has a neutral pH optimum yet is lysosomal [4]. The lysosomal cathepsins are synthesized as pre-proenzymes and acquire N-linked oligosaccharides cotranslationally. Their maturation involves proteolytic processing and modification of the oligosaccharides, processes that occur during their trafficking to the lysosome and that affect their ability to bind to receptors that target them to the lysosomes [5–7]. As indicated earlier, the cathepsins are primarily endopeptidases, hydrolyzing internal peptide bonds. However, cathepsin H is an exopeptidase of the aminopeptidase class [8], and cathepsin B has both endopeptidase and exopeptidase activities, the latter as a carboxydipeptidase [9]. The dual activity of cathepsin B enables this enzyme to participate in degradatory processes directly through degradation of the basement membrane proteins laminin, fibronectin, and type IV collagen [10,11], or indirectly by activating other proteases such as urokinase [12]. The primary intracellular function of lysosomal cathepsins is protein turnover. The evidence for extracellular roles of cathepsins is growing; as an example, cathepsins secreted from macrophages and osteoclasts participate in matrix and bone degradation [13,14].

Cathepsins have also been implicated in several processes, presumably extracellular, that accompany tumor progression: proliferation, angiogenesis, invasion, and metastasis [2]. Surprisingly, the association of cathepsins D and B with malignancy of human breast tumors was first described almost 15 years

R. Dickson and M. Lippman (eds.) MAMMARY TUMOR CELL CYCLE, DIFFERENTIATION AND METASTASIS. 1996. Kluwer Academic Publishers. ISBN 0-7923-3905-3. All rights reserved.

Table 1. General information on cathepsin D and cathepsin B

	Cathepsin D	Cathepsin B
Molecular size		
Proform	43 kD[a] (52 kD[b])	35 kD (43/46 kD)
Mature single chain	38 kD (48 kD)	28 kD (31 kD)
Mature double chain	26 + 12 kD (34 + 14 kD)	22 + 6 kD (25/26 + 5 kD)
Assay substrate	Denatured hemoglobin	Carbobenzyloxy-arginyl-arginyl-4-methylcoumarin
pH optimum	pH 3.0	pH 6.5
Inhibitors		
Endogenous	None	Cystatin superfamily
Exogenous	Pepstatin	E-64, leupeptin, CA074 and CA074Me[c]

[a] Molecular sizes are calculated from amino acid sequences predicted from the nucleotide sequences of human cathepsin D [22] and cathepsin B [49], using an average molecular weight of 110 daltons per amino acid.

[b] Molecular sizes in parentheses represent sizes of glycosylated enzymes immunoprecipitated from metabolically labeled cells [141,142].

[c] E-64 and leupeptin will inhibit cathepsin B, as well as other cysteine proteases, whereas CA074 and CA074Me are selective for cathepsin B.

ago [15–17]. As reviews of earlier literature linking these enzymes to the progression of human cancers are available [2,18–21], we will concentrate in this chapter on the most recent data, with an emphasis on the data linking these enzymes to the progression of human breast cancer. To provide a framework for readers unfamiliar with these two enzymes, in Figure 1 we have diagrammed the gene and protein structures of cathepsins D and B, and in Table 1 we have provided information on the characteristics of both enzymes.

Increased expression of cathepsins D and B

Cathepsin D

The cathepsin D gene is a single copy gene comprised of nine exons and eight introns spanning a region of 11 kb [22,23] (Figure 1). It is located on the short arm of chromosome 11 close to the Ha-*ras* oncogene. This is a region that undergoes frequent rearrangements, including the loss of one c-Ha-*ras* allele, in aggressive breast cancer [24]. The translation initiation site of cathepsin D is encoded by exon 1 and the stop codon by exon 9 [22]. The deduced amino acid sequence [22] indicates that human cathepsin D consists of a pre-proenzyme with a 20-residue signal peptide, a 44-residue propeptide, and a single chain form of 348 residues. The human cathepsin D gene has a compound promoter with features of both housekeeping (high G+C content and potential Sp-1 transcription factor binding sites) and regulated (the presence of a TATA box) promoters [25]. Five transcription start sites (TSSI to V)

Cathepsin D

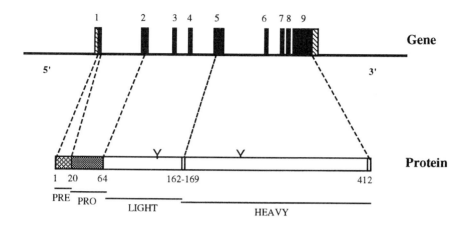

Cathepsin B

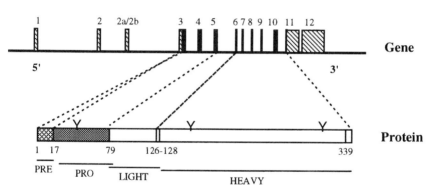

Figure 1. Comparison of the gene and protein structures of cathepsin D and cathepsin B. The human cathepsin D structure is based on Redecker et al. [22], and the human cathepsin B structure is based on Gong et al. [47] and Berquin et al. [48]. Exons are numbered; those encoding the protein are depicted by filled boxes, whereas those representing 5′- and 3′-untranslated regions are depicted by striped boxes. In the protein structures, vertical lines indicate sites of proteolytic processing and Ys indicate putative glycosylation sites. The number of amino acids in the prepeptide, propeptide, and light and heavy chains of mature cathepsin D and cathepsin B are indicated underneath the protein structure.

spanning >52 bp have been identified by RNAse protection assay [25]. In estrogen-dependent breast cancer cells, estradiol induces a 6- to 10-fold increase in cathepsin D transcripts; these transcripts are initiated at TSSI located about 28 bp downstream from the TATA box. Site-directed mutagenesis indicates that the TATA box is essential for initiation of transcription at TSSI [25]. In breast cancer biopsies, high levels of TATA-dependent transcription correlate with overexpression of cathepsin D transcripts (see later). Thus, the cathepsin D gene can behave as either a housekeeping gene with multiple start sites or as a hormone-regulated gene with a single TATA-dependent start site [25].

The major mRNA transcript for cathepsin D, observed in both normal and breast tumor cells, is 2.2 kb [22,23,26]. Estrogen regulates the expression of the cathepsin D gene primarily at the transcriptional level [26–28], as has been observed for other steroid-responsive genes. At least two estrogen-responsive elements are located upstream of TSSI in the cathepsin D gene [29]. In MCF-7 human breast cancer cells, an estrogen receptor-positive (ER⁺) cell line, there is a low constitutive accumulation of cathepsin D mRNA, which is increased about 10-fold by estradiol treatment [26]. The estradiol-induced cathepsin D expression is not inhibited by cycloheximide, suggesting that regulation by estrogen does not involve other effector proteins [26]. Estrogen receptor ligands are the only steroids that induce transcription; the ability of the estrogen receptor ligands to induce transcription parallels their affinity for the estrogen receptor and their mitogenic activity. The promoter has not yet been compared in normal and cancer tissues. Therefore, whether the increased sensitivity to estradiol in breast cancer is due to altered *trans*-acting factors or altered *cis*-acting sequences has not been determined.

The expression of cathepsin D is also increased in estrogen receptor–negative (ER⁻) breast cancers [27]. The mechanism is still unknown, but the constitutive production of autocrine or intracrine factor(s) might be responsible for the induction of cathepsin D. Although Rochefort and coworkers [26–28] have shown that growth factors, such as insulin-like growth factor 1, epidermal growth factor, and basic fibroblast growth factor, acting via a tyrosine kinase pathway, are able to induce cathepsin D mRNA in the ER⁺ MCF-7 cells, the role(s) of growth factors in constitutive overexpression of cathepsin D in ER⁻ breast cancers has not been delineated. The induction of cathepsin D expression by growth factors, in contrast to the induction by estrogen, is inhibited by cycloheximide [27], indicating an indirect mechanism of action.

Increases in the expression of cathepsin D have been observed in breast cancer tissues and cell lines at both the mRNA [26,27,30] and protein [31] levels. Immunohistochemistry [31,32], in situ hybridization and cytosolic immunoassays [33], and northern and western blot analyses [28,34] all indicate that cathepsin D expression is 2- to 50-fold greater in most cases of breast cancer than in normal mammary glands or in fibroblasts. In situ hybridization and immunohistochemistry have established that the increases in expression occur in the breast cancer cells rather than in stromal cells [35–37]; expression in stromal cells has also been reported for urokinase [38] and some metalloproteases [39]. Although macrophages also express cathepsin D at high levels [40], the expression of cathepsin D in macrophages within the breast cancer tissue does not seem to account for the 2- to 50-fold higher expression of cathepsin D [41]. Increases in expression of cathepsin D are not unique to breast cancer; such increases have also been observed in hepatomas [42], brain tumors [43], and thyroid carcinomas [44].

Cathepsin B

The human cathepsin B gene is a single copy gene that maps to chromosome 8p22 [45]. This is a region that is a hot spot in prostate cancer [46]. The human cathepsin B gene is composed of at least 12 exons [47,48], spanning a region of approximately 27 kb [48] (Figure 1). The gene structure of cathepsin B does not correspond to the functional units of the enzyme [2]. The translation initiation site is in exon 3, so that exon 1, 2, and 25 bp of exon 3 are noncoding and constitute the 5'-untranslated region (UTR). Exon 12 and about 80% of exon 11 are also noncoding and make up the 3'-UTR. Alternative splicing of both the 5'- and 3'-UTRs has been observed [47–50]. We recently identified two new exons in the human cathepsin B gene that map between exons 2 and 3 [48]. These two exons can be alternatively spliced and contribute to the diversity of the 5'-UTR of cathepsin B transcripts. The deduced amino acid sequence indicates that cathepsin B transcripts encode a pre-proenzyme with a 17-residue signal peptide, a 62-residue propeptide, and a 254 residue single chain mature form [51] (Figure 1). The single chain form of cathepsin B is processed to the double-chain form by two internal cleavages, which eliminate a dipeptide. Both single and double chain forms of the enzyme have proteolytic activity [52].

The putative promoter region ≤500 bp upstream of exon 1 of the human cathepsin B gene does not have TATA or CAAT motifs, but has a high G+C content and several potential binding sites for the Sp-1 transcription factor [47]. Therefore, the promoter of the human cathepsin B gene has been classified as a housekeeping-type promoter, as has that for the mouse cathepsin B gene [53]. More recent studies suggest that both the mouse [54] and human [48] cathepsin B genes may have more than one promoter. In the mouse, two newly identified putative promoter regions contain a TATA box, with one also containing a CAAT box. The sequence of the two putative promoter regions in the human cathepsin B gene is not yet known. The sequence and exon/intron junctions in the coding region of the human and mouse genes are conserved; however, there is variability in both 5'- and 3'-UTRs, so that there is no direct correspondence of promoter regions in the two genes.

Tissue-, cell-, or differentiation-specific expression of cathepsin B might be due to the existence of several promoters with transcription factors acting differentially on each promoter and the level of those transcription factors dependent on cell type, tissue, stage of differentiation, and/or microenvironment. Recent studies in our laboratory on the putative promoter upstream of exon 1 in the human cathepsin B gene revealed a 20-fold enhancement in expression of a luciferase reporter gene by a segment of the gene >500 bp upstream [55], suggesting that there is a positive regulatory element in that region. To our knowledge, this is the first evidence for transcriptional regulation of the human cathepsin B gene. We have also obtained evidence for post-transcriptional regulation of cathepsin B expression. In vitro transcription of a splice variant in which exon 1 is spliced to exon 3 revealed enhanced stability of this cathepsin B mRNA transcript as compared with the full-length transcript [56].

Increased expression of cathepsin B mRNA and protein correlates with tumor malignancy [2,20,21] (Table 2). In human colorectal carcinoma, cathepsin B mRNA levels are increased compared with matched normal colorectal tissues [57,58]. Immunohistochemical studies demonstrte that increased cathepsin B staining in colorectal carcinomas is predictive of shortened patient survival [59]. Another tumor in which cathepsin B expression is increased is human glioma [60]. Levels of cathepsin B transcripts are from three- to sixfold higher in low-grade astrocytoma and high-grade glioblastoma, respectively, than in normal brain. Increases in cathepsin B activity are even higher: In matched pairs of human brain tissues, cathepsin B activities are 10- and 15-fold higher in the glioblastoma tissues than in normal brain tissues [60]. The greater increase in cathepsin B activity in the gliomas does not appear to be due to a reduction in the endogenous cysteine protease inhibitors in gliomas [Rozhin,

Table 2. Comparative expression of cathepsin B in human cancers

	Breast	Colon	Glioma
mRNA[a]	nd[b]	4-fold	4-fold
Protein[c]	−/+	+++	+++
Activity[d]	8-fold	3-fold	12-fold
Secretion[e]			
Constitutive	+	+	nd
Inducible	+	+	nd
Intracellular distribution[f]	Focal adhesions	Basal/diffuse	Foot processes
Membrane association[g]	External surface	nd	nd
Prognostic value[h]	Yes	Yes	nd

[a] mRNA levels determined by northern blot analyses [58,60].
[b] nd = not determined.
[c] Protein levels determined by immunohistochemical staining [58,60,73].
[d] Activities compared in tumor cells from invasive edges and in matched normal cells [68,69].
[e] Secretion measured from cell lines: Constitutively secreted enzyme is procathepsin B and inducibly secreted enzyme is mature cathepsin B [90].
[f] Intracellular distribution illustrated in Figure 3 or in Campo et al. [59].
[g] Membrane association illustrated in Sameni et al. [92].
[h] Prognostic value illustrated in a poster presented at the Keystone Symposium on Cancer Cell Invasion and Motility in Tamarron, Colorado (Lah TT, Kos J, Krasevec M, Golouh R, Vrhovec I, Turk V: Cathepsin B and L as possible prognostic factors in breast carcinoma) and in Campo et al. [59].
Any unattributed work is unpublished work from our own laboratory.

Mikkelsen, and Sloane, unpublished data], yet may reflect biological variability as mRNA levels were measured in unmatched samples and activities in matched samples. Levels of expression of cathepsin B (mRNA, protein, and activity) parallel the ability of glioblastoma cell lines to invade through Matrigel in vitro [61] and the invasive ability of gliomas in vivo as assessed by magnetic resonance imaging [60]. Thus, the studies on cathepsin B expression in human colon carcinomas and gliomas suggest that this enzyme plays a role in malignant progression of these two tumors.

As has been shown for other proteases [38,39,62–64], increases in expression of cathepsin B are not found uniformly throughout a tumor mass. Often these increases are found in the cells at the invading margins of a tumor, leading us to hypothesize that the expression of cathepsin B is upregulated in these cells in response to interactions between the tumor and surrounding stroma. Such increases in expression of cathepsin B mRNA and protein have been demonstrated at the invading front of bladder and prostate carcinomas by in situ hybridization and immunohistochemistry [65–67]. Furthermore, an inverse correlation between cathepsin B and type IV collagen staining is present at the invading edges of bladder tumors, suggesting that the increases in cathepsin B might be responsible for the local degradation of basement membrane [D.W. Visscher, M. Sameni, and B.F. Sloane, unpublished results].

These measurements of cathepsin B mRNA and protein do not tell us whether the amount of active cathepsin B is increased at the invasive edges, a prerequisite for cathepsin B to play a functional role in tumor growth and invasion. Therefore, we have measured cathepsin B activity in tumor cells isolated from the invasive edges using a microdissection technique. Tumor cells and matched normal epithelial cells have been microdissected from 10 μm frozen sections of human colon tumors [68] and breast tumors [69]. Both cathepsin B and gelatinase A (MMP-2 or 72 kD type IV collagenase) activities are increased in the cells at the invasive edges. Since microdissection studies are labor intensive and not readily applicable to routine pathological analyses, we are attempting to develop monoclonal antibodies that can distinguish active forms of cathepsin B from the inactive pro forms. Such antibodies would be useful for immunohistochemical studies of a large number of samples from a wide variety of human tumors and, thus, for assessment of the importance of observed increases in expression of cathepsin B at the invading margins of human tumors.

Although it has been known since 1980 that breast tumor explants secrete increased amounts of cathepsin B [15], the levels of expression of cathepsin B in human breast cancer have not been as well characterized as those of cathepsin D. To our knowledge, studies on the expression of cathepsin B mRNA in breast cancer have not been performed. Increases in the expression of cathepsin B protein have been demonstrated by immunoassay (ELISA) of cytosolic extracts from breast cancer tissues [70]. Also, using an ELISA, Lah and coworkers [personal communication] have found that cathepsin B protein is 26-fold higher in cytosolic extracts of breast cancer tissue than in non-involved adjacent tissues. Over a 5 year follow-up period, the patients with high levels of cathepsin B protein have a higher risk of recurrence and shortened overall survival. The increases in cathepsin B protein in breast cancer do result in increases in active cathepsin B because cathepsin B activity in breast cancer tissue is 10- to 20-fold higher than in matched pairs of adjacent normal tissues [70,71].

Furthermore, increases in cathepsin B activity are observed in breast cancer cell lines as well as in tissues [70–72]. In contrast, Castiglioni et al. [73] did not demonstrate an increase in staining for cathepsin B in human breast cancer, nor did they demonstrate an increase in staining for cathepsin D or for cathepsin L, another lysosomal cysteine protease. These apparent contradictory results may reflect regional heterogeneities in distribution of the cathepsins in tumors, a phenomenon also reported for other proteases [38,39,62–64]. In this regard, Castiglioni et al. [73] did not evaluate staining in invasive edges of the breast tumors, nor did they indicate whether there was increased staining in stromal cells. Thus, we were unable to assess either regional heterogeneities or the possible contribution of stromal cell cathepsin B to the measurements in tissue extracts of cathepsin B protein and activity [71]. Regional differences in cathepsin B in breast cancer do exist, because cathepsin B activity is eightfold higher in invasive tumor cells than in matched normal cells isolated by microdissection [69].

At present the mechanisms responsible for increases in the expression of cathepsin B in human tumors have not been fully elucidated. However, as discussed earlier, the increases in cathepsin B expression might be regulated transcriptionally and/or post-transcriptionally. In murine B16 melanoma, Qian et al. [74] observed that the transcription rate of the cathepsin B gene is increased and suggested that this is due to the presence of elevated levels of tumor-specific transcription factors. Although this same group found no evidence for a regulated promoter in the mouse cathepsin B gene [53], two other leader sequences are now known to be present [54]. Whether use of an alternative promoter is responsible for the increased rate of transcription in murine B16 melanoma has not been determined. Recent data from our laboratory suggests that the human cathepsin B gene also may have several promoters as well as an enhancer that can increase the expression of a luciferase reporter gene when transfected into a human glioblastoma cell line [55]. In some cells, expression of cathepsin B is dependent on their state of differentiation. For example, phorbol ester and granulocyte-macrophage colony-stimulating factor [75] and interleukin-1 [76] can induce an increase in expression of cathepsin B in parallel with the differentiation of promonocytes to macrophages or synovial fibroblasts, respectively.

Whether similar mechanisms are responsible for increases in expression of cathepsin B in tumors is unknown. Multiple transcript species have been detected in human tumors, arising from alternative splicing of the 5'- and 3'-UTRs [47–50,57,77,78], and therefore increases in expression of cathepsin B in human tumors might reflect changes in post-transcriptional processing. Transcripts arising from splicing of exon 1 to exon 4 [47] or use of a putative alternative transcription initiation site before exon 4 [48] would encode a truncated form of procathepsin B lacking the signal peptide and part of the propeptide by using an in-frame AUG (methionine) codon in exon 4 to initiate translation. Gong et al. [47] proposed that transcripts missing exon 2 and 3 are tumor specific and that truncated procathepsin B contributes to the increase in cathepsin B expression in tumors. This group has expressed recombinant truncated procathepsin B by in vitro transcription/translation and by transfection in COS cells [79]. In addition to affecting the form of cathepsin B synthesized, alternative splicing of the 5'-UTR may result in mature mRNAs that vary in stability and/or translatability. Preliminary data on transcripts missing exon 2 indicate that they are more stable [56]. The presence of additional in-frame AUG codons followed by stop codons in exons 2, 2a, and 2b [48] suggests that transcripts missing these exons might be translated more efficiently. Clearly, more studies on the mechanisms of regulation of cathepsin B expression are needed to determine whether transcriptional and/or post-transcriptional mechanisms are responsible for the increases in cathepsin B expression in human tumors.

Altered trafficking of cathepsins D and B

Secretion

There is an extensive literature on the secretion of procathepsin D by breast cancers [18,19]. As early as 1980, Westley and Rochefort [17] reported that estrogen induces secretion of a 52 kD protein by breast cancer cell lines; however, this protein was not identified as procathepsin D until 1986 [80]. Breast cancer cell lines secrete as much as 50% of their total cathepsin D in the form of procathepsin D: Secretion of procathepsin D by ER⁻ cells is constitutive, whereas that by ER⁺ breast cancer cell lines is induced by estrogen [18,19,35,81]. Mathieu et al. [82] postulated that the secretion of procathepsin D by breast cancer cells results from increased synthesis of cathepsin D overwhelming the mannose-6-phosphate receptors (MPRs) that would normally traffic procathepsin D from the Golgi to the late endosomes. Breast secretions from patients with breast cancer contain high levels of procathepsin D [83], indicating that procathepsin D is also secreted from breast cancer tissue in vivo. Nevertheless, the levels do not correlate with either the levels of procathepsin D in cytosolic extracts nor the estrogen receptor status of the breast cancer tissue.

Interestingly, procathepsin D is only 2–6% of the total cathepsin D in breast cancer extracts rather than the 50% observed in media of breast cancer cell lines [84]. Rochefort and colleagues have suggested that the lesser percentage of procathepsin D observed in cytosolic extracts reflects an in vivo activation of procathepsin D within the tumor. An alternative explanation is that the larger percentage of procathepsin D found in breast cancer cells in culture is due to modifications in trafficking of this enzyme induced by culture conditions. If procathepsin D is secreted in vivo, we do not know whether it is secreted from breast cancer cells or stromal cells. We also do not know whether secreted procathepsin D would be activated extracellularly or intracellularly following its endocytosis by cancer cells or stromal cells. Because activation of procathepsin D requires an acidic pH [85], activation most likely occurs intracellularly in an acidic compartment such as lysosomes or endosomes, perhaps including the large acidic vesicles identified by Rochefort and colleagues in breast cancer cells [86].

Cathepsin B is also secreted by tumors, but often not to the same extent as is cathepsin D [2,20,21]. An early report on secretion of cathepsin B from breast cancer explants did not distinguish between procathepsin B and mature cathepsin B [15]. Increases in the secretion of procathepsin B by human colorectal carcinoma cell lines [87] and hepatomas [88], as well as by human breast cancer explants and cell lines [15,16], have been reported. Secretion of procathepsin B, in apparent contrast to that of procathepsin D, can occur from cell that do not exhibit an increase in mRNA levels for cathepsin B [E. Friedman, M. Ahram, and B.F. Sloane, unpublished data; 89]. Secretion of mature cathepsin B also occurs from human colorectal tumor cells as well as that of procathepsin B [87]. In ras-transformed MCF-10A1neoT cells and murine melanoma and human colorectal carcinoma cell lines, we have shown that secretion of mature cathepsin B can be induced, whereas the secretion of procathepsin B occurs constitutively [90,91] (Table 2). We hypothesize that secretion of procathepsin B occurs via the default pathway and that of mature cathepsin B from an endosomal/lysosomal compartment that is readily mobilized in tumor cells and transformed cells [89,90,92]. A readily mobilized endosomal/lysosomal compartment has been observed in macrophages [93], suggesting that this may be common to the cells that participate in local degradation of extracellular matrices.

Membrane association

In macrophages [94] and hepatocytes [95], endosomes have been observed to contain cathepsin D. Furthermore, Stahl and colleagues [96] have shown that cathepsin D is associated with the membrane of macrophage endosomes. The form of cathepsin D associated with the membrane is the single chain mature form. In breast cancer cells, endosomes have also been shown to contain mature cathepsin D, as demonstrated by double immunofluorescence studies using markers for endocytosis and a monoclonal antibody specific for mature cathepsin D. The endosomal vesicles in this case are large acidic vesicles rather than small vesicles and are heterogeneous in nature. Montcourrier et al. [86] postulate that the function of mature cathepsin D in these large acidic vesicles is the digestion of phagocytosed and/or endocytosed extracellular matrix and consequently the facilitation of tumor cell invasion and metastasis.

In human and animal tumors, tumor cells, and transformed cells, we have consistently found that cathepsin B can be sedimented with a subcellular fraction enriched in plasma membrane and endosomes as well as a subcellular fraction enriched in lysosomes [2,20,21]. Only mature forms of cathepsin B are found in the membrane fractions as assessed by attempting to increase the activity by incubation with pepsin at acidic pH [89,97,99], a procedure that will activate procathepsin B in vitro. That only mature cathepsin B is found in the membrane fractions has been further confirmed by immunoblotting with cathepsin B antibodies [89] and by purifying cathepsin B from these fractions [98].

The presence of active cathepsin B in membrane fractions of tumors coincides with cytochemical observations of cathepsin B activity at the surface of tumor cells [21,99]. For example, in cytochemical studies on malignant breast cancer cells, a microgranular staining pattern indicative of cathepsin B activity is seen both in the perinuclear region (presumably in lysosomes) and throughout the cytoplasm, including in cytoplasmic projections at the cell surface [100]. A similar pattern has also been observed in highly metastatic B16 amelanotic melanoma cells and, in this case, the staining for cathepsin B activity has been shown to be abolished in the presence of E-64, an irreversible inhibitor of cysteine proteases [21,99] (see Table 1). Studies on the localization of cathepsin B protein in tumor cells and tissues confirm the cytochemical observations on the distribution of cathepsin B activity in tumor cells. In a number of human tumors [59,60,67,101,102], including human breast carcinoma [92], cathepsin B protein has been localized to the basolateral region of the cells, to regions adjacent to the cell membrane, to cell processes, and to the cell membrane itself. Immunofluorescent and immunogold studies have established that cathepsin B becomes associated with the cell membrane and cytoplasmic projections of MCF-10A1 human breast epithelial cell subsequent to their transfection with the c-Ha-*ras* oncogene [103–105] (also see chapter by Miller et al. for a further description of these cell lines). Cathepsin D undergoes a similar change in localization [92]. Thus, membrane association of cathepsins B and D occurs at an early stage of malignant progression of breast epithelial cells.

Since cathepsin D and cathepsin B are both lysosomal enzymes, the altered distribution of the two enzymes in *ras*-transformed MCF-10A1neoT cells may simply reflect an altered distribution of the lysosomal compartment or an endosomal compartment. To test this hypothesis, we have performed double-labeling studies for the two enzymes. In parental MCF-10A1 cells, that is, a diploid immortal cell line, cathepsin D and cathepsin B colocalize in perinuclear vesicles [92]. In the *ras*-transformed MCF-10A1neoT cells, perinuclear vesicles label for both cathepsin D and B, and peripheral vesicles label for cathepsin D alone or cathepsin B alone [92]. The fact that the two cathepsins are distributed in different vesicular compartments in transformed cells and tumor cells may be indicative of functional differences.

The presence of cathepsins D and B in distinct vesicles also suggests that the two cathepsins may be trafficked via different pathways [6,7]. Whether a similar mechanism might also be responsible for the membrane association of cathepsin B and cathepsin D is under investigation. Lysosomal enzymes are targeted to lysosomes primarily via the MPR pathway [5]. Both cathepsin D [82] and cathepsin B [106] can be trafficked via the MPR pathway, but whether this pathway is responsible for all of the trafficking of the two cathepsins is not clear. An alternative trafficking pathway, the mannose receptor (MR) pathway, has been identified in macrophages and has been shown to be involved in trafficking of cathepsin D [6].

McIntyre and Erickson [107] have proposed that proforms of two lysosomal proteases, cathepsins D and L, are targeted to the lysosome via two sequential mechanisms: The first is dependent on N-linked carbohydrates (e.g., MPRs or MRs) and the second on a 'targeting signal' or 'proenzyme receptor' binding region in the protein sequence. A lysosomal proenzyme receptor (LPR) responsible for trafficking of procathepsin L has been identified [7]. Mannose 6-phosphate–independent pathways have been identified in macrophages [96] and HepG2 cells, a hepatoma cell line [108]. At this time, Erickson and colleagues have not shown that procathepsin B can be trafficked via the LPR pathway.

Defects in MPRs (an absence or an increased rate of turnover) have been reported in tumor cell lines [109]. A decrease in the number of MPRs or the affinity of MPRs on the cell surface of virally transformed 3T3 fibroblasts has been suggested to be responsible for the secretion of procathepsin B by these cells [110]. Takeshima et al. [111] have shown that in hepatocytes unglycosylated procathepsin D synthesized in the presence of tunicamycin is correctly transported to the lysosomes and is processed to the mature enzyme. However, a deletion mutant of cathepsin D lacking the propeptide, although glycosylated, appears to be accumulated in the endoplasmic reticulum. These observations would suggest that the trafficking of cathepsin D in hepatocytes does not involve either MPRs or MRs, but rather involves a receptor such as the LPR that recognizes the propeptide of cathepsin D. The pathways responsible for targeting procathepsins D and B to lysosomes in normal cells need to be better understood before we can unravel the possible modification in the trafficking of these enzymes to lysosomes in transformed and tumor cells, and how this leads to compartmentalization of cathepsins D and B in distinct vesicles and membrane association of the two cathepsins.

Is cathepsin D a prognostic marker for breast cancer?

Human breast cancers are the leading cause of cancer deaths for women in the United States. Therefore, identifying prognostic factors that will distinguish women at risk for early relapse and metastasis is a critically important goal. Rochefort's group has, for a long time, observed a consistent correlation between cathepsin D and prognosis in patients with breast cancer

Table 3. Prognostic value of cathepsin D in breast cancer cytosols

No. patients	Shortened survival	High risk of relapse	Other information	Ref.
122	+	+	Positive staining correlates with better prognosis, most evident in ER$^+$ or node-positive subsets	112
396	nd	nd	Shorter relapse-free survival in premenopausal and postmenopausal patients	113
140	nd	nd	Independent of *neu/erb*B2 and *int*-2; correlates with c-*myc*	84
397	+	+	Node-negative patients only	34
413	+	+	Shorter survival in node-positive patients	117
139	+	+	All in node-negative patients	116
331	+	nd	Only in ER$^-$ subgroup	119
123	+	+	Only prospective study to date; correlates with axillary lymph node involvement	118

nd = not determined.

[36,81,113,114]. Others, relying primarily on immunohistochemical techniques, have not confirmed this [73,115].

Levels of cathepsin D in cytosolic extracts of breast tissue are measured most frequently by a sandwich ELISA, which uses two monoclonal antibodies. One of these recognizes the 34 kD form of mature cathepsin D, and the other recognizes the 48 and 52 kD proforms of cathepsin D (see Table 1) [113,116]. This assay is simple and reliable; furthermore, >90% of all forms of cathepsin D have been shown to be extracted by the homogenization procedure used to prepare cytosolic extracts of breast tissue. The findings in terms of prognostic value of cathepsin D ELISAs are summarized in Table 3.

In Cox multivariate studies, cathepsin D is one of the three most significant prognostic markers for breast cancer [37,117]. In both retrospective [84,113,114,118] and prospective [119] studies, a high cytosolic level of cathepsin D in breast cancer is associated with shortened patient survival and a higher risk of early relapse and metastasis. If patients are divided into specific subgroups, the published studies support the contention that high cytosolic levels of cathepsin D indicate a poor prognosis for breast cancer patients. A high cytosolic level of cathepsin D does not seem to be related to other important prognostic factors for breast cancer, such as degree of lymph node invasiveness, tumor size, Scarff and Bloom histological grade, DNA ploidy, patient age [34,84,113,114,117,118,120], or amplification of the *neu/erb*B2 or *int*-2 oncogenes [84]. Cathepsin D levels correlate with ER status only in premenopausal patients [114], which is consistent with the high constitutive production of cathepsin D by ER$^-$ cell lines. The prognostic value of cathepsin D, therefore, supplements that of other markers. The independence of cathepsin D from other markers suggests that cathepsin D is associated with a stage

337

of breast cancer progression that differs from that detected by other prognostic parameters of breast cancer.

An important limitation of ELISAs is that neither the cellular origin (cancer cells, macrophages, or fibroblasts) nor the subcellular localization of cathepsin D is determined. Therefore, investigators have performed immunohistochemical analyses of cathepsin D in breast tissues. In contrast to ELISAs, the prognostic value of cathepsin D staining has been found to be negative in some cases and positive in others (Table 4). Although Henry et al. [114] suggest that the difference between the ELISA and immunohistochemistry results may reflect secreted procathepsin D that cannot be determined by immunohistochemistry, this would seem unlikely because the contribution of procathepsin D to total cathepsin D level is generally low (<6%) [84]. Even immunohistochemical studies using the same antibody give contradictory results: Positive staining for cathepsin D indicates a better prognosis in one study [115], yet intense cathepsin D staining is associated with shortened patient survival in two other studies [32,121].

The current controversy over the value of cathepsin D as a prognostic marker in breast cancer is highlighted by two recent independent studies. Castiglioni et al. [73], using a rabbit antiserum to purified human cathepsin D from Dako (Carpenteria, CA), found no evidence for cathepsin D being of prognostic value in breast cancer. In contrast, Roger et al. [36], using the M1G8 mouse monoclonal antibody from Biosys (Gif-sur-Yvette, France) that recognizes procathepsin D, found that immunohistochemical staining for cathepsin D confirmed their ELISAs showing that cathepsin D is an independent prognostic marker for breast cancer. These contradictory results might arise from the fact that, in addition to tumor cells, stromal cells (mainly macrophages and lymphocytes) within breast cancer tissue can express cathepsin D [36,41,121–123]. A further consideration in the immunohistochemical analyses is the distribution within the tumor of the section being stained for cathepsin D (or any other potential prognostic marker). In this regard, we have shown that for cathepsin B, cells at the invasive edges of bladder [65] and prostate [66,67] tumors stain intensely, whereas cells further back in the tumor mass may exhibit no staining. Analyses of cathepsin B activity in tumor cells microdissected from the invasive edges of colorectal [68] and breast [69] cancers also reveal an increased expression of cathepsin B in these regions. Whether the observations on cathepsin B will extend to cathepsin D is not known.

Several recent studies have reported that proteases, including cathepsin D, are present in stromal cells of malignant tumors, suggesting that stromal cells may participate in the process of invasion [122–125]. Unfortunately, many studies, including that of Castiglioni et al. [73], have not provided an independent evaluation of the prognostic importance of tumor cell and stromal cell cathepsin D expression in breast cancer [32,73,120,123]. Visscher et al. [41] have established that cathepsin D staining of stromal fibroblasts, but not of tumor cells, shows a significant correlation with metastasis in breast cancer

Table 4. Immunohistochemical staining for cathepsin D in breast cancer

No. patients	Prognostic value	Antibody[a]	Tumor cells	Stromal cells	Other information	Ref.
103	+	Novocastra polyclonal IgG	69% (criterion of >25% positive cells)	73% (criterion of >25% positive cells)	Increased stromal cell (but not tumor cell) staining correlates with tumor grade and shortened patient survival	121
136	−	Novocastra polyclonal antiserum	60% (criterion of many granules in majority of cells)	73% (criterion of many granules in majority of cells)	No correlation between staining of tumor cells and survival at 5 years	123
245	nd[b]	Dako polyclonal antiserum	49%[c] (staining detectable)	nd	Not an independent marker of survival	32
80	−	Dako polyclonal antiserum	90% (staining detectable)	nd	No correlation between staining and survival or other aggressive behavior	73
562	−	Biosys monoclonal M1G8#	nd	nd	77% positive staining of frozen sections; no relationship between staining and survival	127
41	+	Biosys monoclonal M1G8#	QIC score[d] 65 (2–373)	QIC score[d] 79 (2–220)	Staining intensity in tumor cells, but not macrophages,[e] useful in evaluating risk of metastasis	36
359	+	Polyclonal antiserum	74% (granular cytoplasmic staining detectable)	nd	Correlates with positive nodes; not independent of other tumor variables	120
213	+	Monoclonal 1C11 (IgG1)	77% (staining detectable)	76% (staining detectable)	High stromal cell, but not tumor cell, staining associated with poor survival	122
86	+	Biosys monoclonal	70% (staining detectable)	89% (staining detectable)	Stromal cell staining correlates with positive nodes and metastasis; sum of tumor and stromal cell staining correlates with shortened survival	41

[a] Antibodies in references 121 and 123, references 32 and 73, and references 36 and 127 were from the same origin. The antibodies used in other studies were either prepared in the authors' laboratories [120] or not further described in the publications.

[b] nd = not determined.

[c] Histoscore combining intensity and distribution of staining with the estimated proportion of cells stained.

[d] QIC = computerized quantitative immunohistochemical score (% of stained surface × mean staining intensity × 10×). QIC scores listed from ductal breast carcinoma only.

[e] Macrophages were stained with an anti-CD68 monoclonal antibody (Dakopatts, Glostrup, Denmark).

patients. Recently, two more reports [122,123], using yet another two separate antibodies to cathepsin D (Table 4), demonstrated that increased stromal cell cathepsin D staining is associated with shortened patient survival, but increased tumor cell staining is not. Roger et al. [36] found that macrophages stain heavily for cathepsin D, particularly macrophages in the tumor periphery. In this case, an anti-CD68 monoclonal antibody was used to identify macrophages. Nevertheless, the cytosolic levels of cathepsin D correlate with cathepsin D expression in cancer cells rather than with the number of macrophages.

In another independent study, Isola et al. [37] evaluated cathepsin D expression in macrophages and cancer cells in 262 node-negative breast cancers. In this study, cathepsin D staining in cancer cells, rather than in macrophages, correlates with shortened patient survival. Most studies support the hypothesis that increased expression of cathepsin D in breast cancer cells, rather than the recruitment of macrophages that express cathepsin D, is responsible for the high risk of relapse and development of metastases. This is further substantiated by the increased metastatic capability of tumor cells that overexpress cathepsin D due to transfection with a cathepsin D cDNA [126].

The conflicting results of Castiglioni et al. [73] and Rogers et al. [36] might also be due to the use of different antibodies. Antibodies can differ in their affinity. In addition, as the cathepsin D molecule exists in at least three different protein forms, each of which may differ in glycosylation, antibodies may recognize distinct molecular configurations of the same molecule. However, differences in affinities for cathepsin D and in the specific forms of cathepsin D recognized cannot explain the disparate results obtained in studies using the same polyclonal [121,123] or monoclonal antibody [36,127]. Another possibility is that the use of different fixation procedures and/or methods for quantitation of cathepsin D staining in breast cancer tissue leads to contradictory results (Table 4). Perhaps, given the lack of uniformity in the assays used, contradictory results should be expected. More large-scale cooperative studies in which the pathologists use the same antibody and fixation procedures, as well as the same methods for quantitation, are needed to determine the true prognostic value of cathepsin D staining [121]. Studies using multiple techniques that might provide an internal confirmation of positive or negative findings would also be of value. In such a recent study, Ravdin et al. [127] performed immunohistochemical staining for cathepsin D, but could not confirm their earlier findings by immunoblotting that cathepsin D is a prognostic marker in node-negative breast cancer.

Review of the clinical studies on cathepsin D leads one to the conclusion that the prognostic significance of cathepsin D determinations, although provocative, are still investigational in nature and not yet ready for widespread clinical application. The assays (whether ELISAs, immunohistochemical, or immunoblotting) need to be standardized to ensure quality control. This, together with a deeper understanding of the patient subsets, will be required to fully define the role of cathepsin D in breast cancer.

340

Role of cathepsin D and cathepsin B in breast cancer progression

Both clinical and basic studies on expression of cathepsins D and B in breast cancer indicate that high cathepsin levels are either an epiphenomenon of malignant progression or, more excitingly, play a direct role in at least one step of malignant progression. Several reports have confirmed that increased expression of cathepsins D and B (mRNA, protein and activity) is a marker of the malignant phenotype [2,18,59,60]. Direct evidence that overexpression of cathepsin D in breast cancer cells can promote some steps in metastasis has been obtained in adenovirus-transformed 3Y1 normal rat embryo cells transfected with a cathepsin D cDNA [126].

The mechanisms by which cathepsins are involved in tumor invasion and progression are not clear. Cathepsin B may facilitate invasion directly by degrading extracellular matrix [10] or indirectly by activating other proteases, such as urokinase [12]. Increased expression of cathepsin B at the basolateral surface of colorectal carcinoma cells [59], that is, the surface in direct contact with basement membrane, suggests that this enzyme may be involved in tumor invasion. A strong correlation between overexpression of cathepsin B and a shortened patient survival of colorectal carcinoma indicates that cathepsin B may be a significant prognostic indicator. Briozzo et al. [128] established that the degradation at acidic pH of extracellular matrix by proteases secreted into the conditioned media of breast cancer cells is due primarily to cathepsin D, since it can be completely inhibited by pepstatin, an aspartic protease inhibitor (Table 1). Secreted cathepsin D might also promote the spread of breast cancer by activating other proteases, including procathepsin B or degrading extracellular matrix proteins [21,81,129]. Nevertheless, the pH optimum for cathepsin D is so acidic that a significant extracellular role for this enzyme seems unlikely. Cathepsin D may play a role in digestion of extracellular matrix proteins intracellularly: Matrix proteins have been shown to be degraded by cathepsin D within large acidic vesicles in breast cancer cells [86], presumably following internalization by phagocytosis.

Proteases located on the external cell surface of breast cancer cells might be responsible for extracellular matrix degradation. For cathepsin B, we have shown that the membrane-associated enzyme is a mature active form [89]. Immunofluorescence and immunogold studies indicate that cathepsin B [92] and cathepsin D (Figures 2 and 3) are concentrated on the external surface of the plasma membrane. The localization of these enzymes on the surface of human breast epithelial cells is increased by malignant progression (see Figures 2 and 3; also see Figure 5 in Sameni et al. [92]). There-dimensional reconstructions of optical sections taken through the cells indicate that in *ras*-transformed MCF-10A1neoT cells cathepsin D is localized primarily on the basolateral surface of the cells (Figure 3), as is cathepsin B [130]. We have previously shown that cathepsin B is also on the basolateral surface of MCF-7 and BT20 human breast carcinoma cell lines [92].

Recent studies indicate that cathepsin B is concentrated intracellularly in

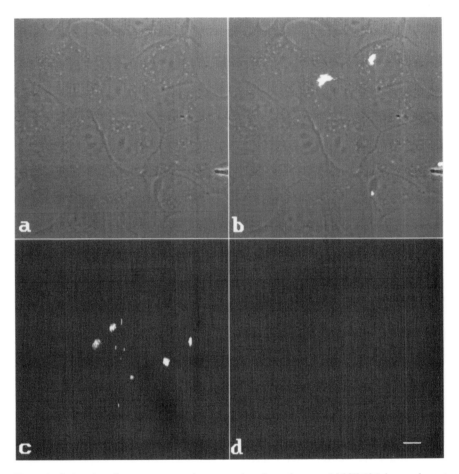

Figure 2. Only a few discrete areas on the external surface of parental MCF-10A human breast epithelial cells exhibit fluorescent labeling for cathepsin D. **a**: Phase contrast image of MCF-10A cells. **b**: Single optical slice of fluorescent labeling for cathepsin D that has been superimposed on the phase contrast image of panel a. **c**: Three-dimensional reconstruction of optical slices of fluorescent labeling for cathepsin D. **d**: Control in which the primary antibody was replaced with nonimmune serum. The primary antibody was rabbit anti-human cathepsin B IgG [52,89], and the secondary antibody was Texas red–conjugated donkey anti-rabbit IgG. Bar, 10 μm.

regions of the cells shown to be involved in matrix degradation (Table 2). Treatment of MCF-7 breast carcinoma cells with tumor necrosis factor α results in the concentration of cathepsin B staining at focal adhesions. In a highly malignant human glioblastoma cell line derived from a glioblastoma that expresses 15-fold more cathepsin B activity than matched normal brain tissue, cathepsin B is concentrated in foot processes. These foot processes resemble invadopodia, highly specialized matrix-degrading structures described by Monsky et al. [131]. Other proteases have been localized to invadopodia [132]. Perhaps this facilitates the proteolytic cascade responsible

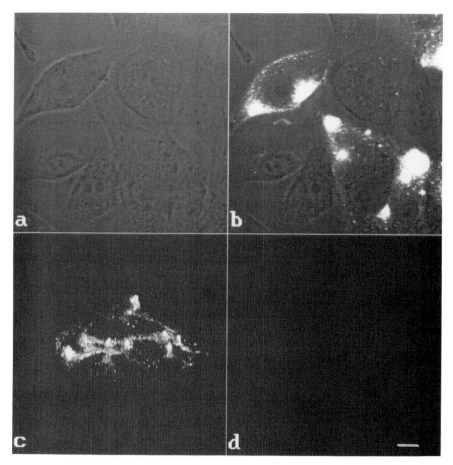

Figure 3. *Ras*-transformation of the MCF-10 human breast epithelial cells resulted in a large increase in labeling for cathepsin D on the external basolateral surface of these cells. **a**: Phase contrast image of MCF-10AneoT cells. **b**: Single optical slice of fluorescent labeling for cathepsin D that has been superimposed on phase contrast image of panel a. **c**: Three-dimensional reconstruction of optical slices of fluorescent labeling for cathepsin D. **d**: Control in which the primary antibody was replaced with nonimmune serum. The primary antibody was rabbit anti-human cathepsin B IgG [52,89], and the secondary antibody was Texas red–conjugated donkey anti-rabbit IgG. Bar, 10 μm.

for degradation of extracellular matrix by invading cells. Many membrane-associated proteases have been identified in breast cancer; these include gelatinase A (MMP-2 or 72 kD type IV collagenase) and its putative membrane receptor [131], stromelysin 3 [133], urokinase and its receptor [134], and cathepsins B and D [89,92]. The localization of proteases on the cell surface will result in an increase in their local concentration to a point that the balance between proteases and their endogenous inhibitors will favor proteolysis [135], thus favoring the degradation of basement membrane and tumor cell

343

invasion. The accessibility of proteases at the surface of tumor cells might be exploited for diagnostic or therapeutic purposes, for example, by the development of specific antibodies to identify micrometastases, by the development of specific antibodies and inhibitors that can block the activities of the proteases, and by the development of specific antibodies that can target cytotoxic agents to kill the targeted cells.

Another possible function for procathepsin D is to promote the proliferation of breast cancer cells by acting as an autocrine mitogen similar to insulin-like growth factor II (IGF II) [136,137]. However, in contrast to IGF II, procathepsin D has a more pronounced mitogenic effect on breast cancer cell lines; proliferation can be inhibited by antibodies specific for the propeptide of cathepsin D [137]. This suggests a specific function for procathepsin D in the progression of breast cancer. The mechanisms for this mitogenic activity of cathepsin D are unknown. However, recent observations suggest that this enzyme may induce cell proliferation by activating latent forms of growth factors or by interacting with growth factor receptors extracellularly or intracellularly [137]. Another possibility is that secreted cathepsin D from breast cancer cells upregulates the activity of IGF by degrading IGF-binding protein-3, a protein that normally binds to IGF peptides and modulates their biological activities [138].

Studies to date support, but do not prove, that cathepsins D and B play functional roles in malignant progression. In breast cancer, cathepsin D appears to play a leading role in progression and metastasis, as indicated by the positive correlation between the level of cathepsin D (protein and activity) and malignant progression, and the high risk of early relapse and metastasis observed in patients with breast cancer [34,84,114]. An important functional role for cathepsin D in breast cancer is further supported by the fact that tumor cells transfected with a mammalian expression vector of human cathepsin D exhibit an increased metastatic potential [126]. In other cancers, for example, in melanoma [47,139,140] and gliomas [60], cathepsin B appears to play a more important role than does cathepsin D. These observations, as well as studies on the roles of metalloproteases and serine proteases in breast cancer and other cancers, suggest that more than one protease is required for malignant progression. The proteases involved appear to depend on the tissue of origin of the cancer. Furthermore, the functional proteases may change depending on the stage of malignant progression. Understanding the roles played by cathepsins D and B and by other proteases will require cooperation among investigators, as we need to evaluate multiple proteases concurrently in a cancer arising in a single tissue, such as breast cancer, and at various stages during the progression of that cancer.

Acknowledgments

The authors thank Dr. Kamiar Moin for his critical reading of the manuscript and Ms. Mansoureh Sameni for providing Figures 2 and 3. This work was

344

supported in part by USPHS grants CA 36481 and CA 56586. Dr. Ren is a fellow of the National Cancer Institute Cancer Center Oncology Research Faculty Development Program of the National Cancer Institute. Development and maintenance of the MCF-10 human breast epithelial cell lines has been supported by a grant from the Elsa U. Pardee Foundation and the core support grant of the Michigan Cancer Foundation/Meyer L. Prentis Comprehensive Cancer Center of Metropolitan Detroit.

References

1. Willstaffer R, Bamann E (1929) Uber die Proteasen der Magenschleimhaut. Erste Abhandlung uber die Enzyme der Leukocyten. *Hoppe-Seylers Z Physiol Chem* 180:127–143.
2. Sloane BF, Moin K, Lah TT (1994) Regulation of lysosomal endopeptidases in malignant neoplasia. In *Aspects of the Biochemistry and Molecular Biology of Tumors*. TG Pretlow, TP Pretlow (eds). New York: Academic Press, pp 411–466.
3. Finley EM, Kornfeld S (1994) Subcellular localization and targetting of cathepsin E. *J Biol Chem* 269:31259–31266.
4. Kirschke H, Wiederanders B, Bromme D, Rinne A (1989) Cathepsin S from bovine spleen. Purification, distribution, intracellular localization and action on proteins. *Biochem J* 264:467–473.
5. Kornfeld S (1990) Lysosomal enzyme targeting. *Biochem Soc Trans* 18:367–374.
6. Stahl P, Schlesinger PH, Sigardson E, Rodman JS, Lee YC (1980) Receptor-mediated pinocytosis of mannose glycoconjugates by macrophages: Characterization and evidence for receptor recycling. *Cell* 19:207–215.
7. McIntyre GF, Erickson AH (1993) The lysosomal proenzyme receptor that binds procathepsin L to microsomal membranes at pH 5 is a 43-kDa integral membrane protein. *Proc Natl Acad Sci USA* 90:10588–10592.
8. Schwartz WN, Barrett AJ (1980) Human cathepsin H. *Biochem J* 191:487–497.
9. Koga H, Yamada H, Nishimura Y, Kato K, Imoto T (1991) Multiple proteolytic action of rat liver cathepsin B: Specificities and pH-dependences of the endo and exopeptidase activities. *J Biochem (Tokyo)* 110:179–188.
10. Buck MR, Karustis DG, Day NA, Honn KV, Sloane BF (1992) Degradation of extracellular-matrix proteins by human cathepsin B from normal and tumour tissues. *Biochem J* 282:273–278.
11. Lah TT, Buck MR, Honn KV, Crissman JD, Rao NC, Liotta LA, Sloane BF (1989) Degradation of laminin by human tumor cathepsin B. *Clin Exp Metastasis* 7:461–468.
12. Kobayashi H, Schmitt M, Goretzki L, Chucholowski N, Calvete J, Kramer M, Gunzler WA, Janicke F, Graeff H (1991) Cathepsin B efficiently activates the soluble and the tumor cell receptor-bound form of the proenzyme urokinase-type plasminogen activator (pro-uPA). *J Bio Chem* 266:5147–5152.
13. Baron R (1989) Molecular mechanisms of bone resorption by the osteoclast. *Anat Rec* 224:317–324.
14. Chapman HA, Munger JS, Shi GP (1994) The role of thiol proteases in tissue injury and remodeling. *Am J Respir Crit Care Med* 150:S155–S159.
15. Poole AR, Tiltman KJ, Recklies AD, Stoker TAM (1980) Differences in the secretion of the proteinase cathepsin B at the edges of human breast carcinomas and fibroadenomas. *Nature* 273:545–547.
16. Recklies AD, Tiltman KJ, Stoker TAM, Poole AR (1980) Secretion of proteinases from malignant and nonmalignant human breast tissue. *Cancer Res* 40:550–556.
17. Westley BR, Rochefort H (1980) A secreted glycoprotein induced by estrogen in human breast cancer cell lines. *Cell* 20:352–362.

18. Rochefort H (1990) Biological and clinical significance of cathepsin D in breast cancer. *Semin Cancer Biol* 1:153–160.
19. Rochefort H, Capony F, Garcia M (1990) Cathepsin D: A protease involved in breast cancer metastasis. *Cancer Metastasis Rev* 9:321–331.
20. Sloane BF (1990) Cathepsin B and cystatins: Evidence for a role in cancer progression. *Semin Cancer Biol* 1:137–152.
21. Sloane BF, Moin K, Krepela E, Rozhin J (1990) Cathepsin B and its endogenous inhibitors: Role in tumor malignancy. *Cancer Metastasis Rev* 9:333–352.
22. Redecker B, Heckendorf B, Grosch H, Mersmann G, Hasilik A (1991) Molecular organization of the human cathepsin D gene. *DNA Cell Biol* 10:423–431.
23. Augereau P, Garcia M, Mattei MG, Cavailles B, Depadova F, Derocq D, Capony F, Ferrara P, Rochefort H (1988) Cloning and sequencing of the 52K cathepsin D complementary deoxyribonucleic acid of MCF7 breast cancer cells and mapping on chromosome 11. *Mol Endocrinol* 2:186–192.
24. Theillet C, Lidereau R, Escot C, Hutzell P, Prunet M, Gest J, Scholm J, Callahan R (1986) Loss of c-H-*ras*-1 allele and aggressive human primary breast carcinomas. *Cancer Res* 46:4776–4781.
25. Cavailles V, Augereau P, Rochefort H (1993) Cathepsin D gene is controlled by a mixed promoter and estrogens stimulate only TATA-dependent transcription in breast cancer lines. *Proc Natl Acad Sci USA* 90:203–207.
26. Cavailles V, Augereau P, Garcia M, Rochefort H (1988) Estrogens and growth factors induce mRNA of the procathepsin D secreted by breast cancer cells. *Nucleic Acids Res* 16:1903–1919.
27. Rochefort H, Cavailles V, Augereau P, Capony F, Maudelonde T, Touitou I, Garcia M (1989) Overexpression and hormonal regulation of pro-cathepsin D in mammary and endometrial cancer. *J Steroid Biochem* 34:177–182.
28. Cavailles V, Garcia M, Rochefort H (1989) Regulation of cathepsin D and pS2 gene expression by growth factors in MCF7 human breast cancer cells. *Mol Endocrinol* 3:552–558.
29. Cavailles V, Augereau P, Rochefort H (1991) Cathepsin D gene of human MCF7 cells contains estrogen-responsive sequences in its 5′ proximal flanking region. *Biochem Biophys Res Commun* 174:816–824.
30. Westley BR, May FEB (1987) Oestrogen regulates cathepsin D mRNA levels in oestrogen responsive human breast cancer cells. *Nucleic Acids Res* 15:3773–3786.
31. Garcia M, Lacombe MJ, Duplay H, Cavailles V, Deroc Delarue JC, Krebs B, Contesso G, Sancho-Garnic, Richer G, Domerque J, Namer M, Rochefort H (1987) Immunohistochemical distribution of the 52-kDa protein in mammary tumors: A marker associated with cell proliferation rather than with hormone responsiveness. *J Steroid Biochem* 27:439–445.
32. Kandalaft PL, Change KL, Ahn CW (1993) Prognostic significance of immunohistochemical analysis of cathepsin D in low-stage breast cancer. *Cancer* 71:2756–2763.
33. Brouillet JP, Theillet G, Maudelonde T (1990) Cathepsin D assay in primary breast cancer and lymph nodes: Relationship with c-myc, c-erb-B-2 and int-2 oncogene amplification and node invasiveness. *Eur J Cancer* 26:437–441.
34. Tandon A, Clark G, Chamness G, Chirgwin J, McGuire WL (1990) Cathepsin D and prognosis in breast cancer. *N Engl J Med* 322:297–302.
35. Capony F, Rougeot C, Montcourrier P, Cavailles V, Salazar G, Rochefort H (1989) Increased secretion, altered processing, and glycosylation of pro-cathepsin D in human mammary cancer cells. *Cancer Res* 49:3904–3909.
36. Roger P, Montcourrier P, Maudelonde T, Brouillet JP, Pages A, Laffargue F, Rochefort H (1994) Cathepsin D immunostaining in paraffin-embedded breast cancer cells and macrophages correlated with cytosolic assay. *Hum Pathol* 25:863–871.
37. Isola J, Weitz S, Visakorpi T (1993) Cathepsin D expression detected by immunohistochemistry has independent prognostic value in axillary node-negative breast cancer. *J Clin Oncol* 11:36–43.

38. Nalton H, Eguchi Y, Ueyama H, Kodama M, Hattort T (1995) Localization of urokinase type plasminogen activator, plasminogen activator inhibitor-1, 2 and plasminogen in colon cancer. *Jpn J Cancer Res* 86:48–56.
39. Polette M, Clavel C, Birembaut P, deClerck YA (1993) Localization by in situ hybridization of messenger RNAs encoding stromelysin-3 and tissue inhibitors of metalloproteinases TIMP-1 and TIMP-2 in human head and neck carcinomas. *Pathol Res Pract* 189:1052–1057.
40. Charpin C, Bonnier P, Khouzami A (1992) Inflamatory breast carcinoma: An immunohis-tochemical study using monoclonal anti-PHER-2/neu, PS2, cathepsin, ER and PR. *Anticancer Res* 12:591–598.
41. Visscher DW, Sarkar F, LoRusso D (1993) Immunohistochemical evaluation of invasion associated proteases in breast carcinoma. *Mod Pathol* 6:302–306.
42. Maguchi S, Taniguchi W, Makito A (1988) Elevated activity and increased mannose-6-phosphate in the carbohydrate moiety of cathepsin D from human hepatoma. *Cancer Res* 48:362–367.
43. Robson DK, Ironside JW, Reid WA, Bogue PR (1990) Immunolocalization of cathepsin D in the human central nervous system and central nervous system neoplasms. *Neuropathol Appl Neurobiol* 16:39–44.
44. Sinadinovic J, Cvejic D, Savin S, Micic JV, Jancic-Zguricas M (1989) Enhanced acid protease activity of lysosomes from papillary thyroid carcinoma. *Cancer* 63:1179–1182.
45. Wang X, Chan SJ, Eddy RL, Byers MG, Fukushima Y, Henry WM, Haley LL, Steiner DF, Shows, TB (1988) Chromosome assignment of cathepsin B (CTSB) to 8p22 and cathepsin H (CTSH) to 15q24–q25. *Cytogenet Cell Genet* 46:710–711.
46. Saka WA, Macoska JA, Benson P, Grignon DJ, Wolman SR, Pontes JE, Crissman JD (1994) Allelic loss in locally metastatic, multisampled prostate cancer. *Cancer Res* 54:3273–3277.
47. Gong Q, Chan SJ, Bajkowski AS, Steiner DF, Frankfater A (1993) Characterization of the cathepsin B gene and multiple mRNAs in human tissues: Evidence for alternative splicing of cathepsin B pre-mRNA. *DNA Cell Biol* 12:299–309.
48. Berquin IM, Cao L, Fong D, Sloane BF (1995) Identification of two new exons and multiple transcriptional start points in the 5'-untranslated region of the human cathepsin B encoding gene. *Gene* 159:143–149.
49. Cao L, Taggart RT, Berquin IM, Moin K, Fong D, Sloane BF (1994) Human gastric adenocarcinoma cathepsin B: Isolation and sequencing of full-length cDNAs and polymorphisms of the gene. *Gene* 139:163–169.
50. Tam SW, Cote-Paulino LR, Peak DA, Sheahan K, Murnane MJ (1994) Human cathepsin B-encoding cDNAS: Sequence variations in the 3'-untranslated region. *Gene* 139:171–176.
51. Chan SJ, San Segundo B, McCormick MB, Steiner DF (1986) Nucleotide and predicted amino acid sequences of cloned human and mouse preprocathepsin B cDNAs. *Proc Natl Acad Sci USA* 83:7721–7725.
52. Moin K, Day NA, Sameni M, Hasnain S, Hirama T, Sloane BF (1992) Human tumour cathepsin B: Comparison with normal human liver cathepsin B. *Biochem J* 285:427–434.
53. Qian F, Frankfater A, Chan SJ, Steiner DF (1991) The structure of the mouse cathepsin B gene and its putative promoter. *DNA Cell Biol* 10:159–168.
54. Rhaissi H, Bechet D, Ferrara M (1993) Multiple leader sequences for mouse cathepsin B mRNA? *Biochimie* 75:899–904.
55. Berquin IM, Ahram M, Sloane BF (1995) Is human cathepsin B expression in human glioblastomas initiated from several promoter regions? *Proc Am Assoc Cancer Res* 36:98.
56. Frosch BA, Berquin IM, Sloane BF (1995) Increased cathepsin B in malignant tissues: The role of post-transcriptional regulation. *Proc Am Assoc Cancer Res* 36:98.
57. Murnane MJ, Sheahan K, Ozdemirli M, Shuja S (1991) Stage-specific increases in cathepsin B messenger RNA content in human colorectal carcinoma. *Cancer Res* 51:1137–1142.
58. Campo E, Munoz J, Nadal A, Jares P, Fernandez PL, Pakein A, Emmert-Buck M, Sloane B, Cardesa A (1995) Cathepsin B mRNA overexpression correlates with tumor progression in colorectal carcinomas. *Lab Invest* 72:A58.

347

59. Campo E, Munoz J, Miquel R, Palacin A, Cardesa A, Sloane BF, Emmert-Buck M (1994) Cathepsin B expression in colorectal carcinomas correlates with tumor progression and shortened patient survival. *Am J Pathol* 145:301–309.

60. Rempel SA, Rosenblum ML, Mikkelsen T, Yan PS, Ellis KD, Golembieski WA, Sameni M, Rozhin J, Ziegler G, Sloane BF (1994) Cathepsin B expression and localization in glioma progression and invasion. *Cancer Res* 54:6027–6031.

61. Mikkelsen T, Spencer D, Nelson K, Rasnick D, Rosenblum ML (1995) Novel cysteine protease inhibitors in the control of glioma cell migration. *Proc Am Assoc Cancer Res* 36:99.

62. Newell KJ, Witty JP, Rodgers WH, Matrisian LM (1994) Expression and localization of matrix-degrading metalloproteinases during colorectal tumorigenesis. *Mol Carcinog* 10:199–206.

63. Nagle RB, Knox JD, Wolf C, Bowden GT, Cress AE (1994) Adhesion molecules, extracellular matrix, and proteases in prostate carcinoma. *J Cell Biochem* 19S:232–237.

64. Romer J, Pyke C, Lund LR, Eriksen J, Kristensen P, Ronne E, Hoyerhasen G, Dano K, Brunner N (1994) Expression of uPA and its receptor by both neoplastic and stromal cells during xenograft invasion. *Int J Cancer* 57:553–560.

65. Visscher DW, Sloane BF, Sameni M, Babiarz JW, Jacobson J, Crissman JD (1994) Clincopathologic significance of cathepsin B immunostaining in transitional neoplasia. *Mod Pathol* 7:76–81.

66. Sinha AA, Gleason DF, DeLeon OF, Wilson MJ, Sloane BF (1993) Localization of a biotinylated cathepsin B oligonucleatide probe in human prostate including invasive cells and invasive edges by in situ hybridization. *Anat Rec* 235:233–240.

67. Sinha AA, Wilson MJ, Gleason DF, Reddy PR, Sameni M, Sloane BF (1995) Immunohistochemical localization of cathepsin B in neoplastic human prostate. *Prostate* 25, 26:171–178.

68. Emmert-Buck MR, Roth MJ, Zhuang Z, Campo E, Rozhin J, Sloane BF, Liotta LA, Stetler-Stevenson WG (1994) Increased gelatinase A (MMP-2) and cathepsin B activity in microdissected human colon cancer samples. *Am J Pathol* 145:1285–1290.

69. Buck MR, Roth MJ, Zhuang Z, Campo E, Rozhin J, Sloane BF, Liotta LA, Stetler-Stevenson WG (1994) Increased levels of 72 kilodalton type IV collagenase and cathepsin B in microdissected human breast and colon carcinomas. *Proc Am Assoc Cancer Res* 35:59.

70. Gabrijelcic D, Svetic B, Spaic D, Skrk J, Budihna M, Dolenc I, Popovic T, Cotic V, Turk V (1992) Cathepsin B, H and L in human breast carcinoma. *Eur J Clin Chem Clin Biochem* 30:69–74.

71. Lah TT, Kokalj-Kunovar M, Strukeli B (1992) Stefins and lysosomal cathepsin B, L and D in human breast carcinoma. *Int J Cancer* 50:36–44.

72. Krepela E, Viacav J, Cernoch M (1989) Cathepsin B in human breast tumor tissue and cancer cells. *Neoplasma* 35:41–52.

73. Castiglioni T, Merino MJ, Elsner B, Lah TT, Sloane BF, Emmert-Buck MR (1994) Immunohistochemical analysis of cathepsins D, B and L in human breast cancer. *Hum Pathol* 25:857–862.

74. Qian F, Chan SJ, Achkar C, Steiner DF, Frankfater A (1994) Transcriptional regulation of cathepsin B expression in B16 melanomas of varying metastatic potential. *Biochem Biophys Res Commun* 202:429–436.

75. Ward CJ, Crocker J, Chan SJ, Stockley RA, Burnett D (1990) Changes in the expression of elastase and cathepsin B with differentiation of U937 promonocytes by GMCSF. *Biochem Biophys Res Commun* 167:659–664.

76. Huet G, Flipo R-M, Colin C, Janin A, Hemon B, Collyn-d'Hooge M, Lafyatis R, Duquesnoy B, Degand P (1993) Stimulation of the secretion of latent cysteine proteinase activity by tumor necrosis factor α and interleukin-1. *Arthritis Rheum* 36:772–780.

77. Corticchiato O, Cajot J-F, Abrahamson M, Chan SJ, Keppler D, Sordat B (1992) Cystatin C and cathepsin B in human colon carcinoma: Expression by cell lines and matrix degradation. *Int J Cancer* 52:645–652.

78. Page AE, Warburton MJ, Chambers TJ, Pringle JAS, Hayman AR (1992) Human osteoclastomas contain multiple forms of cathepsin B. *Biochim Biophys Acta* 1116:57–66.

348

79. Mehtani S, Gong Q, Frankfater A (1995) Expression in COS cells of a cDNA encoding a novel human tumor form of cathepsin B. *J Cell Biochem Suppl* 19B:17.

80. Morisset M, Capony F, Rochefort H (1986) The 52 kDa estrogen-induced protein secreted by MCF-7 cells is a lysosomal acidic protease. *Biochem Biophys Res Commun* 138:102–109.

81. Rochefort H (1992) Cathepsin D in breast cancer: A tissue marker associated with metastasis. *Eur J Cancer* 28A:1780–1783.

82. Mathieu M, Vignon F, Capony F, Rochefort H (1991) Estradiol down-regulates the mannose-6-phosphate/insulin-like growth factor-II receptor gene and induces cathepsin-D in breast cancer cells: A receptor saturation mechanism to increase the secretion of lysosomal proenzymes. *Mol Endocrinol* 5:815–822.

83. Sanchez LM, Ferrandon AA, Diez-Itazu I, Vizoso F, Ruibal A, Lopez-Otin CT (1993) Cathepsin D in breast secretion from woman with breast cancer. *Br J Cancer* 67:1076–1081.

84. Brouillet JP, Spyratos F, Hacene K (1993) Immunoradiometric assay procathepsin D in breast cancer cytosol: Relative prognostic value versus total cathepsin D. *Eur J Cancer* 29A:1248–1251.

85. Rijnboutt S, Stoorvogel W, Geuze HJ, Strous GJ (1992) Identification of subcellular compartments involved in biosynthetic processing of cathepsin D. *J Biol Chem* 267:15665–15672.

86. Montcourrier P, Mangeat PH, Salazar G, Morisset M, Sahuquet A, Rochefort H (1990) Cathepsin D in breast cancer cells can digest extracellular matrix in large acidic vesicles. *Cancer Res* 50:6045–6054.

87. Maciewicz RA, Wardale RJ, Etherington DJ, Paraskeva C (1989) Immunodetection of cathepsin B and L present in and secreted from human pre-malignant and malignant colorectal tumor cell lines. *Int J Cancer* 43:478–486.

88. Ohsawa T, Higashi T, Tsuji T (1989) The secretion of high molecular weight cathepsin B from cultured human liver cancers. *Acta Med Okayama* 43:9–15.

89. Sloane BF, Moin K, Sameni M, Tait LR, Rozhin J, Ziegler G (1994) Membrane association of cathepsin B can be induced by transfection of human breast epithelial cells with c-Ha-*ras* oncogene. *J Cell Sci* 107:373–384.

90. Rozhin J, Sameni M, Ziegler G, Sloane BF (1994) Pericellular pH affects distribution and secretion of cathepsin B in malignant cells. *Cancer Res* 54:6517–6525.

91. Honn KV, Timar J, Rozhin J, Bazaz R, Sameni M, Ziegler G, Sloane BF (1994) A lipoxygenase metabolite, 12-(S)-HETE, stimulates protein kinase C-mediated release of cathepsin B from malignant cells. *Exp Cell Res* 214:120–130.

92. Sameni M, Elliott E, Ziegler G, Fortgens PH, Dennison C, Sloane BF (1995) Cathepsin B and D are localized at surface of human breast cancer cells. *Pathol Oncol Res* 1:43–53.

93. Heuser J (1989) Changes in lysosomal shape and distribution correlated with changes in cytoplasmic pH. *J Cell Biol* 108:855–864.

94. Rodman JS, Levy MA, Diment S, Stahl PD (1990) Immunolocalization of endosomal cathepsin D in rabbit alveolar macrophages. *J Leukocyte Biol* 48:116–122.

95. Casciola-Rosen L, Renfrew CA, Hubbard AL (1992) Lumenal labeling of rat hepatocyte endocytic compartments. Distribution of several acid hydrolases and membrane receptors. *J Biol Chem* 267:11856–11864.

96. Diment S, Leech MS, Stahl PD (1988) Cathepsin D is membrane-associated in macrophage endosomes. *J Biol Chem* 263:6901–6907.

97. Rozhin J, Robinson D, Stevens MA, Lah TT, Honn KV, Ryan RE, Sloane BF (1987) Properties of a plasma membrane-associated cathepsin B-like cysteine proteinase in metastatic melanoma variants. *Cancer Res* 47:6620–6628.

98. Moin K, Cao L, Koblinski J, Rozhin J, Sloane BF (1995) Membrane-associated cathepsin B from murine tumors. *Proc Am Assoc Cancer Res* 36:98.

99. Sloane BF, Rozhin J, Krepela E, Ziegler G, Sameni M (1991) The malignant phenotype and cysteine proteinases. *Biomed Biochim Acta* 50:549–554.

100. Krepela E, Bartek J, Skalkova D, Vicar J, Rasnick D, Taylor-Papadimitriou J, Hallowes RC (1987) Cytochemical and biochemical evidence of cathepsin B in malignant, transformed and normal breast epithelial cells. *J Cell Sci* 87:145–154.

101. Erdel M, Trefz G, Spiess E, Habermaas S, Spring H, Lah TT, Ebert W (1990) Localization of cathepsin B in two human non small lung cancer cell lines. *J Histochem Cytochem* 38:1313–1321.

102. Spiess E, Bruning A, Gack S, Ulbricht B, Spring H, Trefz G, Ebert W (1994) Cathepsin B activity in human lung tumor cell lines: Ultrastructural localization, pH sensitivity, and inhibitor status at the cellular level. *J Histochem Cytochem* 42:917–929.

103. Soule H, Maloney TM, Wolman SR, Peterson WD Jr, Brenz R, McGrath CM, Russo J, Pauley RJ, Jones RF, Brooks SC (1990) Isolation and characterization of a spontaneously immortalized human breast epithelial cell line MCF-10. *Cancer Res* 50:6075–6086.

104. Basolo F, Elliot J, Tait L, Chen QC, Maloney TM, Russo IH, Pauley R, Momiki S, Caamano J, Klein-Szanto AJP, Koszalka M, Russo J (1991) Transformation of human breast epithelial cells by c-Ha-ras oncogene. *Mol Carcinogen* 4:25–35.

105. Miller FR, Soule HD, Tait L, Pauley RJ, Wolman SR, Dawson PJ, Heppner GH (1993) Xenograft model of human proliferative breast disease. *J Natl Cancer Inst* 85:1725–1732.

106. Hanewinkel H, Glossl J, Kresse H (1987) Biosynthesis of cathepsin B in cultured normal and I-cell fibroblasts. *J Biol Chem* 262:12351–12355.

107. McIntyre GF, Erickson AH (1991) Procathepsins L and D are membrane-bound in acidic microsomal vesicles. *J Biol Chem* 266:15438–15445.

108. Rijnboutt S, Aerts HMFG, Geuze HJ, Tager JM, Strous GJ (1991) Mannose 6-phosphate-independent membrane association of cathepsin D, glucocerebrosidase, and sphingolipid-activating protein in HepG2 cells. *J Biol Chem* 266:4862–4868.

109. Dong J, Prence EM, Sahagian GG (1989) Mechanism for selective secretion of lysosomal protease by transformed mouse fibroblasts. *J Biol Chem* 264:7377–7383.

110. Achkar C, Gong Q, Frankfater A, Bajkowski AS (1990) Differences in targeting and secretion of cathepsins B and L by BALB/3T3 fibroblasts and Moloney murine sarcoma virus transformed BALB/3T3 fibroblasts. *J Biol Chem* 264:13650–13654.

111. Nishimura Y, Takeshima H, Himeno M (1994) The function of propeptide region of cathepsin D in the intracellular targeting to the lysosomes. In: Proteases Involved in Cancer. M. Suzuki and T. Hiwasa, eds. (Monduzzi Editore, Bologna, Italy), pp 59–65.

112. Spyratos F, Brouillet J-P, Defrenne A, Hacene K, Rouesse J, Maudelonde T, Brunet M, Andrieu C, Desplaces A, Rochefort H (1989). Cathepsin D: An independent prognostic factor for metastasis of breast cancer. *Lancet* 2:1115–1118.

113. Thorpe SM, Rochefort H, Garcia M, Freiss G, Christensen IJ, Khalaf S, Paolucci F, Pau B, Rasmussen BB, Rose C (1989) Association between high concentration of 52k cathepsin D and poor prognosis in primary breast cancer. *Cancer Res* 49:6008–6014.

114. Henry JA, McCarthy AL, Angus B, Westley BR, May FEB, Nicholson S, Cairns J, Harris AL, Horne CHW (1990) Prognostic significance of the estrogen-regulated protein, cathepsin D, in breast cancer. *Cancer* 65:265–271.

115. Rogier H, Freiss G, Besse MG (1989) Two site imunoenzymatic assay of the 52kDa cathepsin D cytosols of breast cancer tissues. *Clin Chem* 35:81–85.

116. Kute TE, Shao Z-M, Sugg NK, Long RT, Russell GB, Case LD (1992) Cathepsin D as a prognostic indicator for node-negative breast cancer patients using both immunoassays and enzymatic assays. *Cancer Res* 52:5198–5203.

117. Namer M, Ramajoli, Fontana XA, Etienne ME, Hery M, Jourlait A, Milano G, Frenay M, Franccois E, Lapalus F (1991) Prognostic value of total cathepsin D in breast cancer. *Breast Cancer Res Treat* 19:85–93.

118. Pujol P, Maudelonde T, Daaves JP (1993) A prospective study of the prognostic value of cathepsin D levels in breast cancer cytosol. *Cancer* 71:2006–2012.

119. Duffy MJ, Reilly D, Brouillet JP, Mcdermott EWM, Faul C, Ohiggins N, Fennelly JJ, Maudelonde T, Rochefort H (1992) Cathepsin D concentration in breast cancer cytosols — correlation with disease free interval and overall survival. *Clin Chem* 38:2114–2116.

120. Winstanley JHR, Leinster CJ, Cooke TG (1993) Prognosis significance of cathepsin D in patients with breast cancer. *Br J Cancer* 67:767–772.

121. O'Donoghue AEMA, Poller DN, Bell JA, Galea MH, Elston CW, Blamey RW, Ellis IO (1995) Cathepsin D in primary breast carcinoma: Adverse prognosis is associated with expression of cathepsin D in stromal cells. *Breast Cancer Res Treat* 33:137–145.

122. Joensuu H, Toikkanen S, Isola J (1995) Stromal cell cathepsin D expression and long-term survival in breast cancer. *Br J Cancer* 71:155–159.

123. Domagala W, Striker G, Szadowska A (1992) Cathepsin D in invasive ductal NOS breast carcinoma as defined by immunohistochemistry. *Am J Pathol* 141:1003–1012.

124. Grondahl-Hansen J, Ralfkiaer E, Kirkeby LT, Kristensen P, Lund LR, Dano K (1991) Localization of urokinase-type plasminogen activator in stromal cells in adenocarcinomas of the colon in humans. *Am J Pathol* 138:111–117.

125. Hewitt RE, Leach IH, Powe DG, Clark IM, Cawston TE, Turner DR (1991) Distribution pof collagenase and tissue inhibitor of metalloproteinases (TIMP) in colorectal tumours. *In J Cancer* 49:666–672.

126. Garcia M, Derocq D, Pujol P, Rochefort H (1990) Overexpression of transfected cathepsin D in transformed cells increases their malignant phenotype and metastatic potency. *Oncogene* 5:1809–1814.

127. Ravdin PM, Tandon AK, Allred DC, Clark GM, Fuqua SAW, Hilsenbeck SH, Chamness GC, Osborne CK (1994) Cathepsin D by western blotting and immunohistochemistry: Failure to confirm correlations with prognosis in node-negative breast cancer. *J Clin Oncol* 12:467–474.

128. Briozzo P, Morisset M, Capony F, Rougeot C, Rochefort H (1988) In vitro degradation of extracellular matrix with M_r 52,000 cathepsin D secreted by breast cancer cells. *Cancer Res* 48:3688–3692.

129. Pagano M, Capony F, Rochefort H (1990) In vitro activation of procathepsin B by cathepsin D both secreted by cancer cells. *C R Acad Sci Paris III* 309:7–12.

130. Sameni M, Koblinski J, Rozhin J, Ziegler G, Sloane BF (1995) Characterization of the peripheral vesicles staining for cathepsin B in *ras*-transfected human breast epithelial cells. *Proc Am Assoc Cancer Res* 36:98.

131. Monsky WL, Kelly T, Lin C-Y, Yeh Y, Stetler-Stevenson WG, Mueller SC, Chen W-T (1993) Binding and localization of Mr. 72,000 matrix metalloproteinase at cell surface invadopodia. *Cancer Res* 53:3159–3164.

132. Chen W-T, Lee C-C, Goldstein L, Bernier S, Liu CHL, Lin C-Y, Yeh Y, Monsky WL, Kelly T, Dai M, Zhou J-Y, Mueller SC (1994) Membrane proteases as potential diagnostic and therapeutic targets for breast malignancy. *Breast Cancer Res Treat* 31:217–226.

133. Wolf C, Rouyer N, Lutz Y, Adida C, Loriot M, Bellocq J-P, Chambon P, Basset P (1993) Stromelysin 3 belongs to a subgroup of proteinases expressed in breast carcinoma fibroblastic cells and possibly implicated in tumor progression. *Proc Natl Acad Sci USA* 90:1843–1847.

134. Vecchio SD, Stoppelli MP, Caniero MV, Fonti R, Massa O, Li PY, Botti G, Cerva M, D'Aiuto G, Esposito G, Salavatore M (1993) Human urokinase receptor concentration in malignant and benign breast tumors by in vitro quantitative autoradiography: Comparison with urokinase levels. *Cancer Res* 53:3198–3206.

135. Rozhin H, Gomez AP, Ziegler GH, Nelson KK, Chang YS, Fong D, Onoda JM, Honn KV, Sloane BF (1990) Cathepsin B to cysteine proteinase inhibitor balance in metastatic cell subpopulations isolated from murine tumors. *Cancer Res* 50:6278–6284.

136. Mathieu M, Rochefort H, Barenton B, Prebois C, Vignon F (1990) Interactions of cathepsin D and insulin-like growth factor II (IGF-II) on the IGF-II/mannose-6-phosphate receptor in human breast cancer cells and possible consequences on mitogenic activity of EGF-II. *Mol Endocrinol* 4:1327–1335.

137. Vetvicka V, Vektvickova J, Fusek M (1994) Effect of human procathepsin D on proliferation of human cell lines. *Cancer Lett* 79:131–135.

138. Conover CA, Deleon DD (1994) Acid-activated insulin-like growth factor-binding protein-3 proteolysis in normal and transformed cells — Role of cathepsin D. *J Biol Chem* 269:7076–7080.

351

139. Sloane BF, Dunn JR, Honn KV (1981) Lysosomal cathepsin B: Correlation with metastatic potential. *Science* 212:1151–1153.
140. Moin K, Rozhin J, McKernan TB, Sanders VJ, Fong D, Honn KV, Sloane BF (1989) Enhanced levels of cathepsin B mRNA in murine tumors. *FEBS Lett* 244:61–64.
141. Capony F, Morisset M, Barrett AJ, Capony JP, Broquet P, Vignon F, Chambon M, Louisot P, Rochefort H (1987) Phosphorylation, glycosylation and proteolytic activity of the 52K estrogen-induced protein secreted by MCF7 cells. *J Cell Biol* 104:253–262.
142. Sameni M, Rozhin J, Ziegler G, Sloane BF (1993) Alterations in pH affect processing and secretion of cathepsin B by human breast epithelial cells. *Mol Biol Cell* 4:447a.

17. Stromelysin-3 and other stromelysins in breast cancer: Importance of epithelial–stromal interactions during tumor progression

Paul Basset, Jean-Pierre Bellocq, Patrick Anglard, Marie-Pierre Chenard,
Olivier Lefebvre, Agnès Noël, Akiko Okada, Nicolas Rouyer,
Maria Santavicca, Isabelle Stoll, Catherine Wolf, and Marie-Christine Rio

Introduction

Stromelysins belong to the matrix metalloproteinase (MMP, also known as matrixin) family, extracellular proteolytic enzymes that are believed to be physiological mediators of tissue remodeling processes during development, involution, and tissue repair [1,2]. In agreement with this concept, MMPs are capable of degrading most macromolecular components found in or associated with the extracellular matrix (ECM) [1–4]. MMPs have also been implicated in pathological tissue remodeling processes, including those associated with cancer progression [5]. Although it has been proposed that they may be involved in the initiation of oncogenesis [6], MMPs should be better regarded as modulators of cancerous processes, thus contributing to tumor invasion and metastasis [5,7–9].

MMPs have been so far defined as enzymes that (1) degrade at least one component of the ECM, (2) contain a zinc ion and are inhibited by chelating agents, (3) are secreted in a latent form and require activation for proteolytic activity, (4) are inhibited by specific tissue inhibitors of metalloproteinases (TIMPs), and (5) share amino-acid similarities [10]. However, some of the most recently identified members of the MMP family do not fulfill all of these criteria. Thus, it is presently uncertain whether stromelysin-3 [11] and MT-MMP [12] can directly degrade ECM substrates. Second, the major stromelysin-3 form that is found in conditioned media from fibroblasts expressing the endogenous stromelysin-3 gene corresponds to a putative mature enzymic form and not to the zymogen (Figure 1). Finally, it has been recently demonstrated that all MMPs contained not one but two zinc atoms, one being required for catalytic activity and the other for proper protein folding [13]. Taken together, these observations suggest that the MMP family should now be defined solely as a class of zinc proteinases belonging to the metzincin superfamily [14–16], and is characterized by amino acid similarities and inhibition by TIMPs.

R. Dickson and M. Lippman (eds.) MAMMARY TUMOR CELL CYCLE, DIFFERENTIATION AND METASTASIS. 1996. Kluwer Academic Publishers. ISBN 0-7923-3905-3. All rights reserved.

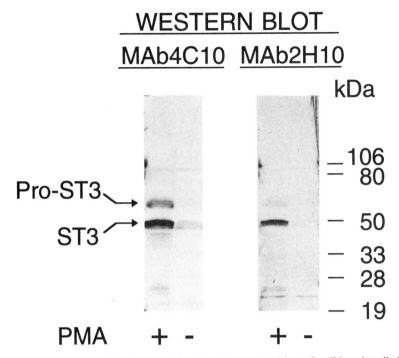

WESTERN BLOT

MAb4C10 MAb2H10

kDa

Pro-ST3

ST3

— 106
— 80

— 50

— 33
— 28

— 19

PMA   + -   + -

Figure 1. Western blot analysis of stromelysin-3 from human fibroblasts. Conditioned media from HFL1 diploid fibroblasts (ATCC CCL 153), cultured in serum-free medium in the absence or presence of 10 ng/ml phorbol 12-myristate 13-acetate (PMA) for 48 hours, were concentrated 100× by ammonium sulfate precipitation and were analyzed by Western blot using monoclonal antibody 5ST-4C10 against the stromelysin-3 catalytic domain, or monoclonal antibody 1ST-2H10 against the 25 C-terminal amino acid residues of stromelysin-3.

Stromelysins

Stromelysins were initially defined as MMPs capable of degrading a broad range of ECM substrates, including proteoglycans, gelatins, fibronectin, laminin, elastin, and collagens of types IV, V, VII, and IX [17]. These activities were first demonstrated for stromelysin-1, and later on for stromelysin-2 and the related enzyme matrilysin [18,19]. However, they are not observed for stromelysin-3, which exhibits unusual functional properties [20,21] (see later). Although more appropriate terminology may be used in the future for stromelysin-3, its present designation is based on the observation that all three stromelysins share a common protein domain organization [11,22,23], and because 'stromelysin-3' is an appropriate designation for a MMP specifically expressed in stromal cells [11] (see later). Thus, in this chapter we review both the observations made in breast cancer for stromelysin-1, stromelysin-2, and matrilysin, which exhibit similar proteolytic activities, and those made for stromelysin-3, which may in fact correspond to a new type of MMP [24].

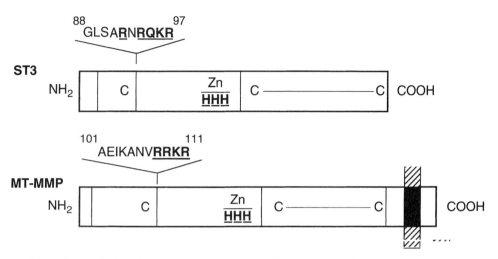

Figure 2. Protein domains of stromelysin-3 and MT-MMP. Both proteins exhibit from N- to C-terminal extremities a predomain, a prodomain (containing a conserved cysteine residue as in other MMPs), a catalytic domain (with the catalytic-zinc atom (Zn) bound to the apoenzyme through 3 histidine residues), and a hemopexin-like domain (in which two cysteine residues form an internal disulfide bridge). MT-MMP, but not stromelysin-3, has, in addition, a transmembrane domain followed by an intracellular domain in its C-terminal portion. However, both stromelysin-3 and MT-MMP are characterized among MMPs by the presence of additional amino acids located at the junction between the prodomain and catalytic domain, and containing a potential cleavage site for convertases of the furin type (amino-acid residues in bold letters). Amino acids are represented using the one-letter code. (From Basset et al. [11] and Sato et al. [12], with permission.)

Stromelysin-3 structural characteristics

Although having four protein domains, like the other stromelysins, stromelysin-3 exhibits a number of structural specificities. First, stromelysin-3 has 10 additional amino acids precisely located at the junction between the prodomain and catalytic domain, and an unusually long hinge region at the junction between the catalytic and hemopexin-like domains (Figure 2) [11]. Furthermore, stromelysin-3 is the only member of the matrixin family that exhibits a threonine instead of a serine C-terminally to the third histidine residue, which is characteristic of catalytic-zinc binding sites of the metzincin family (Table 1). Whether this serine-threonine substitution is functionally important is not known, but it has been observed in human [11], mouse [25], and rat [A. Okada et al., unpublished results] enzymes. Finally, human stromelysin-3 differs from all MMPs so far described, including mouse and rat stromelysin-3, by the presence of an alanine instead of a proline immediately C-terminal to the Met turn characteristic of metzincins (Figure 3). Because of its location in the catalytic environment, this amino acid replacement may be functionally important and could explain some of the differences noted between human and mouse stromelysin-3 [20,21].

Table 1. Comparison of amino acid sequences in the catalytic zinc binding-site region of metzincins

Enzyme family	Sequence[a]						
Astacin	HE	X	XH	XX	G	FX	HE
Serratia	HE	I	GH	AL	G	LX	HP
Reprolysin	HE	X	GH	NL	G	XX	HD
Matrixin							
Other than stromelysin-3	HE	X	GH	XX	G	XX	HS
Stromelysin-3	HE	X	GH	XX	G	XX	HT

[a] Amino acids are represented using the one-letter code.
Data from Basset et al. [11], Bode et al. [15], and Lefebvre et al. [25].

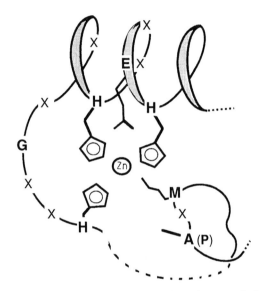

Figure 3. Schematic representation of the catalytic-zinc environment in human stromelysin-3. Human stromelysin-3 differs from all other matrixins, including mouse and rat stromelysin-3, by the presence of an alanine (**A**) instead of a proline (**P**) C-terminally to the 'Met-turn.' The methionine (M) side chain of the Met-turn provides a hydrophobic base beneath the three zinc-liganding histidine (H) side chains. E, glutamic acid; G, glycine; X, non-conserved amino-acid residue; Zn, catalytic zinc atom. (Modified from W. Bode et al. [15], with permission.)

Stromelysin-3 functional properties

Stromelysin-3 differs from previous MMPs both in its activation pattern and its enzymic activity. Stromelysin-3 is the first MMP for which proform maturation cannot be induced by 4-amino phenylmercuric acetate (APMA) treatment [20], suggesting that the removal of the stromelysin-3 propeptide does not involve autolytic cleavage and should rely on another mechanism. In agreement with this possibility, the predominant stromelysin-3 form that is observed in conditioned media from cells in culture corresponds to a form that has lost the N-terminal prodomain (Figure 1) [21], and not to the zymogen, as for other MMPs [4]. This unusual behavior for a MMP possibly relies on the presence of the 10 additional amino acids at the junction between the stromelysin-3 prodomain and catalytic domain (Figure 2). These amino acids comprise a potential cleavage site for furin, a convertase implicated in the processing of various protein precursors [26,27]. Because furin is an ubiquitously expressed convertase associated with membranes of Golgi vesicles, it is possible that stromelysin-3 is processed in these vesicles and then is secreted as an already active enzyme, in contrast to other MMPs, whose proforms must be activated in the extracellular milieu [4]. Interestingly, an activation pathway similar to that proposed for stromelysin-3 could also concern the recently identified MT-MMP, which also contains a potential cleavage site for furin-type enzymes at the junction between the prodomain and catalytic domain (Figure 2) [12].

Stromelysin-3 also differs from other MMPs in its unusual enzymic properties. In particular, both mouse and human stromelysin-3 forms with an intact C-terminal domain do not exhibit caseinolytic activity in zymography and cannot cleave any of the major ECM components [20,21]. The possibility has been raised that stromelysin-3 might represent a member of the MMP family that has lost proteolytic power [28], because this has been observed in some families of proteolytic enzymes [29]. This now appears unlikely because it has been recently demonstrated that human stromelysin-3 could cleave α1 antitrypsin [21], like other MMPs. Furthermore, mouse stromelysin-3 forms that have lost at least part of the C-terminal hemopexin-like domain have been shown to cleave casein and ECM molecules (Figure 4B) [20]. It is unclear, however, whether these C-terminally truncated stromelysin-3 forms, generated during enzyme purification and/or incubation, are physiologically relevant. Although the major stromelysin-3 form found in conditioned media from human diploid fibroblasts expressing the endogenous stromelysin-3 gene is not C-terminally truncated (Figure 1), it cannot presently be ruled out that in other tissues or in other conditions C-terminally truncated stromelysin-3 forms could be also generated. Thus while awaiting additional information, several possibilities must currently be considered for stromelysin-3 function in vivo.

One hypothesis is that stromelysin-3 corresponds to a new type of MMP with specific properties for an as yet undefined substrate, and whose substrate specificity would be in part dictated by the hemopexin-like domain (Figure 5A). A critical role for this domain in controlling MMP substrate specificity has been previously demonstrated for the type I collagenases, which lose the capacity to cleave type I collagen when their hemopexin-like domain is deleted [30–32]. The possibility that the hemopexin-like domain has a critical role in defining stromelysin-3 substrate specificity would be consistent with the observation that the genomic organization corresponding to this domain differs from that of other MMP genes, in ways suggesting that the stromelysin-3 hemopexin-like domain may have a different origin [P. Anglard et al., unpub-

357

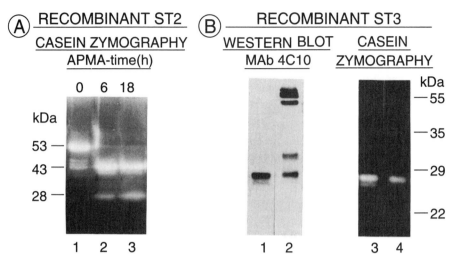

Figure 4. Comparative caseinolytic activities of recombinant stromelysin-2 and stromelysin-3. **A**: Detection of caseinolytic activity for pro–stromelysin-2 (lane 1, protein species at 53kD), and mature forms of stromelysin-2 (lanes 2 and 3) generated by treatment with 4-amino phenylmercuric acetate (APMA) for 6 hours (lane 2) or 18 hours (lane 3). Recombinant stromelysin-2 was recovered from conditioned media of Cos-1 cells transiently transfected with a human stromelysin-2 cDNA cloned into the pSG5 expression vector [23]. **B**: Detection of caseinolytic activity for low molecular weight forms of stromelysin-3. The high molecular species detected using monoclonal antibody 5ST-4C10 against the stromelysin-3 catalytic domain (lane 2) did not cleave casein, in contrast to those of lower molecular weights (lanes 1, 3, and 4). Recombinant stromelysin-3 was obtained by expressing a mouse stromelysin-3 cDNA cloned into the PEE12 vector, and was stably transfected into NSO mouse myeloma cells [20]. Aliquots from the same preparations (lanes 1 and 3, and 2 and 4, respectively) were used for Western blot analysis (lanes 1 and 2) and casein zymography (lanes 3 and 4). (Panel B is a partial reproduction of Figure 2 from Murphy et al. [20], with permission.)

lished results]. In this case, the stromelysin-3 hemopexin-like domain could direct substrate specificity by contributing to the proper orientation of stromelysin-3 substrate(s), so that it (they) can be efficiently processed by the enzyme catalytic site [33,34].

While the reality of this scenario awaits the identification of physiologically relevant stromelysin-3 substrate(s), another possibility is that stromelysin-3 activation would involve both N- and C-terminal processing. In these conditions, the physiologically active stromelysin-3 would correspond to a low molecular weight form exhibiting enzymic properties similar to those of stromelysin-1 and stromelysin-2 (Figure 5B). In this case stromelysin-3 should be regarded as an analog of matrilysin, an MMP characterized both by the absence of a hemopexin-like domain and stromelysin-like activity [19]. Active stromelysin-3 would be generated after proteolytic cleavage from a protein precursor, instead of by direct mRNA translation, as in the case of matrilysin.

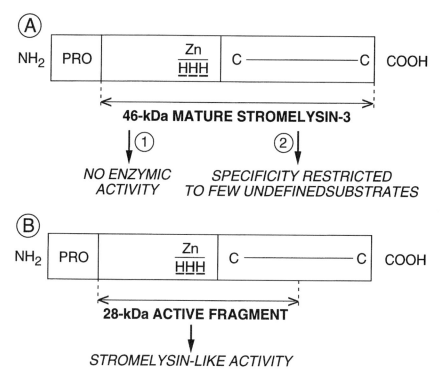

Figure 5. Pro–stromelysin-3 putative activation pathways. In the first model (**A**), the active stromelysin-3 form has lost the N-terminal propeptide and corresponds either to a molecule without proteolytic activity ① or with activity limited to (an) as yet undefined substrate(s) ②. In the second model (**B**), the active stromelysin-3 form has lost both the N-terminal propeptide and the C-terminal portion of the hemopexin-like domain. In this case, stromelysin-3 would be a MMP with stromelysin-like activity [20].

Expression of stromelysin and matrilysin genes in breast carcinoma

Although the stromelysin-3 and matrilysin genes have been found to be expressed in most invasive human breast carcinomas [11,35–40] their expression patterns strikingly differ. The stromelysin-3 gene is specifically expressed in fibroblastic cells surrounding cancer cells (Figure 6) [11,35,38,40]. Stromelysin-3 transcripts are exclusively detected in fibroblastic cells belonging to the tumor stroma, in contrast to gelatinase A and MT-MMP, which are expressed both in fibroblastic cells of tumor stroma and in fibroblasts of surrounding noncancerous tissues [35,40]. The matrilysin gene is specifically expressed in epithelial cells, both in cancer cells and in cells present in the normal tissue surrounding the tumors [35]. Thus, the levels of matrilysin RNA are similar in invasive breast carcinomas and in benign breast fibroadenomas, while stromelysin-3 transcripts are usually not detected in benign breast tumors [11,39]. However, stromelysin-3 expression is not characteristic of invasive

359

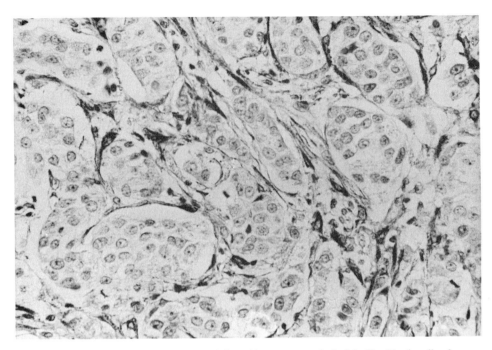

Figure 6. Indirect immunoperoxidase staining of human stromelysin-3 in fibroblastic cells of an infiltrative ductal breast carcinoma. Stromelysin-3 was immunodetected on paraffin-embedded tissue section using monoclonal antibody 5ST-4A9 against the hemopexin-like domain of stromelysin-3. Note that the stromelysin-3–expressing stromal cells are intermixed with the cancer cells inside the tumor mass.

tumors and can be observed in some in situ breast carcinomas, particularly in those of the comedo type [35]. Similarly, stromelysin-3 gene expression has been found in both invasive tumors and high-grade precursor lesions of other types of human carcinomas [41].

In contrast to stromelysin-3 and matrilysin, the stromelysin-1 and stromelysin-2 genes are rarely expressed in human breast cancer. In a study of 10 invasive breast carcinomas performed using in situ hybridization, stromelysin-2 transcripts were detected in only one tumor, and those for stromelysin-1 in none of them [35]. In another study, stromelysin-1 RNA was found in only 2 tumors out of 17 that were examined [42]. The infrequent expression of the stromelysin-2 gene in breast carcinoma can be easily explained because expression of this gene in human carcinomas appears to be specific to squamous cell carcinomas [43–47]. In agreement with these observations, the single breast carcinoma expressing the stromelysin-2 gene in the series examined by Wolf et al. [35] was an adenocarcinoma with an unusual epidermoid differentiation. However, the stromelysin-1 gene appears to be rarely expressed in all types of human carcinomas, including both adenocarcinomas and squamous cell carcinomas [45,46,48].

Role of stromelysin-3 and matrylisin in breast carcinoma

MMPs and other extracellular proteinases were until recently most often regarded as effectors of cancer cell invasion [5,8,9]. This concept was consistent with the capability of these enzymes to degrade ECM components, and with observations demonstrating that in vitro cancer cell invasion could be prevented by proteolytic enzyme inhibitors. However, it is now generally accepted that the contribution of extracellular proteinases to tumor progression is much more complex. Increased expression of extracellular proteinases is not specific to cancer cell invasion, and it has been observed in a number of carcinomas before they become invasive [28,35,40,41], suggesting that extracellular proteolysis may contribute to tissue remodeling processes that precede or are not directly related to cancer cell invasion.

In this regard, one possibility is that in addition to their action on ECM molecules, extracellular proteinases may also control the activities of non-ECM molecules. Thus, it has been recently shown that MMP-like enzymes were implicated in pro-TNFα activation [49,50]. Matrilysin, besides its activity on most ECM components [19], has been shown to catalyze the formation of low molecular weight forms of urokinase [51], which has itself been implicated in controlling the activity of cytokines, including TGF-β and hepatocyte growth factor [8,52]. It is tempting to speculate that this might be also the case for stromelysin-3, which, as discussed earlier, cannot cleave the usual ECM components when it has an intact C-terminal domain. In this case stromelysin-3, which contains a putative cleavage site for a furin-type enzyme (Figure 2), might participate in a cascade of convertases involved in the control of cytokine activities. In any case, observations made in our laboratory indicate that the constitutive expression of the human stromelysin-3 cDNA in human breast cancer cells leads to larger tumors when the cells are subcutaneously injected into nude mice than those observed with the parental cell line (O. Lefebvre and A. Noël et al., unpublished results].

Control of stromelysin-3 gene expression in stromal cells of human carcinomas

It has long been proposed that the tumor stroma is required for growth of most human carcinomas, and particularly for those of the breast [53–56]. The stroma supplies the neovascularization that is required for tumor expansion beyond a certain size, and likely also factors that specifically contribute to tumor growth [57]. The observation that stromelysin-3 and other extracellular proteinases, including gelatinase A and MT-MMP, are expressed in fibroblastic cells of human carcinomas [40] suggests that these proteinases may represent examples of such factors. However, little is known about the mechanisms involved in controlling the stromal expression of these proteinases during cancer progression. Since in all types of human carcinomas examined

PMA-time (h)

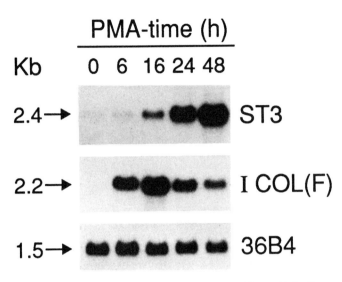

Figure 7. Comparative kinetics of induction of stromelysin-3 and interstitial collagenase RNAs in human fibroblasts. Confluent G47PF human diploid fibroblasts (kindly provided by H. Smith, Geraldine Brush Cancer Research Institute, San Francisco) kept in serum-free medium were stimulated with 10ng/ml 12-phorbol 13-myristate acetate (PMA) and were harvested at the indicated time after PMA addition, for Northern blot analysis using a stromelysin-3 (ST3) or an interstitial collagenase [ICOL(F)] ^{32}P-labeled cDNA probe. The 36B4 probe [69] was used to check for sample loading and RNA tranfer.

so far, stromelysin-3 expression was observed in fibroblastic cells immediately surrounding islands of cancer cells [35,40,41], it is reasonable to believe that stromelysin-3 gene expression is triggered by factors acting in the immediate vicinity of cancer cells. In vitro stromelysin-3 RNA levels in human fibroblasts can be stimulated by treatment with basic fibroblast growth factor or phorbol myristate acetate (PMA) (Figure 7) [11,40]. However, although stromelysin-3 RNA expression can be stimulated at levels comparable with those observed for interstitial collagenase RNA, the kinetics of induction for both RNAs clearly differ. The delayed induction of stromelysin-3 RNA by PMA is unusual among MMPs and suggests that the stromelysin-3 gene may be controlled by specific factors. This possibility is also supported by the observation that the stromelysin-3 gene promoter differs from that of other MMP genes, particularly by not containing an AP1 binding site in the DNA region 5′ to the transcription start (P. Anglard, unpublished results). These findings indicating that the control of stromelysin-3 gene expression differs from that of other MMPs are also consistent with observations made both in human carcinomas [35,40] and during physiological tissue remodeling [58], showing distinct expression patterns for stromelysin-3 as compared with other MMPs. The identification of these factors that may specifically govern stromelysin-3 gene expression is of particular importance for a MMP that is predominantly secreted in a mature form, in contrast to other MMPs, which have to be activated in the extracellular milieu.

Stromelysin-3 as a new prognostic indicator

Only a few studies have been thus far performed to evaluate a possible correlation between stromelysin-3 expression and clinicopathological parameters in breast cancer [36–38]. A unique study in which stromelysin-3 gene expression levels were correlated with breast cancer outcome, was carried out by Engel et al. [38]. They observed that recurrent breast carcinoma was more frequent in patients with tumors with high stromelysin-3 RNA levels than in those with tumors with low stromelysin-3 RNA levels. The possibility that increased levels of stromelysin-3 expression might be used to identify patients at greatest risk for breast cancer recurrence is also consistent with the observations that the stromelysin-3 and urokinase genes exhibit very similar expression patterns in breast carcinoma [35], and that urokinase appears to have prognostic value in breast cancer [59–62]. The next step will be to see whether stromelysin-3 can serve as an independent prognostic variable. Such a study should be carried out in multivariable analyses of significant size in which stromelysin-3 levels in breast tumors are evaluated by immunological assays or semiquantitative immunohistochemistry, and are ranked in importance with other prognostic indicators [63].

Conclusions and future directions

The concept that most human carcinomas are stroma-dependent tumors has been long proposed, but it is only recently that this concept has been supported at the molecular level. A striking finding has been that a number of molecules previously implicated in tumor progression, including some extracellular proteinases, were expressed in stromal cells and not in the cancer cells themselves. This observation has refreshed interest in stromal–epithelial interactions during tumor progression, and has reminded tumor biologists that understanding of human carcinoma progression must involve analysis of both cancer cells and the stroma that they induce. It remains now to be understood how cancer cells gain the capability of inducing the stroma during tumor progression. However, the demonstration that the stroma is an important source of molecules implicated in tumor progression has already opened new therapeutic perspectives. Targeting stromal cells rather than cancer cells, as is the case in conventional chemotherapy, may facilitate drug delivery because the tumor stroma is more easily accessible from the blood stream. Another possible benefit from targeting stromal rather than cancer cells is the decreased likelihood of drug resistance.

In this context, the matrix metalloproteinases are attractive targets, both because they act extracellularly and because it has been possible to success-fully develop synthetic inhibitors for these enzymes. The inhibitors thus far tested were found to be efficient and well tolerated in animal models of cancer [64–68]. The next step will be to identify more specific and/or more potent inhibitors for each of the MMPs usually expressed in human carcinomas. In this respect, stromelysin-3 because of its unusual functional properties and its specific expression pattern in breast and other human carcinomas, represents a particularly attractive target.

Acknowledgments

We are most grateful to P. Chambon for his support and interest in this work, to Yves Lutz for monoclonal antibody preparation, and to J. Byrne for critical reading. This work was supported by funds from the Institut National de la Santé et de la Recherche Médicale, the Centre National de la Recherche Scientifique, the Centre Hospitalier Universitaire Régional, the Mutuelle Générale de l'Education Nationale, the Groupement de Recherches et d'Etudes sur les Génomes (grant 94/50), the Association pour la Recherche sur le Cancer, the Ligue Nationale Française contre le Cancer, the Fondation pour la Recherche Médicale Française, and a grant to P. Chambon from the Fondation Jeantet. M.S. is a recipient of a Ph.D. studentship from the Ligue Régionale du Bas-Rhin contre le Cancer. A.N. is a recipient of postdoctoral fellowships from the European Community and from the Fondations Léon Frédéricq, Rose et Jean Hoguet, Braconier-Lamarche, and the Fondation Cancérologique Saint-Michel, all from Belgium.

References

1. Woessner JF Jr (1991) Matrix metalloproteinases and their inhibitors in connective tissue remodeling. *FASEB J* 5:2145–2146.
2. Matrisian LM (1992) The matrix-degrading metalloproteinases. *BioEssays* 14:455–463.
3. Docherty AJP, O'Connell J, Crabbe T, Angal S, Murphy G (1992) The matrix metalloproteinases and their natural inhibitors: Prospects for treating degenerative tissue diseases. *Trends Biotechnol* 10:200–207.
4. Birkedal-Hansen H, Moore WGI, Bodden MK, Windsor LJ, Birkedal-Hansen B, DeCarlo A, Engler JA (1993) Matrix metalloproteinases: A review. *Crit Rev Oral Biol Med* 4:197–250.
5. Stetler-Stevenson WG, Aznavoorian S, Liotta LA (1993) Tumor cell interactions with the extracellular matrix during invasion and metastasis. *Annu Rev Cell Biol* 9:541–573.
6. Khokka R, Waterhouse P, Lala P, Zimmer M, Denhardt DT (1991) Increased proteinase expression during tumor progression of tissue inhibitor of metalloproteinases cell lines down-modulated for levels: A new transformation paradigm? *J Cancer Res Clin Oncol* 117:333–338.
7. Duffy MJ (1992) The role of proteolytic enzymes in cancer invasion and metastasis. *Clin Exp Metastasis* 10:145–155.
8. Mignatti P, Rifkin DB (1993) Biology and biochemistry of proteinases in tumor invasion. *Physiol Rev* 73:161–195.

364

9. Ponta H, Sleeman J, Herrlich P (1994) Tumor metastasis formation: Cell-surface proteins confer metastasis-promoting or suppressing properties. *Biochim Biophys Acta* 1198:1–10.

10. Matrisian LM (1990) Metalloproteinases and their inhibitors in matrix remodeling. *Trends Genet* 6:121–125.

11. Basset P, Bellocq JP, Wolf C, Stoll I, Hutin P, Limacher JM, Podhajcer OL, Chenard MP, Rio MC, Chambon P (1990) A novel metalloproteinase gene specifically expressed in stromal cells of breast carcinomas. *Nature* 348:699–704.

12. Sato H, Takino T, Okada Y, Cao J, Shinagawa A, Yamamoto E, Seiki M (1994) A matrix metalloproteinase expressed on the surface of invasive tumour cells. *Nature* 370:61–65.

13. Gooley PR, Johnson BA, Marcy AI, Cuca GC, Salowe SP, Hagmann WK, Esser CK, Springer JP (1993) Secondary structure and zinc ligation of human recombinant short-form stromelysin by multidimensional heteronuclear NMR. *Biochemistry* 32:13098–13108.

14. Jiang W, Bond JS (1992) Families of metalloendopeptidases and their relationships. *FEBS Lett* 312:110–114.

15. Bode W, Gomis-Ruth FX, Stöcker W (1993) Astacins, serralysins, snake venom and matrix metalloproteinases exhibit identical zinc-binding environments (HEXXHXXGXXH and Met-turn) and topologies and should be grouped into a common family, the 'metzincins.' *FEBS Lett* 331:134–140.

16. Hooper NM (1994) Families of zinc metalloproteases. *FEBS Lett* 354:1–6.

17. Alexander CM, Werb Z (1991) Extracellular matrix degradation. In *Cell Biology of Extracellular Matrix*, 2nd ed. ED Hay (ed). New York: Plenum Press, pp 255–302.

18. Nicholson R, Murphy G, Breathnach R (1989) Human and rat malignant-tumor-associated mRNAs encode stromelysin-like metalloproteinases. *Biochemistry* 28:5195–5203.

19. Quantin B, Murphy G, Breathnach R (1989) Pump-1 cDNA codes for a protein with characteristics similar to those of classical collagenase family members. *Biochemistry* 28:5327–5334.

20. Murphy G, Segain JP, O'Shea M, Cockett M, Ioannou C, Lefebvre O, Chambon P, Basset P (1993) The 28 kDa N-terminal domain of mouse stromelysin-3 has the general properties of a weak metalloproteinase. *J Biol Chem* 268:15435–15441.

21. Pei D, Majmudar G, Weiss SJ (1994) Hydrolytic inactivation of a breast carcinoma cell-derived serpin by human stromelysin-3. *J Biol Chem* 269:25849–25855.

22. Whitham SE, Murphy G, Angel P, Rahmsdorf HJ, Smith BJ, Lyons A, Harris TJR, Reynolds JJ, Herrlich P, Docherty AJP (1986) Comparison of human stromelysin and collagenase by cloning and sequence analysis. *Biochem J* 240:913–916.

23. Muller D, Quantin B, Gesnel MC, Millon-Collard R, Abecassis J, Breathnach R (1988) The collagenase gene family in humans consists of at least four members. *Biochem J* 253:187–192.

24. Murphy GJP, Murphy G, Reynolds JJ (1991) The origin of matrix metalloproteinases and their familial relationships. *FEBS Lett* 289:4–7.

25. Lefebvre O, Wolf C, Limacher JM, Hutin P, Wendling C, LeMeur M, Basset P, Rio MC (1992) The breast cancer-associated stromelysin-3 gene is expressed during mouse mammary gland apoptosis. *J Cell Biol* 119:997–1002.

26. Nakagawa T, Hosaka M, Torii S, Watanabe T, Murakami K, Nakayama K (1993) Identification and functional expression of a new member of the mammalian Kex-2-like processing endoprotease family: Its striking structural similarity to PACE4. *J Biochem* 133:132–135.

27. Seidah NG, Day R, Marcinkiewicz M, Chretien M (1993) Mammalian paired basic amino acid convertases of prohormones and proproteins. *Ann NY Acad Sci* 680:135–146.

28. Basset P, Wolf C, Chambon P (1993) Expression of the stromelysin-3 gene in fibroblastic cells of invasive carcinomas of the breast and other human tissues: A review. *Breast Cancer Res Treat* 24:185–193.

29. Hecht PM, Anderson KV (1992) Extracellular proteases and embryonic pattern formation. *Trends Cell Biol* 2:197–202.

30. Clark IM, Cawston TE (1989) Fragments of human fibroblast collagenase. Purification and characterization. *Biochem J* 263:201–206.

31. Murphy G, Allan JA, Willenbrock F, Cockett MI, O'Connell JP, Docherty AJP (1992) The

role of the C-terminal domain in collagenase and stromelysin specificity. *J Biol Chem* 267:9612–9618.

32. Hirose T, Patterson C, Pourmotabbed T, Mainardi C, Hasty KA (1993) Structure-function relationship of human neutrophil collagenase: Identification of regions responsible for substrate specificity and general proteinase activity. *Proc Natl Acad Sci USA* 90:2569–2573.

33. Lovejoy B, Cleasby A, Hassell AM, et al. (1994) Structure of the catalytic domain of fibroblast collagenase complexed with an inhibitor. *Science* 263:375–377.

34. Bode W, Reinemer P, Huber R, Kleine T, Schnierer S, Tschesche H (1994) The X-ray crystal structure of the catalytic domain of human neutrophil collagenase inhibited by a substrate analogue reveals the essentials for catalysis and specificity. *EMBO J* 13:1263–1269.

35. Wolf C, Rouyer N, Lutz Y, Adida C, Loriot M, Bellocq JP, Chambon P, Basset P (1993) Stromelysin-3 belongs to a subgroup of proteinases expressed in breast carcinoma fibroblastic cells and possibly implicated in tumor progression. *Proc Natl Acad Sci USA* 90:1843–1847.

36. Hähnel E, Harvey JM, Joyce R, Robbins PD, Sterrett GF, Hähnel R (1993) Stromelysin-3 expression in breast cancer biopsies: Clinico-pathological correlations. *Int J Cancer* 55:1–4.

37. Kawami H, Yoshida K, Ohsaki A, Kuroi K, Nishiyama M, Toge T (1993) Stromelysin-3 mRNA expression and malignancy: Comparison with clinicopathological features and type IV collagenase mRNA expression in breast tumors. *Anticancer Res* 13:2319–2324.

38. Engel G, Heseemeyer K, Auer G, Backdahl M, Eriksson E, Linder S (1994) Correlation between stromelysin-3 mRNA level and outcome of human breast cancer. *Int J Cancer* 58:1–7.

39. Hähnel E, Dawkins H, Robbins P, Hähnel R (1994) Expression of stromelysin-3 and nm23 in breast carcinoma and related tissues. *Int J Cancer* 58:157–160.

40. Okada A, Bellocq JP, Rouyer N, Chenard MP, Rio MC, Chambon P, Basset P (1995) Membrane-type matrix metalloproteinase (MT-MMP) gene is expressed in stromal cells of human colon, breast, and head and neck carcinomas. *Proc Natl Acad Sci USA* 92:2730–2734.

41. Rouyer N, Wolf C, Chenard MP, Rio MC, Chambon P, Bellocq JP, Basset P. Stromelysin-3 gene expression in human cancer: An overview. *Invasion Metastasis* 14:269–275.

42. Polette M, Clavel C, Cockett M, Girod de Bentzmann S, Murphy G, Birembaut P (1993) Detection and localization of mRNAs encoding matrix metalloproteinases and their tissue inhibitor in human breast pathology. *Invasion Metastasis* 13:31–37.

43. Muller D, Breathnach R, Engelmann A, Millon R, Bronner G, Flesch H, Dumont P, Eber M, Abecassis J (1991) Expression of collagenase-related metalloproteinase genes in human lung or head and neck tumours. *Int J Cancer* 48:550–556.

44. Polette M, Clavel C, Muller D, Abecassis J, Binninger I, Birembaut P (1991) Detection of mRNAs encoding collagenase I and stromelysin-2 in carcinomas of the head and neck by in situ hybridization. *Invasion Metastasis* 11:76–83.

45. McDonnell S, Navre M, Coffey RJ, Matrisian LM (1991) Expression and localization of the matrix metalloproteinase pump-1 (MMP-7) in human gastric and colon carcinomas. *Mol Carcinog* 4:527–533.

46. Muller D, Wolf C, Abecassis J, Millon R, Engelmann A, Bronner G, Rouyer N, Rio MC, Eber M, Methlin G, Chambon P, Basset P (1993) Increased stromelysin-3 gene expression is associated with increased local invasiveness in head and neck squamous cell carcinomas. *Cancer Res* 53:165–169.

47. Newell KJ, Witty JP, Rodgers WH, Matrisian LM (1994) Expression and localization of matrix-degrading metalloproteinases during colorectal tumorigenesis. *Mol Carcinog* 10:199–206.

48. Pajouh MS, Nagle RB, Breathnach R, Finch JS, Brawer MK, Bowden GT (1991) Expression of metalloproteinase genes in human prostate cancer. *J Cancer Res Clin Oncol* 117:144–150.

49. Gearing AJH, Beckett P, Christodoulou M, Churchill M, Clements J, Davidson AH, Drummond AH, Galloway WA, Gilbert R, Gordon JL, Leber TM, Mangan M, Miller K, Nayee P, Owen K, Patel S, Thomas W, Wells G, Wood LM, Wooley K (1994) Processing of tumor necrosis factor-α precursor by metalloproteinases. *Nature* 370:555–557.

50. McGeehan GM, Becherer JD, Bast RC Jr, et al. (1994) Regulation of tumour necrosis factor-α processing by a metalloproteinase inhibitor. *Nature* 370:558–561.
51. Marcotte PA, Kozan IM, Dorwin SA, Ryan JM (1992) The matrix metalloproteinase pump-1 catalyzes formation of low molecular weight (pro)urokinase in cultures of normal human kidney cells. *J Biol Chem* 267:13803–13806.
52. Naldini L, Tamagnone L, Vigna E, Sachs M, Hertmann G, Birchmeier W, Daikuhara Y, Tsubouchi H, Blasi F, Comoglio PM (1992) Extracellular proteolytic cleavage by urokinase is required for activation of hepatocyte growth factor scatter factor. *EMBO J* 11:4825–4833.
53. Dvorak HJ. Tumors: Wounds that do not heal (1986) Similarities between tumor stroma generation and wound healing. *N Engl J Med* 315:1650–1659.
54. van den Hoof A (1988) Stromal involvement in malignant growth. *Adv Cancer Res* 50:159–196.
55. Zipori D (1990) Stromal cells in tumor growth and regression. *Cancer J* 3:164–169.
56. Cullen KJ, Lippman ME (1991) Stromal-epithelial interactions in breast cancer. In *Genes, Oncogenes, and Hormones: Advances in Cellular and Molecular Biology of Breast Cancer.* RB Dickson, ME Lippman (eds). Boston: Kluwer Academic, pp 413–431.
57. Folkman J (1995) Angiogenesis in cancer, vascular, rheumatoid and other disease. *Nature Med* 1:27–31.
58. Rodgers WH, Matrisian LM, Giudice LC, Dsupin B, Cannon P, Svitek C, Gorstein F, Osteen KG (1994) Patterns of matrix metalloproteinase expression in cycling endometrium imply differential functions and regulation by steroid hormones. *J Clin Invest* 94:946–953.
59. Duffy MJ, Reilly D, O'Sullivan C, O'Higgins N, Fennelly JJ, Andreasen P (1990) Urokinase-plasminogen activator, a new and independent prognostic marker in breast cancer. *Cancer Res* 50:6827–6829.
60. Foekens JA, Schmitt M, van Putten WLJ, Peters HA, Bontenbal M, Jänicke F, Klijn JGM (1992) Prognostic value of urokinase-type plasminogen activator in 671 primary breast cancer patients. *Cancer Res* 52:6101–6105.
61. Grondahl-Hansen J, Christensen IJ, Rosenquist C, Brünner N, Mouridsen HT, Dano K, Blichert-Toft M (1993) High levels of urokinase-type plasminogen activator and its inhibitor PAI-1 in cytosolic extracts of breast carcinomas are associated with poor prognosis. *Cancer Res* 53:2513–2521.
62. Duffy MJ, Reilly D, McDermott E, O'Higgins N, Fennelly JJ, Andreasen PA (1994) Urokinase plasminogen activator as a prognostic marker in different subgroups of patients with breast cancer. *Cancer* 74:2276–2280.
63. Lippman ME (1993) The development of biological therapies for breast cancer. *Science* 259:631–632.
64. Brown PD (1993) Matrix metalloproteinase inhibitors: A new class of anticancer agent. *Curr Opin Invest Drugs* 2:617–626.
65. Davies B, Brown PD, East N, Crimmin MJ, Balkwill FR (1993) A synthetic matrix metalloproteinase inhibitor tumor decreases burden and prolongs survival of mice bearing human ovarian carcinoma xenografts. *Cancer Res* 53:2087–2091.
66. Chirivi RGS, Garofalo A, Crimmin MJ, Bawden LJ, Stoppacciaro A, Brown PD, Giavazzi R (1994) Inhibition of the metastatic spread and growth of B16-BL6 murine melanoma by a synthetic matrix metalloproteinase inhibitor. *Int J Cancer* 58:460–464.
67. Wang X, Fu X, Brown PD, Crimmin MJ, Hoffman RM (1994) Matrix metalloproteinase inhibitor BB-94 (Batimastat) inhibits human colon tumor growth and spread in a patient-like orthotopic model in nude mice. *Cancer Res* 54:4726–4728.
68. Naito K, Kanbayashi N, Nakajima S, Murai T, Arakawa K, Nishimura S, Okuyama A (1994) Inhibition of growth of human tumor cells in nude mice by a metalloproteinase inhibitor. *Int J Cancer* 58:730–735.
69. Masiakowski P, Breathnach R, Bloch J, Gannon F, Krust A, Chambon P (1982) Cloning of cDNA sequences of hormone-regulated genes from the MCF-7 human breast cancer cell line. *Nucleic Acids Res* 10:7895–7903.

18. Endothelins in breast cancer

Kirti V. Patel and Michael P. Schrey

Introduction

Just how the normally ordered regime of growth and differentiation executed by all cells is over-riden, leading to the transformed phenotype, is as yet not fully understood, but many consider this progression to be a multistep process involving the accumulation of a number of genetic lesions, that is, loss of tumor suppressor genes or proto-oncogene activation [1–3]. Indeed, cytogenetic analysis of human malignant cells has shown that at least 90% of human tumors examined carry some form of cytogenetic alteration [4].

An equally important consideration is the role of regulatory growth substances, which alone probably would not engage a tumorigenic phenotype, but which alongside pre-existing genetic alterations could accelerate tumor growth, invasion, or metastasis. In human breast cancer, 70% of tumors examined were found to be aneuploid or to contain cytogenetic alterations [5]. These abnormalities in the cellular genetic organization may allow cells to respond more favorably to various exogenously derived mitogenic stimuli. In this regard, researchers have for some time now been actively searching for potential growth regulating substances that augment the growth of breast epithelial cells. The ovarian steroid hormone estradiol has long been recognized as just such a substance and has been shown to be essential not only for the normal growth and development of the mammary gland [6] but has promotional effects on the development of hormone-dependent breast tumors [7,8]. Its ability to stimulate the growth of breast cancer cells under both in vivo and in vitro systems has been attributed in part to its ability to stimulate the release of growth factors that can act in an autocrine or paracrine manner. For example, hormone-dependent breast cancer cells in culture treated with estradiol have been shown to release transforming growth factor alpha (TGF)-α and platelet-derived growth factor (PDGF) [9,10], which respectively behave as autocrine and paracrine growth factors.

Paracrine influences of growth factors derived from breast stromal tissue are now considered crucial for normal breast development [11,12] and possibly even play an important part in tumor growth [13–17]. It is not clear if some of the proposed aberrations in stromal fibroblast phenotype are a consequence of

R. Dickson and M. Lippman (eds.) MAMMARY TUMOR CELL CYCLE, DIFFERENTIATION AND METASTASIS. 1996. Kluwer Academic Publishers. ISBN 0-7923-3905-3. All rights reserved.

malignant transformation or represent an additional but vital component that further compounds the existing genetic lesions already in place. In any case, epithelial–mesenchyme interactions involving the bidirectional exchange of growth factors must now be looked upon as an important mechanistic phenomenon that may have a major influence on the differentiation pattern of the mammary gland and on tumor development and growth.

Entering into this area of paracrine regulators of breast development/growth is the recently discovered 21 amino acid peptide called *endothelin* (ET, and later termed ET-1 after the identification of the ET isoforms, see later). Although originally identified by its ability to induce potent longlasting vasoconstriction of vascular smooth muscles [18], it has now emerged that ET-1 has pleiotrophic actions, including the ability to stimulate growth in a variety of different cell types [19]. This mitogenic potential of endothelin has led a number of researchers to examine its role in tumorigenesis, including in breast cancer. The potential importance of this peptide in breast cancer has been recently highlighted by the finding that ET-1 levels are significantly elevated in malignant breast tissue compared with either benign or normal tissue [20]. At the time of writing this chapter, published papers on the role of ET-1 in breast cancer were somewhat limited; hence, in addition to relating all the available information on this topic, we also draw upon other systems in which the ET-1–mediated responses may be of some relevance in breast pathophysiology.

Discovery and distribution

Endothelin-1 is a 21 amino acid peptide with potent vasoactive properties that was isolated in 1989 by Yanagisawa and coworkers [18] from the conditioned medium of porcine aortic endothelial cells. This discovery was fortitous since earlier studies were in fact attempting to identify an endothelium-derived relaxing factor released from endothelial cells [21]. Instead, due to the design of the experiments, a peptidergic agent possessing a potent long-acting vasoconstrictor property was discovered. The challenge of fully identifying this peptidergic vasoconstrictor was taken up by Masaki and his group, and within a very short time they had isolated, purified, sequenced, and cloned this vasoconstrictor peptide, which they named *endothelin*.

On screening of the human genomic cDNA library under low-stringency hybridization with a synthetic ET probe, it was found that there were in fact three distinct ET genes localized on different chromosomes [22]. There appeared to be considerable homology within the portions of the genes encoding the 21 amino acid residues of ET, and they were subsequently referred to as ET-1, ET-2, and ET-3, in which ET-1 corresponded to the ET peptide initially isolated from porcine aortic endothelial cells. Sequence homology was also found with four peptide sarafotoxins, isolated from snake venom of the burrowing snake *Atractaspis engaddensis* [23]. All these ET-like peptides contain 21 amino acids and show complete identity in 10 of these positions. Indeed, all contain two disulphide bonds between Cys^1-Cys^{15} and Cys^3-Cys^{11}, which appear to be necessary for binding to ET receptors [24].

Various studies have indicated that ET isopeptides may be expressed in a differential manner in different tissues. Using essentially Northern analysis, the reverse-transcription–polymerase chain reaction (RT-PCR) and in-situ hybridization techniques, ET expression studies have revealed that ET-1, but not ET-2 nor ET-3, is expressed by endothelial and vascular smooth muscle cells [25,26]. Furthermore, ET-1 expression is not limited to vascular tissues but has been found to be present in other cell types, including macrophages [27], astrocytes [28], neuronal cells [29], decidual cells [30], and normal breast epithelial cells [31]. Several tumor-derived cell lines have also been shown to express ET-1, including colon, pancreas, breast [32], cervix (HeLa) and larynx (HEp-2) [33], and endometrial adenocarcinoma [34]. Data concerning the expression of the ET-2 and ET-3 isoforms in tumor tissues have not been forthcoming. Nonetheless, it has been reported that ET-2 is expressed in a human renal adenocarcinoma cell line [35].

Although breast cancer cell lines were shown to produce ET-1, in order to further investigate a potential role for this peptide in breast cancer, it was necessary to establish if ET-1 concentrations differ between malignant and normal breast tissues. This question was resolved by Yamashita and coworkers [20], who examined 157 breast tumor tissue extracts and found them to have significantly higher ET-1 levels than either benign or normal breast specimens. Furthermore, there appeared to be no apparent trend between the clinical staging of the tumors and ET-1 levels, or an association between ET-1 levels and the classical prognostic factors, including age of patient, tumor size, lymph node involvement, histological type, or estrogen/progesterone (ER/PgR) receptor status. These authors concluded that ET-1 is not related to the growth of breast tumor tissue but may be involved in the process of malignant transformation.

Release of ET-1 from breast epithelial cells

The first reported demonstration of preproET-1 (ppET-1) expression and ET-1 immunoreactivity by normal human breast epithelial cells was communicated by Baley and coworkers [31]. They found that normal human breast epithelial cells expressed low levels of a 2.3 kb mRNA ppET-1 species, which was enhanced significantly by both TGF-β and prolactin. Prolactin also increased immunoreactive ET-1 release, with maximal stimulation occurring at 6 hours, and thereafter ET-1 release remained constant. At the same time, Kusuhara and coworkers [32], using a specific radioimmunoassay, detected ET-1 in the spent medium of four human breast cancer cell lines, MCF-7, BT-20, ZR-75-1, and ZR-75-30. The stage was therefore set for further work to elucidate the possible pathophysiological role for ET-1 in the breast. In our own studies we have found that the glucocorticoids cortisol and dexamethasone, as well as the amphibian-derived peptide bombesin, stimulated ET-1 release from the T47-D human breast cancer cell line [36]. This stimulated release was dose and time dependent, and furthermore was inhibited by cycloheximide treatment, indicating the requirement for de novo protein synthesis.

In our studies, the possiblity that in addition to ET-1 other ET isoforms ET-2 or ET-3 are also released from human breast cancer cell lines was excluded since HPLC fractionation studies revealed the absence of ET-2 or ET-3 immunoreactive peaks. More recently, Yamashita and coworkers [37] have examined the effects of various agents, including estradiol, tamoxifen, TGF-β, and cytokines (IFN-γ, IL-1, tumor necrosis factor (TNF), and IL-6) on ET-1 production in the human breast cancer cells lines MCF-7 and ZR-75-1 cells. They found that IL-6 was the only agent that stimulated ET-1 release by 206% and 314% of control cells during a 6 hour incubation in MCF-7 and ZR-75-1 cells, respectively.

We have examined the effects of various agonists on ET-1 production in several hormone-dependent (MCF-7, T47-D, ZR-75-1) and -independent (MDA-MB-231, BT-20, Hs578T) human breast cancer cell lines. All hormone-dependent and -independent cell lines released ET-1 in a constitutive manner, with hormone-dependent cell lines releasing up to 20 times more ET-1 (Table

Table 1. Effect of various agents on ET-1 production in human breast cancer cell lines

	ET-1 produced fmol/10^6 cells					
Treatment	MCF-7	T47-D	ZR-75-1	MDA-MB-231	Hs578T	BT-20
Control	49.0 ± 1.1	55.6 ± 4.7	50.6 ± 4.2	2.7 ± 0.2	11.8 ± 0.7	14.8 ± 1.5
DEX	97.2 ± 2.4[b]	92.1 ± 4.2[b]	100.3 ± 2.8[b]	10.7 ± 0.9[b]	30.1 ± 3.3[b]	25.5 ± 1.6[a]
TPA	101.4 ± 2.5[b]	91.2 ± 8.7[a]	72.6 ± 1.6[a]	2.2 ± 0.2	57.7 ± 11.7[b]	30.2 ± 1.9[b]
BN	81.3 ± 6.7[a]	79.5 ± 1.1[a]	60.4 ± 3.8	3.3 ± 0.7	10.7 ± 1.0	17.1 ± 1.9
IL-1β	63.4 ± 3.8[a]	58.7 ± 7.5	86.7 ± 8.6[a]	2.7 ± 0.5	41.5 ± 2.4[b]	—
EGF	55.5 ± 4.2	52.2 ± 1.6	50.6 ± 2.6	2.3 ± 0.3	18.1 ± 5.1	17.1 ± 1.6
IGF-1	42.1 ± 7.2	58.2 ± 5.0	55.6 ± 2.3	2.9 ± 1.0	11.4 ± 1.3	15.9 ± 2.6
PGE$_2$	77.5 ± 6.2[a]	146.5 ± 6.7[b]	41.6 ± 6.8	—	—	—
Calcitn	55.3 ± 0.4[b]	62.5 ± 2.9	—	—	—	—

Human breast cancer cell lines grown to subconfluence in 25 cm^2 flasks were incubated for 24 hours in serum-free minimal essential medium containing 0.3% BSA. This medium was then discarded and fresh medium containing treatments [dexamethasone (DEX) 100 nM]; 12-O-tetradecanoylphorbol-13-acetate (TPA) 10 nM; bombesin (BN) 100 nM; interleukin-1β (IL-1β) 20 ng/ml; insulin-like growth factor-1 (IGF-1) 50 ng/ml; epidermal growth factor (EGF) 50 ng/ml; prostaglandin E$_2$ (PGE$_2$) 1 μM; calcitonin (Calcitn) 100 nM was added for a further 24 hours. After this period the overlying medium was collected and assayed for immunoreactive ET-1 using a specific radioimmunometric assay [124]. Results shown represent the mean ± SD, n = 3. Statistical differences were determined by Student's t test. [a] $p < 0.01$; [b] $p < 0.001$ denote significant difference from basal ET-1 release.

1). There were no obvious differences in the behavior of the two groups in terms of responsiveness to various agonists. In general, all cells lines treated with dexamethasone, TPA, or cAMP-elevating agonists (prostaglandin E_2 and calcitonin; see later) significantly increased ET-1 release over a 24 hour incubation period, while most cell lines were unresponsive to IL-1β (except ZR-75-1, MCF-7, Hs578T), IGF-1, and EGF (Table 1). Furthermore, on examining for possible interactions between various agents on ET-1 production in MCF-7 cells, a marked synergistic response was observed after treatment with dexamethasone and TPA or the amphibian-derived peptide bombesin (Figure 1). One possible mechanistic explanation for this cooperative interaction between the glucocorticoid and PKC-stimulated pathways was recently provided by Hansen Ree and coworkers [38], who found that expression of the gluco-

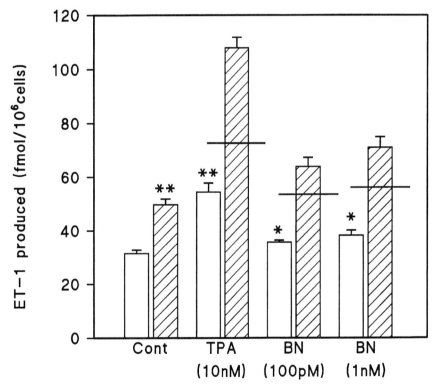

Figure 1. Synergistic interactions between dexamethasone and TPA or bombesin (BN) on ET-1 production in MCF-7 cells. MCF-7 cells grown in 25 cm² flasks were incubated in 2 ml of serum-free Eagle's minimum essential medium containing 0.3% bovine serum albumin with or without TPA or BN, and in the absence (open bars) or presence of dexamethasone (hatched bars). Horizontal lines across bars indicate the expected sum of the responses of the individual agonists. ET-1 production values obtained after the specific immunoradiometric assay were normalized to cell numbers. All data represent the means ± SD of triplicate determinations. *p < 0.01, **p < 0.001 denote significant stimulation compared with untreated cells.

corticoid receptor mRNA and protein in MCF-7 cells was increased after treatment with TPA. Thus, the glucocorticoid-stimulated ET-1 production in breast tissue could be further enhanced by agonists that increase glucocorticoid receptor transcription through interaction with cis-acting elements on the glucocorticoid receptor gene.

As mentioned earlier, screening of a genomic cDNA library revealed that ET-1, ET-2, and ET-3 are encoded by distinct genes, which have been assigned, using somatic cell hybrids and in situ hybridization techniques, to chromosomes 6, 1, and 20, respectively [39,40]. The ppET-1 gene, distributed over 6.8 kb of genomic DNA, contains five exons and four introns, with the mature ET-1 peptide nucleotide sequence present in the second exon. Examination of the 5'-flanking promoter region of the human ppET-1 gene has revealed the presence of TATA and CAAT boxes [41]. Moreover, in endothelial cells two regions in the 5'-flanking region, referred to as *region A* and *region B*, were shown to be necessary to direct the efficient ET-1 gene transcription through cis-acting elements [42]. Region A was found to contain the GATA binding motif, similar to the consensus sequence Eryf-1 identified in erythroid cells, and to which the binding protein GATA-2 binds and regulates ET-1 gene transcription [43]. Region B was found to contain the TPA-responsive element (TRE) to which jun/jun and fos/jun dimers (AP-1 transcriptional factor) bind and mediate ET-1 gene transcription [44]. These dimers interact with the AP-1 promoter binding motif of various genes, leading to cellular responses, such as cell growth and differentiation [45]. Recently, a novel cDNA encoding an extended 5'-flanking region of the ppET-1 gene has been identified from screening a human placental cDNA library [46]. This extended region is thought to contain at least three potential CAP sites, and promoter deletion mutants coupled to reporter genes revealed potential promoter activity within this site. This study also indicated that this novel transcript and the previously identified human endothelial cell ppET-1 transcript may be regulated in a tissue-specific manner.

In addition to the AP-1 promoter element, a number of other cis-acting sequences have been identified that may regulate ET-1 mRNA transcription, possibly in a tissue-specific manner. Thus, the promoter region of the ppET-1 gene is found to contain cis-acting sequences for the nuclear factor-1 and acute phase reaction regulatory factor (APR) transcriptional factors. In addition, intragenic sequences for nuclear factor-1 and APR transcriptional factors are also present. In the MCF-7 and ZR-75-1 breast cancer cell lines, the demonstration that the cytokine IL-6 stimulated ET-1 production suggests that this response may be the result of interaction of the APR transcriptional factor with the APR binding motif within the promoter region of the ET-1 gene [37]. The identification of three putative octanucleotide sequences for the TRE indicates the importance of this sequence in regulating ET-1 mRNA expression. However, it appears that only one of the AP-1 cis-acting elements is essential in regulating ET-1 gene expression. Furthermore, site-directed mutagenesis of the AP-1 site was shown to significantly attenuate promoter activity [44]. In rat-1 fibroblasts ET-1 induced AP-1 transcriptional factor activity, suggesting a potential for ET-1 to regulate its own expression [47]. This finding is consistent with an earlier study that found ET-1 stimulated ppET-1 expression in rat vascular smooth muscle cells [48].

Many studies have shown that one of the first nuclear events initiated by many growth factors and regulatory peptides upon binding to their cell surface receptors is the activation of the immediate-early genes, which include the fos and jun family of genes. One signaling pathway that has been consistently found to be important for AP-1 transcriptional factor activity and ET-1 gene expression has been shown to be dependent on PKC activity. Indeed, many cell types treated with TPA demonstrate increased ppET-1 mRNA transcript and ET-1 peptide synthesis [41,49]. Similarily, increases in intracellular calcium and diacylglycerol, resulting from agonist-stimulated inositol lipid hydrolysis, may augment ET-1 mRNA expression and protein. In line with this proposal, we have found that bombesin stimulated both inositol phospholipid hydrolysis and ET-1 production in the human breast cancer cell lines MCF-7 and T47-D [36,50]. As indicated earlier, most human breast cancer cell lines examined were responsive to TPA treatment, highlighting the potential importance of this signaling pathway in regulating ET-1 production in breast cancers. Indeed, we found that in MCF-7 cells downregulation of PKC by chronic exposure to TPA resulted in the loss of ET-1 production in response to a further challenge to TPA.

We also noted that ET-1 production in response to TPA, in contrast to that induced by glucorcorticoids and cAMP-elevating agonists (see later) did not appear to be dependent on de novo protein synthesis or precursor peptide processing, since treatment of MCF-7 cells with cycloheximide or phosphoramidon only moderatly attenuated the TPA-stimulated ET-1 release. Similar results have been reported in cultured human-vein endothelial cells [51]. These observations are surprising because the TPA-mediated transcription of the fos and jun nuclear proteins is thought to be crucial for ppET-1 gene transcription. It may be that in breast cancer cells two routes for ET-1 release exist, one that utilizes the de novo protein synthesis of ppET-1 followed by rapid processing and release from the cells, and a second, which is dependent on release of the peptide from a preformed store. Another point of regulation of ET-1 mRNA expression appears to be determined by the stability of the mRNA species. In this respect, the 3'-untranslated region of the of the ppET-1 gene contains two AUUUA sequences, which are known to decrease the stability of the mRNA and which probably accounts for the short half-life of the transcript and its superinduction by cycloheximide [41].

Role of cAMP in ET-1 production in human breast cancer cells

In our attempts to identify agents/signaling pathways that can regulate ET-1 production in human breast cancer cells, we found that agonists that elevate intracellular cAMP also stimulated ET-1 production. Treatment of MCF-7 cells with forskolin (Fk), which activates adenylate cyclase or cholera toxin, which stimulates Gs through ADP-ribosylation of the α-subunit of Gs, resulted in a two- to threefold increase in ET-1 release. Similarly, the cell permeable cAMP analogue 8-bromo-cAMP and the cAMP phosphodiesterase inhibitor 3-isobutyl-1-methylxanthine also markedly enhanced ET-1 production. These responses in human breast cancer cells appear to be novel, because similar effects in other cell types have as yet not been reported. Previous reports on the role of cAMP in ET-1 production in other cell types are limited. In cultured endothelial cells, the vasoactive peptide atrial naturetic peptide was found to inhibit the production and secretion of ET-1 by apparently reducing cAMP production [52], indicating that this second messenger does have a role in regulating ET-1 production. However, in the same study addition of a cAMP analogue appeared to have no effect on basal ET-1 release. In contrast, in rat mesangial cells cAMP-elevating agents actually inhibited ET-1 release [49].

Having demonstrated a clear effect of cAMP on ET-1 production in human breast cancer cells, the next step was to identify possible physiological agonists present in breast tissue that could mimic the effect of cAMP elevating agents on ET-1 production. Two potential agents identified were the eicosanoid prostaglandin E_2 (PGE_2) and calcitonin, which have been previously shown to

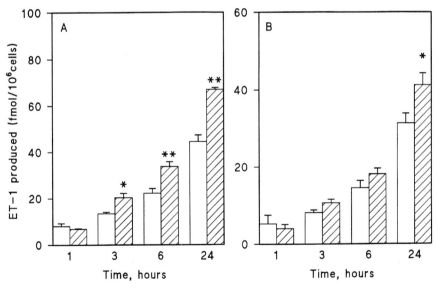

Figure 2. Time course of PGE_2 and calcitonin-stimulated ET-1 production in MCF-7 cells. MCF-7 cells grown in 25 cm² flasks were incubated without (open bars) or with (hatched bars) either (**A**) PGE_2 (1 µM) or (**B**) calcitonin (100 nM) for the times indicated. At the end of each incubation period, the spent medium was removed and assayed for ET-1. Cell numbers were also determined, and the results were subsequently normalized to cell numbers. Results shown represent mean ± SD of triplicate incubations. *p < 0.01 and **p < 0.001 indicate an increase in ET-1 production over respective basal release.

increase cAMP levels in MCF-7 cells [53]. Both PGE_2 and human synthetic calcitonin stimulated ET-1 production in MCF-7 cells during a 24 hour incubation by 150% and 130% of basal levels, respectively (Figure 2). ET-1 production in response to pharmacological and physiological cAMP elevating agents were attenuated both in the presence of the protein translational inhibitor cycloheximide, indicating the requirement of de novo protein synthesis, as well as by the big ET-1 to ET-1 processing enzyme inhibitor phosphoramidon, indicating the activation of the ET-1 synthetic pathway. To further investigate whether the cAMP/PKA or the PKC signaling pathway(s) is responsible for ET-1 production, various experimental procedures were conducted. The PKA inhibitor H-89, at the concentration used, abolished ET-1 production stimulated by cAMP-elevating agents, including Fk and PGE_2, and calcitonin, while the TPA-stimulated response was unaffected (Table 2). Conversely, downregulation of MCF-7 cell PKC through a chronic exposure to TPA resulted in the desensitization of the TPA-stimulated ET-1 release but not that caused by the cAMP-elevating agents FK, PGE_2, or calcitonin.

A cAMP-responsive element (concensus sequence TGACGTCA) within the ppET-1 promoter region appears to be absent. However, on examining the promoter region of the ppET-1 gene for an AP-2 element (consensus sequence CCCCAGGC), which is also known to mediate both cAMP and phorbol ester induction of gene transcription [54], two potential AP-2 sites were found. From the transcriptional start site, these sequences corresponded to

Table 2. Effect of the protein kinase A inhibitor H-89 on TPA- and PKA-mediated stimulation of ET-1 production in MCF-7 cells

Treatment	ET-1 produced fmol/10^6 cells/ 24 hours % of basal release	
	−H-89	+H-89
Forskolin (10 μM)	245 ± 7.6[a]	128 ± 6.5[b]
TPA (10 nM)	228 ± 8[a]	287 ± 32[b]
PGE_2 (1 μM)	183 ± 6[a]	87 ± 14[b]
Calcitonin (100 nM)	129 ± 9.2[a]	119 ± 12

MCF-7 cells grown to approximately 70% confluence in 25 cm² flasks were incubated for 24 hours in serum-free minimum essential medium containing 0.3% bovine serum albumin. Medium was then discarded and cells were pretreated with or without H-89 (30 μM) for 4 hours prior to treatment with forskolin, prostaglandin E_2 (PGE_2), calcitonin, or TPA and in the absence or presence of H-89. Basal ET-1 production values in the absence or presence of H-89 were 33 ± 4 and 13 ± 1.4 fmol/10^6 cells/24 hs, respectively. Results shown represent the mean ± SD, n = 3.
Statistical differences were determined by Student's t test. [a]$p < 0.01$; [b]$p < 0.001$ denote a significant difference from cells not treated with H-89.

(A)CCCAGGC at -2221 to -2228 and (T)CCCAGGC from -2065- to -2072. In this regard, functional studies using promoter-reporter gene constructs will help in identifing specific sequences that regulate transcription of the ppET-1 gene in breast epithelial cells.

Endothelin-1–mediated cell signaling: Potential role in breast fibroblast mitogenesis

Although, ET-1 was originally identified as a potent vasoactive peptide, several studies have shown that this peptide has the ability to act as a mitogen in a variety of cell types. For instance, ET-1 stimulates DNA synthesis and proliferation in vascular smooth muscle cells [55,56], vascular endothelial cells [57,58], murine fibroblast cell lines [59,60], rat mesangial cells [47,61] human melanocytes [62], and glial cells [63]. This long-term response is initiated by the binding of ET-1 to the G-protein–coupled ET receptor. Presently, two ET-receptor subtypes, ETA and ETB, have been identified and cloned [64,65]. A third ET receptor ETc has been proposed based on several studies that have found selective high responsiveness to the ET-3 isopeptide [66]. ETA receptors have higher affinity for ET-1 and ET-2 than for the ET-3 isoform, whereas the ETB receptor demonstrates equal affinity for all ET isoforms. ET-occupied receptors have been shown to activate those signaling pathways that are characteristic of receptors with seven transmembrane-spanning domains coupled to GTP-binding proteins. Treatment of various cell types with ET-1 has been found to elicit rapid phospholipase C–mediated hydrolysis of inositol phospholipids, resulting in the concomitant production of the two second messengers inositol trisphosphate (IP_3) and diacylglycerol (DAG), which mobilize calcium from intracellular stores and activate protein kinase C [57,67], respectively. DAG has also been shown to be generated by ET-1–mediated hydrolysis of phosphatidylcholine through the possible actions of phospholipase C or D [68]. Interestingly, the overexpression of the PKC-β1 isoform in rat 6 fibroblasts [69] or v-src transformed rat-1 fibroblasts cells [70] resulted in enhanced IP_3 production and calcium signaling in response to ET-1 treatment, indicating that cells that demonstrate oncogenic transformation or overexpress key cell signaling components may become more responsive to ET-1. ET- receptors have also been shown to be coupled to the activation of plasma membrane Ca^{2+} channels [24,71], phospholipase A_2 activation leading to the release of the eicosanoid precursor arachidonic acid [24,72] and to adenylate cyclase, mediating either stimulation or inhibition of cAMP production, depending on the ET-receptor subtype activated [24,73].

Activation of these multiple ET-receptor coupled signaling pathways instigates downstream events in the nucleus, resulting in enhanced expression of the immediate early genes c-*fos* and c-*myc* in vascular smooth muscle cells and in Swiss 3T3 cells [56,59,61]. In rat-1 fibroblasts, ET-1 caused the rapid increase in mRNA levels of the c-*fos*, *fos*-B, *fos*-1, c-*jun*, and *jun* B genes [74]. The ET-1–stimulated signaling pathways involved in activation of these genes are still to be fully elucidated. However, both calcium and PKC have been implicated in regulating the expression of these early mitogen-responsive genes. For instance, in rat-1 fibroblasts the ET-1–induced increase in mRNA transcripts of the *jun* and *fos* gene family could be blocked by the calcium chelator EGTA, thereby implicating ET-1–induced elevation in intracellular calcium in fos/jun gene transcription [74]. Similarily, the involvement of PKC in ET-1 induced c-*fos* proto-ongogene expression has been demonstrated in vascular smooth muscle cells and in rat-1 cells in which PKC inhibitors and PKC downregulation inhibited ET-1–induced c-*fos* mRNA expression [56,60].

ET-1 has also been found to stimulate the serine/threonine mitogen-activated protein kinase (MAP kinase) activity in various cells types [75], further demonstrating that ET-1 has the capacity to activate multiple signaling pathways previously associated with mitogenic growth factors. The MAP kinases (p44/p42) have been shown to participate in the phosphorylation of microtuble-associated protein-2 and myelin basic protein [76,77], the ribosomal S6 kinase [78], the *raf*-1 kinase [79], and the c-*jun*, c-*myc* transcriptional factor [80,81]. In human breast fibroblasts, ET-1 was found to stimulate S6 kinase activity [31]. This could be a potentially important signaling pathway through which ET-1 activates nuclear events. For instance, it is known that S6 kinase is capable of phosphorylating the myc, jun and fos [82] nuclear proteins, thereby linking this kinase to a mitogenic response. Presumably, S6 kinase activation is produced by phosphoinositide hydrolysis [31], resulting in the phosphorylation and activation of MAP kinases through the action of both PKC-mediated and or by the MAP kinase kinase (MEK) (see later), since MAP kinase activation is thought to require both threonine and tyrosine phosphorylation. It has also been reported that ET has the ability to stimulate tyrosine phsophorylation of various cellular nonreceptor tyrosine kinases, including the focal adhesion kinase (p125[fak]) in Swiss 3T3 cells [83], as well as stimulating pp60[c-src] in glomerulus mesangial cells [84]. In mesangial cells it has been demonstrated that although PKC is required for DNA synthesis, it is not suffcent. Moreover, it was also found that ET-1–stimulated protein tyrosine kinase activity was required for ET-1 to mediate its mitogenic action, since the use of tyrosine kinase inhibitors successfully blocked growth, c-*fos* induction, AP-1 DNA binding, and the stimulation of AP-1 cis-element directed transcription by ET-1 [84].

Evidence indicates that ET-1 behaves as a paracrine factor in breast tissue; that is, ET-1 released by both normal and malignant breast epithelial cells, which lack ET receptors, appears to bind to high affinity receptors localized on breast fibroblasts, stimulating inositol lipid hydrolysis and S6 kinase activity [31]. The finding that normal breast epithelial cells produce ET-1 but lack ET receptors, whereas breast fibroblasts possess high-affinity ET receptors but do not release ET, suggests that this peptide exerts its action in a paracrine fashion [31]. We investigated the possibility that ET-1 released from breast epithelial cells could act as a paracrine mitogen for breast fibroblasts. In serum-starved quiescent breast fibroblasts obtained from either normal breast or from malignant breast tumors, we found that ET-1 alone had little effect on

DNA synthesis. However, in combination with the IGF-1, EGF, or PDGF, there was a significant synergistic effect on DNA synthesis (Table 3). This mitogenic effect was most apparent in the presence of IGF-1, with DNA synthesis being stimulated at ET-1 concentrations as low as 10 pM [36]. This suggests that in human breast fibroblasts ET-1 is acting as a competence-type growth factor, allowing the transition from G_0 to G_1, a point in the cell cycle where progression growth factors act to drive the cell cycle from the G_1 to S phase. Similar results have been demonstrated with ET-1 acting synergistically with growth factors in stimulating DNA synthesis in other cell types [59,85,86].

This concerted interaction of ET-1 with breast fibroblasts in the presence of IGF-1, which has also been shown to be expressed by breast fibroblasts [87,88], may play an important role in regulating the growth of these cells. Furthermore, it is suggested from this model that as a consequence of the increased proliferation of the stromal fibroblast cell population, which is adjacent to the tumor cells, there is an increased production of mitogenic growth factors, such as IGF-1 and IGF-II, by the fibroblasts, resulting in the increased proliferation of both epithelial and stromal components of the tumor. An indication that this may be the case has recently been demonstrated in human breast phyllodes tumors. These rare tumors, which account for less than 2.5% of breast cancers, are characterized as fibroepithelial tumors that exhibit an abundant stromal component. The malignant form of these tumors is even less common than the benign tumors and generally exhibit hypercellularity and an increased mitotic rate [89–91]. Yamashita and coworkers [89] examined 4 phyllodes tumors and 10 fibroadenomas for their ET-1 content. They found that the phyllodes tumors had an 18-fold higher ET-1 concentration than the fibroadenomas. Furthermore, these elevated levels were also considerably higher than the ET-1 concentrations found in breast tumors.

Interestingly, in human placental fibroblasts it was shown that ET-1 stimulated the production of both IGF-binding proteins and of IGF-II, but not IGF-I [92]. This finding may be of importance if this effect of ET-1 is also reproduced in the human breast, since Cullen and coworkers [87] have reported that fibroblasts grown from normal or benign breast tumours express predominantly IGF-1 mRNA, whereas fibroblasts grown from malignant breast tumors express largely the IGF-II message. Moreover, in situ hybridization studies have confirmed this change from IGF-1 expression in normal and benign breast tissue to IGF-II expression in malignant tumors [93]. Thus, the high levels of ET-1 found in malignant breast tumor tissue may be instrumental in the increased IGF-II expression observed in the firoblasts surrounding these tumours.

Prostaglandin E2: A paracrine mediator of ET-1 action and production

We have recently identified breast stromal fibroblasts as a potential source for the raised levels of PGE_2 associated with breast tumors [94]. Since several

Table 3. Synergistic stimulation of DNA synthesis in human breast fibroblasts by ET-1 and various polypeptide growth factors

Treatment	[³H] Thymidine incorporation (cpm/well)					
	B-FIB-M1	B-FIB-M2	B-FIB-M3	B-FIB-N1	B-FIB-N2	B-FIB-N3
Control	736 ± 48	2192 ± 223	657 ± 8	2380 ± 600	1239 ± 68	2991 ± 77
FCS	1712 ± 170[b]	5486 ± 250[b]	8569 ± 249[b]	17986 ± 365[b]	10369 ± 572[b]	18404 ± 698[b]
ET-1	723 ± 164	1645 ± 290[b]	706 ± 89	4839 ± 372[b]	1097 ± 113[b]	2775 ± 323
IGF	2063 ± 203[b]	3441 ± 40[b]	4956 ± 384[b]	12346 ± 262[b]	3953 ± 379[b]	9728 ± 1192[b]
IGF+ET–1	4011 ± 395[b]	6804 ± 98[b]	15673 ± 581[b]	21180 ± 2362[b]	6794 ± 65[b]	15674 ± 785[b]
EGF	931 ± 137[b]	2529 ± 59	2358 ± 95[b]	5985 ± 611[b]	1893 ± 89[b]	5581 ± 166[b]
EGF+ET–1	1524 ± 276[b]	3904 ± 123[b]	3989 ± 187[b]	13041 ± 1239[b]	2896 ± 37[b]	4406 ± 263[b]
PDGF	1611 ± 40[b]	3089 ± 235[a]	1205 ± 58[b]	11603 ± 698[b]	2996 ± 32[b]	3574 ± 163[a]
PDGF+ET–1	2350 ± 390[b]	4578 ± 393[b]	1287 ± 98[b]	16967 ± 989[b]	4524 ± 63[b]	5810 ± 589[b]

Human breast fibroblasts obtained from breast tumors (B-FIB-M1 to M3) or reduction mammoplasties (B-FIB-N1 to N3) were cultured as described previously [36]. Fibroblasts grown in 75 cm² flasks were split into 3.8 cm² 12-well tissue culture plates at a density of approximately 5 × 10⁴ cell per well and on reaching 70% confluence were washed with phosphate buffered saline and incubated in serum-free Eagle's minimum essential medium for 48 hours. After this period, the medium was removed and treatments were added [ET-1 (10 nM); IGF (50 ng/ml); EGF (50 ng/ml); PDGF (5 ng/ml)] in a final volume of 1 ml. Fibroblasts were incubated for a further 14 hours, at which time [³H] thymidine (1 μC/ml) was added to each well. Cells were incubated for a further 4 hours, after which time incorporation of radiolabeled thymidine into trichloroacetic acid precipitable material was assessed, as described previously [36]. Results shown represent the mean ± SD, n = 3. Statistical differences were determined by Student's t test. [a] p < 0.01; [b]p < 0.001 denote a significant difference from untreated cells.

studies have previously shown that ET-1 can induce eicosanoid production in various tissues [95–97], we have also investigated whether ET-1 may have a similar action in the breast by stimulating PGE_2 production in breast fibroblasts. Early passage breast fibroblasts obtained from reduction mammoplasties were unresponsive to ET-1. However, when the breast fibroblasts were pretreated with the cytokine interleukin-1β (IL-1β), there was a marked synergistic increase in PGE_2 production in response to ET-1 and other inflammatory peptides, such as bradykinin or des-Arg[9] bradykinin (Figure 3). Although the cellular mechanisms mediating this potentiated PGE_2 production are uncertain, an increase in substrate availability via phospholipase A_2 activation by ET-1 or bradykinin, coupled with induction of cyclooxygenase by the cytokine, has been previouly reported in other cells [98,99]. These in vitro effects of ET-1 and other inflammatory mediators on PGE_2 production in breast fibroblasts may explain in part why PGE_2 levels are elevated in malignant breast tumors [100–102], as well as in experimental murine mammary tumor models [103].

In view of our earlier observation that PGE_2 can increase ET-1 production in human breast cancer cells, we propose that under in vivo conditions a potential exists for a bidirectional paracrine loop. This crosstalk would involve breast cancer epithelial cell–derived ET-1 acting on proximal breast fibroblasts resulting in proliferation and increased PGE_2 production, in the respective presence of IGF-1 and IL-1β, while breast fibroblast–derived PGE_2

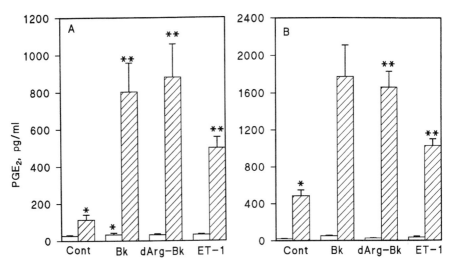

Figure 3. Effect of IL-1β pretreatment on breast fibroblast PGE_2 production in response to ET-1, BK, and des-Arg[9]BK in two different human breast fibroblast cell lines (**A**, HBF-12; **B**, HBF-10). Fibroblasts were preteated with (hatched bars) or without (open bars) IL-1β (1 ng/ml) prior to incubation in the presence or absence of BK (1 μM), des-Arg[9]BK (1 μM), and ET-1 (0.1 μM). All values represent means ± SD, n = 3. *p < 0.01 for stimulation compared with basal control values. **p < 0.001 for potentiation of responses in the presence of IL-1β.

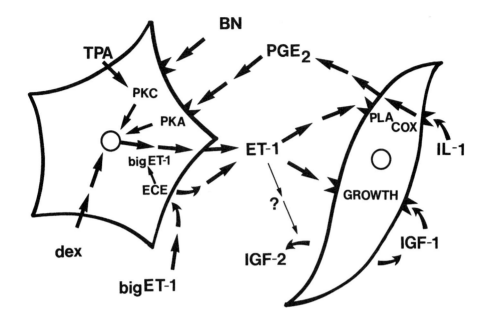

cancer cell   **fibroblast**

Figure 4. Potential role for ET-1 in the regulation of breast tumor cell growth and function. ET-1 production by breast cancer cells is regulated by diverse signaling pathways, including glucocorticoids (dex)-, and PKA- and PKC-mediated mechanisms. PGE_2 and bombesin (BN) represent two candidate agonists for activation of these pathways. Breast cancer cells also exhibit the potential to regulate tissue ET-1 levels by processing exogenous big ET-1 via endothelin converting enzyme (ECE). ET-1 acts in concert with other growth factors, such as IGF-1, as a paracrine mitogen on tumor mesenchyme. ET-1 may also upregulate PGE_2 and IGF-II production by breast fibroblasts. These factors may, in turn, exercise a reciprocal paracrine influence on cancer cell growth and function.

acts on breast epithelial cells, stimulating ET-1 production (Figure 4). Whether this proposed positive paracrine feedback mechanism is indeed instrumental in mediating the raised levels of PGE_2 and ET-1 seen in breast tumors remains to be established.

Role of proteolytic enzymes in regulation of ET-1 in breast tissue

Circulating plasma concentrations of ET-1 have been found to be in the range of 2–5 pM in normal subjects [104], but under certain pathophysiological conditions these levels have been found to be elevated [104]. It is not presently known if precancerous lesions or malignancy leads to an elevation of circulating ET-1 concentrations. However, in a rare skin ET-1–secreting tumor hemangioendothelioma, which is associated with hypertension, plasma levels were found to be 15- to 20-fold higher than of normal subjects [105,106]. Moreover, surgical removal of the tumor resulted in decreases in blood pressure and plasma ET-1 levels; however, recurrence was associated with increases in both these parameters. Thus, some tumors may have a significant effect on circulating levels of ET-1. Nonetheless, it is unlikely that plasma concentrations of ET-1 play a significant role in the development and/or growth of various tumors, since it is rapidly metabolized by the kidney and lung [107,108], probably though the actions of proteolytic enzymes, such as the neutral endopeptidase 24.11 [(also called *common acute lymphoblastic leukemia antigen* CD 10 (CALLA)] [109,110]. In the adult breast, this enzyme has been shown to be expressed by the myoepithelial cells [111] and possibly in stromal fibroblasts associated with some breast tumors [112]. It is possible that under in vivo conditions, the actions of ET-1 upon its target cell type is tightly regulated by various proteolytic ectoenzymes. In this respect it will be important to determine whether these ectoenzymes are downregulated in certain breast pathologies, allowing greater availability of growth regulating peptide hormones to receptor-expressing cell types [113].

It is becoming increasing apparent that within a particular tissue that contains cell types expressing ET-receptors, the major source of ET-1 is probably derived from proximal cell types. In colonic cancer tissues, it has been found that whereas the colon cancer cell produce ET-1, specific ET-1 binding sites are localized prodominantly in stromal tissue fibroblasts adjacent to the cancer cell nests [114]. In breast phyllodes tumors, immunocytochemical staining for ET-1 was clearly demonstrated on the epithelial but not the stromal component of the tumor [89], and ET-1 receptors have been shown to be present on breast fibroblasts but not on breast epithelial cells [31].

Although, epithelial cell–derived ET-1 probably represents the major source of local tissue ET-1 in the breast, we have to consider the possibility that the ET-1 precursor big ET-1, derived from the circulation, where its concentrations are generally two- to fourfold higher than ET-1, may be utilized by breast epithelial cell endothelin-converting enzyme (ECE) as an additional source of mature ET-1. The processing steps for the production of mature ET-1 have been proposed. Initially the conversion of the 212 amino acid prepro ET-1 to big ET-1 is thought to involve a pair of dibasic endopeptidases and carboxypeptidases. This is followed by the conversion of big ET-1 to ET-1 by an unidentified ECE that catalyzes an unusual proteolytic cleavage between the Trp^{21} and Val^{22} bond of big ET-1. This unusual processing step has also been reproduced in heterologous systems, such as in COS cells [115] and baculovirus-infected insect cells [116].

This putative ECE has been intensely studied in the past 4–5 years in many different cell types, and it appears to have properties characteristic of previously identified proteolytic enzymes. These include the cathepsin D–like [117] or cathepsin E–like aspartic protease [118], the soluble phosphoramidon-sensitive [119] and -insensitive metalloproteinase [120], and a membrane-bound phosphoramidon-sensitive metalloproteinase [121]. From these and numerous other studies conducted so far, the emphasis now appears to be directed toward the neutral phosphoramidon-sensitive metalloproteinase described by Ohnaya et al. [121] as being the likely physiological relevant enzyme involved in big ET-1 processing. An ECE from rat endothelial cells has been recently cloned and functionally expressed [122]. This enzyme appears to be a highly glycosylated protein containing 10 possible N-linked glycosylation sites, a zinc-binding domain, and a single membrane spanning region. Similarities also exist between properties of this enzyme and those purified to near homogeneity from porcine aortic endothelium [121] and rat lung microsomes [123], that is, all enzymes were inhibited by phosphoramidon, EDTA, and O-phenanthroline. Moreover, all the enzymes had an optimal activity between 6.6 and 6.8. However, differences were evident in their ability to process the various ET isopeptides.

We have examined the biochemical characteristics of the breast ECE in both hormone-dependent (MCF-7 and T-47D) and hormone-independent (MDA-MD-231) breast cancer cell lines, and have found that all cell lines processed exogenously added big-ET-1 to ET-1 as measured by a sensitive ET-1 radioimmunometric assay [124]. This converting activity was inhibited by phosphoramidon but not by other classes of protease inhibitors, including thiorphan. Inhibition was also achieved by the use of metal chelating agents such as EDTA and O-phenanthroline. Optimal activity of the breast ECE was observed between pH 6.2 and 7.2, indicating a neutral metalloproteinase-like activity similar to that previously observed in porcine aortic endothelial [121] and rat lung microsomes [123]. Michaelis-Menten kinetics of big-ET-1 to ET-1 converting activity in the MCF-7, T-47D, and MDA-MB-231 breast cancer cell lines revealed respective apparent Km values of 7.0, 6.22, and 15.7 nM, and Vmax values of 11.36, 4.43, and 145 fmol/10^6 cells. These studies revealed that the enzyme in MCF-7 and T47-D cell lines appears to have a twofold greater affinity for the substrate than the hormone-independent MDA-MD-231 cells, while Vmax rates indicated that the hormone-independent cell line possess more ECE activity than the hormone-dependent cell lines, although this may just reflect differences in the availability of the precursor to the cell lines. As shown from our results in Table 1, differences in the basal production of ET-1 between hormone-dependent and -independent cell lines do not fall in line with the findings of Yamashita and coworkers [20], in which no association was found between ET-1 production by breast tumors and their ER/PgR receptor status. However, our present kinetic study on the breast ECE indicates that hormone-independent tumors may compensate for low basal ET-1 release by processing more exogenous big-ET-1. It is still not known how the ECE is regulated in various cells. Presumably, regulation of ECE production could represent another important control mechanism in ET-1 synthesis.

Conclusions and future directions

From the evidence available at present, we cannot as yet assign a definitive role for endothelins in the human mammary gland or its involvement in the process to tumorigenesis. It is clear, however, that in the breast ET-1 is derived from the parenchymal tissues and acts in a paracrine fashion on neighboring stromal cells. From our own in vitro studies we have found that ET-1 acts as a mitogen in breast fibroblasts but only in the presence of other growth factors, such as IGF-1, EGF, and PDGF. These findings have important implications with regard to the possible role of ET-1 in breast morphogenesis, growth, and development. Of particular interest was the recent report of ET-1 gene targeting in mice, in which homozygous disruption of the ET-1 gene resulted in lethal malformations of the craniofacial tissues, a consequence of a disturbance in the development of the pharyngeal arches [125]. In addition to highlighting the importance of ET-1 on developmental processes, this study also proposed a role for paracrine actions of ET-1 in the development of the pharyngeal arches–derived tissues.

It is now increasingly evident, largely from rodent mammary gland studies, that the mesenchyme is crucial for the development of the mammary gland and may also contribute to the growth of breast tumors. Therefore, the ability of breast epithelial cell–derived endothelin peptide to interact with other local growth factors on breast fibroblasts may contibute to the control of mesenchyme growth and function: This process presumably could lead to the increased production of fibroblast-derived growth factors, such as the IGFs, which would have a mitogenic action on both the breast epithelial and stromal components. Although the developmental role of ET-1 in the breast is not known, there is evidence that this mitogenic peptide may contribute to stomal expansion, an event commonly associated with breast carcinomas. Indeed, high ET-1 levels have been found in human breast phyllodes tumors, which are also characterized by an abundant stoma [89].

There are a number of areas relating to possible actions of ET-1 in the breast that require urgent investigation if we are to establish whether ET-1 induces responses that may be related to the process of malignant transformation and/or to events that lead to greater invasineness of tumors. For instance, can ET-1 induce growth factor production in breast fibroblasts or the ability to stimulate angiogenesis or invasion/metastasis? Alas, very little is known about the role of ET-1 in any of these processes, either in the breast or other tissues. Nonetheless, there are indications that ET-1 may directly or indirectly participate in these unfavorable tumor-mediated events.

Evidence supports a role for tumors in stimulating angiogenesis through the action of soluble factors [126,127]. Purely on a speculative basis, it can be proposed that ET-1, in the presence of other growth factors, such as basic fibroblast growth factor, which is known to induce endothelial cell migration, proteolysis, and proliferation, may contribute to tumor angiogenesis [127,128]. At present reports of the ability of ET-1 to stimulate endothelial cell proliferation are confined to brain endothelial capillary cells [57] and human vascular endothelial cells [58]. The pathological preturbations within normal tissues that lead to tumor angiogenesis have been likened to the invasion/metastatic processes that occur around the tumor microenviroment, since in both cases there are components that require the degradation of basement membranes/

extracellular matrixes and migratory responses [129,130]. In this regard, the dissolution of the primary blood vessel basement membrane barrier followed by the sprouting of new venules is thought to involve the actions of proteolytic enzymes, including the type IV collagenase and plasminogen-type activator. Interestingly, ET-1 has been shown to stimulate the release of tissue-type plasminogen activator in endothelial cells [131], which has the ability to process plasminogen to plasmin and which, in turn, can convert the type IV procollagenase to type IV collagenase and may also play a part in the activation of some latent forms of growth factors, for example, TGF-β.

It is not yet known if ET-1 has chemotactic properties, although strong chemotactic effects of ET-1 have been reported on blood monocytes [132]. The ability of tumor cells to migrate is a crucial part of the invasion/metastatic process, and to date there is no clear evidence that ET-1 is involved in this life-threatening phenomenon. However, it is possible that ET-1 may effect this response through secondary mediators. For example, the cytokine IL-6, which is produced by various cells types, including breast fibroblasts [133], and after treatment of rat aortic endothelial cells with ET-1 [134], has been recently demonstrated to stimulate ET-1 production from human breast cancer cell lines [37]. IL-6 has also been reported to induce shape change in ZR-75-1 human breast cancer cells from an epithelial to a fibroblastoid-like morphology, accompanied by a loss in cell–cell interaction and an increase in cell motility [135,136]. Here, again, we are confronted with another hypothetical paracrine loop. The cytokine IL-6 stimulates ET-1 production in human breast cancer cells and, correspongingly, ET-1 induces IL-6 release from endothelial and/or breast fibroblasts. The IL-6 generated may then stimulate cell motility. In addition, IL-6 is also known to increase vascular permeability [137], thereby possibly enhancing the release of angiogenic factors, growth factors, and/or proteolytic enzymes.

A role for ET-1 has also been recently proposed as a regulator of fibroblast-mediated extracellular matrix contraction [138] and myofibroblast contraction during wound healing [139]. Hence, in view of the high proportion of myofibroblasts associated with malignant breast tissue [140] in conjunction with raised tumor ET-1 levels, such a mechanism may also lead to tissue contracture in breast cancer. Various signaling pathways have been identified in human breast cancer cells that upon activation lead to the ET-1 production. Amongst these, the most prominent appear to involve PKC and PKA-mediated responses. A role for the PKA-stimulated pathway in breast epithelial cells appears novel with regard to agonists known to stimulate ET-1 production in various cell types. Whether this finding has any relevence to breast cancer pathophysiology is at present unclear. It remains to be examined if activation of the PKA-mediated pathway similarily increases ET-1 production in normal breast epithelial cells. A novel paracrine loop has also been identified that involves the respective bidirectional exchange of ET-1 from breast cancer cells and PGE_2 from breast fibroblasts. This finding may have important implications if previous reports of elevated PGE_2 levels present in mammary tumors are confirmed, and are positively associated with elevated levels of ET-1 in breast tumors. A considerable amount of work is still required to establish the role(s) of ET-1 in breast pathophysiology. It is hoped that this chapter will alert readers to recent developments in this area and perhaps encourage further work to help eludidate where ET-1 fits into this complex disease of breast cancer.

Acknowledgments

We gratefully acknowledge financial support from the Cancer Research Campaign.

References

1. Bishop JM (1987) The molecular genetics of cancers. *Science* 235:305–311.
2. Marshall CJ (1991) Tumor suppressor genes. *Cell* 64:313–326.
3. Cantly LC, Auger KR, Carpenter C, Duckworth B (1991) *Cell* 64:281–302.
4. Croce CM (1986) Chromosomal translocation and human cancer. *Cancer Res* 46:6019–6023.
5. Trent JM (1985) Cytogenetic and molecular biologic alterations in human breast cancer: A review. *Breast Cancer Res Treat* 5:221–229.
6. Laidlaw IJ, Clarke RB, Howell A, Owen AWMC, Potten CS, Anderson E (1995) The proliferation of normal breast tissue implanted into athymic nude mice is stimulated by estrogen but not progesterone. *Endocrinology* 136:164–171.
7. Dickson RB, Lippman ME (1986) Hormonal control of human cancer cells. *Cancer Surv* 5:617–624.
8. Darbre PD, Daly RJ (1989) Effects of oestrogen on human breast cancer cells in culture. *Proc R Soc Edin* 95B:119–132.
9. Bates SE, Davidson NHE, Valverius EN, Freter CE, Dickson RB, Tam JP, Kudlow JE, Lippman ME, Salomon DS (1988) Expression of transforming growth factor-α and its mRNA in human breast cancer; its regulation by estrogen and its possible functional significance. *Mol Endocrinol* 2:543–555.
10. Bronzert DA, Pantazis P, Antoniades HN, Kasid A, Davidson N, Dickson RB, Lippman ME (1987) Synthesis and secretion of platelet-derived growth factor by human breast cancer cell lines *Proc Natl Acad Sci USA* 84:5763–5767.
11. Sakakura T, Nishizuka Y, Dawe CJ (1976) Mesenchyme-dependent morphogenesis and epithelium-specific cyto-differentiation in mouse mammary gland. *Science* 19:1439–1441.
12. Sakakura T (1991) New aspects of stroma-parenchyma relations in mammary gland differentiation. *Int Rev Cytol* 125:165–202.
13. Mukaida H, Hirabayashi N, Hirai T, Iwata T, Saeki S, Toge T (1991) Significance of freshly cultured fibroblasts from different tissues in promoting cancer cell growth. *Int J Cancer* 48:423–427.
14. Van Roozendaal CEP, van Ooijen B, Klijn JGM, Claasen C, Eggermont AMM, Henzen-Logmans SC, Foekens JA (1992) Stromal influences on breast cancer cell growth. *Br J Cancer* 65:77–81.
15. Horgan K, Jones DL, Mansel RE (1987) Mitogenicity of human fibroblasts in vivo for human breast cancer cells. *Br J Surg* 74:227–229.
16. Ryan MC, Orr DJA, Horgan K (1993) Fibroblast stimulation of breast cancer cell growth in a serum-free system. *Br J Cancer* 67:1268–1273.
17. Clarke R, Dickson RB, Lippman ME (1992) Hormonal aspects of breast cancer: Growth factors, drugs and stromal interactions. *Crit Rev Oncol Hematol* 12:1–23.

18. Yanagisawa M, Kurihara H, Kimura S, Tomobe Y, Kobayashi M, Mitsui Y, Yazaki Y, Goto K, Masaki T (1988) A novel potent vasoconstrictor peptide produced by vascular endothelial cells. *Nature* 332:411–415.
19. Battistini B, Chailer P, D'Orleans-Juste P, Briere N, Sirois P (1993) Growth regulatory properties of endothelins. *Peptides* 14:385–399.
20. Yamashita J-I, Ogawa M, Inada K, Yamashita S-I, Matsuo S, Takano S (1991) A large amount of endothelin-1 is present in human breast cancer tissue. *Res Commun Chem Pathol Pharmacol* 74:363–370.
21. Hickey KA, Rubanyi GM, Paul RJ, Highsmith RF (1985) Characterization of a coronary vasoconstrictor produced by cultured endothelial cells. *Am J Physiol* 248:C550–C556.
22. Inoue A, Yanagisawa M, Kimura S, Kasuya Y, Miyauchi T, Goto K, Masaki T (1989) The human endothelin family: Three structurally and pharmacologically distinct isopeptides predicted by three separate genes. *Proc Natl Acad Sci USA* 86:2863–2867.
23. Kloog Y, Sokolorsky M (1989) Similarities in mode and sites of action of sarafotoxins and endotoxins. *Trends Pharmacol Sci* 10:212–214.
24. Polokoff MA, Rubanyi GM (1994) Endothelins: Molecular biology, biochemistry, pharmacology, physiology and pathphysiology. *Pharmacol Rev* 46:325–415.
25. Firth JD, Ratcliffe PJ (1992) Organ distribution of the three rat endothelin messenger RNAs and the effects of ischemia on renal gene expression. *J Clin Invest* 90:1023–1031.
26. Shiba R, Sakurai T, Yamada G, Morimoto H, Saito A, Masaki T, Goto K (1992) Cloning and expression of rat preproendothelin-3 cDNA. *Biochem Biophys Res Commun* 186:588–594.
27. Ehrenreich H, Anderson RW, Fox CH, Rieckmann P, Hoffman GS, Travis WD, Coligan JE, Kehr LJH, Fauci AS (1990) Endothelins, peptides with potent vasoactive properties, are produced by human macrophages. *J Exp Med* 172:1741–1748.
28. Ehrenreich H, Costa T, Clouse KA, Pluta PM, Ogino Y, Coligan JE, Burd PR (1993) Thrombin is a regulator of astrocytic endothelin-1. *Brain Res* 600:201–207.
29. Giaid A, Gibson SJ, Ibrahim BM, Legon S, Bloom SR, Yanagisawa M, Masaki T, Varndell IM, Polak JM (1989) Endothelin-1, an endothelium derived peptide, is expressed in neurons of the human spinal cord and dorsal root ganglia. *Proc Natl Acad Sci USA* 86:7634–7638.
30. Kubota T, Kamada S, Hirata Y, Eguchi S, Imai T, Marumo F, Aso T (1992) Synthesis and release of endothelin-1 by human decidual cells. *J Clin Endocrinol Metab* 75:1230–1234.
31. Baley PA, Resink TJ, Eppenberger U, Hahn AW (1990) Endothelin messenger RNA and receptors are differentially expressed in cultured human breast cancer epithelial and stromal cells. *J Clin Invest* 875:1320–1323.
32. Kusuhara M, Yamaguchi K, Nagasaki K, Hayashi C, Suzaki A, Hori S, Handa S, Nakamura Y, Abe K (1990) Production of endothelin in human cancer cell lines. *Cancer Res* 50:3257–3261.
33. Shichiri M, Hirata Y, Nakajima T, Ando K, Imai T, Yanagisawa M, Masaki T, Marumo F (1991) Endothelin-1 is an autocrine/paracrine growth factor for human cancer cell lines. *J Clin Invest* 87:1867–1871.
34. Economos K, MacDonald PC, Casey ML (1992) Endothelin-1 gene expression and biosynthesis in human endometrial HCE-1A cancer cells. *Cancer Res* 52:554–557.
35. Tokito F, Susuki N, Hosoya M (1991) Epidermal growth factor (EGF) decreased endothelin 2 (ET-2) production in human renal adenocarcinoma cells. *FEBS Lett* 295:17–22.
36. Schrey MP, Patel KV, Tezapsidis N (1992) Bombesin and glucocorticoids stimulate human breast cancer cells to produce endothelin, a paracrine mitogen for breast stromal cells. *Cancer Res* 52:1786–1790.
37. Yamashita J-I, Ogawa M, Norura K, Matsuo S, Inada K, Yamashita S-I, Nakashima Y, Saishoji T, Takano S, Fujita S (1993) Interleukin 6 stimulates the production of immunoreactive endothelin 1 in human breast cancer cells. *Cancer Res* 53:464–467.
38. Hansen Ree A, Tasken K, Hansson V (1994) Regulation of glucocorticoid receptor (GR) mRNA amd protein levels by phorbol ester in MCF-7 cells. Mechanism of GR mRNA induction and decay. *J Steriod Biochem Mol Biol* 48:23–29.

389

39. Bloch KD, Friedrich SP, Lee M-E, Eddy RL, Shows TB, Quertermous T (1989) Structural organisation and chromosomal assignment of the gene encoding endothelin. *J Biol Chem* 264:10851–10857.
40. Arinimi T, Ishikawa M, Inoue M, Yamagisawa M, Masaki T, Yoshida MC, Hamaguchi H (1991) Chromosomal assignments if the human endothelin family genes: The endothelin-1 gene (EDN1) to 6p23–p24, the endothelin-2 gene (EDN2) to 1p34, and the endothelin-3 gene (EDN-3) to 20q13.2–q13.3. *Am J Hum Genet* 48:990–996.
41. Inoue A, Yanagisawa M, Takuwa Y, Mitsui Y, Kobayashi M, Masaki T (1989) The human preproendothelin 1 gene. Complete nucleotide sequence and regulation of expression. *J Biol Chem* 264:14954–14959.
42. Lee ME, Block KD, Clifford JA, Quertermous T. (1990) Functional analysis of the endothelin-1 gene promoter. Evidence for an endothelial cell specific cis acting sequence. *J Biol Chem* 265:10446–10450.
43. Dorfman DM, Wilson DB, Bruns GA, Orkins SH (1992) Human transcriptional factor GATA 2. Evidence for regulation of preproendothelin 1 gene expression in endothelial cells. *J Biol Chem* 267:1279–1285.
44. Lee ME, Dhadly MS, Temizer DH, Clifford JA, Yoshizumi M, Quertermous T (1991) Regulation of endothelin-1 gene expression by fos and jun. *J Biol Chem* 266:19034–19039.
45. Herschman HR (1991) Primary response genes induced by growth factors and tumor promoters. *Ann Rev Biochem* 60:281–319.
46. Benatti L, Bonecchi L, Cozzi L, Sarmientos P (1993) Two preproendothelin 1 mRNAs transcribed by alternative promoters. *J Clin Invest* 91:1149–1156.
47. Simonson MS, Jones JM, Dunn MJ (1992) Differential regulation of fos and jun gene expression and AP-1 cis-element activity by endothelin isopeptides: Possible implications for mitogenic signaling by endothelin. *J Biol Chem* 267:8643–8649.
48. Hahn AWA, Resink TJ, Scott-Burden T, Powell J, Dohi Y, Buhler FR (1990) Stimulation of endothelin mRNA secretion in rat vascular smooth muscle cells: A novel autocrine function. *Cell Regul* 1:649–659.
49. Sakamoto H, Sasaki S, Nakamura Y, Fushimi K, Marumo F (1992) Regulation of endothelin-1 production in cultured rat mesangial cells. *Kidney Int* 41:350–355.
50. Patel KV, Schrey MP (1990) Activation of inositol phospholipid signalling and Ca^{2+} efflux in human breast cancer cells by bombesin. *Cancer Res* 52:334–340.
51. Yanagisawa M, Inoue A, Takuwa Y, Mitsui Y, Kobayashi M, Masaki T (1989) The human preproendothelin-1 gene: Possible regulation by endothelial phosphoinositide turnover signaling. *J Cardiovasc Pharmacol* 13(Suppl 5):S13–S17.
52. Ming Hu R, Levin ER, Pedram A, Frank HJL (1992) Atrial natriuretic peptide inhibits the production and secretion of endothelin from cultured endothelial cells. *J Biol Chem* 267:17384–17389.
53. Yasutomo Y, Shimada N, Kimura N, Nagata N (1993) Estradiol up-regulates the stimulatory GTP-binding protein expression in MCF-7 human mammary carcinoma cell line. *FEBS Lett* 322:25–29.
54. Imagawa I, Chiu R, Karin M (1987) Transcription factor AP2 mediates induction by two different signal-transduction pathways: Protein kinase C and cAMP. *Cell* 51:251–260.
55. Komuro I, Kurihara H, Sugiyama T, Takuka F, Yazaki Y (1988) Endothelin stimulates c-fos and c-myc expression and proliferation in vascular smooth muscle cells. *FEBS Lett* 238:249 252.
56. Bobik A, Grooms A, Millar JA, Mitchell A, Grinpukel S (1990) Growth factor activity of endothelin on vascular smooth muscle. *Am J Physiol* 258:C408–C415.
57. Vigne P, Marsault R, Breitmayer JP, Frelin C (1990) ET stimulates phosphatidylinositol hydrolysis and DNA synthesis in brain capillary endothelial cells. *Biochem J* 266:415–420.
58. Takagi Y, Fukasa M, Takata S, Yoshimi H, Tokunaga O, Fujita T (1990) Autocrine effect of endothelin on DNA synthesis in human vascular endothelial cells. *Biochem Biophys Res Commun* 168:537–543.
59. Takuwa N, Takuwa Y, Yanagisawa M, Yamashita K, Masaki T (1989) A novel vasoactive

peptide endothelin stimulates mitogenesis through inositol lipid turnover in Swiss 3T3 fibroblasts. *J Biol Chem* 264:7856–7861.

60. Muldoon L, Pribnow D, Rodland KD, Magun BE (1990) Endothelin-1 stimulates DNA synthesis and anchorage-independent growth of Rat-1 fibroblasts through a protein kinase C-dependent mechanism. *Cell Regul* 1:379–390.

61. Simonson MS, Wann S, Mene P, Dubyak GR, Kester M, Nakazato Y, Sedor JR, Dunn MJ (1989) Endothelin stimulates phospholipase C, Na$^+$/H$^+$ exchange, c-fos expression, and mitogenesis in rat mesengial cells. *J Clin Invest* 83:708–712.

62. Yada Y, Higuchi K, Imokawa G (1991) Effects of endothelins on signal transduction and proliferation in human melanocytes. *J Biol Chem* 266:18352–18357.

63. MacCumber MW, Ross CA, Snyder SH (1990) Endothelin in brain: Receptors, mitogenesis, and biosynthesis in glial cells. *Proc Natl Acad Sci USA* 87:2359–2363.

64. Arai H, Hori S, Aramori I, Ohkubo H, Nakarishi S (1990) Cloning and expression of a cDNA encoding an endothelin receptor. *Nature* 348:730–732.

65. Sakurai T, Yanagisawa M, Takuwa Y, Miyazaki H, Kimuras, Goto K, Masaki T (1990) Cloning of a cDNA encoding a non isopeptide selective subtype of the endothelin receptor. *Nature* 348:732–735.

66. Warner TD, Schmidt HHHW, Murad F (1992) Interactions of endothelin and EDRF in bovine native endothelial cells: selective effects of endothelin-3. *Am J Physiol* 262:H1600–H1650.

67. Muldoon LL, Rodland KD, Forsythe ML, Magun BE (1989) Stimulation of phosphatidylinositol hydrolysis, diacylglycerol release, and gene expression in response to endothelin, a potent new agonist for fibroblasts and smooth muscle cells. *J Biol Chem* 264:8529–8536.

68. Resink TJ, Scott-Burden T, Buhler FR (1990) Activation of multiple signal transduction pathways by endothelin in cultured human vascular smooth muscle cells. *Eur J Biochem* 189:415–421.

69. Pachter JA, Mayer-Ezell R, Cleven RM, Fawzi AB (1993) Endothelin (ETA) receptor number and calcium signalling are up-regulated by protein kinase C-β1 overexpression. *Biochem J* 294:153–158.

70. Mattingly RR, Wasilenko WJ, Woodring PJ, Garrison JC (1992) Selective amplification of endothelin-stimulated inositol 1,4,5-trisphosphate and calcium signaling by v-src transformation of rat-1 fibroblasts. *J Biol Chem* 267:7470–7477.

71. Goto K, Kasuya Y, Matsuki N, Takuwa Y, Kurihara H, Ishikawa T, Kimura S, Yanagisawa M, Masaki T (1989) Endothelin activates the dihydropyridine-sensitive, voltage-dependent Ca^{2+} channel in vascular smooth muscle. *Proc Natl Acad Sci USA* 86:3915–3918.

72. Resink TJ, Scott-Burden T, Buhler FR (1989) Activation of phospholipase A2 by endothelin in cultured vascular smooth muscle cells. *Biochem Biophys Res Commun* 158:279–286.

73. Eguchi S, Hirata Y, Imai T, Marumo F (1993) Endothelin receptor subtypes are coupled to adenylate cyclase via different guanyl nucleotide-binding proteins in vasculature. *Endocrinology* 132:524–529.

74. Pribnow D, Muldoon LL, Fajardo M, Theodor L, Chen LY, Magun BE (1992) Endothelin induces transcription of fos/jun family genes: A prominent role for calcium ion. *Mol Endocrinol* 6:1003–1012.

75. Wang Y, Simonson MS, Pouyssegur J, Dunn MJ (1992) Endothelin rapidly stimulates mitogen activated protein kinase activity in rat mesengial cells. *Biochem J* 287:589–594.

76. Ray LB, Sturgill TW (1987) Rapid stimulation by insulin of a serine/threonine kinase in 3T3-L1 adipocytes that phosphorylates microtubule-associated protein 2 in vitro. *Proc Natl Acad Sci USA* 84:1502–1506.

77. Thomas G (1992) MAP kinase by any other name smell just as sweet. *Cell* 68:3–6.

78. Sturgill TW, Ray LB, Erikson E, Maller JL (1988) Insulin-stimulated MAP-2 kinase phosphorylates and activates ribosomal protein S6 kinase II. *Nature* 334:715–718.

79. Anderson NG, Maller JL, Tonks NK, Strurgill TW (1981) Requirement for integration of signals from two distinct phosphorylation pathways for activation of MAP kinase. *Nature* 343:651–653.

80. Pulverer BJ, Kyriakis JM, Avruch J, Nikolakaki E, Woodgrett JR (1991) Phosphorylation of c-jun mediated by MAP kinases. *Nature* 353:670–674.
81. Alvarez NG, Northwood IC, Gonzalez FA (1991) Pro-Leu-Ser/Thr-Pro is a consensus primary sequence for substrate protein phosphorylation. Characterization of the phosphorylation of c-myc and c-jun proteins by an epidermal growth factor receptor threonine 669 protein kinase. *J Biol Chem* 266:15277–15285.
82. Chen-RH, Abate C, Blenis J (1993) Phosphorylation of the c-fos transrepression domain by mitogen-activated protein kinase and 90-kDa ribosomal S6 kinase. *Proc Natl Acad Sci USA* 90:10952–10956.
83. Zachary I, Sinnett-Smith J, Rozengurt E (1992) Bombesin, vasopressin, and endothelin stimulation of tyrosine phosphorylation in Swiss 3T3 cells. Identification of a novel tyrosine kinase as a major substrate. *J Biol Chem* 267:19031–19034.
84. Simonson MS, Herman WH (1993) Protein kinase C and protein tyrosine kinase activity contributes to mitogenic signalling by endothelin-1. *J Biol Chem* 268:9347–9357.
85. Brown KD, Littlewood CL (1989) Endothelin stimulates DNA synthesis in Swiss 3T3 cells. *Biochem J* 263:977–980.
86. Yeh Y-C, Burns ER, Yeh J, Yeh H-W (1991) Synergistic effects of endothelin-1 (ET-1) and transforming growth factor alpha (TGF-α) or epidermal growth factor (EGF) on DNA replication and G1 to S phase transition. *Bioscie Rep* 11:171–180.
87. Cullen KJ, Smith HS, Hill S, Rosen N, Lippman ME (1991) Growth factor mRNA expression by human breast fibroblasts from benign and malignant tissues. *Cancer Res* 51:4978–4985.
88. Cullen KJ, Allison A, Martire I, Ellis M, Singer C (1992) Insulin-like growth factor expression in breast cancer epithelium and stroma. *Breast Cancer Res Treat* 22:21–29.
89. Yamashita J-I, Ogawa M, Egami H, Matsuo S, Kiyohara H, Inada K, Yamashita S-I, Fujita S (1992) Abundant expression of immunoreactive endothelin 1 in mammary phyllodes tumors: Possible role of endothelin 1 in the growth of stromal cells in phyllodes tumor. *Cancer Res* 52:4046–4049.
90. Pietruszka M, Barnes L (1978) Cytosarcoma phyllodes: A clinicopatholoic analysis of 42 cases. *Cancer* 41:1974–1983.
91. Auger M, Hanna W, Kahn HJ (1989) Cytosarcoma phyllodes of the breast and its mimics: An immunohistochemical and ultrastructure study. *Arch Pathol Lab Med* 113:1231–1235.
92. Fant ME, Nanu L, Word RN (1992) A potential role for endothelin-1 in human placenta growth: Interactions with the insulin-like growth factor family of peptides. *J Clin Endocrinol Metab* 74:1158–1163.
93. Paik S (1992) Expression of IGF-1 and IGF-II mRNA in breast tissue. *Breast Cancer Res Treat* 22:31–38.
94. Schrey MP, Patel KV (1995) Prostaglandin E$_2$ production and metabolism in human breast cancer cells and breast fibroblasts. Regulation by inflammatory mediators. *Br J Cancer* 72:1412–1419.
95. Schrey MP, Hare A (1992) Endothelin-1 stimulates phospholipid hydrolysis and prostaglandin F2α production in primary human decidua cell cultures. *Prostaglandins Leukot Essent Fatty Acids* 47:321–325.
96. Barnett RL, Ruffini L, Hart D, Mancuso P, Nord EP (1994) Mechanism of endothelin activation of phospholipase A2 in rat renal medullary interstitial cells. *Am J Physiol* 266:F46–F56.
97. Stanimirovic DB, Bacic F, Uematsu S, Spatz M (1993) Profile of prostaglandins induced by endothelin −1 in human brain capillary endothelium. *Neurochem Int* 23:385–393.
98. Lerner UH, Modeer T (1991) Bradykinin B$_1$ and B$_2$ receptor agonists synergistically potentiate interleukin-1 induced prostaglandin biosynthesis in human gingival fibroblasts. *Inflammation* 15:427–436.
99. Bathon JM, Proud P, Krackow K, Wigley FM (1989) Pre-incubation of human synovial cells with interleukin-1 modulates prostaglandin E$_2$ release in response to bradykinin. *J Immunol* 143:579–586.

100. Karmali RA, Welt S, Thaler HT, Lefevre F (1983) Prostaglandins in breast cancer: Relationship to disease stage and hormone status. *Br J Cancer* 48:689–693.

101. Rolland PH, Martin PM, Jacquemier J, Rolland AM, Toga M (1980) Prostaglandins in human breast cancer: Evidence suggesting that an elevated prostaglandin production is a marker of high metastatic potential for neoplastic cells. *J Natl Cancer Inst* 64:1061–1070.

102. Watson J, Chuah SY (1985) Prostaglandins, steroids and human mammary cancer. *Eur J Cancer Clin Oncol* 2:1051–1055.

103. Tan WC, Privett OS, Goldyne ME (1974) Studies of prostaglandins in rat mammary tumours induced by 7, 12-dimethylbenz(a)anthracene. *Cancer Res* 34:3229–3231.

104. Battistini B, D'Orleans-Juste, Sirois P (1993) Endothelin: Circulating plasma levels and presence in other biolgic fluids. *Lab Invest* 68:600–628.

105. Yokawa K, Tahara H, Kohno M, Murakawa K, Yasunari K, Nakagawa K, Hamada T, Otani S, Yanagisawa M, Takeda T. (1991) Endothelin secreting tumor. *J Cardiovasc Pharm* 17(Suppl 7):S398–S401.

106. Yokawa K, Tahara H, Kohno M, Murakawa K, Yasunari K, Nakagawa K, Hamada T, Otani S, Yanagisawa M, Takeda T (1991) Hypertension associated with endothelin sececreting malignanat hemangioendothelioma. *Ann Intern Med* 114:213–215.

107. Pernow J, Hemsen A, Lundberg JM (1989) Tissue specific distribution, clearance and vascular effects of endothelin in the pig. *Biochem Biophys Res Commun* 161:647–653.

108. De Nucci G, Thomas R, D'Orleans-Juste P, Antunes E, Walder C, Warner TD, Vane JR (1988) Pressor effects of circulating endothelin are limited by its removal in the pulmonary circulation and by the release of prostacyclin and endothelium-derived relaxing factor. *Proc Natl Acad Sci USA* 85:9797–9800.

109. Vijaraghavan J, Scichi AH, Careterio OA, Slaughter C, Moomaw C, Hersch LB (1990) The hydrolysis of endothelins by neutral endopeptidase 24.11 (encephalinase). *J Biol Chem* 265:14150–14155.

110. Sokolovsky M, Galron R, Kloog Y, Bdolah A, Indig FE, Blumberg S, Fleminger G (1990) Endothelins are more sensitive than sarafotoxins to neutral endopeptidase: Possible physiological significance. *Proc Natl Acad Sci USA* 87:4702–4706.

111. Gusterson BA, Monaghan P, Mahendran R, Ellis J, O'Hare MJ (1986) Identification of myoepithelial cells in human and rat breasts by anti-common acute lymphoblastic leukaemia antigen antibody A12. *J Natl Cancer Inst* 77:343–349.

112. Atherton A, Anbazhangan R, Monaghan P, Bartek, Gusterson B (1994) Immunolo calisation of cell surface peptidases in the developing human breast. *Differentiation* 56:101–106.

113. Kenny AJ, O'Hare MJ, Gusterson B (1989) Cell surface peptidases as modulators of growth and differentiation. *Lancet* 2:785–787.

114. Inagaki H, Bishop AE, Eimoto T, Polack JM (1992) Autoradiographic localization of endothelin-1 binding sites in human colonic cancer tissue. *J Pathol* 168:263–267.

115. Dilelli AG, Ohlstein E, Elshourbagy N, Bhatngar PK, Nambi P, Dewolf WE, Caltabiano MM (1991) Expression of human preproendothelin-1 cDNA in COS cells results in the production of mature vasoactive endothelin-1. *Biochem Biophys Res Commun* 175:697–705.

116. Benatti L, Cozzi L, Zamai M, Tamburin M, Vaghi F, Caiolfa VR, Fabbrini MS, Sarmiento SP (1992) Human preproendothelin-1 is converted into the active endothelin-1 by baculovirus-infected insect cells. *Biochem Biophys Res Commun* 186:753–759.

117. Sawamura T, Kimura T, Shinmi O, Sugita Y, Yanagisawa M, Goto K, Masaki T (1990) Purification and characterization of putative endothelin converting enzyme in bovine adrenal medulla: Evidence for a cathepsin D-like enzyme. *Biochem Biophys Res Commun* 168:1230–1236.

118. Lees WE, Kalinka S, Meech J, Capper SJ, Cook ND, Kay J (1990) Generation of human endothelin by cathepsin E. *FEBS Lett* 273:99–102.

119. Takada J, Okada K, Ikenaga T, Matsuyama K, Yano M (1991) Phosphoramidon-sensitive endothelin-converting enzyme in the cytosol of cultured bovine endothelial cells. *Biochem Biophys Res Commun* 176:860–865.

120. Matsumara Y, Ikeyawa R, Tskahara Y, Takoaka M, Morimoto S (1991) Conversion of big endothelin-1 to endothelin-1 by two types of metalloproteinases of cultured porcine vascular smooth muscle cells. *Biochem Biophys Res Commun* 178:899–905.

121. Ohnaya K, Takayanagi R, Nishikawa M, Haji M, Nawata H (1993) Purification and characterization of a phosphoramidon-sensitive endothelin-converting enzyme in porcine aortic endothelium. *J Biol Chem* 268:26759–26766.

122. Shimida K, Takahashi M, Tanzawa (1994) Cloning and functional expression of endothelin-converting enzyme from rat endothelial cells. *J Biol Chem* 269:18275–18278.

123. Takahashi M, Matsumoto H, Kitada S, IIjima Y, Tazawa K (1993) Purification and characterisation of endothelin-converting enzyme from rat lung. *J Biol Chem* 268:21394–21398.

124. Patel KV, Schrey MP (1995) Human breast cancer cells contain a phosphoramidon-sensitive metalloproteinase which can process big endothelin-1 to endothelin-1: A proposed mitogen for human breast fibroblasts. *Br J Cancer* 71:442–447.

125. Kurihara Y, Kurihara H, Suzuki H, Kodama T, Maemura K, Nagi R, Oda H, Kuwaki T, Cao W-H, Kamada N, Jishage K, Ouchi Y, Azuma S, Toyoda Y, Ishikawa T, Kumada M, Yazaki Y (1994) Elevated blood pressureand craniofacial abnormalities in mice deficent in endothelin-1. *Nature* 368:703–710.

126. Shing Y, Folkman J, Haudenschild C, Lund D, Crum D, Klagsburn M (1985) Angiogenesis is stimulated by a tumor-derived endothelial cell growth factor. *J Cell Biol* 29:275–287.

127. Pepper MS, Belin D, Montesano R, Orci L, Vassalli J-D (1990) Transforming growth factor-beta 1 modulates basic fibroblast growth factor-induced proteolytic and angiogenic properties of endothelial cells in vitro. *J Cell Biol* 111:743–755.

128. Beauchamp RD, Coffey RJ, Lyons RM, Perkett EA, Townserd CM, Moses HL (1991) Human carcinoid cell production of paracrine growth factors that can stimulate fibroblast and endothelial cell growth. *Cancer Res* 51:5253–5260.

129. Klagsburn M, D'Amore PA (1991) Regulators of angiogenesis. *Ann Rev Physiol* 53:217–239.

130. Liotta LA, Steeg PS, Stetler-Stevenson G (1991) Cancer metastasis and angiogenesis: An imbalance of positive and negative regulation. *Cell* 64:3279–336.

131. Pruis J, Emeis JJ (1990) Endothelin-1 and endothelin-3 induce the release of tissue-type plasminogen-activator and von Willebrand factor from endothelial cells. *Eur J Pharmacol* 187:105–112.

132. Hanggono Achmad T, Govind RS (1992) Chemotaxis of human blood monocytes towards endothelin-1 and the influence of calcium channel blockers. *Biochem Biophys Res Commun* 189:994–1000.

133. Adams EF, Rafferty B, White MC (1991) Interleukin 6 is secreted by breast fibroblasts and stimulates 17β-oestradiol oxidoreductase activity of MCF-7 cells: Possible paracrine regulation of breast 17β-oestradiol levels. *Int J Cancer* 49:118–121.

134. Xin X, Cai Y, Matsumoto K, Agui T (1995) Endothelin-induced interleukin-6 production by rat aortic endothelial cells. *Endocrinology* 136:132–137.

135. Tamm I, Cardinale I, Krueger J, Murphy JS, May LT, Sehgal PB (1989) Interleukin 6 decreases cell-cell association and increased motility of ductal breast carcinoma cells. *J Exp Med* 170:1649–1669.

136. Tamm I, Cardinale I, Murphy JS (1991) Decreased adherence of interleukin 6-treated breast carcinoma cells can lead to seperation from neighbors after mitosis. *Proc Natl Acad Sci USA* 88:4414–4418.

137. Maruo N, Morita I, Shirao M, Murota S-I (1992) IL-6 increases endothelial permeability in vitro. *Endocrinology* 131:710–714.

138. Guidry C (1992) Extracellular matrix contraction by fibroblasts: Peptide promoters and second messengers. *Cancer Metast Rev* 11:45–54.

139. Thiemermann C, Corder R (1992) Is endothelin-1 the regulator of myofibroblast contraction during wound healing? *Lab Invest* 67:677–679.

140. Ronnov-Jessen L, Van-Deurs B, Nielsen M, Petersen OW (1992) Identification, paracrine generation, and possible function of human breast carcinoma myofibroblasts in culture. *In Vitro Cell Dev Biol* 28A:273–283.

19. Breast cancer immunology

Wei-Zen Wei and Gloria H. Heppner

Introduction

Breast cancer is a multifactorial, clinically, and, quite probably, etiologically heterogeneous disease that manifests itself only after a long and largely obscure latency period. Breast cancer is also a systemic disease, responding to and causing changes in the host well beyond the sites of cancer growth per se. Given these complexities, it is not surprising that, despite the efforts of numerous investigators, the field of breast cancer immunology has yet to have a major impact on either the understanding or control of the disease. Perhaps this lamentable situation results, at least in part, from the majority of research in breast cancer immunology being directed toward investigations of what — in terms of natural history — are actually the *later* stages of the disease, that is, the 'earliest' evidence of clinical cancer. Perhaps by this time, the momentum of the neoplastic process has reached a stage where it blunts the finely regulated inflammatory and immune systems to the extent that whatever immune growth-regulatory influences have been operative during preclinical cancer development are swamped by the combined effects of the disease and its treatment. The purposes of this review are to summarize the current state of knowledge about breast cancer immunology and to present our perspective on the most promising areas of future research. We have not attempted to be all inclusive in the literature reviewed and apologize to any colleagues whose work is slighted.

General immune status of breast cancer patients

In preparing the present review, the senior author (GHH) stepped back in time and reread a review she had written on the same topic in 1976 [1]. It was both personally and professionally distressing to realize how small has been the advance in *solid* and *useful* knowledge over the past 20 years. Then, as now, there was the general impression that lymphocytic infiltration of the primary tumor is usually a favorable sign [2–4], as is draining node 'sinus histiocytosis' and follicular hyperplasia [5–8]. These observations suggest a

R. Dickson and M. Lippman (eds.) MAMMARY TUMOR CELL CYCLE, DIFFERENTIATION AND METASTASIS. 1996. Kluwer Academic Publishers. ISBN 0-7923-3905-3. All rights reserved.

possible protective effort of the immune response against breast cancer. However, it is evident that in cancer patients such an immune response must be failing. According, in 1976 a great deal of effort was being expended on assessment of the overall immune competence of breast cancer patients, with the general consensus that, except in advanced cases, breast cancer patient values were most often within the normal range (which is quite broad and variable) for assays of T-cell competence (peripheral lymphocyte counts, skin testing, in vitro blastogenesis assays, etc.) [9–12], and that B-cell competence was essentially normal [1]. Furthermore, in those patients whose T immunity values did fall below the normal range, there was no evidence of an association with generally accepted clinicopathological correlates of prognosis, nor, except for terminal patients, of clinical outcome.

Essentially similar results were reported in a 1993 paper by Head and associates [13], who performed T and B blastogenesis assays on peripheral lymphocytes from a series of 142 breast cancer patients before surgery and 2–4 weeks after chemotherapy. Lymphocytes from 58% of the patients, preoperatively, were judged to have deficient reactivity to phytohemagglutin, a general T-cell mitogen, a frequency that was statistically different from normal donor lymphocytes. However, this deficiency was defined as being at the 25th percentile or below of the values for normal donors, so there was extensive overlap between the two groups. Using the same criterion there was no difference in reactivity to the B-cell mitogen, pokeweed. Among the cancer patients, there were no relationships betwexen low PHA reactivity and age, tumor size, local invasion, or metastasis, although there was a weak, statistical association with nodal status. Following chemotherapy, some patients exhibited a rebound in these general measures of immune competence. Thus, it appears that the immune status of breast cancer patients is not grossly abnormal, at least for the greater part of the disease course.

Breast tumor–infiltrating lymphocytes

Skin test and blastogenesis assays of peripheral lymphocytes reveal only the most global picture of immune competence and say little of the status of immunity at the sites of neoplastic growth. Numerous investigators have approached this problem by isolating lymphocytes from primary breast cancers and testing their functionality in a variety of in vitro assays. Vose and Moore [14] reported that tumor infiltrating lymphocytes (TIL) from seven breast cancers were predominantly T cells but that these cells were not only functionally deficient, they were also able to suppress the reactivity of peripheral lymphocytes in blastogenesis or cytotoxicity assays. Similarly, Eremin and coworkers [15] reported little natural killer (NK) activity in breast TIL, but significant NK suppression when TIL were added to peripheral lymphocyte assays.

More recently, the same overall conclusions were presented by Whiteside and associates [16] as a result of their detailed analysis of the clonal proliferation potential of TIL isolated from 10 breast cancer patients. As in the previous studies, T cells were found to predominate, with CD8 cells being more frequent than CD4. Few T cells appeared to be activated (i.e., expressing HLA-DR antigens or IL-2 receptor) and, compared with peripheral lymphocytes, blastogenesis in response to PHA stimulation was depressed. Whiteside and associates took the analysis a step further by expanding and analyzing 170 TIL clones isolated after PHA exposure. In contrast to the starting population, most of the clones were CD4+, and over half of these were cytolytic in a lectin-dependent assay for murine P815 cells. Only a few clones were cytolytic for MCF-7 (allogeneic breast cancer) or for K562 cells (NK activity). About half of the tested clones produced IL-2. These promising results indicate that breast TIL may include potentially cytolytic cells, but it appears that the unmodified tumor environment is not conducive to the expression of effective immunity.

Special considerations in breast cancer immunology: An editorial comment

Although this chapter is a review, not an editorial, we feel compelled to present some commentary on the basic facts about breast cancer:
1. Breast cancer occurs in the breast; that is, in a complex organ that contains a number of different cell types arranged in organized structures.
2. Breast cancer undergoes phenotypic progression over the course of time, and its biological behavior (including its relationship to the inflammatory/ immune systems) might be expected to be highly dependent on the stage of progression.
3. Breast cancer, like normal breast, is a tissue with interacting cellular components and with major responsiveness to the endocrine system, as well as to peptide growth factors.
4. The systems that influence the breast and breast cancer development, including the endocrine and perhaps the immune system, are themselves interdependent networks that often use the same signals to communicate [17].
5. It is perilous to view breast cancer as some sort of generic CANCER, without paying attention to the biological and physiological characteristics of the site.

The breast is a complex organ — mostly fat and connective tissue stroma with a minor epithelial compartment, except during lactation [18]. It is an organ that has been physiologically 'engineered' for proliferative extremes, with the capacity to undergo extensive and prolonged hyperplasia, followed by the re-establishment of an almost quiescent state. The cellularity and cellular composition of the breast change both with age and parity. As part of its normal function during lactation, the breast plays an immunological role, being the source of immunoglobulins, and possibly T-cell immunity, that are transmitted from mother to infant, and therefore lymphocytes must be capable of functioning within the normal breast environment [19]. It is against this backdrop of normal physical and physiological change that breast cancer develops and, also, that the influences of the immune response are played out.

The origins of breast cancer are still somewhat obscure, but they appear to involve a continuum of hyperplastic, 'high-risk' alterations, collectively referred to as *proliferative breast disease* and associated neoplastic phenotypes, *carcinoma-in-situ* [20]. These various microscopic evidences of proliferation/differentiation abnormalities may coexist, along with normal breast epithelium, for long periods of time, during which the influence, if any, of the inflammatory/immune system is unknown. Although it may be logistically impossible to study the natural evolution of the relationship of the immune system to preclinical breast cancer, it is hazardous to try to guess at that natural history from the assessment of immune competence, general or specific, in clinical breast cancer patients. As an approach to resolving this dilemma, we suggest that it is possible to come to understand the most relevant biological principles by investigations in focused animal models and defined human populations, for example, women who bear the epidemiological or genetic stigmata of being at high risk for breast cancer development. It may be no accident that the most persuasive indication of the existence of effective immunity to breast cancer remains the early work of Black and Leis [21], who used an in vivo, skin-window technique to detect inflammatory responses to cryostat sections of patients' own tumors. They found positive reactivity in 82% of patients whose disease was limited to precancerous lesions or in situ carcinoma, as contrasted to 47% of patients with node-negative, invasive cancer and 20% of node-positive patients. Their observations do not allow judgments about either the specificity of the response or the causal relationship between response and disease status, but they do call attention to the importance of evaluating breast tumor immunity in the context of early disease progression.

Immunology of breast cancer progression

The published literature on the immunology of breast cancer development, since the work of Black and Leis, is, however, discouraging, both in terms of scope and of results. Many investigators, including ourselves, have employed syngeneic, transplantable mouse mammary tumor models to demonstrate that such cancers *may*, but often do not, induce cell-mediated immunity, as detected either by in vitro assays or by transplantation immunity. However, since the work of Weiss and associates [22] in the 1960s, few investigators have studied the immune reactions to autochthonous mammary tumors, that is, to untransplanted tumors, in their original host. It is instructive to recall the

398

overall results of Weiss's work: About one third of the cancers he investigated produced no detectable response in the host of origin, whereas about one third grew less well and another one third grew better when transplanted into naive, syngeneic mice. Although Weiss' studies were logistically difficult and statistically problematic, it is clear that, even in an inbred strain of mice, the immunological relationship between mammary cancers and their own hosts is heterogeneous and not necessarily protective.

We have utilized another mouse mammary tumor model to attempt to understand the role of the immune response in the development of breast cancer. The model we chose is the preneoplastic C4 hyperplastic alveolar nodule (HAN) line developed by Medina [23]. In this model the C4 HAN line is transplanted into 'cleared' (epithelium-free) mammary fat pads of syngeneic, strain BALB/c mice. The HAN implants grow out to fill the pads, and eventually, after periods of many months, focal tumors arise within the HAN tissue. Thus, in this model, tumor development is spontaneous and within the mammary site, although it occurs in transplanted HAN tissue. There are a number of different HAN models available; we chose the C4 line because C4 tumors tend to be immunogenic in transplantation tests, suggesting that the immune response is engaged in this system. The system is an imperfect model of the human disease, however, in that the preneoplastic lesion is alveolar, rather than ductal, and the HAN implant produces a rather uniform outgrowth, not the discrete, multilesional–normal epithelial mixture seen in human breasts.

Our experiments have been directed to investigating the role of the immune response during HAN $\rightarrow$ tumor progression. The results can be stated briefly: There is no evidence for a protective immune response during this transition. If anything, the host response appears to stimulate the development of the cancers. We believe that the mechanism of the enhancement involves the NK cell. Activated NK cells are present in enhanced numbers (as compared with normal mammary epithelium) [24]; suppression of NK activity is accompanied by lengthening of the latency period and a reduction in the frequency of tumor formation, whereas NK stimulation correlates with shortening of the latency and increased tumor formation [25].

Initially, these results were unexpected and disconcerting. As stated earlier, NK activity has been reported to be low in human breast cancers, and breast cell infiltrates have been found to be capable of suppressing NK activity [15]. However, we have found that although the numbers of NK cells remain elevated in C4 tumors, their activity is depressed, probably due to the presence of suppressor cells. Perhaps of more relevance to our work is a 1984 paper by Pross and coworkers [26], who found that a subset of women, characterized as being of high risk for developing breast cancer due to a mammographic pattern defined as *benign breast syndrome*, had a history of abnormally high peripheral NK activity. Pross and associates speculated that prolactin, reported to be at high levels in patients with proliferative breast disease [27,28], might contribute to NK stimulation. Indeed, recent work from our laboratory has shown that inhibition of pituitary prolactin production by bromocriptine simultaneously decreases both C4 HAN → tumor progression and HAN-infiltrating NK activity [29] and that prolactin may stimulate NK activity in vitro [30]. Taken together, these results suggest a possible influence at the level of the interface of the immune and endocrine systems during the early progression of breast cancer. A very recent report [31] suggests that tamoxifen might have inhibitory effects on NK activity in breast cancer patients treated with postsurgical telecobalt radiotherapy, although correlations with clinical outcome were not presented. The idea that NK activity may be a stimulatory factor in mammary tumor growth is supported by results in another animal model, the androgen-responsive Shionogi's mouse mammary tumor, in which Rowse and associates [32] have demonstrated a positive correlation between tumor size and NK activity as a function of stress variation due to the number of mice housed per cage.

'Immune stimulation' of breast cancer

The association of increased NK activity with increased risk of developing breast cancer or increased breast cancer growth brings to mind the issue of the 'immune stimulation' of cancer, as proposed by Prehn and Lappe [33] 25 years ago. In a 1994 perspective [34], Prehn has returned to this theme and makes several points of significance to the present review. He emphasizes that the behavior of autochthonous tumors may be very different than that of the transplanted tumors upon which so many of our ideas about tumor immunology are based. He presents data showing that 'weak' immune responses might result in tumor enhancement, but he points out that this is actually 'good news' in that even a weak response may offer the possibility of eventual success in the immunoprevention or immunotherapy of cancer.

That the inflammatory/immune system may be growth enhancing in at least some subsets of breast cancer patients has been reviewed recently by Stewart and Tsai [35]. These authors stress the importance of the specific clinicopathological characteristics of the patient groups in regard to whether a lymphocytic infiltration carries a favorable prognosis (see earlier) or whether it has negative implications. They also review clinical studies in which immunosuppression by chemotherapy or stimulation by Bacille, Calmette, Guerin (BCG) 'paradoxically' had a good or deleterious effect, respectively, on treatment outcome. They further point out, as has been also done by others [36–38], that lymphocytes (T cells, NK cells, etc.) are sources of a variety of cytokines, lymphokines, and peptide hormones, (including prolactin-like molecules [39]) for which cells, including normal, preneoplastic and cancerous breast epithelial cells, may have receptors and to which these cells may respond by proliferation. For example, TNF-α, a cytokine produced by T cells and NK cells, is a positive growth factor for mammary epithelial cells in the rat

400

[40]. Theoretically, it would seem to make little difference whether a lymphocytic tumor infiltrate was present due to a 'nonspecific' inflammatory stimulus or in response to a 'specific' tumor antigen; the potential for the production of growth-enhancing cytokines might be the same. However, to echo Prehn [34], the fact that breast cancer cells react *at all* to the influx of inflammatory cells presents the possibility that the reaction can form the basis for therapeutic intervention. Again, theoretically it would seem that a specific immune stimulus, that is, a tumor antigen, would offer the best opportunity, in terms of optimal control and targeting, with the least toxicity, for development of effective interventions.

Breast cancer associated antigens

Significant effort has been devoted to the identification of breast cancer associated antigens. Monoclonal antibodies (mAb) with varying degree of specificity for breast cancer cells have been produced in a number of laboratories [41,42]. These mAbs, some of which recognize carcinoembryonic antigen (CEA), hormone receptor, transferrin receptor, or growth factor receptors, may be useful in the analysis of disease progression. However, the most pervasive finding is the demonstration of breast cancer associated immunogenic epitopes on high molecular weight glycoproteins that have the properties of mucins. At least 70 mAbs have been shown to interact with either mucin peptide or associated carbohydrates [43].

Mucins are normal components of glandular epithelial cells and secretory products of these cells. They are glycoproteins with repetitive peptide segments of 20 amino acids and numerous glycans that are predominantly O-linked to the abundant Ser or Thr residues [43–45]. In breast epithelial cells, the mucin encoded by the MUC1 gene is a transmembrane protein with a large extracellular domain and a cytoplasmic domain of 69 amino acids. The rigid extracellular structure protrudes from the membrane and can reach several hundred nanometers above the cell surface, greatly exceeding the height of other membrane-associated proteins, including the major histocompatibility complex (MHC). On normal glandular cells, the distribution of mucin is polarized toward the apical surface, which may provide protection from the extracellular environment to the underlying epithelial cells. In transformed cells, the polarity is often lost and the level of expression is increased. Altered architecture and prolific expression in malignant tissue lead to greatly elevated levels of mucin in the circulation and may contribute to anti-mucin humoral immune reactivity in cancer patients [43]. Mucin-reactive mAbs recognize either carbohydrate moieties or protein backbones. Of particular interest are mAbs that interact with all, or part, of the peptide epitope PDTRP, which corresponds to the tandem repeat domain of the MUC1 mucin product. Exposure of this epitope appears to be the result of aberrant glycosylation of mucin on cancer cells and mAb SM-3, which recognizes this epitope, and identifies breast cancer cells with a high level specificity [46].

Cytolytic T lymphocytes induced by the MUC1 epitope

A real surprise was the observation that cytolytic T lymphocytes (CTL) induced with either allogeneic or autologous breast cancer cells recognize the MUC1 peptide epitope in an MHC unrestricted fashion [47–49]. T cell immunogenicity of MUC1 protein was indicated by the ability to induce anti–breast cancer CTL with soluble mucin or MUC1 transfected B cells as well as the blockage of such CTL activity by mAb SM-3. The anti–breast CTL express CD3 and α/β T-cell receptors (TCR). In general, α/β TCR recognize antigenic peptides bound to a cleft formed by the extracellular domains of the MHC heterodimers [50]: CD8+ T cells recognize peptides in class I MHC [51] and CD4+ T cells recognize peptides in class II MHC [52], a result of binding between the MHC I constant region with CD8 and that of the MHC II with CD4 [53–56]. Peptides associated with class I MHC are of 8–10 amino acids, synthesized endogenously, degraded in the cytosol, and transported into the endoplasmic reticulum. Most solid tumor associated antigens fall into this category. The MHC independence of antimucin CTL was, therefore, unexpected. It was suggested to be the result of simultaneous engagement of multiple T-cell receptors by multiple identical epitopes on the mucin molecule, thus bypassing the need for MHC stabilization [47]. The MHC independence of MUC1 reactive CTL presents a significant advantage for attempts to induce anti–breast cancer T-cell reactivity. The same MUC1 molecule could be used to activate CTL in patients from any HLA background, thereby being an ideal vaccine candidate. A possible drawback, however, is that the binding of MUC1 epitope with TCR without accessary molecules may be weak and may induce incomplete signal transduction. Whether the immunogenicity of the MUC1 epitope can be potentiated needs further investigation.

There is another, and potentially more serious, down side to the massive presence of immunogenic mucin. The rigid structure of mucin may hinder the interaction of T cells with MHC associated antigenic peptides lying at the foot of the mucin. Expression of mucin by gene transfection in fibroblasts and melanoma cells has been shown to result in reduced adhesion and sensitivity to allogenic CTLs [45,58], indicating reduced recognition of MHC. The masking effect of mucin may contribute to the poor record, to date, in generating breast cancer reactive MHC restricted CTL. However, newer techniques now offer opportunities to reveal previously obscure, potentially immunogenic peptides.

Breast cancer associated, MHC restricted peptide antigens

Even with the difficulty of generating breast cancer–specific CTL, several breast cancer associated antigenic molecules and their MHC I restricted peptides have been characterized and the list is growing. This good fortune is due to the identification of antigenic peptides in other tumor systems. Identification of MHC restricted peptides from known immunogenic molecules has been accelerated with knowledge of peptide binding motifs. The peptides presented by individual MHC I molecules have unique amino acid motifs, defined primarily by the terminal amino acid residues that anchor the peptides to the particular presenting MHC. The center groups of the peptides protrude to interact with T-cell receptors [58]. The antigenic peptides of each cell are, therefore, determined by its MHC and can only be recognized by T cells of the same MHC type. Peptide motifs of several human and mouse MHC I have been determined by eluting and sequencing peptides from specific MHC I [59] and by testing the binding and immunogenicity of synthetic peptides corresponding to the eluted peptides. The establishment of the basic rules of MHC-peptide interaction opened the gate to the unequivocal identification of tumor associated T cell epitopes. Therefore, tumor peptides have been determined by testing the MHC binding and the immunogenicity of peptides predicted from the candidate protein sequences and the established MHC I binding motifs [60–64].

Several human tumor-associated antigens and their MHC restricted peptides have been determined [60,65]. Most notable are antigens found on melanoma cells, including MAGE 1, MAGE3 [66,67], and BAGE1. It has been possible to generate autologous, MHC restricted CTL from melanoma patients. These CTL lines are effective probes in the identification and cloning of melanoma antigens. MAGE and BAGE genes identified by cDNA cloning appear to be silent in normal tissues except in testis. CTL specific for MAGE or BAGE peptides recognize approximately 10% of breast cancer specimens, indicating the presence of the same or similar peptide epitopes on breast cancer cells. The function of these gene products is not yet clear. A possible physiological role of MAGE was suggested by its reported expression during would healing [68].

An alternative approach to identify tumor associated antigenic peptides is to induce primary CTL in vitro with synthetic peptides predicted from the protein sequences of potentially antigenic molecules. Oncogene products, which are often expressed at elevated level in cancer cells, are candidate molecules. At least two HLA-A2.1 restricted ERBB-2 peptides have been defined, and anti–ERBB-2 CTL have been shown to lyse breast, ovarian, and small cell lung carcinoma cells that overexpress ERBB-2 [69,70]. Since peptide reactive CTL recognize and lyse breast cancer cells, the expression of MHC restricted antigens on breast cancer cells is beyond question.

Human model systems for studying breast cancer immunology

For the purpose of vaccine development and for the analysis of host immune reactivity during the course of disease, it will be of clear advantage to establish a panel of breast cancer associated antigenic peptides. It will be prudent to identify these molecules directly from breast cancer cells rather than indirectly from other tumor types. Although difficulty in generating MHC restricted

403

breast cancer specific CTL remains, it should be feasible to identify candidate antigenic molecules that are new or overexpressed proteins in breast cancer cells and to define the antigenic peptides in these molecules. The first task is to identify candidate antigens that are present on both preneoplastic and neoplastic breast epithelial cells, and to determine their immunogenic peptides. Short of a large-scale population study, the most direct approach is to compare the gene products of a normal breast epithelial cell line with its transformed preneoplastic or neoplastic derivatives. A breast cancer progression model system, MCF-10, which has been developed at the Michigan Cancer Foundation, is an ideal system for such direct comparisons [71–75]. The human breast epithelial cell line MCF-10M (mortal) was established from the breast tissue of a patient with mild hyperplasia. MCF-10M cells undergo senescence after about 20 passages in culture; however, spontaneous immortalizations have occurred on several occasions.

Two immortalized lines, MCF-10A and MCF-10F, have been used to develop models of preneoplasia and carcinoma. MCF-10A was transfected with the T24 HRAS oncogene to yield MCF-10AneoT cells, which form persistent, small flat nodules in immunodeficient nu/nu beige mice. Histologically, these nodules contain simple or complex ducts. About 30% of the nodules eventually develop into carcinomas. One of the carcinomas was cultured and the cells (TG1) were again injected into nu/nu beige mice. The process of in vivo growth and in vitro culture was repeated and cell lines TG2, TG3, etc., were established. The TG lines differ from the parent MCF-10AneoT cells in forming hyperplastic lesions, including atypical hyperplasia, which resemble proliferative breast disease in women at high risk of developing breast cancer [71]. As in women, the complete spectrum of normal, hyperplastic, carcinoma in situ (CIS), and cancerous growth can be found within a single specimen. With each successive transplant generation, there is an increased the percent of hyperplastic lesions as well as CIS or invasive carcinoma. The MCF-10A derived TG lines, therefore, comprise a transplantable xenograft model of slowly progressing premalignant lesions, with a 30% chance of developing into carcinoma. The model is unique in that it recapitulates the histological picture of early breast cancer progression.

The immortalized MCF-10F line was exposed to 0.2 µg/ml benzo[a]pyrene for 24 hours and a clone, BP1, was established. BP1 has a reduced doubling time in culture and an increased colony size in soft agar compared with MCF-10F, but does not form tumors in immune deficient mice. BP1 cells were transfected with the T24 HRAS oncogene and a BP1-Tras subclone was established. When injected into mammary fatpads, BP1-Tras cells form palpable tumors within 10–15 weeks. Therefore, BP1-Tras cells demonstrate direct tumor growth, in contrast to MCF-10AneoT and the TG lines, which exhibit a preneoplastic phenotype prior to the development of carcinoma. Together, cells from the MCF-10 series provide the biological tools with which to define antigens associated with neoplastic progression of the breast.

404

Development of breast cancer vaccines

Since products from ERBB-2, MAGE, and BAGE have been shown to generate antigenic peptides in breast cancer cells, it should be possible to identify additional breast cancer antigens and peptides from new or overexpressed gene products. It is also realistic to expect the development of breast cancer vaccines with these antigenic peptides. With the available MCF-10 cell series, this exciting prospect can be explored. Various strategies may be used to identify genes that are overexpressed in preneoplastic lesions, as well as in breast cancers. For example, mRNA differential display, which allows direct comparison of mRNA species from normal and transformed cells [76,77], may be useful for this purpose.

Differential display followed by sequence comparison with data in Genbank has been informative in analyzing molecular responses to exogenous agents and molecular alterations during tumorigenesis. Metalloproteinase was detected in preneoplastic, but not neoplastic, mouse epidermal JB6 cells [78]. A novel gene product TM2H-8 was identified in highly tumorous preneoplastic mouse mammary epithelial cell lines but not the poorly tumorigenic variant nor pregnant mouse mammary gland [79]. Identification of transformation associated mRNA in heterogenous cancer specimens or cell lines of different genetic origin is problematic because of their intrinsic differences, for example, HLA polymorphisms, which are independent of transformation events. Most human breast cell lines are derived from advanced disease, and their normal cell origin is not available for comparison. The MCF-10 cell line series allows direct comparison of breast cancer cells with their parental 'normal' cells and the potential for identifying tumor associated antigens. Our laboratory is currently utilizing differential display technology to identify potential candidates for vaccine development.

Mouse mammary tumor progression as a model for testing breast cancer vaccines

Active immunization of high risk asymptomatic women may provide long-term protection. However, before this can be attempted, it is necessary to develop a detailed understanding of the optimal form of peptide vaccines, as well as the efficacy, limitations, and possible toxicity. As described earlier, mouse mammary tumor progression is an excellent model for testing tumor vaccine because there are distinct, transplantable preneoplastic lesions, HAN, that precede the tumors [80]. The efficacy of peptide vaccination in preventing spontaneous tumorigenesis from preneoplasia is readily measurable in mice bearing preneoplastic lesions.

The well-characterized mouse mammary tumor virus (MMTV) associated antigens are realistic model tumor antigens. Endogenous MMTV related sequences (*Mtv*) are present in the germline DNA of most inbred strains of mice and wild mice [81]. MMTV and endogenous *Mtv* genomes are highly homologous (90–95%) [82,83]. RNA and protein products from endogenous *Mtv* are expressed in proliferating mammary epithelial cells and activated lymphocytes [84,85]. In the preneoplastic and neoplastic mammary epithelial cells, MMTV mRNA and protein products are elevated. MMTV peptides, therefore, represent overexpressed self-antigens, which can serve as tumor antigens. Based on peptide motif prediction, Wei et al. identified mouse mammary tumor associated MMTV antigenic epitopes [86]. With this murine model system, it is now possible to address critical questions regarding in vivo peptide specific T-cell reactivity during mammary tumor progression.

Future directions

At the outset of this review, we discussed the present state of knowledge and stressed the general lack of meaningful progress to date in the field of breast cancer immunology. We believe, however, that this pessimistic view is rapidly becoming history. Although the role of the immune response in the natural history of breast cancer may, if anything, be facilitatory in nature, it would appear that the host's immune/inflammatory system does recognize and respond to breast cancer development. Can this response be turned to a therapeutic, perhaps even preventative, advantage? Recent technological advances have given us both the understanding and tools to make the attempt. We know a great deal about how antigenic epitopes are processed and recognized by T cells, and we are now able to turn this knowledge around and use the mechanism of T-cell recognition to identify candidate antigens. We also have new techniques to pinpoint molecular differences among normal, preneoplastic, and cancerous breast cells, differences that also offer candidate targets for immunological attack. We have a better understanding of the progression of human breast cancer, and we have experimental models that mimic the process in fine detail. Finally, we have workable animal models with which we can test the feasibility of immunoprevention strategies. Surely, some future author writing 20 years hence will be able to present a very different, and much more heartening, picture of breast cancer immunology than is possible today. The future has never looked better.

Acknowledgments

We wish to acknowledge the generous support of Concern and Concern II Foundation, and NIH grants CA 61217 and CA 57831.

References

1. Heppner GH (1976) Immunology: breast cancer. *Recent Results Cancer Res* 57:95–108.

2. Berg JW (1959) Inflammation and prognosis in breast cancer. A search for host resistance. *Cancer* 12:714–730.
3. Lane N, Goksel H, Salerno RA, Haagensen CD (1961) Clinico-pathologic analysis of the surgical curability of breast cancers: A minimum ten-year study of a personal series. *Ann Surg* 153:483–498.
4. Black MM (1972) Cellular and biologic manifestations of immunogenicity in precancerous mastopathy. *Natl Canc Inst Monogr* 35:73–82.
5. Dipaola M, Angelini L, Bertoletti A, Colizza S (1974) Host resistance in relation to survival in breast cancer. *Br Med J* 4:268–270.
6. Hunter RL, Ferguson DJ, Coppleson LW (1975) Survival with mammary cancer related to the interaction of germinal center hyperplasia and sinus histocytosis in axillary and internal mammary lymph nodes. *Cancer* 36:528–539.
7. Tsakraklides V, Olson P, Kersey JH, Good RA (1974) Prognostic significance of the regional lymph node histology in cancer of the breast. *Cancer* 34:1259–1267.
8. Catalona WJ, Chretien PB (1973) Abnormalities of quantitative dinitro-chlorobenzene sensitization in cancer patients: Correlation with tumor stage and histology. *Cancer* 31:353–356.
9. Mitchell RJ (1972) The delayed hypersensitivity response in primary breast carcinoma as an index of host resistance. *Br J Surg* 59:505–508.
10. Roberts MM, Jones Williams W (1974) The delayed hypersensitivity reaction in breast cancer. *Br J Surg* 61:549–552.
11. Nemoto T, Han T, Minowada J, Angkur V, Chamberlain A, Dao TL (1974) Cell-mediated immune status of breast cancer patients: Evaluation by skin tests, lymphocyte stimulation, and counts of rosette-forming cells. *J Natl Cancer Inst* 53:641–645.
12. Catalona WJ, Sample WF, Chretien PB (1973) Lymphocyte reactivity in cancer patients: Correlation with tumor histology and clinical stage. *Cancer* 31:65–71.
13. Head JF, Elliott RL, McCoy JL (1993) Evaluation of lymphocyte immunity in breast cancer patients. *Breast Cancer Res Treat* 26:77–88.
14. Vose BM, Moore M (1979) Suppressor cell activity of lymphocytes infiltrating human lung and breast tumours. *Int J Cancer* 24:579–585.
15. Eremin O, Coombs RRJ, Ashby (1981) Lymphocytes infiltrating human breast cancers lack K-cell activity and show low levels of NK-Cell activity. *Br J Cancer* 44:166–176.
16. Whiteside TL, Miescher S, Hurlimann J, Moretta L, von Fliedner V (1986) Clonal analysis and in situ characterization of lymphocytes infiltrating human breast carcinomas. *Cancer Immunol Immunother* 23:169–178.
17. Blalock JE (1992) *Neuroimmunology*. Basel: Karger, pp 1–190.
18. Osborne MP (1987) Breast development and anatomy. In *Breast Diseases*. JD Harris, S Hellman, IC Henderson, DW Kinne (eds). Philadelphia: JB Lippincott, pp 1–14.
19. Eglinton BA, Roberton DM, Cummings AG (1994) Phenotype of T-cells, their soluble receptor levels, and cytokine profile of human breast milk. *Immunol Cell Biol* 72:306–313.
20. Page DL, Anderson JJ (1987) *Diagnostic Histopathology of the Breast*. Edinburgh: Churchill Livingston, pp 120–192.
21. Black MM, Leis HP (1973) Cellular responses to autologous breast cancer tissue. Sequential observations. *Cancer* 32:384–389.
22. Weiss DW, Faulkin LJ, De Ome KB (1964) Acquisition of heightened resistance and susceptibility to spontaneous mouse mammary carcinomas in the original host. *Cancer Res* 24:732–741.
23. Medina D (1976) Mammary tumorigenesis in chemical carcinogen-treated mice. VI. Tumor-producing capabilities of mammary dysplasias in BALB/cCrgl mice. *J Natl Cancer Inst* 57:1185–1189.
24. Wei W-Z, Heppner G (1987) Natural killer activity of lymphocytic infiltrates in mouse mammary lesions. *Br J Cancer* 55:589–594.
25. Wei W-Z, Fulton A, Winkelhake J, Heppner G (1989) Correlation of natural killer activity with tumorigenesis of a preneoplastic mouse mammary lesion. *Cancer Res* 49:2709–2715.

407

26. Pross HF, Sterns E, MacGillis DR (1984) Natural killer cell activity in women at 'high risk' for breast cancer, with and without benign breast syndrome. *Int J Cancer* 34:303–308.

27. Cole EN, Sellwood RA, England PC, Griffiths K (1977) Serum prolactin concentrations in benign disease throughout the menstrual cycle. *Eur J Cancer* 13:597–603.

28. Franks S, Ralphs DNL, Seagroatt V, Jacobs HS (1974) Prolactin concentrations in patients with breast cancer. *Br Med J* 2:320–321.

29. Tsai SJ, Loeffler DA, Heppner GH (1992) Assorted effects of bromocriptine on neoplastic progression of mouse mammary preneoplastic hyperplastic alveolar nodule (HAN) line C4 and on HAN-infiltrating and splenic lymphocyte function. *Cancer Res* 52:2209–2215.

30. Tsai J, Heppner GH (1994) Immunoendocrine mechanisms in mammary tumor progression direct prolactin modulation of peripheral and preneoplastic hyperplastic-alveolar-nodule infiltrating lymphocytes. *Cancer Immunol Immunother* 39:291–298.

31. Lukac J, Kusic Z, Kordic D, Koncar M, Bolanca A (1994) Natural killer cell activity, phagocytosis, and number of peripheral blood cells in breast cancer patients treated with tamoxifen. *Br Cancer Res Treat* 29:279–285.

32. Rowse G, Weinberg J, Emerman J (1995) Role of natural killer cells in psychosocial stressor-induced changes in mouse mammary tumor growth. *Cancer Res* 55:617–622.

33. Prehn RT, Lappe MA (1971) An immunostimulation theory of tumor development. *Transplant Rev* 7:26–54.

34. Prehn RT (1994) Stimulatory effects of immune reactions upon the growths of untransplanted tumors. *Cancer Res* 54:908–914.

35. Stewart THM, Tsai S-C J (1993) The possible role of stromal cell stimulation in worsening the prognosis of a subset of patients with breast cancer. *Clin Exp Metastasis* 11:295–305.

36. Whiteside TL, Jost LM, Heberman RB (1992) Tumor infiltrating lymphocytes. Potential and limitations to their use for cancer therapy. *Crit Rev Oncol Hematol* 12:25–47.

37. Schwartzentruber D, Solomon D, Rosenberg S, Topalian S (1992) Characterization of lymphocytes infiltrating human breast cancer: Specific immune reactivity detected by measuring cytokine secretion. *J Immunother* 12:1–12.

38. Panerai AE (1993) Lymphocytes as a source of hormones and peptides. *J Endocrinol Invest* 16:549–557.

39. Montgomery DW, Le Fevre JA, Ulrich ED, Adamson CR, Zukoski CF (1990) Identification of prolactin-like proteins synthesized by normal murine lymphocytes. *Endocrinology* 127:2601–2603.

40. Ip MM, Shoemaker SF, Darcy KM (1992) Regulation of rat mammary epithelial cell proliferation and differentiation by tumor necrosis factor-α. *Endocrinology* 130:2833–2844.

41. Taylor-Papadimitriou J (1991) Report on the first international workshop on carcinoma-associated mucins. *Int J Cancer* 49:1–5.

42. Tjandra JJ, McKenzie IF (1988) Murine monoclonal antibodies in breast cancer: An overview. *Br J Surg* 75:1067–1077.

43. Hayes D, Sekine H, Ohno T, Abe M, Keefe K, Kufe D (1985) Use of a murine monoclonal antibody for detection of circulating plasma DF3 antigen levels in breast cancer patients. *J Clin Invest* 75:1671–1678.

44. Hilkens J, Ligtenberg MJL, Vos HL, Litvinov SV (1992) Cell membrane-associated mucins and their adhesion-modulating property. *Trends Biochem Sci* 17:359–363.

45. Longenecker BM, MacLean G (1993) Prospects for mucin epitopes in cancer vaccines. *Immunologist* 1:89–93.

46. Girling A, Bartkova J, Burchell J, Gendler S, Gillett C, Taylor-Papadimitriou J (1989) A core protein epitope of the polymorphic epithelial mucin detected by the monoclonal antibody SM-3 is selectively exposed in a range of primary carcinomas. *Int J Cancer* 43:1072–1076.

47. Jerome KR, Barnd DL, Bendt KM, Boyer CM, Taylor-Papadimitriou J, McKenzie IFC, Bast RC, Finn OJ (1991) Cytotoxic T-lymphocytes derived from patients with breast adenocarcinoma recognize an epitope present on the protein core of a mucin molecule preferentially expressed by malignant cells. *Cancer Res* 51:2908–2916.

48. Jerome KR, Bu D, Finn OJ (1992) Expression of tumor-associated epitopes on Epstein-Barr

virus-immortalized B-cells and Burkitt's lymphoma tansfected with epithelial mucin complementary DNA. *Cancer Res* 52:5985–5990.

49. Jerome KR, Domenech N, Finn OJ (1993) Tumor-specific cytotoxic T cell clones from patients with breast and pancreatic adenocarcinoma recognize EBV-immortalized B cells transfected with polymorphic epithelial mucin complementary DNA. *J Immunol* 151:1654–1662.

50. Davis MM, Bjorkman PJ (1988) T-cell antigen receptor genes and T-cell recognition. *Nature* 334:395–402.

51. Monaco JJ (1992) Pathways of antigen processing: A molecular model of MHC class-I-restricted antigen processing. *Immunol Today* 13:173–176.

52. Neefjes JJ, Ploegh HL (1992) Intracellular transport of MHC class II molecules. *Immunol Today* 13:179–183.

53. Salter RD, Benjamin RJ, Wesley PK, Buxton SE, Garrett TP, Clayberger C, Krensky AM, Norment AM, Littman DR, Parham P (1990) A binding site for the T-cell co-receptor CD8 on the α3 domain of HLA-A2. *Nature* 345:41–46.

54. Cammarota G, Scheirle A, Takacs B, Doran DM, Knorr R, Bannwarth W, Guardiola J, Sinigaglia F (1992) Identification of a CD4 binding site on the β2 doamin of HLA-DR molecules. *Nature* 356:799–801.

55. Clayberger C, Lyu S-C, Dekruyff R, Parham P, Krensky AM (1994) Peptides corresponding to the CD8 and CD4 binding domains of HLA molecules block T lymphocyte immune responses in vitro. *Immunol* 153:946–951.

56. Nisco S, Farfan F, Hoyt G, Lyu S-C, Pouletty P, Krensdky A, Claybergeogy C (1994) Induction of allograft tolerance in rats by an HLA class I-derived peptide and cyclosporine A. *Immunol* 152:3786–3792.

57. Kemenade E, Ligtenberg MJL, de Boer AJ, Buijs F, Vos HL, Melief CJM, Hilkens J, Figdor CG (1993) Episialin (MUC1) inhibits cytotoxic lymphocyte-target cell interaction. *J Immunol* 151:767–776.

58. Guo HC, Jardetzky TS, Garrett TPJ, Lane WS, Strominger JL, Wiley DC (1992) Different length peptides bind to HLA-Aw68 similarly at their ends but bulge out in the middle. *Nature* 360:364–366.

59. Falk K, Rotzschke O, Stevanovic S, Jung G, Rammensee HG (1991) Allele-specific motifs revealed by sequencing of self-peptides eluted from MHC molecules. *Nature* 351:290–296.

60. Kawakami Y, Eliyahu S, Delgado CH, Robbins PF, Sakaguchi K, Appella E, Yannelli JR, Adema GJ, Miki T, Rosenberg SA (1994) Identification of a human melanoma antigen recognized by tumor-infiltrating lymphocytes associated with in vivo tumor rejection. *Proc Natl Acad Sci USA* 91:6458–6462.

61. Kawakami Y, Eliyahu S, Sakaguchi K, Robbins PF, Rivoltini L, Yannelli JR, Appella E, Rosenberg SA (1994) Identification of the immunodominant peptides of the MART-1 human melanoma antigen recognized by the majority of HLA-A2-restricted tumor infiltrating lymphocytes. *J Exp Med* 180:347–352.

62. Robbin PF, El-Gamil M, Kawakami Y, Rosenberg SA (1994) Recognition of tyrosinase by tumor-infiltrating lymphocytes from a patient responding to immunotherapy. *Cancer Res* 54:3124–3126.

63. Bakker ABH, Schreurs MWJ, de Boer AJ, Kawakami Y, Rosenberg SA, Adema GJ, Figdor CG (1994) Melanocyte lineage antigen gp 100 is recognized by melanoma-derived tumor-infiltrating lymphocytes. *J Exp Med* 179:1005–1009.

64. Celis E, Tsai V, Crimi C, DeMars R, Wentworth PA, Chesnut RW, Grey HM, Sette A, Serra HM (1994) Induction of anti-tumor cytotoxic T lymphocytes in normal humans using primary cultures and synthetic peptide eiptopes. *Proc Natl Acad Sci USA* 91:2105–2109.

65. Gaugler B, Van den Eynde B, van der Bruggen P, Romero P, Gaforio JJ, De Plaen E, Lethe B, Brasseur F, Boon T (1994) Human gene MAGE-3 codes for an antigen recognized on a melanoma by autologous cytolytic T lymphocytes. *J Exp Med* 179:921–930.

66. van der Bruggen P, Traversari C, Chomez P, Lurquin C, De Plaen E, Van den Eynde B, Knuth

A, Boon T (1991) A gene encoding an antigen recognized by cytolytic T lymphocytes on a human melanoma. *Science* 254:1643–1647.

67. Brasseur F, Marchand M, Vanwijck R, Herin M, Lethe B, Chomez P, Boon T (1992) Human gene MAGE-1, which codes for a tumor rejection antigen, is expressed by some breast tumors. *Int J Cancer* 52:839.

68. Becker JC, Gillitzer R, Brocker E-B (1994) A member of the melanoma antigen-encoding gene (BAGE) family is expressed in human skin during wound healing. *Int J Cancer* 58:346–348.

69. Disis ML, Smith JW, Murphy AE, Chen W, Cheever MA (1994) In vitro generation of human cytolytic T cells specific for peptides derived from the Her-2/neu protooncogene protein. *Cancer* 54:1071–1076.

70. Fisk B, Chesak B, Ioannides MC, Wharton JT, Ioannides CG (1994) Sequence motifs of human HER-2 proto-oncogene important for peptide binding to HLA-A2. *Int J Oncol* 5:51–63.

71. Miller FR, Soule HD, Tait L, Pauley RJ, Wolman SR, Dawson PJ, Heppner GH (1993) Xenograft model of progressive human proliferative breast disease. *J Natl Cancer Inst* 85:1725–1732.

72. Pauley RJ, Soule DH, Tait L, Miller FR, Wolman SR, Dawson PJ, Heppner GH (1993) The MCF-10 family of spontaneously immortalized human breast epithelial cell lines: Models of neoplastic progression. *Eur J Cancer Prev* 2:67–76.

73. Soule HD, Maloney TM, Wolman SR, Peterson WD, Brenz R, McGrath CM, Russo J, Pauley RJ, Jones RF, Brooks SC (1990) Isolation and characterization of a spontaneously immortalized human breast epithelial cell line, MCF-10. *Cancer Res* 50:6075–6086.

74. Calaf G, Zhang PL, Alvarado MV, Estrada S, Russo J (1995) c-Ha-ras enhances the neoplastic transformation of human breast epithelial cells treated with chemical carcinogens. *Int J Oncol* 6:5–11.

75. Calaf G, Russo J (1993) Transformation of human breast epithelial cells by chemical carcinogens. *Carcinogenesis* 14:483–492.

76. Liang P, Pardee AB (1992) Differential display of eukaryotic messenger RNA by means of the polymerase chain reaction. *Science* 257:967–971.

77. Liang P, Averboukh L, Pardee AB (1993) Distribution and cloning of eukaryotic mRNAs by means of differential display: Refinements and optimization. *Nucleic Acids Res* 21:3269–3275.

78. Sun Y, Hegamyer G, Colburn NH (1994) Molecular cloning of five messenger RNAs differentially expressed in preneoplastic or neoplastic JB6 mouse epidermal cells: One is homologous to human tissue inhibitor of metalloproteinases-3. *Cancer Res* 54:1139–1144.

79. Zhang L, Medina D (1993) Gene expression screening for specific genes associated with mouse mammary tumor development. *Mol Carcinog* 8:123–126.

80. Medina D (1973) Preneoplastic lesions in mouse mammary tumorigenesis. *Methods Cancer Res* 7:3–53.

81. Kozak C, Peters G, Pauley R, Morris V, Michalides R, Dudley J, Green M, et al. (1987) A standard nomenclature for endogenous mouse mammary tumor viruses. *J Virol* 61:1651–1654.

82. Michalides R, Schlom J (1975) Relationship in nucleic acid sequences between mouse mammary tumor virus variants. *Proc Natl Acad Sci USA* 72:4635–4639.

83. Ringold GM, Blair PB, Bishop JM, Varmus HE (1976) Nucleotide sequence homologies among mouse mammary tumor viruses. *Virology* 70:550–553.

84 Acha-Orbea H, Palmer E (1991) Mls — a retrovirus exploits the immune system. *Immunol Today* 12:356–361.

85 Pauley RJ, Lopez DM (1991) Expression of endogenous Mtv provirus transcripts in BALB/c splenic lymphocytes. *Proc SEBM* 196:316–320.

86. Wei WZ, Gill RF, Jones RF, Lichlyter D, Abastado J-P (In press) Induction of cytotoxic T lymphocytes to mouse mammary tumor cells with a K^d-restricted immunogenic peptide. *Int J Cancer.*

87. Gill RF, Abastado JP, Wei WZ (1994) Systematic identification of H-2Kd binding peptides and induction of peptide specific CTL. *J Immunol Methods* 176:245–253.

Index

276–278, 280, 283–284, 288, 289–
290, 291–292, 313
168FARN cells, 257, 259
Fetal calf serum (FCS), 152, 237
Fetal fibroblasts, 310–311
FGF, *see* Fibroblast growth factor
FGF3 gene, *see int*-2 gene
FGF4 gene, *see hst/FGF4* gene
γ-Fibrinogen, 11
Fibroadenomas, 43, 359
Fibroblast growth factor (FGF), 57, 58,
61, *see also* Acidic fibroblast
growth factor; Basic fibroblast
growth factor
Fibroblasts
endothelin role in mitogenesis of,
378–380
fetal, 310–311
stromelysin-3 and, 362
Fibronectin
apoptosis and, 10–11, 18–19
cathepsin B and, 325
cell motility and, 317
stromelysin and, 354
Fibronectin III, 121
Flk-1 receptor, 268
Focal atypical hyperplasia, 56
Folliculostellate-derived growth factor
(FSDGF), 271, 272
Forskolin, 376, 377
fos-1 gene, 379
fos-B gene, 174, 379
Fos protein, 213, 217
Fourier analysis, 306, 308
fra-1 gene, 174
fra-2 gene, 174
Frank carcinoma, 29
F8RA/vWF, *see* Factor VIII-related
antigen/von Willebrand's factor
FSK4 cells, 42
Fumagillin, 267
Furin, 357, 361

G418, 113–114
β-Galactosidase gene, 256
GATA, 374
GC cells, 132
G_0 cell cycle phase, *see* G_0/G_1 cell cycle
phase boundary
G_1 cell cycle phase, 141, 142, 148–149,
150, *see also* G_0/G_1 cell cycle phase
boundary
antiprogestins and, 207

estrogen and, 153, 178, 213
nuclear oncogenes and, 172
oscillation of cyclin in breast cancer
cells and, 151–153
p27 and, 161
p53 and, 175–176
pRb interaction with, 147–148
progestins and, 154, 180
role of cyclin in, 144–146
UCN-01 and, 100
G_2 cell cycle phase, *see* G_2/M cell cycle
phase
Gelatinase A, 331, 343, 359, 361
Gelatins, 354
Gene amplification, cyclin, 149–150
Gene expression
involution and, 11–12
matrilysin in, 359–360
stromelysin-3 in breast carcinoma,
359–360
stromelysin-3 in stromal cells of
carcinoma, 361–363
transgenic gland method for, 23–27
Genes, *see also* specific types
cell motility, 311–313
changes in during carcinoma
development, 71–72
MMTV-related in preneoplasia, 49–
51
Gentamicin, 109
Gestoden, 205
G_0/G_1 cell cycle phase boundary, 159,
207, 306, 380
Gliomas, 330–331
D-Gluco-D-galactan sulfate (DS4152),
267
Glucose-6-phosphate dehydrogenase,
177
Gly-CAM-1, 11
Glycogen synthase kinase-3 (GSK-3),
181
G_2/M cell cycle phase, 141, 142, 143–
144, 151, 207
Granulocyte colony stimulating factor,
271
Granulocyte-macrophage colony-
stimulating factor, 332
Growth factor receptors, 401
Growth factors, *see also* specific types
ductal hyperplasia and, 42
nuclear oncogene regulation by, 181
preneoplasia and, 56–58, 61
Growth hormone, 16
GR virus, 49, 50

417

Guanosine triphosphate-activating
protein (GAP), 120–121

H7, 95
H-89, 377
Haptotaxis, 304, 305–306, 317
  cytokine stimulation of, 311
  defined, 305
  methods of measuring, 308
Ha-*ras* gene, 43, 158, 160, 326
HBL-100 cells, 149, 151
HDH4 outgrowth line, 42–43
Heat shock protein 90 (hsp90), 214
HEGO, 201
HeLa cells, 131, 132, 151, 201
Heparin, 271
Hepatocyte growth factor, 271–272, 361
Hepatocyte growth factor/scatter factor
  (HG/SF), 237–238, 305, 309–310,
  317
Hepatomas, 329, 334
HepG2 cells, 336
HER2 gene, 271, *see also neu* gene
HG/SF, *see* Hepatocyte growth factor/
  scatter factor
HLA-A2.1, 403
HLA-DR, 397
18-Hn1 cells, 109, 112, 114–116, 117,
  118, 119–120
Hormone-independent growth
  of epithelium expressing *wnt*-1, 31–
  32
  of preneoplasia, 43, 45
H-RAS gene, 136, 244, 404
Hs578t cells, 94, 100, 372, 373
hst/FGF4 gene, 32, 49, 157
Hyaluronic acid degradation products,
  272
Hydrocortisone, 11, 109, 237
4-Hydroxytamoxifen, 99, 153, 218–219
Hyperplasia, 44–45, 46, 48–49
  atypical, 71, 244, 248–250, 252
  cell cycle control in, 58–60
  ductal, 38, 39–42, 44
  fetal fibroblasts and, 311
  focal atypical, 56
  MCF10AneoT.TGn cells and, 252
  MMTV-related genes in, 49
  neu and, 29
  proto-oncogene expression in, 51–53
  wnt-1 and, 30–31
Hyperplastic alveolar nodule (HAN),
  38, 44, 46–47, 49, 55, 243

apoptosis and, 5, 16
breast cancer vaccine testing and,
  405
ductal hyperplasia compared with,
  42
immunology and, 399–400
lesions of, 244–245
MMTV-related genes and, 50
Hyperplastic outgrowth lines (HOG/
  HPO), 38–39, 45, 51
Hyperproliferative disorders, 72–74

ICI 164384, 50, 201, 203, 221
  cyclin and, 153
  mechanism of action, 219–220
  role of, 218
ICI 182780, 154, 218, 219–220
IGF, *see* Insulin-like growth factor
Immortalization, 46, 48–49, 53, 60
  defined, 44
Immune stimulation, 400–401
Immunofluorescence analysis, 110
Immunohistochemistry, 328, 331, 338
Immunology, 395–406
  human model systems for, 403–404
  of tumor progression, 398–400
Infants, breast development in, 229–
  231
Inhibitors of kinases (INK), 58
Inositol trisphosphate (IP$_3$), 378
In situ hybridization, 328, 331, 371
Insulin, 109, 154, 174, 179, 180
Insulin-like growth factor I (IGF-I),
  183
  antiestrogens and, 219
  c-fos and, 174
  c-jun and, 174
  cyclin and, 152
  endothelins and, 373, 380, 383, 386
  estrogen and, 177, 213
  nuclear oncogene regulation by, 181
  preneoplasia and, 56, 58
Insulin-like growth factor II (IGF-II)
  angiogenesis and, 268
  endothelins and, 380
  estrogen and, 177
  nuclear oncogene regulation by, 181
  preneoplasia and, 56, 58
  procathepsin D and, 344
Integrin, 268
Interferon-α, 267
Interferon-γ, 372
Interleukin-1, 332, 372

MMEC cells, 53
MMP, *see* Matrix metalloproteinase
MMTV, *see* Mouse mammary tumor virus
MNU, *see* Methylnitrosourea
Monoclonal antibodies, 401
   c-*erb*B-2, 110
   Ki-67, 132, 272
   LAR-PTPase, 110, 113
   M1G8, 338
   PTP1B, 110
   SM-3, 401, 402
Motility, *see* Cell motility
Motility factors, 308
Mouse mammary tumor virus (MMTV), 25, 27, 33, 72, 73, 76, 81
   breast cancer vaccine testing and, 405–406
   c-*myc* fusion, 174
   genes related to in preneoplasia, 49–51
   hst/*FGF-4* fusion, 32
   hyperplastic alveolar nodule and, 38, 46
   hyperproliferative disorders and, 74
   polyomavirus middle T antigen fusion, 78–80
   preneoplasia and, 52, 53, 55
   tumorigenesis and, 74, 75
   wnt-1 and, 30
Mouse models, *see also* Transgenic mouse models
   apoptosis and neoplasia in, 3–19
   for breast cancer vaccines, 405–406
   cell motility in, 311, 312
   of immunology, 398–400
   of melanoma, 312, 332
   of metastasis, 255–261
   of preneoplasia, 37–43, 44–49
mts-1 gene, 311–312, 317
MUC1 gene, 401, 402
Mucins, 401, 402
Multidrug resistance, 97
Multiple myeloma, 287, 289, 293
MXT mammary carcinoma, 194, 196, 199, 202, 203
myc gene, 30, 142, 158, 160, 181, 213

Natural killer (NK) cells, 396, 397, 399–400
neo gene, 28
Neoplasia, 3–19, 43
   apoptosis and, *see* Apoptosis

MMTV-related genes in, 49
neu deletion mutants (NDL), 77
neu gene, 25, 80, 109
   angiogenesis and, 271
   cathepsin D and, 337
   in metastasis, 75–77, 81–82
   preneoplasia and, 53, 55
   in transgenic glands, 56
   in tumorigenesis, 75–77
   types of lesions caused by, 28–29
neu gene-transformed 184B5 cells, 109, 120
   expression of *neu* and PTPases in, 114–116
   LAR-PTPase in LAR-PTPase-transfected, 117
   LAR-PTPase transfection into, 116–117
   proliferation of, 113–114
   proliferation of LAR-PTPase-transfected, 118–119
   tumorigenicity of, 114
   tumorigenicity of LAR-PTPase-transfected, 119
Neural cell adhesion molecules (N-CAM), 121–122
Neutral endopeptidase (NEP), 230, 233, 235
Nicotinamide, 272
NIH 3T3 cells, 46, 122, 130, 132, 144, 145, 336, 379
Nitric oxide, 272
Nitrosomethylurea, 44
nm23-H1 gene, 312–313, 317
nm23-H2 gene, 312–313
N-*myc* gene, 172
Non-small-cell lung carcinoma, 286, 293
Northern blot analysis
   of apoptosis, 11, 18
   of cathepsin D, 328
   of endothelins, 371
   of protein tyrosine phosphateses, 110–111, 115
67NR cells, 257
NRK cells, 144
Nuclear factor-1, 374
Nuclear matrix, 127–138
   defined, 129
Nuclear matrix breast (NMB), 133, 137
Nuclear matrix breast cancer (NMBC), 133, 137, 138
Nuclear matrix normal breast (NMNB), 133, 137

in human mammary glands, 43–44
MCF10AneoT.TGn cells as model
of, 243–254
MMTV-related genes in, 49–51
molecular alterations in, 49–58
mouse models of, 37–43, 44–49
phenotype as model system, 37–44
proto-oncogene expression in, 51–56
in rat mammary glands, 43–44
in transgenic glands, 56, 60–61
in transgenic models, 55–56
Procathepsin B, 333, 334
Procathepsin D, 279, 333–334, 344
Progesterone, 38
Progesterone antagonists, *see*
Antiprogestins
Progesterone receptors
angiogenesis and, 279
endothelins and, 371, 385
estrogen receptors and, 178
protein kinase C and, 92
Progestins, 39
cyclin and, 154–155
nuclear oncogene regulation by,
179–180
Prognostic indicators
cathepsin D, 336–340
intratumoral microvessel density,
276–285
stromelysin-3, 363
Programmed cell death, *see* Apoptosis
Prolactin, 273, 399–400
hyperplastic alveolar nodules and, 38
involution and, 11
preneoplasia and, 45
Prolactin receptors, 95–96
Proliferating cell nuclear antigen
(PCNA), 59, 160, 286
Proliferation, *see* Cell proliferation
Proliferative breast disease (PBD),
244, 245, 398, 399–400
Prostaglandin E_1, 272, 314
Prostaglandin E_2
angiogenesis and, 272, 314
endothelins and, 373, 377, 382–383,
388
Prostate cancer, 133
angiogenesis in, 286–288, 293
cathepsin B and, 331
cell motility in, 306, 308
Protein A, 144
Proteinases
fibronectin and, 18–19
involution and, 13–14

Protein kinase A (PKA), 221, 377,
387–388
protein kinase C (PKC), 91–102
activity in human breast cancer cell
lines, 93
activity in human breast tumors, 91–
93
endothelins and, 377, 378, 379, 387
metastasis and, 96–97
multidrug resistance and, 97
as a therapeutic target, 99–101
Protein kinase C-α (PKC-α), 92–93, 97,
98–99, 100, 101
Protein kinase C-β (PKC-β), 92, 98, 99
Protein kinase C-$β_I$ (PKC-β-$_I$), 91
Protein kinase C-$β_{II}$ (PKC-β-$_{II}$), 91
Protein kinase C-δ (PKC-δ), 92–93, 97
Protein kinase C-ε (PDC-ε), 92-93, 97,
98
Protein kinase C-η (PKC-η), 98
Protein kinase C-γ (PKC-γ), 92, 97, 98
Protein kinase C-ζ (PKC-ζ), 92, 98,
101
Protein tyrosine kinases (PTKs), 107
Protein tyrosine phosphatases
(PTPases), 107–123, *see also* LAR-
PTPase
Proteoglycans, 354
Proteolytic enzymes, 383–385
Proto-oncogenes, 51–56
pS2, 99
PTP1B, 107, 108, 110, 114–116, 120,
122–123
Puberty, breast development in, 229–
231

raf-1 gene, 379
ras gene
cyclin and, 142
MCF10AneoT.TGn cells and, 252
metastasis and, 261
preneoplasia and, 52–53, 55
Rat models, 233
of preneoplasia, 43–44
of prostate cancer, 306, 308
Rb gene, 53, 172
antiprogestins and, 155
characteristics of, 176
cyclin and, 142, 150
estrogen and, 178
Receptor binding studies, of
antiprogestins, 192–195
Rectal carcinoma, 287, 293, *see also*